Hot Topics in Acute Ca and Trauma

MW00990637

Series Editors

Federico Coccolini
Pisa, Pisa, Italy

Raul Coimbra
Riverside, USA

Andrew W. Kirkpatrick
Calgary, AB, Canada

Salomone Di Saverio
Cambridge, Cambridgeshire, UK

Editorial Board

This series covers the most debated issues in acute care and trauma surgery, from perioperative management to organizational and health policy issues. Since 2011, the founder members of the World Society of Emergency Surgery's (WSES) Acute Care and Trauma Surgeons group, who endorse the series, realized the need to provide more educational tools for young surgeons in training and for general physicians and other specialists new to this discipline: WSES is currently developing a systematic scientific and educational program founded on evidence-based medicine and objective experience. Covering the complex management of acute trauma and non-trauma surgical patients, this series makes a significant contribution to this program and is a valuable resource for both trainees and practitioners in acute care surgery.

More information about this series at http://www.springer.com/series/15718

Emmanouil Pikoulis • Jay Doucet
Editors

Emergency Medicine, Trauma and Disaster Management

From Prehospital to Hospital Care and Beyond

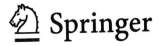 Springer

Editors
Emmanouil Pikoulis
Department of Surgery
National and Kapodistrian University
of Athens
Athens
Greece

Jay Doucet
Department of Surgery
University of California
San Diego, CA
USA

ISSN 2520-8284   ISSN 2520-8292   (electronic)
Hot Topics in Acute Care Surgery and Trauma
ISBN 978-3-030-34118-3   ISBN 978-3-030-34116-9   (eBook)
https://doi.org/10.1007/978-3-030-34116-9

This Springer imprint is published by the registered company Springer Nature Switzerland AG
The registered company address is: Gewerbestrasse 11, 6330 Cham, Switzerland

Foreword to the Series April 2019

Research is fundamentally altering the daily practice of acute care surgery (trauma, surgical critical care, and emergency general surgery) for the betterment of patients around the world. Management for many diseases and conditions is radically different than it was just a few years previously. For this reason, concise up-to-date information is required to inform busy clinicians. Therefore, since 2011 the World Society of Emergency Surgery (WSES), in a partnership with the American Association for the Surgery of Trauma (AAST), endorses the development and publication of the "Hot Topics in Acute Care Surgery and Trauma," realizing the need to provide more educational tools for young in-training surgeons and for general physicians and other surgical specialists. These new forthcoming titles have been selected and prepared with this philosophy in mind. The books will cover the basics of pathophysiology and clinical management, framed with the reference that recent advances in the science of resuscitation, surgery, and critical care medicine have the potential to profoundly alter the epidemiology and subsequent outcomes of severe surgical illnesses and trauma.

Pisa, Italy
Riverside, CA, USA
Calgary, AB, Canada
Cambridge, Cambridgeshire, UK

Federico Coccolini
Raul Coimbra
Andrew W. Kirkpatrick
Salomone Di Saverio

Foreword by Bernd Domres and Norman Hecker

Emergency and Disaster Medicine

Medical Ethics[1]

The discipline of medical ethics is concerned with morality, moral obligations, and the principles of proper professional conduct concerning the rights and duties of the physician himself, his patients, and fellow practitioners, as well as his actions in the care of patients and in relation to their families. Its foundations lie in the philosophical traditions of Eastern and Western thought and have strongly shaped modern codes of conduct and conventions.

One of the first statements of a moral conduct explicitly for physicians is found in a text from Ionian Greece: the Hippocratic Oath (Hippocrates of Cos, ca. 460–370 BC), which states: "To the law of medicine my life as physician shall be for the benefit of my patients according to my ability and judgment, and not for their hurt or for any wrong!"[2]

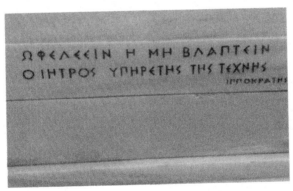

---

[1] See: Domres B, Koch M, Manger A, Becker HD: Ethics and triage. Prehosp Disast Med 2001; 16(1): p. 53–58.
[2] Kollesch J, Nickel D: Antike Heilkunst. Ausgewählte Texte aus den medizinischen Schriften der Griechen und Römer, Stuttgart, 1994. p. 53–55.

Geneva Conventions

The first attempt for the establishment of a more codified way of conduct was initiated on 22 August 1864 by Henry Dunant (1828–1910). After the shock of seeing the battlefield of Solferino (1859) and the agony of a great number of wounded soldiers lying unattended, he suggested that the governments of Europe and several American States come to a conference for the purpose of adopting a "Convention for the Amelioration of the Condition of the Wounded in Armies in the Field."

Triage and Its Ethical Dimension

In disasters,[3] where the sheer number of injured or ill may overwhelm the capacities of medical responders, priorities must be established as to who should be treated and in which order they should be treated and/or transported. This process is called triage. Triage is defined as the selection and categorization of the victims of a disaster aiming at appropriate treatment according to the degree of severity of illness or injury and the availability of medical and transport facilities.[4] The principle concerning the interest of the subject, which is supposed to prevail over the interest of the society, under these circumstances cannot be followed. In disasters the physician, while remaining responsible for the well-being of each of the victims, must on the other hand decide who should get help urgently with regard to the outcome, i.e., survival.

In 1994, the World Physician Association released a statement on ethics and disaster medicine declaring that under disaster conditions it is acceptable to abandon one's commitment of treatment of a single person in favor of stabilizing the vital functions of many patients. It continues to point out that it is unethical for a physician to persist, at all costs, at maintaining the life of a patient beyond hope, thereby wasting scarce resources needed elsewhere. Even, and especially, in disasters, the physician needs to demonstrate the highest degree of personal moral integrity and responsibility.

A clear classification and training in triage will create a system in which the ultimate instance[5] in decision making—the individual conscience—will not have to serve as the chief point of reference. Only in extreme cases, in which the standard of triage does not apply and where a huge moral dilemma appears, will the physician have to rely on his or her personal conscience. These cases do occur, though, and thus conscience has to be considered as the complementary factor in triage.

---

[3] A more general definition of a disaster can be found in: Gunn SWA: *Multilingual Dictionary of Disaster Medicine and International Relief.* Kluwer Academic Publishers: Dordrecht, Boston, London 1990. p. 81. It defines a disaster as "the result of a vast ecological breakdown in the relation between man and his environment, a serious and sudden event (or slow, as in drought) on such as scale that the stricken community needs extraordinary efforts to cope with it, often with outside help or international aid."

[4] Gunn (see Note 10).

[5] Wolbert, W: *Das fehlbare Gewissen. Gesammelte Studien*, Herder: Freiburg, 2008. p. 157.

Conscience as a Last Resort

However, it needs to be pointed out that classification can only be an instrument, lightening a burden that cannot completely be taken away from the physician: To make the final moral decision on treatment or deferral, thus deciding to possibly lose a life in favor of another whose chances for survival are considered higher. Conscience is not a norm. A norm is shared by a number of people (usually one society or one group within society), whereas conscience is per definition located in the individual. The individual and their conscience are shaped by the social norm, but it still has the power to decide against the norm. It is the core freedom of conscience to—on moral grounds—disagree with social norms and make a different decision. Sometimes this even serves as a forerunner of a new norm.[6] Both aspects clearly point out that decisions based on personal conscience are highly dependent upon a single individual making the decision. Responsibility is involved, as is power. Neither the patient nor the physician hopes to solely rely on such decisions with the psychological insecurity they pose for the patient, and the huge burden that repeated conscience-based decision making poses for the physician.[7]

We would like to thank the editors and contributors, who have written this book with the aim to teach students in this global specialty; furthermore it is hoped that this book accompanies the experts during their work in field missions worldwide and that their insight and attention are always guided by the conscience of ethical aspects!

Tübingen, Germany

Bernd Domres
Norman Hecker

---

[6] See Note 17 (above).

[7] In this context it is worth noting that legally the categorization into T-4 is highly problematic, since "non-treatment" is primarily considered as failure to render assistance and thus punishable.

Foreword by Norman Rich

Emergency Medicine, Trauma and Disaster Management: From Prehospital to Hospital Care and Beyond is a result of annual courses on the Island of Rhodes organized and conducted by Professor Manos Pikoulis, Chairman of Surgery at Athens University in Greece and Adjunct Professor of Surgery at the Uniformed Services University of the Health Sciences in Bethesda, Maryland, in the USA. For this very comprehensive and valuable contribution to Global Medicine and Surgery he is joined by Professor Jay Doucet of the University of California in San Diego as co-editor. With more than 25 years of experience each, these two world leaders in Surgery and Trauma Care provide vast exposure from both civilian and military perspectives as well as those from governments and universities. They are joined by other global leaders in a wide variety of specialties from many countries in addressing how best to assist those who are in harm's way and/or have the misfortune to be injured whether by man-made or natural disasters.

There are 49 chapters covering multiple responses to managing disasters and those who are injured allowing rapid access to areas of specific interest ranging from the overall Principles of Disaster Medicine by Professor Pikoulis to the Art of Triage by Professor Ari Leppaniemi of Helsinki, Finland, to the Basics of Trauma Management by Professor Kluger Yorham of Tel Aviv, Israel, to Incidents Caused by Fire and Toxic Gases, Hazardous Material, Chemicals and Irradiation by Director of the Catastrophe Center in Tubingen, Germany, and to Ethical Dilemmas in Disaster Health Management by Professor Boris Sakakustev of Sofia, Bulgaria.

With armed conflict continuing in numerous areas in the world, with earthquakes and tsunamis, with forest fires, with hurricanes, tornadoes, and typhoons, with volcanic eruptions, with gas explosions, with airplane, car, railroad, and boat crashes,

---

The opinions or assertions contained herein are the private ones of the authors and are not to be construed as official or reflecting the views of the Department of Defense, the Uniformed Services University of the Health Sciences or any other agency of the U.S. Government.

with global warming and flooding, with migration and famine, with urban gunshot wounds, with mine and other industrial accidents, and with a rapidly expanding world population with many living in harm's way, there is an increasing need for appropriate response by experienced individuals. This important book by Pikoulis, Doucet, and colleagues helps meet that challenge.

Bethesda, MD, USA

Norman Rich

Foreword by James Ryan

Introduction to the Manual: The World in the Twenty-First Century

The introduction to the manual is being written in October 2017 at a time when the world has become increasingly unstable and dangerous. We are beset by war, including the threat of nuclear war, insurrection, terrorism, political upheavals, mass migration into Europe on a scale not seen since the aftermath of the Second World War, and natural disasters. Natural disasters are of increasing concern. Disasters have been defined as "a situation or event, which overwhelms local capacity, necessitating a request to a national or international level for external assistance" (Centre for Research on the Epidemiology of Disasters—CRED). As we head towards the third decade of the twenty-first century, the numbers and scale of disasters facing the world's population are increasing in severity and complexity.

Complex Humanitarian Emergencies (CHEs) are currently the most common human-generated disasters. These emergencies are characterized by widespread violence with large-scale injury and loss of life, extensive damage to societies and their economies, massive population displacement, and mass famine or food shortage. Large-scale humanitarian assistance is needed, but this may be hindered or prevented by military, religious, or political constraints. Even if a response is possible significant security risks may face expatriate humanitarian aid workers reacting to the crisis. CHEs are also a fertile nursery for terrorism, both local and international.

Thus they have major political, public health, and security features and account for more morbidity and mortality than all natural and technological disasters combined. CHEs have occurred or are ongoing in every continent. Ongoing examples include Afghanistan, Somalia, Sierra Leone, Sudan, Myanmar, Colombia, Haiti, and Congo. Countries or regions recovering from such events include the Balkans, the Caucasus, Rwanda, Azerbaijan, Angola, Mozambique, and many territories in South East Asia and South America.

A review of the current world political situation is also quite sobering. Kim Jong Um of North Korea and President Donald Trump appear to be on the verge of launching nuclear missiles at each other, which if it comes to pass will engulf us all. The threat of terrorism hangs over every society. Isil or Daesh, while close to defeat in Iraq and Syria, has turned its sights beyond the Middle East. It now has a global reach with the ability to commit atrocities in the UK, France, Spain, Italy, Germany, Turkey, Greece, and even the USA. Affiliates of Isil have emerged in Africa and Asia and employ similar tactics. Terrorist war is now being fought in our streets, sporting arenas, concert halls, and restaurants. It seems that nowhere is safe.

A relatively new humanitarian crisis affecting Europe in particular is mass migration. More than a million migrants and refugees crossed into Europe in 2015, compared with just 280,000 the year before. The scale of the crisis continues and there is no end in sight. Among the forces driving people to make the dangerous journey are the conflicts in Syria, Iraq, and Afghanistan. The vast majority—more than 80%—of those who have reached Europe by boat come from those three countries. In addition, poverty, human rights abuses, and deteriorating security are also prompting people to set out from countries such as Eritrea, Pakistan, Morocco, Iran, and Somalia in the hope of a new life in somewhere like Germany, Sweden, or the UK.

The population of the world is growing fast, and ever-increasing numbers of people are forced to live in marginal areas. These may be areas where growing food is difficult due to climate, water shortages, or adverse environments, or they may be areas that are particularly vulnerable to the effects of sudden impact natural disasters. Already more than 90% of those who die in natural disasters live in the developing world, and the economic impact of such disasters is far more serious in deprived countries than in the developed world.

In addition to all of the above political and religious extremism is resulting in high levels of social instability, violence, and mass killing in many of those countries that are least able to cope with such situations. For example Isil is recognized by the UN as the perpetrator of genocide of Yazidis in Iraq starting in 2014. This has led to the expulsion, flight, and effective exile of the remaining Yazidis from their ancestral lands in *Northern Iraq*. In recent weeks, half a million people—mostly Rohingya women and children—have fled violence, including murder in Myanmar's Rakhine Province. They are seeking refuge in Bangladesh, where they urgently need water, food, shelter, and medical care in a country least able to help them.

There are other aspects of conflict, which concern humanitarians.

These include routine violence against women, the proliferation of narcotics, transnational criminal activity, human trafficking, ethnic cleansing, and the widespread use of kidnapped children as child soldiers.

The world indeed has become a very dangerous place and there is little room for optimism.

There is now a growing international realization that those responding to these events whether man-made such as terrorist bombings and forced migration or natural disasters need much more than technical competency in their primary field—in most cases the provision of health and medical care. Organizing, planning, executing, and sometimes surviving missions to difficult and often dangerous environments require knowledge and skills not acquired during traditional education and practice.

The question is how should we prepare, train, and credential humanitarian volunteers to work in the dangerous and complex environment that characterizes humanitarian aid work in the twenty-first century? In the case of medical personnel should appropriate training be included in the medical school curriculum?

The truth is there is no easy one-size-fits-all solution. Progress however has been made in many European countries, particularly in the Netherlands, Greece, and the UK.

The required training curriculum to prepare humanitarian volunteers is considerable and growing. The Society of Apothecaries of London have in place an examination called The Diploma in the Medical Care of Catastrophes (DMCC) since 1994 supported by a yearlong training course. A perusal of their course program for 2107 is illustrative of the scale and complexity of the training need. The DMCC is taught in the UK, the Netherlands, and the USA, and discussions are taking place with Australia with a view to licensing the examination in South Australia.

There is a growing view that medical volunteers, including doctors, biomedical scientists, dentists, nurses, and professionals allied to medicine, should be offered training and education at undergraduate level with continuation training at postgraduate level. There are now many avenues open for medical students and allied students to gain skills, experience, and deployment in humanitarian medicine. The earliest opportunity is to select a humanitarian module as a component of an intercalated Bachelor of Science degree. At the time of writing, these are available in the UK at St George's University of London, Kings College London, University College London, and the University of Birmingham. Oxford University will offer modules from 2018.

In Greece annual conferences have taken place in Rhodes over the last 8 years. The Global health—disaster medicine—health crisis management manual being edited by Professor Manos Pikoulis in Athens is in the planning stage and will support a Master of Science qualification.

There has never been a more urgent need for these important initiatives led by Professor Pikoulis and his colleagues in Greece. Their efforts in Greece and internationally will insure that future humanitarian volunteers will be fully trained and appropriately educated for deployment missions to the most challenging of environments. They are to be congratulated and deserve widespread audience in Greece and the international community.

London, UK   James M. Ryan

Further Reading

1. Course timetable for 2017. http://www.apothecaries.org/faculty-of-the-conflict-catastrophe-medicine/course-in-conflict-catastrophe-medicine.
2. Centre for Research on the Epidemiology of Disasters. http://www.cred.be.

Foreword by Eric Elster and Kyle Remick

Since the dawn of the twenty-first century, US Military surgical teams have deployed in support of combat operations to provide lifesaving care to US and coalition nation service members. In July 2008, one such team arrived to a US Army base in Jalalabad, Afghanistan. With a capacity of four resuscitation beds and two operating room tables with the requisite surgeons, nurses, and medics, this team had trained to provide combat casualty care for multiple casualties in austere conditions. However, war has a strange way of testing a team's readiness despite many months of preparation. It is commonly said that in war the best plans do not survive the first contact with the enemy. This applies equally to mass casualty events from any cause.

Early in this team's deployment, there was enemy contact at a nearby base with a vehicle explosion and a direct enemy attack. There were 10–20 casualties inbound by helicopter with more casualties possible within the hour. The 20-person team quickly huddled and activated its mass casualty plan, the equivalent of a "disaster plan" for a small military surgical team. This involved calling on the help of other base medical personnel, assigning triage duties and locations, and ensuring we had positive command and control for patient movement through our surgical team.

Twelve injured service members arrived on the first chinook helicopter with little prehospital care. They were sorted and the immediately urgent patients were brought into the facility for care. Two patients were noted to be surgical and so the two operating rooms were rapidly occupied. Our capacity was overwhelmed immediately, and we were forced to make life and death decisions based on limited availability of personnel and resources in order to save the most lives. Lifesaving interventions were carried out both inside and outside our facility with the extra personnel we had mustered. Inside the operating room, anesthesiologists frantically scrambled to provide damage control resuscitation and surgeons made difficult operative decisions. The least possible interventions needed to stabilize patients to fly to the larger combat hospital were done in order to make space for the next round of casualties.

The opinions or assertions contained herein are the private ones of the authors and are not to be construed as official or reflecting the views of the Department of Defense, the Uniformed Services University of the Health Sciences or any other agency of the U.S. Government.

In the end, this team received 25 total patients within an hour and completed final lifesaving care in 6 h. Physically and mentally fatigued, this team then reset the trauma area, the operating room, and the critical care area for future patients, conducted a team debrief, and released personnel to rest for whatever was next. Although rehearsed countless times prior to deployment, the mass casualty event was physically and emotionally challenging. This team would have similar mass casualty incidents several times per month for the next 15 months.

Many who have cared for the injured in war have learned through trial and repetition the principles of disaster management. The response to this scenario is not unique to this team or to this war or even to the military. It demonstrates how we must prepare and train for large-scale disaster and mass casualty events at home. The twenty-first century has already proven to require our heightened vigilance and attention to be prepared to respond to these scenarios. It is acutely evident that the need to prepare for intentional mass casualty events is not only for armies but also for the sake of our global civilization as these incidents continue to spill into civilian settings. In addition, natural disasters over the same time period have caused us to recognize the need to be prepared for the good of humanity.

September 11th, 2001, scarred US history with a horrific act of intentional terrorism and has caused the world community to be intensely aware of the need for preparation. In addition to the historic terrorist attack on the World Trade Center and the Pentagon in the United States, there have also been a significant number of other intentional terrorism events around the world. In 2004, terrorists killed 193 people and injured 2000 in a coordinated attack on the train system in Madrid. In 2005, a coordinated terrorist attack resulted in the detonation of 3 home-made bombs in the London Underground train system killing 52 and injuring 700. The Mumbai attack in India by 10 terrorists using automatic weapons and grenades resulted in 164 deaths in 2008. In 2015, a coordinated terrorist attack in Paris killed 130 people and wounded 494 using automatic weapons and explosives. In 2017, a terrorist ran over pedestrians on the London Bridge and then proceeded to stab numerous people in the area killing 8 and injuring 48. In addition since 2001, there have been numerous planned terrorist attacks that have been thwarted by law enforcement, but could have resulted in similar mass casualty events if unchecked.

At the same time, our global community has been equally affected by natural disasters. In 2001, thousands were killed by the Gujarat Earthquake in India as well as thousands more in Bangladesh. In 2003, an earthquake in southeastern Iran caused an estimated 40,000 deaths. The Indian Ocean Tsunami of 2004 caused the death of over 200,000 in multiple countries with Indonesia being most affected. The Kashmir earthquake in 2005 is estimated to have caused 100,000 deaths in Afghanistan, Pakistan, and the adjacent region of China. Hurricane Katrina flooded the city of New Orleans in the USA and along the gulf coast causing thousands of deaths in the same year. Cyclone Nargis caused destruction and over 100,000 deaths in Myanmar in 2008. The Sichuan Earthquake in China caused over 60,000 deaths also in the same year. The earthquake in Haiti in 2010 left that nation with over 100,000 deaths and with millions injured and otherwise affected. The Tohoku earthquake in 2011 caused a tsunami that hit Japan with an over 15,000 deaths and damage to include most notably the meltdown of the Fukushima Daiichi Nuclear Power Plant reactors affecting the region.

Greece itself has been plagued with earthquakes throughout its history to include one as recently as 2017 that caused destruction and killed 2 people on the tourist island of Kos. Recognizing the importance of preparation for disaster and mass casualty events, military and civilian experts in Greece, led by Dr. Manos Pikoulis, Professor of Surgery at the University of Athens, created a curriculum and hands-on practical course titled the "Management of Disaster Victims" which has provided training to enhance preparedness for the last 8 years. The Department of Surgery at the Uniformed Services University as the academic hub of military medicine and surgery in the United States has been honored to participate in this effort for the last several years.

This text provides a written foundation for the disaster course. Experts in disaster management and mass casualty patient care throughout the world have contributed. The textbook is divided into five sections. *Part I—Prehospital Emergency Services* deals with initial response on scene, patient triage, transport, initial stabilization, and resuscitation priorities. *Part II—Hospital Response* includes a host of topics of trauma management for the spectrum of injuries. *Part III—Management of Incidents* discusses leadership and management principles of various types of disaster and mass casualty events. *Part IV—After the Disaster* describes critical issues to address after the response is complete. Lastly, *Part V—Evaluation, Ethical Issues, Education and Research* deals with disaster-specific ethics, the critical component of education in preparation for these events, and research specific to advancing disaster and mass casualty care.

At this juncture in world history, it is imperative that we come together in an effort to effectively prevent, prepare, respond, and recover from these devastating events. This textbook provides a solid foundation necessary to provide the optimal response in our new global environment and provides a platform from which to launch this international effort.

Bethesda, MD, USA   Eric Elster
                                                                                                                            Kyle Remick

Preface

The number of natural and man-made disasters has risen dramatically over the last decade. Natural disasters, industrial accidents, terrorist attacks, and last but not least the COVID-19 pandemic are all events involving multiple casualties that threaten to overwhelm health systems.

In these events, health professionals face multiple challenges because the type and standard of care to be provided may change from what they were taught or how they practice, and may require the adoption of new standards of care. The aim of this book is therefore to inform and prepare healthcare professionals for the challenges posed by disasters, so that they can act effectively in medical teams whether sent on humanitarian missions, working in conflict zones, or even while in their own hospital systems at threat of being overwhelmed, as in the current pandemic.

This book offers an interdisciplinary and interprofessional approach covering all stages of the disaster management cycle and is divided into five sections: Part I: Prehospital Emergency Services; Part II: Hospital Response; Part III: Management of Incidents; Part IV: After the Disaster; and Part V: Evaluation, Ethical Issues, Education and Research.

With authors and coauthors that include more than 100 prominent academics, researchers, and experienced practitioners from multiple medical disciplines in 15 countries, this one of a kind book has as a vision to promote a common universal understanding and a common language of the hybrid field of Disaster Medicine. We believe this book underlines not only its humanitarian aspects but also the field's very practical and "lcts think outside of the box" character.

Athens, Greece
San Diego, CA, USA

Emmanouil Pikoulis
Jay Doucet

Contents

Part I

Prehospital Emergency Services

Principles of Disaster Medicine

Emmanouil Pikoulis, Anastasia Pikouli, and Eleni Pavlidou

1.1 What Is a Disaster?

Catastrophic events are frequently mentioned in the media nowadays. It seems that disasters occur with increasing frequency (four times more in the last 20 years in contrast to the previous 20) and they have a larger negative impact on the population and on their everyday lives. The main explanations for this are the growth of the population, urbanization, living in hazardous areas due to poverty, poor living conditions, climate change, and also due to systematic reports of such events with the optimization of surveillance tools [1, 2].

In general the term "disaster" is used differently by different professions, organizations, and people, as we are lacking a common definition of this specific word. The most accurate definition of a generalized catastrophic event, in relation to one community, includes the inability to respond to a disaster by its own means [3].

According to the World Health Organization(WHO) and the United Nations International Strategy for Disaster Reduction(UNISDR), a disaster is "a serious disruption of the functioning of a community or a society causing widespread human, material, economic or environmental losses which exceed the ability of the affected community or society to cope usingits own resources." [4, 5].

E. Pikoulis (✉)
Third Department of Surgery, Attikon University Hospital, National and Kapodistrian University of Athens, School of Medicine, Athens, Greece
e-mail: mpikoul@med.uoa.gr

A. Pikouli
Third Department of Surgery, Attikon University Hospital, National and Kapodistrian University of Athens, Athens, Greece

E. Pavlidou
University General Hospital of Patras, Patras, Greece

Global Health-Disaster Medicine, School of Medicine, National and Kapodistrian University of Athens, Athens, Greece

© Springer Nature Switzerland AG 2021
E. Pikoulis, J. Doucet (eds.), *Emergency Medicine, Trauma and Disaster Management*, Hot Topics in Acute Care Surgery and Trauma,
https://doi.org/10.1007/978-3-030-34116-9_1

From a medical perspective, a disaster is a multi-casualty incident (MCI) which has occurred in a specific area, where the number of victims and the severity of their trauma overwhelm the availability of our resources so that we are unable to provide effective therapy [6].

When the quantity of victims is between 10 and 50 (in a hospital ED), this defines a small-scale MCI. A quantity of 50–250 defines a moderate-scale MCI and more than 250 indicates a severe-scale MCI. Specific importance is placed on the location and the type of MCI because we have significantly more resources available when an MCI occurs in an urban area compared to when an MCI occurs in a rural or remote area. It is clear that seriously traumatized victims in a remote environment have less chances of survival. This is due to difficulties in reaching the victims in a timely manner and fewer resources available. In relation to the type of accidents, aviation accidents have lower survival rates, therefore fewer victims to attend to [7].

1.2   Disaster Medicine: Evolving Medical Field

Education is the basis of effective management of a disaster. In 2015, we had 34 complete academic postgraduate long-term training programs in disaster medicine on a global level, mainly in high-income countries (HIC). Also we have a lot of short-term educational programs (without a degree). The absence of such programs is characteristic in low- and middle-income countries (LMICs) located in Asia and Africa, areas with great vulnerability to disasters [8].

With regard to a disaster, health workers are concerned with all the phases of the disaster cycle specifically the immediate response to the event, the phase of recovery and reconstruction, and also the phases of preparation, planning and mitigation of the consequences.

The education and competency of health workers responding to a disaster are predominantly divided into the following domains: planning and preparation for catastrophic events, searching for victims, effective communication, appropriate initial medical management of the casualties, safety issues, estimation of the consequences on public health, and appropriate response taken, legal matters, and social aspects which concern the affected area [9, 10].

Disaster medicine fuses together specific areas of disaster management and emergency medicine specialty. The handling of a disaster demands that health care personnel are incorporated into non-medical multidiscipline response teams. Effective collaboration has a profound effect on achieving their goal: the reduction of the consequences of a disaster in terms of loss of life and in terms of physical and psychological health. Practical education in disaster management often relies on simulated situations. It is through the decision-making process that we teach and evaluate the trainees in every stage of the simulation. The trainees learn through the consequences of their decisions in this learning procedure [11].

Worldwide, emergency medicine as a medical specialty dedicates a large portion of its educational curriculum specifically to disaster medicine [12].

Education in disaster medicine is also included in the university curriculum of many pre-graduate medical programs, mainly in Europe and the United States [13].

Education in disaster management, even in the setting of the European Union, is deficient. It is rare in certain countries for health workers to be exposed to a real disaster. It should be mandatory to have a universal educational program which would apply to all professionals who are involved in the three different levels of disaster management (strategic, tactical, and operational) on a national and international scale [14].

1.3   Public Health and Emergency Management Systems

The CDC (Center for Disease Control and Prevention) defines public health as "The science and art of preventing disease, prolonging life, and promoting health through the organized efforts and informed choices of society, organizations, public and private communities and individuals." With regard to public health, the main aim is to provide services which (a) have the most positive impact on the health of the population as a whole, and (b) ensure that living conditions allow the population to be healthy. A public health system must be designed with the purpose of improving the health of a certain population and must take measures to prevent diseases, trauma, and disability (health campaigns, public health information, primary health care, etc.). When approaching a specific public health problem, the methodology is as follows: (1) implementation of surveillance systems which detect the problem, (2) identify the specific cause, (3) evaluate one specific and appropriate intervention, and (4) implement this intervention. The determining factors of the health of a population are behavioral choices (40%), genetics (30%), social circumstances(15%), medical care (10%), and physical environment (5%) [15, 16].

Disasters have very serious consequences on public health systems. The consequences depend mainly on the specific type of disaster which has occurred but also on the structure and quality of the affected area's pre-existing health system. The existence of efficient emergency preparedness practices plays a significant role as it increases the affected communities' ability to endure the disaster. In floods, for example, which are the most frequent natural disasters today, a large number of deaths are caused by drowning as well as multi-cause trauma due to the transfer of debris, and also pneumonia and hypothermia. Specific problems arise from resulting water pollution and the destruction of sewage disposal systems in the area. This exacerbates communicable diseases [17].

The destruction of health facilities, the inability to provide immediate medical care when access to the victims is reduced and when communication collapses, and possible trauma to or loss of health workers are all universal problems across the majority of natural disasters, despite their differences. The danger of an epidemic and the loss of basic amenities (water, food, sanitation, and shelter) are also serious consequences on public health which demands immediate intervention to ensure the protection of the affected population. The provision of health in areas of armed conflicts is also very challenging and the International Red Cross is the major organization responsible [18–20].

The influence of a disaster on the mental health of victims is also very important. Biological, social, and economic factors point towards an increase in mental health morbidity [21].

Disaster victims such as those with a low socio-economic and educational level, those without family support (mainly women), as well as all children, old-aged pensioners, people with pre-existing psychiatric history and also those who have been repeatedly exposed to traumatic events, have increased probability of developing psychiatric pathology after a disaster [22].

Disasters, where the existing health system and government is lacking formal organization, have been named by the humanitarian community as "complex emergencies." In such disasters, there is a large-scale population displacement and a huge increase in the percentage of mortality (sometimes tenfold) and morbidity, for the specific population. These increases are mainly due to a lack of food supplies and outbreaks of infectious diseases. In 2016, 6.53 million people were displaced due to armed conflicts. The involvement of Public Health Systems on Disaster Management concerns all the phases of the cycle of disaster.

The existence of a national emergency management plan is of great importance. The actions of public health practitioners are incorporated into this plan. As far as the response phase is concerned, public health services (a) make contact to determine the immediate needs of the affected population, (b) assess the whole situation of the affected area, (c) coordinate the provision of immediate care to the victims, (d) receive and provide information to all the participants in the management of the situation, (e) give instructions regarding possible threats, (f) gather and analyze epidemic data, and (g) are leaders in implementing appropriate measures to control the situation. In the recovery phase, Public Health Systems boost communities' abilities to return to normal, ensuring public health programs resume and also monitoring the affected population for possible long-term consequences in their physical and mental health [23].

1.4   Types of Disaster

There are three main types of disasters: natural, man-made, and hybrid (both humanly involved and natural forces). We also separate disasters into sudden onset disasters and long-term disasters. As far as natural disasters are concerned, they usually occur due to geological (i.e., earthquakes) and weather-related events (storms and hurricanes).

Man-made disasters not only include all types of technological disasters but also war-type conflicts. Examples of hybrid disasters are usually floods and landslides. According to CRED (Centre of Research on Epidemiology of Disasters), responsible for the surveillance of disasters on a global level, to record an actual disaster, it is necessary to fulfill at least one of the following criteria:

- Causing death to more than 10 people.
- Affecting everyday life of more than 100 people.
- Requesting international help for managing the incident.
- Declaring an emergency situation [24].

1.5   Disaster Epidemiology

Since 1970 the establishment of The Centre for Disease Control (The CDC) formed the existing epidemiology of disasters. Prior to 1970, scientific reports depended mainly on military data from the two previous World Wars [25].

Disaster epidemiology focuses on providing scientific data in relation to the health aspects of a disaster and is useful for the more efficient management of short- and long-term consequences. The moment of disaster impact—and ideally within a 72-h period—a rapid needs assessment must be made which will guide the response of rescuers and also reveal (to some level) the importance of the specific incident, so that all the required supplies are scheduled. It is also especially important to emphasize the significance of the knowledge of the previous epidemiological characteristics of the affected population [26].

Natural disasters have increased in frequency every decade since 1970. For the period of 1996 until 2015 7056 disasters were recorded, with a progressive increase in weather-related disasters (floods, storms, extreme temperatures). The occurrence of earthquakes was stable in this period. The total number of deaths was 1,346,196. During this 20-year period, two massive-scale disasters were responsible for the largest proportion of victims, namely, the Haiti earthquake of 2010 and the tsunami in the Indian Ocean in the year 2004. Tsunamis are the deadliest natural disasters. The second position is occupied by storms, for example, the cyclone 'Nargis' in Myanmar in 2008 which resulted in 138,000 deaths. The reality is that the possibility of death in a disaster is 200 times higher in low-middle-income countries (LMICs) in comparison to OECD countries. During the period of 2006–2015, we experienced a reduction in the death toll from weather-related disasters compared to the previous decade 1996–2005. In high-income countries (HIC), we have real threats from nuclear accidents and extreme temperatures. In Europe in 2003, due to heatwaves, we had 70,000 deaths [27].

The financial consequences of disasters have been studied systematically in the last decade, as far as the relationship and the impact on the economic status of a country are concerned. The financial loss of a disaster can be measured in a macro-economic level (GPD, tax revenue, trade balance) as well as in a microeconomic level (households, local authority performance) [28].

The year with the largest financial loss was 2011 (US 400 billion) due to the earthquake/tsunami in Japan (Pacific Ocean). In 2017 the major economic damage was due to weather-related disasters [29].

1.6   Risk, Hazard, Vulnerability: Main Terms and Definitions

Preparation for a possible disaster gives us the chance to minimize its consequences or the opportunity to avoid it. Experience from previous disasters has shown us that terms such as hazard, probability, risk, susceptibility, vulnerability, and risk acceptance, all play an important role in planning and implementing measures for the mitigation of consequences of a given catastrophe. The risk, meaning the possibility of losses in a catastrophe, has a direct connection with the type of hazard and the vulnerability (human–structural–economical) of a population in a specific time and place. The degree of repetition of this phenomenon is also crucial. A specific hazard does not necessarily always lead to a disaster. For example, a cyclone that strikes a deserted area has little a consequence. The vulnerability and susceptibility of people and structures are what dictates whether a hazard will have catastrophic results. We define vulnerability as a weakness in implementing adequate responses to a disaster [30, 31].

The assessment of vulnerability of a certain population and place is an especially complex process with a lot of parameters. Climate change, the interaction of humans on their environment, specifically the impact our advances in technology have on the environment, and also the degree of risk acceptance from the specific society for a substantial hazard (for instance living in close proximity to an active volcano), all play a vital role in a vulnerability study. On a global level, we have developed indexes for risk assessment and vulnerability. Examples are: Disaster Risk Index (DRI) from the United Nations Developing Program which connects vulnerability and the level of development for a certain country. The Disaster Deficit Index (DDI) from Inter-American Development Bank which connects the possible economical losses from a disaster with financial capacity of a country. As health workers, our focus is on the level of vulnerability of a certain population in connection with the possible human losses. It is important to recognize that the exposure of the least developed countries in a given hazard will produce a much higher number of victims in comparison with the most developed countries [32, 33].

1.7   Global Goals for Resilience in Disasters

In the World Conference on Disaster Reduction in January 2005 in Hyogo, Japan, the United Nations, after recognizing a global increase in catastrophic events, presented the Framework for Action 2005–2015 aimed at reducing vulnerability and the risk from certain hazards. Specific challenges were first of all a catastrophe in a certain place has consequences on other places on the global map (for example, immigration, epidemics.) Secondly, in the effort to reduce the risk of a catastrophe, we must incorporate politics and programs for a sustainable development and the elimination of poverty through local and international corporations. The major action areas were (a) government level (laws and policies), (b) recognition and follow-up of specific disasters and development of early warning systems, (c) education for the public and government agencies, (d) development of specific measures taken to reduce the risks, and (e) improving disaster response systems through the establishment of effective plans on a national and local level. It is important to mention that the provision of economical help to developing countries is mandatory after a disaster for the recovery and the establishment of prevention strategies through a development course [34].

In March 2015, The Sendai Framework for Disaster Reduction 2015–2030 was presented for the first time during the third United Nations World Conference in Sendai, Japan. Primarily, they evaluated the results of implementation of Hyogo

Framework for Action 2005–2015 across different countries. It was clear there was a significant reduction of mortality for certain disasters. Taking measures to reduce the disaster risk is a cost-effective investment in order to avoid future losses, therefore ensuring the positive contribution for sustainable development. This enhancement of smaller communities is of vital importance. Small-scale disasters and slow onset disasters are a very important portion of the total losses of a specific country, especially in the case of developing countries. The Sendai Framework sets seven global targets for disaster resilience for the decade of 2020–2030. In brief, this framework includes efforts to reduce: the 100,000 Global Mortality Rate, the global number of affected people, and the direct economic loss from a disaster. Further aims were to enhance the resilience of a country through the restoration of important structures ('Build Back Better'), international collaborations, educational programs, and provide access to disaster information and a multi-hazard warning system. It is important to highlight that the whole community needs to participate in the management of a disaster in order to ensure its resilience [35].

References

1. Alexander D. Globalization of disaster: trends, problems and dilemmas. J Int Affairs. 2006;59(2)
2. Helmer M, Hilhorst D. Natural disaster and climate change. Disasters. 2006;30(1):1–4.
3. Mayner L, Arbon P. Defining disaster: the need for harmonization of terminology. Australas J Disaster Trauma Stud. 2015;19
4. Humanitarian Health Action. World Health Organization (WHO). Definitions: emergencies. http://www.who.int/hac/about/definitions/en/.
5. Terminology. United Nations Office for Disaster Risk Reduction (UNISDR). Terminology on disaster risk reduction. 2009. https://www.unisdr.org/we/inform/terminology.
6. Sztajnkrycer MD, Madsen BE, Baez AA. Unstable ethical plateaus and disaster triage. Emerg Med Clin North Am. 2006;24(3):749–68.
7. Advanced Life Support Group (ALSG). Chapter 1: Introduction. In: Major Incident Medical Management and Support (MIMMS). 3rd ed. UK: Wiley-Blackwell; 2012.
8. Algaali KYA, Djalali A, Corte FD, Ismail MA, Ingrassia PL. Postgraduate education in disaster health and medicine. Front Public Health. 2015;3:185.
9. Subbarao I, Lyznicki JM, Hsu EB, Gebbie KM, Markenson D, Barzansky B, et al. A consensus-based educational framework and competency set for the discipline of disaster medicine and public health preparedness. Disaster Med Public Health Prep. 2008;2(1):57–68.
10. Hsu EB, Thomas TL, Bass EB, Whyne D, Kelen GD, Green GB. Healthcare worker competencies for disaster training. BMC Med Educ. 2006;6:19.
11. Lennquist S. Education and training in disaster medicines. Scand J Surg. 2005;94:300–10.
12. Counselman FL, Borenstein MA, Chisholm CD, Epter ML, Khandelwal S, Kraus CK, et al. The 2013 model of the clinical practice of emergency medicine. Acad Emerg Med. 2014;21(5):574–98.
13. Pfenninger EG, Domres BD, Stahl W, Bauer A, Houser CM, Himmelseher S. Medical student disaster medicine education: the development of an educational resource. Int J Emerg Med. 2010;3(1):9–20.
14. Khorram-Manesh A, Lupesco O, Friedl T, Arnim G, Kaptan K, Djalali AR, et al. Education in disaster management: what do we offer and what do we need? Proposing a new global program. Disaster Med Public Health Prep. 2016;10(6):854–73.
15. Introduction to Public Health. Centers for Disease Control and Prevention. Handout of key public health terms. https://www.cdc.gov/publichealth101/public-health.html.

16. The Public Health System & The 10 Essential Public Health Services. Centers for Disease Control and Prevention. Public Health 101. https://www.cdc.gov/stltpublichealth/publichealthservices/essentialhealthservices.html.
17. Jonkman SN, Kelman I. An analysis of the causes and circumstances of flood disaster deaths. Disasters. 2005;29(1):75–97.
18. Noji EK. The public health consequences of disasters. National Center for Infectious Diseases (CDC). April 1999.
19. Noji EK. Public health issues in disasters. Crit Care Med. 2005;33(1):S29–33.
20. Leaning J, Guha-Sapir D. Natural disasters, armed conflict, and public health. N Engl J Med. 2013;369:1836–42.
21. Davidson JR, AC MF. The extent and impact of mental health problems after disaster. J Clin Psychiatry. 2006;67(Suppl 2):9–14.
22. Benjet C, Bromet E, et al. The epidemiology of traumatic event exposure worldwide: results from the World Mental Health Survey Consortium. Psychol Med. 2016;46(2):327–43.
23. Rose DA, Murthy S, Brooks J, Bryant J. The evolution of public health emergency management as a field of practice. Am J Public Health. 2017;107(S2):S126–33.
24. Shaluf IM, Disaster types, disaster prevention and management: an international journal. vol 16, no 5. UK: Emerald Publishing, pp 704–17.
25. Kano M, Wood MM, et al. Chapter 1: Disaster research and epidemiology. In: Disaster medicine: comprehensive principles and practices. 2nd ed. Cambridge: Cambridge University Press; 2014. p. 5–6.
26. Malilay J, Heumann M, et al. The role of applied epidemiology methods in the disaster management cycle. Am J Public Health. 2014;104(11)
27. Poverty & Death: Disaster Mortality. Center for Research on the Epidemiology of Disasters (CRED). 1996–2015. https://www.preventionweb.net/files/50589_creddisastermortalityallfinalpdf.pdf.
28. Lazzaroni S, van Bergeijk PAG. Natural disasters' impact, factors of resilience and development: a meta-analysis of the macroeconomics literature. Ecol Econ. 2014;107:333–46.
29. CRED CRUNCH. Natural disasters in 2017: lower mortality, higher cost. USAID, Issue No. 50. https://cred.be/downloadFile.php?file=sites/default/files/CredCrunch50.pdf.
30. Introduction to Disaster Preparedness, International Federation of Red Cross and Red Crescent Societies. http://www.ifrc.org/Global/Publications/disasters/all.pdf.
31. Cardona OD. The need for rethinking the concepts of vulnerability and risk from a holistic perspective: a necessary review and criticism for effective risk management. Columbia: National University of Columbia; 2004. https://www.researchgate.net/publication/254267457_The_Need_for_Rethinking_the_Concepts_of_Vulnerability_and_Risk_from_a_Holistic_Perspective_A_Necessary_Review_and_Criticism_for_Effective_Risk_Management1.
32. Fuchs S, Birkmann J, Glade T. Vulnerability assessment in natural hazard and risk analysis: current approaches and future challenges. Nat Hazards. 2012;64(3):1969–75.
33. Peduzzi P, Dao H, et al. Assessing global exposure and vulnerability towards natural hazards: the Disaster Risk Index. Nat Hazards. 2009;9:1149–59.
34. Hyogo Framework for Action 2005–2015: building the resilience of nations and communities to disasters, United Nations. https://www.unisdr.org/files/1037_hyogoframeworkforactionenglish.pdf.
35. Sendai Framework for Disaster Risk Reduction 2015–2030, United Nations. https://www.preventionweb.net/files/43291_sendaiframeworkfordrren.pdf.

The Role of the First Responder

2

Dimitrios Jannussis, Georgia Mpompetsi,
and Kollaras Vassileios

"Make a habit of two things: to help; or at least to do no harm"

—Hippocrates (460–c. 370 BC)

Real testimony: Socratis Doukas, MD Gen Surgeon, HELIOS AIRWAYS FLIGHT ACCIDENT, 14 August 2005.

"My shift as an emergency doctor on the ambulance of EKAB (Greek National Medical Unit for Emergency Response) starts at 8 o' clock in the morning. Along with my crew, the rescuer-paramedic Haris Kapnopoulos, we leave the central EKAB station and head towards the Schinias coastal region to start duty there.

The instruction to be stationed there is given by the EKAB headquarters, to cover the coastal front where many visitors are expected during summertime.

Upon arrival, we notify the radio that we have been stationed at our duty location and we are on standby. I receive a phone call from the head of medicine service of EKAB who informs me that arrangements have been made for a TV crew to film a hypothetical scenario of drowning and the way we deal with a case like that. The intention is that the film will be broadcasted on the news as an information report for the public.

We are on standby and the temperature has already risen above 30–32 °C even though it is before midday.

Sometime later, the radio reports:

D. Jannussis (✉)
National Center for Emergency Care (EKAB), MSF Greece volunteer member,
Athens, Greece

G. Mpompetsi · K. Vassileios
University General Hospital "Attikon", National and Kapodistrian University of Athens,
Athens, Greece

© Springer Nature Switzerland AG 2021
E. Pikoulis, J. Doucet (eds.), *Emergency Medicine, Trauma and Disaster Management*, Hot Topics in Acute Care Surgery and Trauma,
https://doi.org/10.1007/978-3-030-34116-9_2

"Vehicle 1 heading towards Grammatiko."

My crew and I are surprised by the broadcast since we receive no further information. Immediately we conclude that since we expect a drill at the airport, this broadcast is about such a drill but with a change in location.

We set off for the Grammatiko region and ask the operator for further information.

"Vehicle 1 to Center, please inform us about the message."

We are taken aback by the reply.

"Vehicle 1, this is a commercial airplane crash."

For a few seconds, we try to take in the information, and as we confirm that this is not a drill, we get permission to use "siren and lights."

Within 8 minutes, we reach the village square at Grammatiko Village (50 km from Athens) and try to detect the possible location of the plane crash looking for fire or smoke on the horizon.

Unfortunately, we are quite far as the plane has crashed on Grammatiko Mountain and we are still at the foot of it. There, we are met by a local resident on his motorbike, who is clearly upset, and tells us he has seen where the crash is, and he can lead us there.

We tell him to go ahead and we will follow.

We ascend the mountain of Grammatiko through dirt roads which are clearly used as firebreaks.

After some time, we reach the top of the mountain, where we encounter an unforgettable but chilling sight.

It is the tail of the plane.

It was the flight Helios of the Cypriot airlines.

We notify arrival on the spot and confirm the operator that this is a commercial flight.

From this moment onwards, time seems to have stopped and the relativity theory gets its essence.

Everything takes place at incredible speeds and time stands still.

I get off the vehicle holding the radio and move towards the tail of the aircraft, seeing the crash site for the first time.

I quickly check the surrounding area, moving about 100 m further back. I can see two of the aircraft wheels and luggage scattered around.

I deduce that this is possibly the impact location, and I head towards the opposite direction to look for the airframe or what is left of it.

I realise that there lie two big gorges where wreckage can be seen. I descend the first gorge where, among wires, metal, luggage ... I can see people.

Resembling a wheat field and having become one with the metal, they are lying there, some disfigured, some dismembered, others stuck on the seats ... headless.

I keep moving, trying to detect signs of life, anyone alive. I reach the second gorge where there is a bigger piece of the airplane, as well as one the wings.

Unfortunately, no sign of life.

I report to the operation center.

Barely breathing because of the tension, running, and the temperature well over 38 °C, I describe what I see for the EKAB operation center.

I can hear the radio operator, relentlessly transmitting to EKAB ambulances and mobile units to move towards Grammatiko.

I keep investigating the wreck site, trying to define the area of the crash and detect any sign of life.

To no avail. The same sight everywhere. A picture of war. Many young children. Appalling tragedy.

My thoughts are interrupted by the operator.

His voice changes! It is not as strict.

"Doctor," I can hear him saying.

"Center," I reply.

"Doctor, tune in channel 3". This is a frequency on which the rest of the vehicle network cannot listen to the transmission. I tune into the channel.

"Doctor … well, there is a possibility that this might have been a terrorist attack and there may be radioactive materials on the airplane. You are to move away from it and wait for Demokritos (specialized center which measures radioactivity) to arrive."

This is the moment when I go weak at the knees.

I am thinking of my own children. I am thinking that I have been exposed to radioactive material and whatever life I have left is going to be short.

I am tearing up as I slowly go up the gorge and I sit on a rock looking back and realizing that I am not going to see my children grow up.

Soon, ambulances arrive as well as the fire brigade, the police, civil protection assistance units, and the army.

Forty minutes after my arriving at the crash site, a fire breaks out due to the high temperature and leaked fuel.

Panic spreads as the number of people in the scene is great, making leaving the area difficult. We are in danger of getting burnt ourselves because of the fire spreading fast.

We evacuate the area by descending to a lower spot and wait for the fire to be extinguished. Hours later, and after the fire brigade uses ground and air means, the fire is under control and collection of the bodies from the crash site starts.

What we see, can only be described as tragedy.

It is now evening, and the operation is almost complete. I signal "end" for the dispatch center and I return to the EKAB base.

It was 14 august 2005. The worst aviation accident that had ever happened in Greece.

Helios Airways Flight-522. 121 dead; 22 children among them."

Doctor Doukas and his paramedic were in the middle of a very bad and difficult situation with many possible hazards:

- Kerosene fires
- Twisted sharp metals
- Composite fibers (sharp puncture and inhalation hazards)

- High-pressure hydraulic lines (1000 PSI. Plus)
- High-pressure oxygen cylinders and accumulators
- Electrical wiring

And if this had been a terroristic attack, there was the risk of high explosive devices and radioactive substances existing on site.

In the chaos of a large mass-casualty event, one person or one crew can make the difference between the complete disorder and the right approach of the situation.

This crew or the one person who is the first responder and their role, is critical for the effective outcome of the EMS operation.

The first responder is the most important player, having the responsibility of keeping the scene of the accident under control and giving the victims more chance to be safe and the injured people, major possibility to survive.

Even a minor mistake of the first responder can prove fatal for the operation.

E.g., Wrong parking, of first responder-vehicle which blocks the other vehicles to arrive, or the placement of the vehicle very close to the wreckage fire, can be catastrophic for the development of the operation.

Many of the pre-hospital medical workers, paramedics, or firefighters have never been involved as first responders in a true disaster, and most of them will only respond to one or two mass-casualty events during their professional life.

This means that the first-arriving crew, with no previous real experience, must deal with major, chaotic and dangerous events.

In recent years, there has been an increase in terrorist attacks in the Western world and the location of the terrorist attacks is an extremely unstable and dangerous environment.

In a large-scale accident, cooperation of the first responders is the key to the successful outcome of the rescue operation.

The first responders need to be able work together and to have good coordination during the initial critical time (Vital First Minutes) to manage a well-run accident scene and to minimize the risk of loss of life for the victims.

The safety of the first responder is of primary importance during the arrival to the location of the accident and it is important for them to stay calm.

A calm mind in a chaotic environment saves lives and the calm mind can be 'contagious'.

2.1   Scene Safety

Scene safety begins immediately after the initial dispatch information.

It is essential to request further information so you will know the extent of the accident.

For example, if it is a plane crash, information such as the type of the aircraft, ultralight, small frame, large frame airplane; if it is a road accident, traffic and access information, type of vehicles, for example vehicles with flammable materials, hybrid vehicles with the use of electricity for power (high-voltage risk), are all important information.

A probable number of casualties, access difficulties, and, in case of an industrial accident, risk of hazardous substance release must be estimated. In case of terroristic attack, consider that the first responders can be eventual victims, without the correct information of the potential threats; the first responder is unable to evaluate the risks to personal safety on arrival at a terrorist incident.

2.2 On the Arrival

Assess the situation quickly, rapid check for secondary threats, and size-up and assess the scene from all angles.

Check if there is any danger to yourself, the casualty, or others before rendering any assistance.

Consider the geographical features of the place of the accident, plan how to deal with the scene safety, estimate the fend-off distances, and establish outer and inner perimeters of the scene.

Pass the information to the operational center with simple clear language. Clear communications and standardization of terminology are the golden standard for the correct communications.

Rapid check for the need of calling for special reinforcements, such as law enforcement, special antiterrorist units, mine specialists, and any other special units.

If it is a road accident, arrive with careful approach, and park the emergency vehicle in fend-off position 10 m from the incident. Warning signs have to be placed approximately 200–400 m from each side of the incident. Avoid the use of siren. The noise can increase the stress and the confusion of the responders and make the communication between them more difficult. The siren is useful if you transport critical patients. It is better to have the red lights of the vehicle on. **The emergency vehicle must be ready to move, and never to block** the movement of other emergency vehicles which could be catastrophic and dangerous, in case of rapid evacuation.

2.3 Secure the Staging Area

The parked ambulance or other emergency vehicles, next to the scene of accident, represent potential targets during a suspected terrorist attack, and moreover a "potential target" for the media people, and bystanders, who can prevent the rescue operation and pose a major security risk.

It is important to restrict vehicle and pedestrian access to the accident area, and to engage immediately the law enforcement, if they are in proximity, or call them immediately with reinforcement if they are not present. Create a secure perimeter around the staging area, and ask the non-uniformed people to leave the place.

2.4   One-Way Entry

Find a safe staging area for incoming units and stabilize as soon as possible the one-way entry to the emergency vehicles' parking area. Think and find the correct place for the next rescue vehicles that will arrive, and secure the continuous flow for all the ambulance in one-way direction, and have an evacuation and rapid evacuation route and plan in mind if the situation worsens.

2.5   Stop the Killing in Mass Shooting Incident

In the United States, more than 33,000 people are killed each year by guns.

The total incidents of gun violence have increased in recent years, including the number of deaths, mass shooting incidents, and the number of patients with multi-compartmental injuries (due to extensive use of weapons with higher magazine capacity).

Seventy percent of active shooter incidents are over within 5 min. However, about 30% of active shooter incidents ended by the arrival of the police or military enforcement personnel.

For this reason, in case of continuing terrorist shooting incident, it is important that the first responder officer has military experience and carry a gun to enter immediately the shooting place and try to disarm the perpetrators, by carefully monitoring the situation without forgetting the self-protection measures.

At the same time the armed forces, in close cooperation with the unarmed first responders, must secure safe corridors of rapid access to victims, despite ongoing threats.

The victims need immediate care at the point of wounding within the shortest time possible.

At this stage, the treatment of victims is based on the principles of military experience with the minimal hemorrhage and airway control, before the rapid evacuation to a more secure zone.

If the incident is a bomb attack, it is highly recommended to use appropriate personal protective equipment (PPE) and to check for danger of a second bomb which may be placed to cause casualties to the personnel responding to the first attack.

The secondary attack can be done with chemical dispersal devices, secondary explosive devices, or booby traps (terrorist pretending to be a relative of the victims).

Also ensure that personal protective measures and shielding are used for the incoming rescuers.

In case of a massive or uncommon terrorist attack, check for warning signs of WMD (weapons of mass destruction) threats (chemical, radiological, biological) like unexplained sickness or convulsions of the victim and order the decontamination requirements.

2.6   Stop the Bleeding

The role of the first responders with the immediate hemorrhage control is crucial in the chain of survival for the victims.

Remember "run, hide, fight", particularly those in locations vulnerable to terrorism (schools, political institutions, religious institutions) and to use tourniquets and minimal airway protection and improve this concept to rapidly respond to stop the killing and stop the dying from severe bleeding. (Some times civilians can also make life and death decisions.)

The medical approach of the situation is based on the priorities of care and immediate hemorrhage control, and differs from the classical approach of immediate correction of airway and breathing problems.

The rescue personnel must be trained also in the principles of self-care in case of injury during the emergency operation in hostile environment.

The methodology is based to the Hartford Consensus and the THREAT algorithm.

*H*emorrhage control *R*apid *E*xtrication to safety *A*ssessment by medical providers *T*ransport to definitive care.

Finally, the first responder must hand over to the leader officer after having informed all cooperating partners involved in the rescue operation. This needs to be carried out in a spirit of cooperation and composure. It might be necessary for them to work together for some more time.

Bibliography

1. Lockey DJ, Mackenzie R, Redhead J, Wise D, Harris T, Weaver A, Hines K, Davies GE. London bombings July 2005: the immediate pre-hospital medical response. Resuscitation. 2005;66:9–12. https://doi.org/10.1016/j.resuscitation.2005.07.005.
2. Maguire BJ, Hunting KL, Smith GS, Levick NR. Occupational fatalities in emergency medical services: a hidden crisis. Ann Emerg Med. 2002;40:625–32. https://doi.org/10.1067/mem.2002.128681.
3. Calland V. A brief overview of personal safety at incident sites. Emerg Med J. 2006;23:878–82. https://doi.org/10.1136/emj.2004.022624.
4. Vernon A. Explosive devices: what every responder should know about IEDs. JEMS. 2010;35:42–7.
5. Sollid SJ, Rimstad R, Rehn M, Nakstad AR, Tomlinson AE, Strand T, Heimdal HJ, Nilsen JE, Sandberg M. Collaborating group Oslo government district bombing and Utoya island shooting July 22, 2011: the immediate prehospital emergency medical service response. Scand J Trauma Resusc Emerg Med. 2012;20:3. https://doi.org/10.1186/1757-7241-20-3.
6. Benedek DM, Fullerton C, Ursano RJ. First responders: mental health consequences of natural and human-made disasters for public health and public safety workers. Annu Rev Public Health. 2007;28:55–68. https://doi.org/10.1146/annurev.publhealth.28.021406.144037.
7. Fattah S, Rehn M, Lockey D, Thompson J, Lossius HM, Wisborg T. A consensus based template for reporting of pre-hospital major incident medical management. Scand J Trauma Resusc Emerg Med. 2014;22:5. https://doi.org/10.1186/1757-7241-22-5.
8. 10 tips for ambulance staging at mass casualty incidents Greg Friese, MS, NRP.

9. Olchin L, Krutz A. Nurses as first responders in a mass casualty: are you prepared? J Trauma Nurs. 2012;19(2):122–9. https://doi.org/10.1097/JTN.0b013e3182562984.

10. Committee for Tactical Emergency Casualty Care guidelines. www.c-tecc.org. Accessed 17 June 2015.

11. U.S. Fire Administration, FEMA. Fire/Emergency Medical Services Department operational considerations and guide for active shooter and mass casualty incidents. September 2013. https://www.usfa.fema.gov/downloads/pdf/publications/active_shooter_guide.pdf. Accessed 30 June 2015.

12. Maryland Institute for Emergency Medical Services Systems. 2015 Maryland medical protocols for emergency medical services providers. http://meiss.org/home/EMSProviderProtocol/tabid/106/default.aspx. Accessed 17 June 2015.

13. Mass-Casualty Response: The vital first few minutes https://emsworld.com/node/173782. Article 31 Mar 2009.

14. How to respond to plane crashes, 16 Mar 2009 by Chief Bob Lindstrom Aircraft Rescue and Fire Fighting Working Group.

15. Thompson J, Rehn M, Lossius HM, Lockey D. Risks to emergency medical responders at terrorist incidents: a narrative review of the medical literature. Crit Care. 2014;18:521. https://doi.org/10.1186/s13054-014-0521-1. PMCID: PMC4422304. PMID: 25323086.

16. Xu J, Murphy SL, Kochanek KD, Bastian BA. Final data for 2013. Nat Vital Rep. 2016;64(2):1–119. https://www.cdc.gov/nchs/products/nvsr.htm. Published 30 June 2016. Accessed 11 2017.

17. Gun Violence Archive. Gun violence archive summary ledgers 2014. 2015 and 2016, Washington DC. http://www.gunviolencearchive.org/past-tolls. Accessed 11 Jan 2017.

18. Tasigiorgos S, Economopoulos KP, Winfield RD, Sakran JV. Firearm injury in United States an overview of an evolving health problem. J Am Coll Surg. 2015;221(6):1005–14.

19. Livingston DH, Lavery RF, Lopreiato MC, Lavery DF, Passanante MR. Unrelenting violence an analysis of 6322 gunshot wound patients at a Level 1 trauma center. J Trauma Acute Care Surg. 2014;76(1):2–9.

20. Jacobs L. The Hartford Consensus: how to maximize survivability in active shooter and intentional mass casualty events. World J Surg. 2014;38(5):1007–8. https://doi.org/10.1007/s00268-014-2481-7.

Prehospital Fluid Resuscitation, Pain Relief and Stabilization

3

Maria Diakomi

3.1 Introduction

The concept of emergency medical transport originated from the need to move wounded soldiers from the battlefield to medical facilities [1]. However, it was not until the mid-1950s in the United States that the emergency medical service (EMS) systems began to mature in parallel with the interstate highway system and the associated increasing number of serious vehicular crash accidents [2]. The crash accidents' victims necessitated the need for standards for prehospital care concerning provider education, scope of practice, equipment, and system design [3, 4]. This was the beginning of the dramatic improvement in prehospital care.

3.2 Prehospital Stabilization

Prehospital medicine typically consists of two levels of care: basic life support (BLS) and advanced life support (ALS). Wide variation exists in the level of treatment provided in the prehospital setting [5]. It is also uncertain whether the patient will benefit from the on-site ALS protocol or not. However, regardless of the level of care, the main principle of any EMS system is to deliver quality patient care in the briefest period of time following injury, minimizing transport time to the hospital [6]. Rapid transport is especially beneficial for the hemodynamically unstable patient with penetrating trauma, as well as for the patient suffering neurotrauma [7].

Additionally, prehospital trauma care is governed by three basic principles: (1) examination with the recognition of severe injuries and injuries with potential to cause rapid decompensation, (2) triage in case of multiple victims, and (3) stabilization and transport to a hospital capable of coping with the identified injuries. The

M. Diakomi (✉)
Anesthesiology Department, Asklepieion Hospital of Voula, Athens, Greece

© Springer Nature Switzerland AG 2021
E. Pikoulis, J. Doucet (eds.), *Emergency Medicine, Trauma and Disaster Management*, Hot Topics in Acute Care Surgery and Trauma,
https://doi.org/10.1007/978-3-030-34116-9_3

highly qualified person in charge that ensures the implementation of protocols for appropriate prehospital medical care, triage, and hospital notification is called the EMS medical director.

Triage of trauma victims is the process of rapidly and accurately evaluating patients to determine the extent of their injuries and the appropriate level of medical care required [8]. Trauma specialists have developed a number of prehospital triage scoring systems in an effort to accurately differentiate between major and minor injuries. The majority of these scoring systems assess neurologic, respiratory, and circulatory function, as well as anatomy and mechanism of injury [9].

Once triage is completed, the most viable patients are managed first aiming at stabilization and transport to the appropriate medical facility. The initial evaluation of the trauma patient follows the "ABCDE" pattern, provided by the Advanced Trauma Life Support (ATLS) guidelines by the American College of Surgeons: Airway, Breathing, Circulation, Disability (Neurologic status) and Exposure. So, prioritizing the necessary actions to be undertaken, the prehospital care provider secures the patient's airway and establishes manual in-line stabilization of the cervical spine simultaneously, assists ventilation whenever breathing is labored or absent, obtains vital signs and controls any hemorrhage with direct pressure, assesses neurologic status, and exposes critical areas of the body for obvious and occult injuries. Spinal immobilization is continuously maintained by rigid cervical collar and backboard placement, which requires special skill and technique to prevent any secondary injury. Moreover, patients trapped in a vehicle pose challenging problems for safe extrication, which may require the use of special devices that may prolong scene time, but the benefit may outweigh the risk for patients with potentially unstable spinal injuries. The final primary assessment is an evaluation of the entire patient.

After the completion of the initial assessment and stabilizing treatments, the prehospital provider performs a quick but thorough review of the entire body, referred to as the secondary survey. The goal is to discern and manage as appropriate any injuries missed during the primary survey. Following the secondary survey, the patient should be prepared for transport [10].

3.3 Fluid Resuscitation

In the setting of prehospital care, several questions have been raised over time regarding fluid resuscitation, but no definite answer has been given yet. In the era of "evidence based medicine," there is limited information suggesting the benefit of prehospital fluid resuscitation, although it is considered to be standard of care in hospital setting. The advocates of "scoop and run" method support the timely transfer of the patient to a definite care facility without unnecessary and potential harmful interventions, while the advocates of "stay and play" method focus in prehospital interventions that could improve the patient's outcome and survival. For instance, in the case of hemorrhagic hypovolaemic shock, prehospital fluid resuscitation could minimize the risk of tissue and organ damage, but any delay reaching hospital could result in exacerbation of hemorrhage outweighing any benefit of prehospital care.

In medicine, following guidelines has been an efficient method of dealing with difficult problems. So, several trauma societies have launched guidelines for prehospital fluid resuscitation. This chapter will deal with NICE and EAST guidelines and will point out the questions that authors try to answer and the actions that the prehospital care provider has to undertake.

NICE guidelines included seven studies and dealt with the following questions: (1) Should we give fluids? (2) To which patients? (3) If so how much? (4) What type?

- Fluids in boluses of ≤250 ml should be given in the absence of radial pulse in adults.
- The fluid bolus is repeated until radial pulse is felt while continual reassessment of the patient takes place.
- Radial pulse guides intervention in blunt injuries, but central pulse in torso penetrating injuries.
- There is insufficient evidence for pediatric patients.
- Crystalloid solutions are recommended to be administered [11].

On the other hand, EAST guidelines included 42 studies and dealt with the following questions: (1) Should injured patients have vascular access attempted prehospital? (2) What location is preferred for access? (3) Should intravenous fluids be given? (4) Which solution is preferred? (5) At what volume and rate?

- Placement of intravenous access should be made en route, because venous access attempted at the scene delays transport.
- Intraosseous access can be attempted.
- There is no preferred access site.
- Fluids should not be given in patients with penetrating injury and short transit time (<30 min) when brachial pulse is palpable.
- Fluids should only be given: (a) in 250 ml boluses (b) to return the patient to coherent mental status (c) to return radial pulse (d) in traumatic brain injury to maintain systolic blood pressure >90 mmHg or mean arterial pressure >60 mmHg.
- Normal saline is the preferable solution to be administered.
- Rapid infusion systems and pressurized devices should be avoided [12].

Recent data suggest that prehospital fluid therapy should be goal directed based on the presence or absence of hypotension and that excessive IV fluid infusion may lead to adverse outcomes including coagulopathy and death [13]. Volumes more than 1 L might be associated with increased likelihood of blood transfusion in the emergency department, but further research is required to determine any causal relationship [14]. Bores et al. found no significant difference in mortality between patients who did or did not receive prehospital fluid resuscitation after penetrating trauma [15]. Additionally, a systematic review of nine randomized trials involving 3490 trauma patients concluded that prehospital fluid resuscitation using hypertonic saline does not improve survival compared to resuscitation using isotonic crystalloid [16].

3.4   Pain Therapy

The American College of Emergency Physicians has clearly stated that ALS-capable EMS systems should provide analgesia and sedation with appropriate physician oversight and quality improvement programs [17]. However, oligoanesthesia and oligoanalgesia are a common practice in prehospital setting, in all age groups, especially children [18, 19]. Insufficient pain management has been associated with variable factors, including short time at the scene (below 10 min), moderate pain scores at the scene, nontrauma patients and concerns about the patient's condition, for example, blunting respiratory drive in a patient with breathing difficulty [20].

Prehospital pain management aims at reducing pain to a tolerable level without causing serious side effects. Evaluation of pain, the first step in pain treatment, is carried out by means of standard questions, regarding "Onset, Provoking factor, Quality, Radiation, Severity and Time Sequence (OPQRST –pain assessment mnemonic)." Numeric Rating Scale is another useful and efficacious tool, grading pain from 0—no pain to 10—the worst pain [21].

The evaluation of pain is followed by pain control modalities. Controlling pain is an issue of more than drug administration. For instance, extremity injury pain due to fracture requires, except for medication, immobilizing or splinting the extremity, elevating the immobilized extremity and application of ice to painful areas. Communication with the patient is another basic component of pain treatment, as it contributes to breaking pain anxiety cycle [21].

There are variable medications to treat prehospital pain. The health care provider should be familiar with the pharmacodynamics principles of each agent, especially the indications and adverse effects. Pain relief should be rapid (within 10 min) and the patient should be able to respond to verbal stimuli without requiring ventilatory support. Opioids are considered safe analgesics, as sedation and cardiovascular instability are uncommon [22]. Another feature that makes opioids favorable for use in the prehospital setting is naloxone, which readily reverses their effects.

The results of several observational studies suggest that fentanyl can be given safely to trauma patients in the prehospital setting [23, 24]. Except for the intravenous and intramuscular route of administration, subcutaneous route is also available [25]. In pediatric patients fentanyl can be effective intranasally [26]. Morphine may also be used, but it has a longer duration of action and is more likely to cause hypotension and respiratory depression [27, 28]. So, prehospital providers should carefully monitor the respiratory and hemodynamic status of all patients receiving opioids.

Common parenteral analgesic agents used in US Combat Theater in Afghanistan battlefield include fentanyl, morphine, hydromorphone, ketamine, and ketorolac [30]. There is little evidence regarding the prehospital use of ketamine [22]. Better results are expected when ketamine is combined with an opioid compared to opioid or ketamine monotherapy. Disorientation of the patient is an expected adverse effect of ketamine [20, 29]. In addition, the use of nonsteroidal anti-inflammatory drugs (NSAIDs) is associated with a reduced incidence of trauma-induced coagulopathy [31].

References

1. Shah MN. The formation of the emergency medical services system. Am J Public Health. 2006;96(3):414–23. Epub 2006 Jan 31.
2. Boyd DR. The conceptual development of EMS systems in the United States, Part I. Emerg Med Serv. 1982;11(1):19.
3. Law of the 89th Congress: National Highway Safety Act of 1966, Public Law 89-564, Washington, DC. 1966.
4. Law of the 93rd Congress: Emergency Medical Services Systems Act of 1973, Public Law 93-154, Washington, DC. 1973.
5. Bulger EM, Nathens AB, Rivara FP, MacKenzie E, Sabath DR, Jurkovich GJ. National variability in out-of-hospital treatment after traumatic injury. Ann Emerg Med. 2007;49(3):293.
6. Liberman M, Mulder D, Sampalis J. Advanced or basic life support for trauma: meta-analysis and critical review of the literature. J Trauma. 2000;49(4):584.
7. Harmsen AM, Giannakopoulos GF, Moerbeek PR, Jansma EP, Bonjer HJ, Bloemers FW. The influence of prehospital time on trauma patients outcome: a systematic review. Injury. 2015;46(4):602–9. https://doi.org/10.1016/j.injury.2015.01.008. Epub 2015 Jan 16. Review.
8. Lossius HM, Rehn M, Tjosevik KE, Eken T. Calculating trauma triage precision: effects of different definitions of major trauma. J Trauma Manag Outcomes. 2012;6(1):9. https://doi.org/10.1186/1752-2897-6-9.
9. Sasser SM, Hunt RC, Faul M, et al. Guidelines for field triage of injured patients: recommendations of the National Expert Panel on Field Triage, 2011. MMWR. 2012;61:1.
10. National Association of Emergency Medical Technicians. Prehospital trauma life support. 8th ed. United States of America: Jones and Bartlett Learning, LLC; 2016.
11. Prehospital initiation of fluid replacement therapy in trauma. National Institute for Health and Care Excellence, Technology Appraisal 74, January 2004.
12. Cotton BA, Jerome R, Collier BR, Khetarpal S, Holevar M, Tucker B, Kurek S, Mowery NT, Shah K, Bromberg W, Gunter OL, Riordan WP Jr, Eastern Association for the Surgery of Trauma Practice Parameter Workgroup for Prehospital Fluid Resuscitation. Guidelines for prehospital fluid resuscitation in the injured patient. J Trauma. 2009;67(2):389–402. https://doi.org/10.1097/TA.0b013e3181a8b26f.
13. Brown JB, Cohen MJ, Minei JP, Maier RV, West MA, Billiar TR, Peitzman AB, Moore EE, Cuschieri J, Sperry JL, Inflammation and the Host Response to Injury Investigators. Goal-directed resuscitation in the prehospital setting: a propensity-adjusted analysis. J Trauma Acute Care Surg. 2013;74(5):1207.
14. Geeraedts LM Jr, Pothof LA, Caldwell E, de Lange-de Klerk ES, D'Amours SK. Prehospital fluid resuscitation in hypotensive trauma patients: do we need a tailored approach? Injury. 2015;46(1):4–9. https://doi.org/10.1016/j.injury.2014.08.001. Epub 2014 Aug 11. Review.
15. Bores SA, Pajerowski W, Carr BG, Holena D, Meisel ZF, Mechem CC, Band RA. The association of prehospital intravenous fluids and mortality in patients with penetrating trauma. J Emerg Med. 2018; https://doi.org/10.1016/j.jemermed.2017.12.046. pii: S0736–4679(17)31212-X [Epub ahead of print].
16. de Crescenzo C, Gorouhi F, Salcedo ES, Galante JM. Prehospital hypertonic fluid resuscitation for trauma patients: a systematic review and meta-analysis. J Trauma Acute Care Surg. 2017;82(5):956.
17. American College of Emergency Physicians Policy Statement. Out-of-hospital use of analgesia and sedation. Ann Emerg Med. 2016;67(2):305–6.
18. McEachin CC, McDermott JT, Swor R. Few emergency medical services patients with lower-extremity fractures receive prehospital analgesia. Prehosp Emerg Care. 2002;6(4):406.
19. Hewes HA, Dai M, Mann NC, Baca T, Taillac P. Prehospital pain management: disparity by age and race. Prehosp Emerg Care. 2018;22(2):189–97. https://doi.org/10.1080/10903127.2017.1367444. Epub 2017 Sep 28.

20. Oberholzer N, Kaserer A, Albrecht R, Seifert B, Tissi M, Spahn DR, Maurer K, Stein P. Factors influencing quality of pain management in a physician staffed helicopter emergency medical service. Anesth Analg. 2017;125(1):200–9. https://doi.org/10.1213/ANE.0000000000002016.
21. Phrampus PE, Paris P. The science of pain. A guide to prehospital pain management. JEMS. 2016;41(11):53–6. Review.
22. Park CL, Roberts DE, Aldington DJ, Moore RA. Prehospital analgesia: systematic review of evidence. J R Army Med Corps. 2010;156(4 Suppl 1):295–300. Review.
23. Garrick JF, Kidane S, Pointer JE, Sugiyama W, Van Luen C, Clark R. Analysis of the paramedic administration of fentanyl. J Opioid Manag. 2011;7(3):229–34.
24. Soriya GC, McVaney KE, Liao MM, Haukoos JS, Byyny RL, Gravitz C, Colwell CB. Safety of prehospital intravenous fentanyl for adult trauma patients. J Trauma Acute Care Surg. 2012;72(3):755–9.
25. Lebon J, Fournier F, Bégin F, Hebert D, Fleet R, Foldes-Busque G, Tanguay A. Subcutaneous fentanyl administration: a novel approach for pain management in a rural and suburban prehospital setting. Prehosp Emerg Care. 2016;20(5):648–56. https://doi.org/10.3109/10903127.201 6.1162887. Epub 2016 Apr 8.
26. Murphy AP, Hughes M, Mccoy S, Crispino G, Wakai A, O'Sullivan R. Intranasal fentanyl for the prehospital management of acute pain in children. Eur J Emerg Med. 2017;24(6):450–4. https://doi.org/10.1097/MEJ.0000000000000389.
27. Fleischman RJ, Frazer DG, Daya M, Jui J, Newgard CD. Effectiveness and safety of fentanyl compared with morphine for out-of-hospital analgesia. Prehosp Emerg Care. 2010;14(2):167–75. https://doi.org/10.3109/10903120903572301.
28. Smith MD, Wang Y, Cudnik M, Smith DA, Pakiela J, Elerman CL. The effectiveness and adverse events of morphine versus fentanyl on a physician-staffed helicopter. J Emerg Med. 2012;43(1):69–75.
29. Jennings PA, Cameron P, Bernard S, Walker T, Jolley D, Fitzgerald M, Masci K. Morphine and ketamine is superior to morphine alone for out-of-hospital trauma analgesia: a randomized controlled trial. Ann Emerg Med. 2012;59(6):497–503. Epub 2012 Jan 13.
30. Schauer SG, Mora AG, Maddry JK, Bebarta VS. Multicenter, prospective study of Prehospital Administration of Analgesia in the U.S. Combat Theater of Afghanistan. Prehosp Emerg Care. 2017;21(6):744–9. https://doi.org/10.1080/10903127.2017.1335814. Epub 2017 Aug 22.
31. Neal MD, Brown JB, Moore EE, Cuschieri J, Maier RV, Minei JP, Billiar TR, Peitzman AB, Cohen MJ, Sperry JL. Inflammation and host response to injury investigators. Prehospital use of nonsteroidal anti-inflammatory drugs (NSAIDs) is associated with a reduced incidence of trauma-induced coagulopathy. Ann Surg. 2014;260(2):378–82. https://doi.org/10.1097/SLA.0000000000000526.

Resuscitation in Limited Resources Environments

4

Theodoros Xanthos and Athanasios Chalkias

4.1 Introduction

Cardiac arrest (CA) can be the end outcome of many categories of critically unwell patients. This is also applicable in the setting of major incidents, where many of the critically injured will develop CA as their disease or injury pathophysiology can result in multi-organ failure. Primary CA due to cardiac pathophysiology is thought to be rare in the setting, despite the fact that no studies have addressed this issue. A patient with CA will not take priority in the setting of a major incident, given that despite recent advances in resuscitation, survival to hospital discharge remains low in patients developing CA [1]. More specifically, the overall survival rates after cardiac arrest range from 1% to <20% for out of hospital non-traumatic cardiac arrest and <40% for in-hospital cardiac arrest [2]. Published studies report a 10–50% poor neurological outcome of CA survivors [3, 4].

Cardiopulmonary Resuscitation (CPR) is complex procedure, which does not only involve chest compressions and ventilation. CPR requires a team of dedicated health care professionals, which will perform various tasks and will work in a coordinated manner not only to achieve return of spontaneous circulation (ROSC), but also to ascertain that the neurological outcome of the CA patient will be as optimal, as it can possibly be [5]. In the setting of a major incident, where many casualties

T. Xanthos (✉)
Physiology and Pathophysiology, Chair Department of Medicine, European University Cyprus, Nicosia, Cyprus

Hellenic Society of Cardiopulmonary Resuscitation, Athens, Greece
e-mail: t.xanthos@euc.ac.cy

A. Chalkias
Hellenic Society of Cardiopulmonary Resuscitation, Athens, Greece

Anesthesiology, Faculty of Medicine, University of Thessaly, Volos, Greece

© Springer Nature Switzerland AG 2021
E. Pikoulis, J. Doucet (eds.), *Emergency Medicine, Trauma and Disaster Management*, Hot Topics in Acute Care Surgery and Trauma,
https://doi.org/10.1007/978-3-030-34116-9_4

are involved, patients requiring CPR should not take priority over other patients who have better chances of survival.

This chapter will discuss the procedures of proper CPR both in out-of-hospital and in-hospital settings, with the understanding that enough resources can be allocated to patients developing CA. It goes without saying that all critically ill patients, who have not yet developed CA should be actively resuscitated and they should take priority in the allocation of resources.

4.2   Cardiac Arrest

Recent studies have identified that the pathophysiology of cardiac arrest is not uniform. In fact, there appear to be two types of arrest with distinct pathophysiology, the asphyxia CA and the Ventricular Fibrillation CA. These two types of arrest, not only exhibit distinct pathophysiologies, but also differences in the post-resuscitation brain injury and the ensuing post-resuscitation myocardial dysfunction [6]. The underlying rhythm of CA due to cardiac causes is reported to be ventricular fibrillation (VF) in about 25–50% of the cases [7], however when an automated external defibrillator is attached immediately after arrest, the proportion of patients in VF can be as high as 75% [8]. These numbers signify the importance of early defibrillation. In fact, defibrillation, which is delivered 3–5 min of collapse can produce survival rates as high as 50–70%; this signifies the importance of the availability of defibrillators (automated or manual) in the deployment of any team after a major incident. CA can also be the outcome of non-cardiac causes (such as asphyxia). In this setting early initiation of rescue ventilation and chest compressions are of utmost importance for the improvement of survival of these patients. In the setting of a major incident a patient who has developed CA does not take priority over a patient who is critically ill. If a critically ill patient develops CA, prompt defibrillation along with chest compressions and ventilation will increase survival.

Recognition of CA can be challenging in any setting, given that carotid pulse check can be inaccurate in determining the presence or absence of circulation. This is why, the current European Resuscitation Council (ERC) guidelines recommend the determination of the presence of absence of breathing or the presence of agonal breathing to determine whether a patient is in CA or not [9]. In the setting of a major incident, any critically unwell patient, who suddenly develops seizures, should be considered to be in CA, until proven otherwise. Despite the fact that no studies have addressed the issue in the setting of major incidents, recent studies have shown a positive association between seizures and the development of CA [10], leading the ERC 2015 guidelines to recommend "Bystanders should be suspicious of cardiac arrest in any patient presenting with seizures" and to emphasize that "the call taker should be highly suspicious of cardiac arrest, even if the caller reports that the victim has a prior history of epilepsy." Seizures develop because of brain hypoxia and in the case of a major incident, the team needs to be aware that sudden onset of seizures can be a sign of CA.

4.3   Adult Basic Life Support (BLS)

In the setting of a major incident, it is absolutely necessary to highlight the importance of the providers' safety. Only when the safety of the providers has been ascertained, should the BLS sequence be followed. The 2015 ERC guidelines have recommended a specific BLS sequence [9]. This sequence will be valid until the revised 2020 guidelines on resuscitation are published. Given that CA is not immediately recognized, the guidelines highlight the recognition of an unresponsive patient, who is not breathing normally, as the first link of the adult BLS sequence. The second link is the activation of the emergency medical service system (EMS), but in the setting of a major incident, the EMS has already been activated and as result this step needs to be taken for granted. In the unlikely event that the EMS has not been activated, the people who are the first responders in a major incident, should activate the EMS immediately and in this case the EMS activation should be the first step in the resuscitation sequence, as the EMS will be needed for all the victims involved in the incident.

In case of CA in this setting, the cause is unlikely to be cardiac in origin, unlike the cases of CA which occur unexpectedly. In the case of sudden CA, the blood remains oxygenated for some minutes and thus the next step in the BLS sequence is immediate initiation of chest compressions in the middle of a chest with a rate of 100–120/min, allowing for full chest recoil. In the case of a major incident, the cause of the arrest is unlikely to be cardiac in origin and it is unlikely that there is still sufficiently oxygenated blood in the arterial blood system and in the lungs. The 2015 ERC guidelines have not addressed this issue, but it is logical for a healthcare provider to provide other life-saving interventions in CA patients involved major incidents along with chest compressions.

Chest compressions should be delivered in the center of the chest, with the CPR provider kneeling next to the victim. When the CA patient is found in a confined space (which may well be the case in any major incident), over the head and straddle CPR can be considered as an acceptable alternative [11]. This alternative has also been mentioned in the 2015 ERC guidelines in resuscitation.

The next step in the adult BLS sequence is the delivery of rescue breaths of rescue ventilations. The 2015 ERC guidelines recommend a tidal volume of 500–600 ml to be delivered over a period of 1 s, basically because this is the amount of air which can cause the chest to rise visibly [12]. There is insufficient data to suggest the optimal volume and timing of ventilation in resuscitation [13]. The recommended compression to ventilation ratio is 30 compressions to 2 ventilations, despite the fact that the optimal compression to ventilation ratio is unknown. The 2015 recommendation was based on a few observational studies which showed improvement with this ratio compared to the previous recommended ratio of 15 compressions to 2 ventilations [14].

The next step is early defibrillation. Automated external defibrillators (AED) can be safely used by lay people to deliver defibrillation in shockable rhythms. The 2015 ERC guidelines recommend minimal interruption in the delivery of chest

Table 4.1 Recommended BLS/AED sequence for out-of-hospital non-traumatic cardiac arrest by a lay rescuer	Unresponsive and no breathing normally *then*
	Call emergency services *then*
	Deliver 30 high-quality chest compressions *then*
	Provide two rescue breaths (or two ventilations)
	Continue CPR 30 compressions to 2 ventilations *until*
	AED arrives, switch on and follow instructions

compressions during the use of an AED. Despite the fact that public access defibrillation programs have been proven successful, the use of AEDs in the hospital setting has reduced survival. This may be due to the fact that AEDs cause harmful delays in starting CPR, or interruptions in chest compressions in patients with non-shockable rhythms [15]. It appears reasonable that in the case of a major incident where a fully deployed team of healthcare professionals is in place, the use of manual defibrillators should be preferred. This however should take into consideration the teams' ability of interpreting ECG recordings. The adult BLS/AED sequence can be seen in Table 4.1, which is based on the 2015 ERC guidelines on resuscitation.

4.4 Advanced Life Support

Despite the fact that the 2015 ERC guidelines address the in-hospital arrest and the Advanced Life Support (ALS) for the hospital setting, it appears reasonable that certain ALS providers in major incidents can have the resources and the skill to provide ALS support. As a result, this chapter will continue discussion with the ALS techniques as these can be provided on site of the major incident. The ALS treatment algorithm is a universal algorithm but certain specific interventions may be needed in special circumstances. In cases of major incidents special circumstances is the rule and not the exception and it is logical that these healthcare providers who perform advance techniques in the site of major incident possess the clinical reasoning skills to perform additional life-saving procedures. The universal ALS treatment algorithm can be found in the 2015 ERC guidelines and will not be repeated in this chapter.

In non-traumatic CA there is little doubt that the only interventions that improve the outcome are early initiation of bystander CPR, uninterrupted high-quality chest compressions and early defibrillation for the shockable rhythms. The shockable rhythms in CA is VF and pulseless ventricular tachycardia (PVT). The ALS treatment algorithm uses the 2-min cycle despite the fact that there is not enough evidence to fully support this cycle. In fact, regional differences with other timings do exist [16]. The ALS treatment algorithm uses as a prerequisite the use of a manual defibrillator and as a result this implies that the healthcare providers know how to recognize shockable versus non-shockable rhythms.

When in a major incident, the team decides to change to the ALS treatment guidelines, it is expected that the team is trained according to the current guidelines and complies to local protocol policies. When CA has been diagnosed, one member of the team needs to provide uninterrupted chest compressions as another member of the team prepares the manual defibrillator. The person using the manual defibrillator should use it as quickly as possible to determine whether the underlying CA rhythm is shockable or non-shockable. This can be done by a technique called "quick look." This technique allows the operator of the manual defibrillator to quickly assess the underlying rhythm. This is the only time where the chest compressions need to stop and this time should be less than 10 s. The operator charges the defibrillator to the recommended energy. The minimum energy for biphasic defibrillators is at least 150 J. There is not enough evidence to suggest that this is the optimal defibrillation energy and as a result the current guidelines state that "it is appropriate to consider escalating the shock energy if feasible, after a failed shock and for patients where re-fibrillation occurs" [9].

Immediately after the delivery of the first shock, there should be no interruption in chest compressions in order to assess if a shock has been successful. The 2015 ERC guidelines on resuscitation recommend immediate initiation of chest compressions following the delivery of the shock to limit the post-shock pause and the total peri-shock pause [17]. This cycle of resuscitation and defibrillation is repeated every 2 min, provided that the patient remains in a shockable rhythm. Unlike the adult BLS sequence the ALS treatment algorithm is linear in the sense that multiple tasks should be performed simultaneously. The team providing ALS should be able to secure an intravenous or an intraosseous line. There is not enough evidence to suggest that the use of any supraglottic device increases the possibilities of survival [18]. However, if the team is trained in the insertion of any supraglottic device, this should be inserted. Routine endotracheal intubation is not recommended by non-anesthetists as it entails a high level of skill and training. When an anesthetist is available, endotracheal intubation and mechanical ventilation should be preferred. The use of automated ventilator during CPR is associated with several favorable effects, such as pulmonary recruitment, minimal thoracic volume reduction, reduced ventilation/perfusion mismatch, and improved oxygenation, which increase the possibilities of ROSC [19, 20].

When a supraglottic device has been inserted, chest compressions should be delivered uninterrupted at a rate of 100–120/min and ten breaths should be delivered asynchronously. The 2015 ERC guidelines emphasize on the use of capnography, as a tool to monitor CPR quality and to enable early detection of ROSC without pausing chest compressions and may be used as a way of avoiding a bolus injection of adrenaline after ROSC has been achieved. There is no evidence that routine use of adrenaline at any dose improves survival. Adrenaline 1 mg is given in shockable rhythms after the third unsuccessful defibrillation attempt. There is evidence suggesting that adrenaline is associated with improved ROSC, but may be associated with worse neurological outcomes [21]. Adrenaline can be administered every other 2 cycles (fifth, seventh, ninth cycle, etc.). After the third unsuccessful defibrillation attempt, 300 mg of amiodarone should be administered IV with another 150 mg administered after the fifth attempted defibrillation. There is no sufficient data to support the use of amiodarone for in-hospital arrest and a recent meta-analysis, which was published after the 2015 guidelines revealed that Amiodarone significantly improves survival to hospital admission, but neither survival to hospital

Table 4.2 Reversible causes in cardiac arrest

The 4 Hs	The 4 Ts
Hypoxia	Tension pneumothorax
Hypovolemia	Tamponade (cardiac)
Hypothermia	Toxins
Hypokalemia/hyperkalemia (and other metabolic disturbances)	Thrombosis (cardiac or pulmonary)

discharge nor neurological outcome compared to placebo or nifekalant [22]. All drugs which are administered peripherally must be followed by a flush of at least 20 ml of fluid and elevation of the extremity for 10–20 s to facilitate drug delivery to the central circulation.

Non-shockable rhythms of CA include pulseless electrical activity (PEA) and asystole. PEA in CA is the presence of electrical activity (other than ventricular tachyarrhythmia), which is normally associated by the presence of a palpable pulse [23]. In case of non-shockable rhythms, the team needs to administer 1 mg of adrenaline and try and identify the reversible causes of cardiac arrest (Table 4.2), without interrupting high-quality resuscitation. Again each cycle lasts for 2 min, after which a rhythm check should be performed in order to identify whether a patient is still in non-shockable rhythm. Several studies have examined the use of ultrasound during cardiac arrest to detect potentially reversible causes [24]. Despite the paucity of evidence to suggest that this imaging modality improves outcome, the ERC 2015 guidelines on resuscitation recommend its use to exclude various causes. In case of traumatic CA, resuscitative thoracotomy should be considered in pulseless patients with chest/upper abdominal wounds not responsive to thoracostomy. Survival rates for resuscitative thoracotomy have been reported approximately 15% for all patients with penetrating wounds and 35% for patients with a penetrating cardiac wound. In contrast, survival from resuscitative thoracotomy following blunt trauma remains dismal (0–2%) [9]. The success of resuscitative thoracotomy depends on expertise, equipment, environment, and elapsed time. The procedure may be performed also in the prehospital setting, provided that the time from loss of pulse is less than 10 min [25].

4.5 Monitoring During ALS

Clinical signs, such as opening of the eyes, breathing efforts and movement can be a sign of ROSC, but can also be due to the fact that high-quality CPR can produce sufficient blood flow to restore signs of life. A recent meta-analysis identified nine reports, describing ten patients. Six of the patients had CPR performed by mechanical devices, three of these patients were sedated. Four patients arrested in the out-of-hospital setting and six arrested in hospital. There were four survivors. Varying levels of consciousness were described in all reports, including purposeful arm movements, verbal communication, and resuscitation interference [26]. Feedback devices should be used as part of a broader system of improvement of CPR quality.

Capnography is a new tool which monitors interventions during ALS One of the major challenges regarding capnography may be its implementation and correct interpretation during resuscitation. Although changes and trends in $ETCO_2$ values during CPR are more important than absolute $ETCO_2$ levels, current data suggest that certain cutoff values may be targeted; although an $ETCO_2 > 10$ mmHg is correlated with increased possibility for ROSC, rescuers should target a 20-min $ETCO_2$ of at least 20 mmHg. However, the value of a trend more than absolute values may be most important in the presence of a treatable cause [27]. Pulse checks are not routinely recommended to record CPR quality. Moreover, continuous monitoring is the standard of care during ALS. Motion artifacts prevent reliable heart rhythm assessment during chest compressions forcing rescuers to stop chest compressions to assess the rhythm, and preventing early recognition of recurrent VF/pVT. Some modern defibrillators have filters that remove artifacts from compressions but there are no human studies showing improvements in patient outcomes from their use [9]. Blood gas analysis is not recommended as a routine procedure during resuscitation because arterial gas values may be misleading and bear little relationship to the tissue acid–base state. Since 1986, we know that arterial blood does not reflect the marked reduction in mixed venous (and therefore tissue) pH, and thus arterial blood gases may fail as appropriate guides for acid–base management in CA [28]. Cerebral oximetry using near-infrared spectroscopy measures regional cerebral oxygen saturation noninvasively. Other similar techniques such as bispectral index monitoring (BIS) has the potential to offer information about the adequacy of cerebral blood flow and oxygenation, although changes in BIS readings often lag behind changes in arterial pressures. When BIS monitoring is used during CPR, it can be used as a potential predictor of cerebral perfusion, therefore helping the resuscitating team in assessing the cerebral response to the CPR. BIS is of limited value during the early phase of post-resuscitative care. BIS values of zero help predict a poor neurologic outcome after CA and induced hypothermia. However, a non-zero BIS is insufficient as a sole predictor of good neurologic survival. Despite the promising results in other settings, the use of this technology needs further evaluation in the CPR setting [29].

4.6 Post Cardiac Arrest Treatment

Successful ROSC is the first step toward the goal of complete recovery from cardiac arrest. The complex pathophysiological processes that occur following whole body ischemia during cardiac arrest and the subsequent reperfusion response during CPR and following successful resuscitation have been termed the post-cardiac arrest syndrome. Post-resuscitation myocardial stunning is the mechanical dysfunction that persists after the ROSC and is characterized by the absence of irreversible damage, as well as by normal or near-normal coronary flow [30]. Cardiovascular failure accounts for most deaths in the first 3 days, while brain injury accounts for most of the later deaths. Post-cardiac arrest brain injury may be exacerbated by microcirculatory failure, impaired autoregulation, hypotension, hypercarbia, hypoxemia, hyperoxemia, pyrexia, hypoglycemia, hyperglycemia and seizures. Given the complexity of the syndrome during the immediate ROSC period, several aspects of the unstable patient need to be addressed. Hypoxemia and hypercarbia both increase the likelihood of a further cardiac arrest and may contribute to secondary brain injury. Despite the common attitude to administer high level oxygen in all CA patients who have achieved ROSC, several studies have addressed the possibility that hyperoxemia can be equally life threatening. In the immediate post-resuscitation period, titrate the oxygen concentration to the patients' arterial blood gases. Every patient post-arrest who has not achieved sufficient level of consciousness needs sedation, intubation and ventilation. Despite the lack of prospective evidence, there have been studies associating hypocapnia with poor neurological outcome [32]. The current guidelines recommend normocarbia and active monitoring of the patients' CO_2 in the arterial blood gases and $ETCO_2$.

In the setting of a major incident, the ERC 2015 recommendations regarding percutaneous coronary intervention should be considered in all non-traumatic cardiac arrest. An ALS team should pharmacologically stabilize the circulation of all post-arrest patients. Hemodynamic instability, possibly multifactorial in origin, is common after cardiac arrest with abnormalities of cardiac rate, rhythm, systemic blood pressure, and organ perfusion. Adequate fluid resuscitation in patients with low central venous pressure or pulmonary artery occlusion pressure and treatment of associated arrhythmia, myocardial ischemia and electrolyte abnormalities are essential. During post-resuscitation care it may be necessary to augment blood pressure and cardiac output by one of three ways: (1) pharmacological vasoactive support, (2) intra-aortic balloon counterpulsation (3) revascularization with thrombolysis, percutaneous intervention or coronary artery bypass surgery [31]. There is a strong association between high blood glucose after resuscitation from cardiac arrest and poor neurological outcome. Based on the available data, following ROSC maintain the blood glucose 180 mg/dl and avoid hypoglycemia [9]. For more than a decade, mild induced hypothermia (32–34 °C) has been the cornerstone of post–cardiac arrest care. Mild to moderate hypothermia induced after global brain ischemia or cardiac arrest was initially evaluated in animal models that showed improved neurological function for those receiving induced hypothermia. The Temperature Task Force issued a statement recommending targeted temperature management for adults with out-of-hospital cardiac arrest with an initial shockable rhythm at a constant temperature between 32 and 36 °C for at least 24 h. Similar suggestions are made for out-of-hospital cardiac arrest with a non-shockable rhythm and in-hospital cardiac arrest. The task force recommends against prehospital cooling with rapid infusion of large volumes of cold intravenous fluid [9].

4.7   Conclusion

In the setting of a major incident or a massive destruction, resources should not be allocated to people who do not have signs of life. All resources should be targeted to people who are critically ill and have better chances of survival. In case of CA, the standard ERC 2015 algorithm should be followed, but the providers should bear in mind, that the underlying cause in the setting is rarely cardiac in origin. Other reversible causes of arrest should be identified and treated.

References

1. Perkins GD, Jacobs IG, Nadkarni VM, Berg RA, Bhanji F, Biarent D, Bossaert LL, Brett SJ, Chamberlain D, de Caen AR, Deakin CD, Finn JC, Gräsner JT, Hazinski MF, Iwami T, Koster RW, Lim SH, Ma MH, BF MN, Morley PT, Morrison LJ, Monsieurs KG, Montgomery W, Nichol G, Okada K, Ong ME, Travers AH, Nolan JP, Collaborators Utstein. Cardiac arrest and cardiopulmonary resuscitation outcome reports: update of the utstein resuscitation registry templates for out-of-hospital cardiac arrest: a statement for healthcare professionals from a task force of the International Liaison Committee on resuscitation (American Heart Association, European Resuscitation Council, Australian and New Zealand Council on Resuscitation, Heart and Stroke Foundation of Canada, InterAmerican Heart Foundation, Resuscitation Council of Southern Africa, Resuscitation Council of Asia); and the American heart association emergency cardiovascular care committee and the council on cardiopulmonary, critical care, perioperative and resuscitation. Resuscitation. 2015;96:328–40.
2. Cave DM, Gazmuri RJ, Otto CW, Nadkarni VM, Cheng A, Brooks SC, Daya M, Sutton RM, Branson R, Hazinski MF. Part 7: CPR techniques and devices: 2010 American Heart Association Guidelines for Cardiopulmonary Resuscitation and Emergency Cardiovascular Care. Circulation. 2010;122(18 Suppl 3):S720–8.
3. Stiell IG, Brown SP, Christenson J, Cheskes S, Nichol G, Powell J, Bigham B, Morrison LJ, Larsen J, Hess E, Vaillancourt C, Davis DP, Callaway CW, Resuscitation Outcomes Consortium (ROC) Investigators. What is the role of chest compression depth during out-of-hospital cardiac arrest resuscitation? Crit Care Med. 2012;40:1192–8.
4. Ebell MH, Jang W, Shen Y, Geocadin RG, Get With The Guidelines-Resuscitation Investigators. Development and validation of the good outcome following attempted resuscitation (GO-FAR) score to predict neurologically intact survival after in-hospital cardiopulmonary resuscitation. JAMA Intern Med. 2013;173:1872–8.
5. Griffith DM, Salisbury LG, Lee RJ, Lone N, Merriweather JL, Walsh TS, RECOVER Investigators. Determinants of health-related quality of life after ICU: importance of patient demographics, previous comorbidity, and severity of illness. Crit Care Med. 2018;46:594–601.
6. Varvarousis D, Varvarousi G, Iacovidou N, D'Aloja E, Gulati A, Xanthos T. The pathophysiologies of asphyxial vs dysrhythmic cardiac arrest: implications for resuscitation and post-event management. Am J Emerg Med. 2015;33:1297–304.
7. Ringh M, Herlitz J, Hollenberg J, Rosenqvist M, Svensson L. Out of hospital cardiac arrest outside home in Sweden, change in characteristics, outcome and availability for public access defibrillation. Scand J Trauma Resusc Emerg Med. 2009;17:18.
8. Berdowski J, Blom MT, Bardai A, Tan HL, Tijssen JG, Koster RW. Impact of onsite or dispatched automated external defibrillator use on survival after out-of-hospital cardiac arrest. Circulation. 2011;124:2225–32.
9. Monsieurs KG, Nolan JP, Bossaert LL, Greiff R, Maconochie IK, Nikolaou NI, Perkins GD, Soar J, Truhlárl A, Wyllie J, Zideman DA, on behalf of the ERC Guidelines 2015 Writing Group. European Resuscitation Council guidelines for resuscitation 2015 Section 1. Executive summary. Resuscitation. 2015;95:1–80.
10. Stecker EC, Reinier K, Uy-Evanado A, et al. Relationship between seizure episode and sudden cardiac arrest in patients with epilepsy: a community-based study. Circ Arrhythm Electrophysiol. 2013;6:912–6.
11. Perkins GD, Stephenson BT, Smith CM, Gao F. A comparison between over-the-head and standard cardiopulmonary resuscitation. Resuscitation. 2004;61:155–61.

12. Baskett P, Nolan J, Parr M. Tidal volumes which are perceived to be adequate for resuscitation. Resuscitation. 1996;31:231–4.
13. Chalkias A, Xanthos T. Timing positive-pressure ventilation during chest compression: the key to improving the thoracic pump? Eur Heart J Acute Cardiovasc Care. 2015;4:24–7.
14. Olasveengen TM, Vik E, Kuzovlev A, Sunde K. Effect of implementation of new resuscitation guidelines on quality of cardiopulmonary resuscitation and survival. Resuscitation. 2009;80:407–11.
15. Gibbison B, Soar J. Automated external defibrillator use for in-hospital cardiac arrest is not associated with improved survival. Evid Based Med. 2011;16:95–6.
16. Lexow K, Sunde K. Why Norwegian 2005 guidelines differs slightly from the ERC guidelines. Resuscitation. 2007;72:490–2.
17. Cheskes S, Schmicker RH, Verbeek PR, et al. The impact of peri-shock pause on survival from out-of-hospital shockable cardiac arrest during the Resus-citation Outcomes Consortium PRIMED trial. Resuscitation. 2014;85:336–42.
18. Stiell IG, Wells GA, Field B, et al. Advanced cardiac life support in out-of-hospital cardiac arrest. N Engl J Med. 2004;351:647–56.
19. Chalkias A, Pavlopoulos F, Koutsovasilis A, d'Aloja E, Xanthos T. Airway pressure and outcome of out-of-hospital cardiac arrest: a prospective observational study. Resuscitation. 2017;110:101–6.
20. Gazmuri RJ, Ayoub IM, Radhakrishnan J, Motl J, Upadhyaya MP. Clinically plausible hyperventilation does not exert adverse hemodynamic effects during CPR but markedly reduces end-tidal PCO_2. Resuscitation. 2012;83:259–64.
21. Xanthos T, Pantazopoulos I, Demestiha T, Stroumpoulis K. Epinephrine in ventricular fibrillation: friend or foe? A review for the Emergency Nurse. J Emerg Nurs. 2011;37:408–12.
22. Laina A, Karlis G, Liakos A, Georgiopoulos G, Oikonomou D, Kouskouni E, Chalkias A, Xanthos T. Amiodarone and cardiac arrest: systematic review and meta-analysis. Int J Cardiol. 2016;221:780–8.
23. Myerburg RJ, Halperin H, Egan DA, et al. Pulseless electric activity: definition, causes, mechanisms, management, and research priorities for the next decade: report from a National Heart, Lung, and Blood Institute workshop. Circulation. 2013;128:2532–41.
24. Flato UA, Paiva EF, Carballo MT, Buehler AM, Marco R, Timerman A. Echocardiography for prognostication during the resuscitation of intensive care unit patients with non-shockable rhythm cardiac arrest. Resuscitation. 2015;92:1–6.
25. Chalkias A, Xanthos T. Should prehospital resuscitative thoracotomy be incorporated in advanced life support after traumatic cardiac arrest? Eur J Trauma Emerg Surg. 2014;40:395–7.
26. Olaussen A, Shepherd M, Nehme Z, Smith K, Bernard S, Mitra B. Return ofconsciousness during ongoing cardiopulmonary resuscitation: a systematic review. Resuscitation. 2014;86C:44–8.
27. Pantazopoulos C, Xanthos T, Pantazopoulos I, Papalois A, Kouskouni E, Iacovidou N. A review of carbon dioxide monitoring during adult cardiopulmonary resuscitation. Heart Lung Circ. 2015;24:1053–61.
28. Weil MH, Rackow EC, Trevino R, Grundler W, Falk JL, Griffel MI. Difference in acid–base state between venous and arterial blood during cardiopulmonary resuscitation. N Engl J Med. 1986;315:153–6.
29. Pothitakis C, Ekmektzoglou KA, Piagkou M, Karatzas T, Xanthos T. Nursing role in monitoring during cardiopulmonary resuscitation and in the peri-arrest period: a review. Heart Lung. 2011;40:530–44.
30. Chalkias A, Xanthos T. Pathophysiology and pathogenesis of post-resuscitation myocardial stunning. Heart Fail Rev. 2012;17:117–28.
31. Kakavas S, Chalkias A, Xanthos T. Vasoactive support in the optimization of post-cardiac arrest hemodynamic status: from pharmacology to clinical practice. Eur J Pharmacol. 2011;667:32–40.
32. Roberts BW, Kilgannon JH, Chansky ME, Mittal N, Wooden J, Trzeciak S. Association between postresuscitation partial pressure of arterial carbon dioxide and neurological outcome in patients with post-cardiac arrest syndrome. Circulation. 2013;127:2107–13.

Anesthesia for Critically Injured in Limited Resources Environments

5

Theodosios Saranteas, Iosifina Koliantzaki,
Paraskeui Matsota, and Georgia Kostopanagiotou

5.1 Introduction

Disaster settings are typically associated with high numbers of casualties and calamitous consequences for the victims, particularly in contexts where the healthcare systems' infrastructures are damaged. Consequently, the management of disaster-related trauma is less efficient in developing countries, where the infrastructures network is wobbly and deficient. Additionally, the contingent fallouts from disasters are very likely to be large scale in developing countries, because the healthcare systems are frequently already lacking in human resources, and health care providers have not got sufficient medical expertise [1–3].

Electronic monitoring may not be present, or the electricity may not be sufficient (forcing the anesthesia provider to manually monitor the patient), and oxygen supply as well as drugs provision may be difficult and in some cases even impossible [4]. Even if the conditions are very hard and hostile during disasters, safe administration of anesthesia techniques (regional and general anesthesia) remains possible and should be of the best possible quality. That's to say the principle of "do not harm" must define the anesthesia provision and ought to be applied at all times [1–5].

Pain evaluation and management in disaster settings should also be emphasized. The notion of evaluating pain as a vital sign has been previously presented [6]. In emergency settings, healthcare providers prioritize and provide pain treatments, often suboptimal, relative to the severity of the conditions. Next, critical patients are immediately sent to hospitals to continue therapy in a more precise and individualized fashion. In disaster setting, this sequence is disrupted. Patients must be treated at the site of the disaster, or better yet in designated-improvised areas converted into

T. Saranteas · I. Koliantzaki · P. Matsota · G. Kostopanagiotou (✉)
Second Department of Anesthesia, National & Kapodistrian University of Athens, Medical School, Athens, Greece
e-mail: gkostopan@med.uoa.gr

© Springer Nature Switzerland AG 2021
E. Pikoulis, J. Doucet (eds.), *Emergency Medicine, Trauma and Disaster Management*, Hot Topics in Acute Care Surgery and Trauma,
https://doi.org/10.1007/978-3-030-34116-9_5

operating theaters [3, 4]. Nevertheless, the premise of early and aggressive pain treatment is inevitable and vital. In fact, apart from the administration of the traditional analgesic pharmacotherapy, local-regional anesthesia techniques [7–9] are effective and may be in order, when resuscitating these patients. It is apparent, therefore, that the evaluation and management of pain must be considered throughout the trauma assessment in disaster settings. Pain evaluation and management is paramount; the letter "P" merits attention as much as the other letters of the algorithm of ATLS and should probably be added to this protocol, especially in these trauma cases [1, 6, 10, 11].

From the wake of these findings, it is acknowledged that in disaster settings, the anesthetic and pain management must be always considered throughout the trauma assessment. Therefore, in this chapter, we set out to discuss the different types of anesthetic techniques which can be implemented in precarious situations, in addition to emphasizing on the decisive and vital role of pain management in multi-trauma victims.

5.2 Regional Anesthesia Techniques

5.2.1 Rationale for Regional Anesthesia in Massive Disasters Trauma

At the site of the disaster, regional anesthesia (RA) is extremely useful to provide analgesia, operative anesthesia, and postoperative analgesia. RA techniques deliver local anesthetic close to a nerve structure in order to block sensation and subsequently pain at the specific injured anatomic region [1, 7, 11].

Taking into consideration that cardio-respiratory depression and neuro-muscular relaxation should be avoided, and limited dependence on oxygen and biomedical monitoring should be maintained, RA techniques take on significant dimensions in the analgesia/anesthesia management of trauma patients in massive disaster settings [7, 12].

In patients with lower and upper limb trauma, authoritative hospital-based studies have advocated RA to be more effective in alleviating pain as compared to opioids alone. In hospitals, however, trauma patients having sustained multiple and complex injuries are treated in an organized medical environment; thereby conclusions drawn from these studies have limited generalizability in disaster settings [13, 14]. Nevertheless, the role of RA in trauma is considered indispensable, and extrapolations to massive disaster settings seem to be imperative and in order when managing patients in this extreme context.

In fact, there are reports supporting the feasibility of RA techniques for the management of massive disaster-related trauma; however, there have been no randomized controlled trials to evaluate the effectiveness and safety of RA after a major disaster [15, 16].

RA includes neuraxial (epidural and spinal anesthesia) and peripheral nerve block techniques. Wound infiltration constitutes a remedy; nevertheless, as some risks are present (e.g., local anesthetic intravenous injections), it should be performed in designated areas where specific kits for resuscitation are available [17, 18].

Peripheral nerve blocks can be achieved using either anatomic landmarks or ultrasound (US) guidance. In fact, US-guided nerve blocks should be performed by emergency physicians, who have undergone adequate training and have the capacity to provide adequate pain control, with safety to patients with traumatic injuries in disaster settings [18].

Regional nerve blocks offer many characteristics of a supreme analgesic technique. Major advantages comprise excellent analgesia, reduction of stress response, patients' cooperation, and chronic pain prevention; also, RA techniques facilitate transport from the accident site to the hospital. Difficult airway cases, aggravation of cervical spine injury, and pneumothorax enlargement are common problems encountered in general anesthesia and should be avoided in a disaster setting by implementing RA techniques [1, 11, 17, 18].

5.2.2   RA Applications in Massive Disasters Trauma

5.2.2.1 Thoracoabdominal Trauma
Blunt thoracic injuries such as rib fractures and pulmonary contusions are common, with significant morbidity and mortality. RA modalities include thoracic epidural analgesia (TEA), thoracic paravertebral block (TPVB), and intercostal nerve blocks [19–21].

In trauma, TEA is utilized for managing multiple fractures which are associated with severe pain [19–21]. In hazardous settings, there are no reports for the role of TEA in thoracic trauma. Although this technique seems to be very effective to alleviate chest pain in multi-trauma patients, its implementation might be difficult or infeasible, and may not be the optimal approach of anesthesia or pain management in massive disaster conditions.

TPVB and intercostal nerve blocks have lately exhibited a resurgence of interest [21]. Although these techniques confer supreme analgesic effects on trauma patients, their role in disaster settings has been neglected thus far.

5.2.2.2 Upper and Lower Extremities Trauma
Extremity injuries are particularly suited to RA techniques. Brachial plexus nerve blocks, axillary, infraclavicular and interscalene approaches, femoral nerve, fascia iliaca, ankle foot, and sciatic nerve blocks have been employed in the disaster setting to provide optimal anesthesia/analgesia conditions [15, 16, 22, 23]. Although a clinical trial is underway setting out to investigate the impact of regional anesthesia techniques on disaster settings [24], report cases have already pointed out their contribution to effective analgesia/anesthesia for painful injuries after disaster [15, 16, 22, 23].

Brachial plexus interscalene and axillary nerve blocks have been proposed for upper limb trauma. Both stimulation and US-guided approaches have been utilized successfully [25–29]. US allows visualization of the brachial plexus from roots to the terminal branches [25]. US techniques can minimize needle attempts and local anesthetic volumes in addition to providing higher success rate brachial plexus nerve blocks with respect to neuro-stimulation techniques [25]. By using US techniques, nerves can be traced to their origin where they pass through the intervertebral foramen as they run in the interscalene groove and further down until they reach the axillary cavity [25, 27].

Femoral and sciatic nerve blocks have been used either in isolation or in combination to provide anesthesia/analgesia in a lower limb trauma. There is a variety of methods available for the performance of a femoral nerve block [19–21]. The femoral nerve can be anesthetized using stimulation, US or a fascia iliaca-pop technique [29–31]. In the absence of available ultrasound machines or nerve stimulators, the fascia iliaca compartment block can be easily performed using a simple blunt needle and local anesthetic [32–34].

Sciatic nerve blocks become more important in more distal femur fractures and fractures of the leg and ankle. US and neurostimulation techniques have been widely performed along the anatomic course of the sciatic nerve in the gluteal region, posterior thigh and the popliteal fossa [15, 19, 35, 36]. Lateral and anterior approaches of sciatic nerve block have been put forth in trauma patients as they do not need to turn in the lateral position with the affected leg uppermost; that way less pain and patients' comfort are assured [36, 37].

Spinal anesthesia is an anesthetic technique for any patient requiring surgery below the umbilicus who is not hemodynamically unstable. Injection of a local anesthetic in the subarachnoid space yields excellent anesthetic state for any procedure in the lower extremities [34].

5.2.2.3 Limitations and Challenges of RA Techniques

In terms of safety, the usage of epidural/spinal anesthesia/analgesia entails complications that could very likely outweigh its possible benefits. In these settings, analgesia/anesthesia with the aid of epidural catheters and/or with spinal technique can be invariably difficult to achieve; patients' posture and complications such as hematomas, not easily reversed hemodynamic perturbations, can be detrimental for the patients, as well as an additional burden for the already-exhausted anesthesia providers. Epidural catheters can also pose risks in that their implementation exhibit extreme difficulties in the postoperative surveillance of patients [34].

Although there are no studies to compare US and neuro-stimulation nerve block techniques at the site of the disaster, extrapolation and previous experience from trauma patients in the emergencies and/or hospital theaters can enable disaster response teams to incorporate these techniques in the disaster settings. For example, the application of neuro-stimulation may result in severe pain, and short but strong systemic analgesia may be required for patients' relief. US-guided nerve blocks cannot easily be performed in patients with emphysema and tissue edema [38].

US systems should also be available at the site of the disaster. That's to say that a US system should be portable and durable, set up by a team of well-educated personnel with rapid readiness to respond to other rescue interventions, and by all means electric supply is a prerequisite [22, 25].

The potential infectious risks of practicing RA in a nonsterile setting, as well as the conceivable risk of delaying the diagnosis of compartment syndrome, must be investigated. The interscalene nerve block, in particular, presents the possibility of higher-risk complications, such as pneumothorax, high epidural block, and phrenic nerve paralysis; hence it should not be employed in trauma cases with compromised pulmonary function [18, 29].

Additionally, local anesthetic toxicity (LAST) is a rare complication (0.2%) of RA which is frequently associated with an inadvertent intravascular injection. LAST presents with both central nervous system and cardiovascular system effects that should be immediately perceived and treated accordingly [18, 29].

Last but not least, in massive disaster conditions, anesthesiologists with experience in RA techniques cannot be sufficient to deal with the massive burden of casualties. To circumvent this downside, rescue units should be properly educated to provide analgesia/anesthesia; RA techniques must be easy to learn and to perform in a way that they would be safe and effective. More to the point, Randall et al. reported the results of a successful initiative to educate orthopedic nurses in the performance of fascia iliaca blockade in orthopedic wards [39]. The concept of a "physician extender" that can ameliorate patient access to successful pain control with the use of a simple, safe, and easily taught procedure can be a template for disaster settings as well.

5.3 General Anesthesia

5.3.1 Oxygen Supply

Anesthesia practice from the Haiti earthquake showed that H cylinders are the only source of oxygen and were supplied by trucks from a distant location. These oxygen tanks were attached to a flow regulator for use with anesthesia machines, but there was no pressure gauge on any of them. Tanks were inconsistently color coded and varied in hue: green, partially green, partially blue, brown, and white [40, 41]. From the Nepal earthquakes, high experience was gained and it is pointed out that all heavy apparatus, such as oxygen cylinders, should be secured and tied down. In most disasters, oxygen cylinders are not operational and, in some cases, even dangerous [23]. Oxygen concentrators are a substitute, but they require an electric supply and deliver oxygen at a pressure approximately of one bar, not sufficient for Boyles-type anesthetic machines and subsequently for inhalation anesthesia [34]. From the above mentioned, hence, many authors have reasoned RA techniques (do not require supplemental oxygen and afford quicker and safer evacuation of everyone from the site of the disaster) to be the mainstay of anesthesia in austere settings [23].

5.3.2 General Anesthesia Techniques and Sedation

This technique can be performed with intravenous or inhaled anesthetics, supplemented by muscle relaxants. General anesthesia requires the availability of mechanical ventilation, which, in precarious situations, is not always available. Because of the absence of anesthesia machines and ventilators, maintaining patients in spontaneous ventilation during long periods of the intervention is vital, and drugs such as ketamine, can be administered [40–43]. Although ketamine is a remedy in a precarious situation, more complex trauma cases (requiring airway management, general anesthesia with Propofol/muscle relaxants, and maintenance by a volatile anesthetic or Propofol) should be transferred to designated areas converted into well-organized operating rooms to meet surgical demands. In most cases, the operating theaters are improvised areas, not affording basic medications and equipment in the least.

Ketamine in a dose 1–2 mg/kg still remains a significant agent for intravenous anesthesia in disaster settings [23, 40–42]; it has analgesic and anesthetic effects that limit or avoid the use of opioids during the surgical intervention; Ketamine does not suppress ventilation, as well as the laryngeal reflexes; thus, it allows performing operations without intubation. In fact, there are occasions with anesthesia providers not being highly skilled in general intravenous anesthesia techniques, where ketamine is successfully used for Cesarean sections. Additionally, ketamine possesses sympathomimetic action, and thus, it is recommended in trauma cases with significant hemodynamic perturbations [8, 42].

Low dose of IV midazolam (0.05–0.10 mg/kg) can also be used: augmentation by locally administered anesthesia if possible has also been suggested. Although propofol can effectively suppress ventilation and laryngeal reflexes, minimal bolus doses (0.3 mg/kg) of the drug are necessary as a supplement for its hypnotic effects [40–42].

In the disaster settings, inhalational anesthesia seems to be difficult as the lack of anesthesia circuits, constraints in the supply of volatile anesthetics, hardships to properly evacuate these anesthetic agents from improvised operating rooms are the main impediments [3]. However, the use of inhaled analgesic nitrous oxide (N_2O) can be an alternative option as portable, commercially available; cylinders containing 50/50 gas mixture of N_2O with oxygen can deliver N_2O to patients through a facemask. The N_2O is a rapid-acting, innocuous, and active nonnarcotic analgesic which has been successfully employed in emergency prehospital cases [44–46]. The administration of N_2O is unproblematic and its portability entails many advantages under emergency circumstances in distant or difficult-to-reach locations or in massive disaster situations. In the management of trauma patients, the use of N_2O is contraindicated. In pneumothorax, air embolism, pneumocephalus, or any other case where expansion of trapped air into the body occurs, the anesthetic provision with N_2O can be detrimental. Additionally, N_2O should be avoided in traumatic brain injury, in that it may increase the intracranial pressure.

5.4 Pain Therapy and Challenges in Opioids Use

In 2011, the IASP (International Association for the Study of Pain) dedicated the year to acute pain study. In this regard, worldwide scientific discussion has been commenced on pain management throughout emergency triage in hospital and pre-hospital disaster medicine states. The treatment of pain and the use of adequate analgesia was then reckoned an indispensable human right that joins ethics with clinical medicine [9, 47].

Many drugs have been put forward for pain management in precarious situations. Paracetamol, diclofenac, tramadol, titrated doses of opioids, and ketamine have been extensively used for pain control, either individually or in combination with RA [40–42].

Multimodal analgesia is implemented by combining different analgesics (paracetamol, non-steroid anti-inflammatory drugs, opioids, ketamine, and local anesthetics) with different pharmacodynamics, at different sites in the nervous system, resulting in synergistic analgesia, with less adverse effects than those that may occur after the administration of each individual analgesic. Pain management in trauma exhibits a pyramid configuration; regional anesthesia techniques constitute the basis of the pyramid where the other analgesic regiments are built upon [6]. Although modern pain management dictates the multimodal use of both drugs and techniques, the applicability and the concept of multimodal analgesia in disaster settings have not been widely introduced thus far.

More significantly, in a disaster setting, shortage of painkilling drugs, either opioids or non-opioids, tops out in the first hours after a massive disaster and is related to internal transport difficulties in transferring medications to the site of the disaster. Moreover, insufficient administration of strong opioids may also be contingent on hardships not only in finding, but in prescribing, controlling, and dispensing these drugs as well [9, 40]. Consequently, in the presence of natural disasters, opioids in various formulations appear to be less available, yet essential for the treatment of patients with acute pain [9, 48]. The terms "opiophobia" and "oligoanalgesia" along with "oligoanesthesia" are also used interchangeably, to present the circumstances under which pain treatment takes place in austere environments. The need of regulation changes that will allow the instant, but supervisory allocation and administration of these medications in the site of the disaster is more ethically essential than ever before.

As far as pain is considered a vital sign, it becomes an independent and autonomous pathology heavily affecting the psychological and physical integrity of a person in the aftermath. For that reason, under disaster settings, the pain mitigation should be an ultimate intention of health systems; opioids and other pain medications or treatment techniques unavailability is unreasonable and preposterous. Consequently, taking into consideration that in massive disaster settings, the suboptimally treated and poorly controlled severe pain can infringe on the psycho-physical status of individuals and inflict cognitive and behavioral dysfunctions in the long term, it is all the more important, therefore, for teams highly trained in pain management to undertake patients care [9]. Once more, the concept of a "physician extender" that can properly and safely dispense and use these medications in precarious and unsound settings should be thoroughly considered.

5.5   Conclusions

There are no established guidelines or validated and authoritative protocols which could provide adequate indications either for the type of anesthesia or pain management, in the context of massive disasters settings. Under these circumstances, the pylon of any improvised intervention must be conditioned by ethos. Phronesis (practical skills and wisdom), arete (virtue), and eunoia (goodwill) toward the patient should be established as an interplay in the nucleus of which is the patient whose well-being must be the guiding force of our clinical decision-making at all times.

References

1. Missair A, Gebhard R, Pierre E. Surgery under extreme conditions in the aftermath of the 2010 Haiti earthquake: the importance of regional anesthesia. Prehosp Disaster Med. 2010;25(6):487–93.
2. Zaracostas J. Syrian crisis: aid delivery becoming increasingly difficult. Lancet. 2016;388:49.
3. DeVille C. What should we learn from recent earthquakes in Asia? Prehosp Disaster Med. 2008;23(4):305–7.
4. Tordrup D, Ahmed W, Bukhari KS. Availability of medical supplies during the 2010 Pakistan floods. Lancet. 2013;1:e13.
5. Helminen M, Saarela E, Salmela J. Characterization of patients treated at the red cross field hospital in Kashmir during the first three weeks of operation. Emerg Med J. 2006;23:654–6.
6. Mavrogenis AF, Igoumenou VG, Kostroglou A, Kostopanagiotou K, Saranteas T. The ABC and pain in trauma. Eur J Orthop Surg Traumatol. 2018;23
7. Buckenmaier C, Lee E, Shields C. Regional anesthesia in austere environments. Reg Anesth Pain Med. 2003;28:321–7.
8. Mulvey J, Qadri A. Maqsood. Earthquake injuries and the use of ketamine for surgical procedures: the Kashmir experience. Anaesth Intensive Care. 2006;34:489–94.
9. Guetti C, Angeletti C, Paladini A, Varrassi G, Marinangeli F. Pain and natural disaster. Pain Pract. 2013;13(7):589–93.
10. Jian J, Xu H, Liu H, et al. Anaesthetic management under field conditions after the 12 may 2008 earthquake in Wanchuan, China. Injury. 2010;41:e1–3.
11. Sinatra R. Causes and consequences of inadequate management of acute pain. Pain Med. 2010;11(12):1859–71.
12. Adenunkanmi A. Where there is no anaesthetist: a study of 282 consecutive patients using intravenous, spinal and local infiltration anaesthetic techniques. Trop Dr. 1999;29(2):56–7.
13. Beaudoin FL, Haran JP, Liebmann O. A comparison of ultrasound-guided three-in-one femoral nerve block versus parenteral opioids alone for analgesia in emergency department patients with hip fractures: a randomized controlled trial. Acad Emerg Med Off J Soc Acad Emerg Med. 2013;20(6):584–91.
14. Christos SC, Chiampas G, Offman R, Rifenburg R. Ultrasound-guided three in-one nerve block for femur fractures. West J Emerg Med. 2010;11(4):310–3.

15. Trelles Centurion M, Van Den Bergh R, Gray H. Anesthesia provision in disasters and armed conflicts. Curr Anesthesiol Rep. 2017;7(1):1–7.
16. Shah S, Dalal A, Smith RM, Joseph G, Rogers S, Dyer GS. Impact of portable ultrasound in trauma care after the Haitian earthquake of 2010. Am J Emerg Med. 2010;28(8):970–1.
17. Hell K. Local anesthesia in war and in a disaster area. Schweizerische Zeitschrift Militar Katastrophenmedizin. 1974;51:129–37.
18. Lippert SC, Nagdev A, Stone MB, Herring A, Norris R. Pain control in disaster settings: a role for ultrasound-guided nerve blocks. Ann Emerg Med. 2013;61(6):690–6.
19. Carrier FM, Turgeon AF, Nicole PC, et al. Effect of epidural analgesia in patients with traumatic rib fractures: a systematic review and meta-analysis of randomized controlled trials. Can J Anaesth. 2009;56:230–42.
20. Karmaker MK, Chui PT, Joynt GM, Ho AMH. Thoracic paravertebral block for management of pain associated with multiple fractured ribs in patients with concomitant lumbar spinal trauma. Reg Anesth Pain Med. 2001;26:169–73.
21. Wang Z, Sun Y, Wang Q, et al. Anesthetic management of injuries following the 2008 Wenchuan, China earthquake. Eur J Trauma Emerg Surg. 2011;37:9–12.
22. Saranteas T, Mavrogenis AF. Holistic ultrasound in trauma: an update. Injury. 2016;47(10):2110–6.
23. Dumont L, Khanal S, Thüring D, Junod JD, Hagon O. Anaesthesia in the wake of the Nepal earthquake: experience and immediate lessons learnt. Eur J Anaesthesiol. 2016;33(5):309–11.
24. Levine AC, Teicher C, Aluisio AR, Wiskel T, Valles P, Trelles M, Glavis-Bloom J, Grais RF. Regional Anesthesia for Painful Injuries after Disasters (RAPID): study protocol for a randomized controlled trial. Trials. 2016;17(1):542.
25. McCartney CJ, Lin L, Shastri U. Evidence basis for the use of ultrasound for upper-extremity blocks. Reg Anesth Pain Med. 2010;35(2 Suppl):S10–5.
26. Choi JJ, Lin E, Gadsden J. Regional anesthesia for trauma outside the operating theatre. Curr Opin Anaesthesiol. 2013;26(4):495–500.
27. Gros T, Delire V, Dareau S, Sebbane M, Eledjam JJ. Interscalene brachial plexus block in prehospital medicine. Ann Fr Anesth Reanim. 2008;27(10):859–60.
28. Lopez S, Gros T, Deblock N, Capdevila X, Eledjam JJ. Multitruncular block at the elbow for a major hand trauma for prehospital care. Ann Fr Anesth Reanim. 2002;21(10):816–9.
29. Gadsden J, Warlick A. Regional anesthesia for the trauma patient: improving patient outcomes. Local Reg Anesth. 2015;12(8):45–55.
30. Marhofer P, Schrogendorfer K, Wallner T, Konig H, Mayer N, Kapral S. Ultrasonographic guidance reduces the amount of local anesthetic for 3-in-1 blocks. Reg Anesth Pain Med. 1998;23(6):584–8.
31. Abou-Setta AM, Beaupre LA, Rashiq S. Comparative effectiveness of pain management interventions for hip fracture: a systematic review. Ann Intern Med. 2011;155(4):234–24.
32. Lopez S, Gros T, Bernard N, Plasse C, Capdevila X. Fascia iliaca compartment block for femoral bone fractures in prehospital care. Reg Anesth Pain Med. 2003;28(3):203–7.
33. Monzon DG, Iserson KV, Vazquez JA. Single fascia iliaca compartment block for post-hip fracture pain relief. J Emerg Med. 2007;32(3):257–62.
34. Craven RM. Managing anaesthetic provision for global disasters. Br J Anaesth. 2017;119(Suppl 1):i126–34.
35. Saranteas T, Chantzi C, Paraskeuopoulos T, Alevizou A, Zogojiannis J, Dimitriou V, Kostopanagiotou G. Imaging in anesthesia: the role of 4 MHz to 7 MHz sector array ultrasound probe in the identification of the sciatic nerve at different anatomic locations. Reg Anesth Pain Med. 2007;32(6):537–78.
36. Saranteas T, Chantzi C, Zogogiannis J, Alevizou A, Anagnostopoulou S, Iatrou C, Dimitriou V. Lateral sciatic nerve examination and localization at the mid-femoral level: an imaging study with ultrasound. Acta Anaesthesiol Scand. 2007;51(3):387–8.
37. Chantzi C, Saranteas T, Zogogiannis J, Alevizou N. Dimitriou V Ultrasound examination of the sciatic nerve at the anterior thigh in obese patients. Acta Anaesthesiol Scand. 2007;51(1):13.

38. Saranteas T, Karakitsos D, Alevizou A, Poularas J, Kostopanagiotou G, Karabinis A. Limitations and technical considerations of ultrasound-guided peripheral nerve blocks: edema and subcutaneous air. Reg Anesth Pain Med. 2008;33(4):353–6.
39. Randall A, Grigg L, Obideyi A, Srikantharajah I. Fascia iliaca compartment block: a nurse-led initiative for preoperative pain management in patients with a fractured neck of femur. J Orthop Nurs. 2008;12:69–7.
40. Ariyo P, Trelles M, Helmand R, et al. Providing anesthesia care in resource-limited settings. A 6-year analysis of anesthesia services provided at Médecins Sans Frontières facilities. Anesthesiology. 2016;124(3):561–9.
41. Missair A, Pretto E, Visan A, et al. A matter of life or limb? A review of traumatic injury patterns and anesthesia techniques for disaster relief after major earthquakes. Anesth Analg. 2013;117(4):934–41.
42. Craven R. Ketamine. Anaesthesia. 2007;62(S1):48.
43. Mellor A. Anaesthesia in austere environments. J R Army Med Corps. 2005;151:272–6.
44. Faddy SC, Garlick SR. A systematic review of the safety of analgesia with 50% nitrous oxide: can lay responders use analgesic gases in the prehospital setting? Emerg Med J. 2005;22:901–6.
45. Ducassé JL, Siksik G, Durand-Béchu M, Couarraze S, Vallé B, Lecoules N, Marco P, Lacombe T, Bounes V. Nitrous oxide for early analgesia in the emergency setting: a randomized, double-blind multicenter prehospital trial. Acad Emerg Med. 2013;20(2):178–84.
46. Porter KM, Siddiqui MK, Sharma I, Dickerson S, Eberhardt A. Management of trauma pain in the emergency setting: low-dose methoxyflurane or nitrous oxide? A systematic review and indirect treatment comparison. J Pain Res. 2017;11:11–21. https://doi.org/10.2147/JPR.S150600. eCollection 2018.
47. Reinhardt O, Oldroyd DR. Kant's theory of earthquakes and volcanic action. Anna Sci. 1983;40:247–72.
48. Angeletti C, Guetti C, Papola R, et al. Pain after earthquake. Scand J Trauma Resusc Emerg Med. 2012;20:43–7.

Media and Disaster Scene Management

6

Theomary Karamanis

6.1 Introduction

Disasters are not new to our world but they seem to be increasing in recent years causing concern and alarm globally. A 2018 report by the Centre for Research on the Epidemiology of Disasters and the United Nations Office for Disaster Risk Reduction found that between 1998 and 2017, climate-related and geophysical disasters killed 1.3 million people and left a further 4.4 billion injured, homeless, displaced, or in need of emergency assistance. While the majority of fatalities were due to geophysical events, mostly earthquakes and tsunamis, 91% of all disasters were caused by floods, storms, droughts, heatwaves, and other extreme weather events. In 1998–2017, disaster-hit countries experienced direct economic losses valued at almost US$ 3 billion. Overall, reported losses from extreme weather events rose by 150% between this 20-year period, and although absolute economic losses seem to be concentrated more in high-income countries, lower-income countries suffer more from the human cost of disasters [1].

Disasters are potentially traumatic events that are collectively experienced, have an acute onset, and seriously disrupt the functioning of a community, causing human, material, and economic losses that exceed the community's ability to cope using its own resources [2]. Disasters may have natural causes (earthquakes, hurricanes, tsunamis, floods, draughts, disease epidemics, etc.) or human causes (terrorist attacks, industrial and transport accidents, displaced populations, etc.). The world is now facing serious challenges that also constitute aggravating factors for disasters, such as climate change, population growth, unplanned urbanization, poverty, the threat of pandemics, as well as an increasing dependency on complex yet

T. Karamanis (✉)
Management Communications, Cornell SC Johnson College of Business, Cornell University, Ithaca, NY, USA

© Springer Nature Switzerland AG 2021
E. Pikoulis, J. Doucet (eds.), *Emergency Medicine, Trauma and Disaster Management*, Hot Topics in Acute Care Surgery and Trauma, https://doi.org/10.1007/978-3-030-34116-9_6

vulnerable technological systems. For some it is a fear, for others a certainty that these factors will result in increased frequency, complexity, and severity of disasters worldwide.

It is not surprising therefore that building and maintaining effective disaster prevention and management systems and processes is a global priority. A core component of disaster planning, response, and recovery is communication. Effective disaster communication may prevent a disaster or lessen its impact, while ineffective disaster communication may cause a disaster or make its effects worse [3]. Disasters often cause damage to the communication information infrastructure, leading to reduced availability and decreased flow of information. This diminished communication capacity occurs at a time when uncertainty, fear, and risks/threats are unusually high and people need a steady and reliable information flow to make informed decisions and protect themselves. Finding ways in which to disseminate accurate information quickly can save lives in emergency situations. Therefore, developing effective disaster communication processes and systems should be a priority for government organizations, communities, and citizens [3, 4].

Disasters typically constitute major media events, and governments and other officials have traditionally relied on media to disseminate information during emergencies, especially when those are catastrophic or the first of their kind. Mainstream media such as TV and radio have traditionally been the main sources of information during disasters, and continue to be today. However, with the advent of social media we now have the possibility of more efficient and effective disaster communication with increased information capacity and interactivity [5, 6].

This chapter examines the importance of effective communication before, during, and after disasters and its impact on affected and non-affected populations. It discusses the role of the media during emergencies and how agencies and response organizations should work with the media to more effectively address the unique challenges presented by crisis events. Finally, it explores best practices in crisis communication strategy and implementation targeted at optimizing disaster response.

6.2   Conceptual Framework: Risk, Crisis, Emergency, and Disaster Communication

Disaster communication is often related in the literature with risk and crisis communication, as well as emergency communication. Although narrowly defining these concepts and analyzing their differences is beyond the scope of this chapter, it is useful to establish a common conceptual framework to facilitate the discussion. Risk communication has typically been associated with health communication and efforts to warn the public about the risks pertaining to particular behaviors. Risk communication has largely been conceptualized as a problem of getting the public and/or specific target audiences to understand identifiable risks, such as smoking, unsafe sex, or drinking and driving, and adjusting their behavior accordingly [7]. WHO [8] defines risk communication as the exchange of real-time information, advice, and opinions between experts and people facing threats to their health, economic, or social well-being. The ultimate purpose of risk communication is thus to enable people at risk to take informed decisions to protect themselves. Risk communication uses many communications techniques ranging from media and social media communications, mass communications, and community engagement. It requires a sound understanding of people's perceptions, concerns, and beliefs, as well as their knowledge and practices. It also requires the early identification and management of rumors, misinformation, and other challenges.

Crisis communication, on the other hand, is more typically associated with strategic communication and public relations and the need for organizations to repair damaged images after a crisis or disaster [9]. Crisis in this context is any event that threatens a company's reputation, image, or credibility among its stakeholders and/ or any event that hinders or threatens a company's operations in the short run or long run. Crisis communication therefore aims at safeguarding the organization's reputation, maintain positive brand associations to the extent possible, curtail financial impact, and restore trust in the organization.

In another context, crisis communication is associated with emergency management and the need to inform and alert the public about an event. In this case, the crisis is not associated with a company's image or reputation, but constitutes a sudden and threatening event which requires an immediate response. Crisis communication then refers to the government's or other public authorities' efforts to inform the public. For example, community leaders might need to evacuate a community in advance of a hurricane. The content, form, and timing of the communication can help reduce and contain the harm or make the situation worse [10].

It should be rather obvious then that disasters are crises and therefore require crisis communication, while in most cases they entail communication about risk. Further, almost always disasters require an emergency response from the community involving disaster warning messages. As such, a more comprehensive approach toward these scholarly traditions of risk and crisis communication would be fruitful. For the purposes of this chapter, the author favors the merged approach of the crisis and emergency risk communication (CERC) model [10, 11]. This merged approach is, in part, a larger acknowledgment of the developmental features of risks and crisis, and recognition that effective communication must be an integrated and ongoing process [12].

As explained by the Centers for Disease Control and Prevention [10], CERC combines the elements of crisis communication and risk communication as they are used during an emergency response. CERC involves the dissemination of information that allows people to make the best possible decisions about their well-being, but also accept the imperfect nature of choices during a crisis. CERC differs from pure risk communication in that a decision must be made within a narrow time constraint. The decision may be irreversible, the outcome of the decision may be uncertain, and the decision may need to be made with imperfect or incomplete information. Therefore, communicators must inform and persuade the public in the hope that they will plan for and respond appropriately to risks and threats. Further, Houston [13] has followed a similar merged approach, proposing the Disaster Communication

Intervention Framework (DCIF), which concentrates on broader outcomes, such as improving community disaster preparedness; increasing individual and community resilience; and promoting wellness, coping, and recovery.

In this chapter, we shall be using the terms "disaster communication," "crisis communication," and "emergency communication" almost interchangeably, with the understanding that a CERC definitional approach has been adopted.

6.3 The Media's Role in Disaster Management and Prevention

Can you imagine any emergency response with the absence of mass media? How would public officials be able to quickly communicate to citizens both the nature of the crisis and any risk mitigation measures? Most developed nations nowadays have emergency alert systems which inform the public of an imminent or current emergency directing them to sources of additional information so that they can limit their exposure to threat. And while text alert systems and email alert systems are becoming more and more standard, traditional media continue to play a critical role as a source for information following an alert.

In fact, the media continue to serve as an important emergency information system during a crisis and they do this very well. Professional media representatives that recognize their role in public safety serve their communities in a significant manner during a crisis [10]. Further, as Nair [14] points out, for the affected population information provided by the mass media can enable people to prepare for the disaster, act reasonably during it, and recover after it. For the non-affected audience, the role of the mass media is to mobilize help from communities that have not been affected by the disaster—in some cases, even elicit international help.

Because of their immediacy and traditional high impact, television and radio are particularly important in crises that develop quickly. Nowadays all mainstream media have their own social media channels, through which they can get pictures, videos, and updates both from citizens and from public officials. This has increased the demand on media organizations to keep pace with information delivery, but at the same time, it has allowed them to provide information and crisis updates immediately and continuously.

Social media have definitely changed the landscape for disaster communications and operations. According to The Pew Research Center, following the Boston Marathon bombings in 2013, one quarter of Americans looked to Facebook, Twitter, and other social networking sites for information. What's more, when the Boston Police Department posted its final "captured!!!" tweet of the manhunt, more than 140,000 people retweeted it [15]. More and more researchers, policy makers, and security experts are examining the use of social media in disasters and its potential to improve disaster communication and management.

Social media are thought to be more advantageous for disaster communication because of their unique characteristics. Mills et al. [16] argue that an ideal emergency communication system is low cost, easy to use, mobile, reliable, and fast and provides capacity for one-to-one communications. Social media platforms usually have these traits. There are many different aspects of social media use and application. Houston et al. [3] have offered a comprehensive framework on the topic and describe the functions of disaster social media as follows:

- Provide and receive disaster preparedness information/warnings.
- Signal and detect disasters.
- Send/receive requests for assistance.
- Inform others of own condition during a disaster.
- Document what is happening in the disaster.
- Deliver and consume news coverage of the disaster.
- Raise awareness and donations.
- Express emotions and concerns; memorialize victims.
- Provide and receive information about recovery.
- Reconnect with community members.

Despite all the optimism about social media use and improved disaster communication, there are still inherent risks with using social media in emergency situations. An important one is the potential rapid spread of misinformation. False information can easily go viral and in an environment of uncertainty and high risk/threat when multiple organizations disseminate messages, it is not clear who polices the cyber space to correct errors.

As much as social media have made it possible for disaster response organizations to disseminate their own messages unfiltered and provide guidance and information directly to the community, it is indisputable that one cannot achieve adequate information flow before, during, and after disasters to all affected (and nonaffected) populations without news organizations. During crises, public authorities and agencies must work with the media to gather and disseminate information to serve the public interest. This symbiosis, however, is not always without challenges. The latter derive from the role of media in society and the sometimes competing priorities they have vis-à-vis the government.

According to the social value school, the media's role is to help the development of a democratic society; they do so when they play the role of the watchdog and report on the activities of public institutions and government, informing the public so that officials can be held accountable [17]. During a crisis, this may translate into investigative reporting which centers around assigning responsibility and blame, and assessing the adequacy of the disaster response [10]. On top of that, media are profit-maximizing enterprises. Above and beyond their democratic duty, they need to survive. Therefore, they need a story to capture their audience; sound bites and scandals that sell; quick and easy to digest information to stir emotions and raise viewership. That goal often leads to sensationalism, exaggeration of blame, political bias, or coverage mainly for entertainment rather than for informational purposes.

This role of the media is therefore often a source of conflict between them and different organizations and public institutions. Especially during crises when outrage and fear are high and uncertainty is paramount, public officials and organizations feel threatened by the media and blame them as sources of gossip, misinformation, and false accusations. However, as the old adage goes, "although tempting, a war with the media is a war you will never win." They key is to establish a relationship of integrity and trust with the media whereby all stakeholders' interests are being served. Journalists have a responsibility to report information they believe is honest and objective. Emergency management professionals cannot just assume that the media will report in a way that supports public officials' goals. The media are obviously not affiliated with public emergency response organizations and have their own commitment to the public. Emergency management planners should acknowledge the media's role in a crisis and plan to meet reasonable media requests [10]. It is imperative that public officials, emergency operation centers, and all organizations involved in crisis response understand the appropriate needs of the media and how to fulfill those needs as an ongoing and well-thought-out part of the response plan. This approach deliberately includes the media as an indispensable ally to disaster management.

6.4 Effective Crisis and Emergency Risk Communication

The principles of and best practices for effective crisis communication described below are drawn from research literature and crisis response/emergency training manuals, with the focus primarily on widespread public crises or disasters. They are guided by and fully aligned with prior work published—also widely accessible online—by the World Health Organization (WHO), the Pan-American Health Organization (PAHO), the Centers for Disease Control and Prevention (CDC), and the Federal Emergency Management Administration (FEMA).[1] The purpose here is not to offer an in-depth review or analysis of the academic discipline, but rather to provide a succinct overview of widely accepted and proven strategies and tactics of effective communication during emergencies and other crises.

6.4.1 Stages of Crisis Communication

One of the most common mistakes in crisis communication is the conceptualization of the need to communicate only at the beginning of a crisis. However, a crisis is a dynamic situation, which in turn renders crisis communication dynamic. Preparation of appropriate messages is an ongoing task during the different crisis phases, depicted in Fig. 6.1.

Most people conceptualize crisis communication at the beginning of the crisis, the "Start" phase. However, crisis communication entails much more than that. Even before a crisis hits, organizations and communities need to be prepared. They need to monitor and recognize emerging risks, and educate and prepare the public for the possibility of adverse events. This is the time when trust should be built

---

[1] It is recognized that a series of scholars, scientists, practitioners and crisis experts have collaborated to produce these manuals and publications.

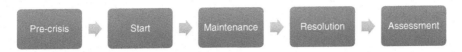

Fig. 6.1 Stages of a crisis

between institutions communicating risk and their different stakeholders. It is also prudent at this stage to form alliances with other partner organizations, create communication plans, and build and test communication systems. Effective crisis communication really starts before the advent of a crisis.

At the start of the crisis, one needs to quickly communicate the nature of the crisis and any other factual and warning messages to affected groups and the general public. Messages during this stage should aim at reducing emotional turmoil, convey reassurance, and promote self-efficacy. The initial phase of a crisis is characterized by confusion and intense media interest. Information is usually incomplete, and the facts are sparse. In this stage, it is appropriate to accept uncertainty, acknowledge limitations in information gathering, and explain that investigations are underway. The "don't know" answer from response organizations at this initial phase is effective and well received.

However, as the crisis goes into the maintenance phase, people and the media will be expecting more facts, solutions, and actions. Response organizations need to be able to communicate the causes of the crisis and steps taken to mitigate negative consequences, as well as any steps to prevent this type of crisis from happening in the future (if and when possible). This is a phase when showing you are in control is crucial in building trust with one's publics. Communication objectives during the crisis maintenance phase include ensuring that the public is updated, understanding ongoing risks, and knowing how to mitigate these risks. It also entails a dialogue with the affected public and filling gaps in communication (such as correcting misunderstandings or clarifying guidelines).

The resolution stage of a crisis is often a missed opportunity for organizations. This is the time when the crisis is largely behind them. It is the time to celebrate the wins and reflect on what has occurred. Communication objectives for the resolution phase include explaining recovery and facilitating broader-based discussions on causes, responsibility, resolutions, and adequacy of the response. This is the stage when continued messages for preparedness should be communicated, along with positive brand images for response agencies and organizations. Finally, the assessment stage involves evaluating the effectiveness of response and going full circle again to the pre-crisis stage, so that lessons learned can feed crisis communication plans.

As such, crisis communication never stops; it is a never-ending activity, with different messages directed to different stakeholders in each stage of the crisis. Since the communication loop is continuous, there is also continuous improvement in terms of responding to future crises.

6.4.2   Elements of Effective Crisis Communication

As Fig. 6.2 shows, there are four core elements to effective crisis communication: transparency, speed, accuracy, and empathy. Once an organization achieves the right

Fig. 6.2 Elements of
effective crisis
communication

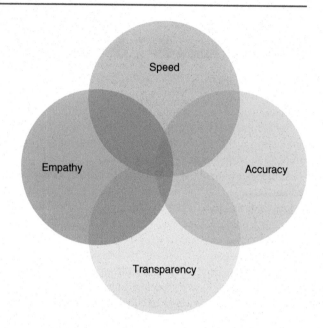

balance of these core elements, it establishes credibility and trust, which guarantees success in its communication with the public.

Transparency has traditionally been the most difficult to tackle, as there are a number of barriers to public organizations being open and transparent. Those include real or perceived competing interests (usually economic); spokespersons who do not wish to share bad news; fear that the media will use the information in a negative or sensational way; concern that the bad news will cause panic; and the (almost always false) hope that "if you say nothing, nothing will happen." Experience has again and again shown that the result of this approach is loss of control. Especially nowadays with increased media convergence, connectivity, and interactivity, audiences expect openness and candor. In cases where crisis communication also entails risk communication, the element of transparency is paramount, since affected populations are not likely to follow guidelines by organizations or officials whom they do not trust.

Speed of communication is equally important. Being first to communicate establishes the organization as the primary source of information and gives the opportunity to control the narrative from early on. Speedy responses suggest that there is a crisis response system in place and that appropriate actions are being taken by the appropriate experts and staff. In the absence of an organization's early announcement of a crisis, the public will look to other sources of information, which may spread rumors and/or promote different agendas.

One of the primary dilemmas of effective crisis communication therefore is to be speedy without sacrificing accuracy. It is obvious that responding quickly with the wrong information or poorly developed messages damages credibility. The factual content of the message needs to be carefully crafted and double-checked for accuracy, especially when it comes to specific recommendations for action. Further, coordination and monitoring of other communication partners become very important, as all credible sources need to speak with one voice. Inconsistent messages tend to cause confusion, increase anxiety, and quickly undermine the credibility of response disaster agencies.

Last, but certainly not least, crisis communication messages should convey empathy. There is a saying that perfectly applies in this case: "They don't care how much you know, until they know how much you care." Oftentimes during a crisis spokespersons are so focused on showing they are in control that they forget the human dimension. Disasters in particular are associated with loss of life, injuries, and large-scale financial losses. Showing caring in communications is thus very important in establishing trust with your audience. When one communicates during a crisis, it is important that he/she acknowledge fear, pain, suffering, and uncertainty. Early on in the message, organizations through their spokespersons need to share in the sacrifice and discomfort of the emergency situation. This will also help them to be viewed as part of the community and ultimately create a tighter bonding among stakeholders.

6.4.3   Developing Key Messages for the Media

Accepting and involving the public and the media as legitimate partners in times of crisis increases the effectiveness of a disaster response. A best practice for developing communication messages is the 3 × 3 rule: prepare three key points that communicate your core messages, each accompanied by three "proof points" or supporting messages. Although the 3 × 3 is just a guideline, what is important to remember is that a multitude of messages and a lot of details will dilute the core message and may disorient the public. Key messages for the media should be designed to address the most common public and media concerns during emergencies:

- Risks (personal, family, and community).
- Information (who, what, where, why, and how).
- Process of decision making.
- Equality and fairness.
- Accountability (cause, blame, responsibility).
- Sensitivity to cultural norms and practices.

Along with the factual information disseminated, it is also important to recognize and acknowledge anger, frustration, fear, outrage, or concern. It has also been shown that it is effective to provide a few positive points to counter negative information, while trusted third-party endorsements make messages more credible. Regular press briefings and continuous open dialogue with the community are also elements of success.

6.5　Conclusion

No disaster response is ever perfect and crisis events can develop in unexpected and often dramatic ways. This chapter has provided an overview for the need of effective crisis and emergency risk communication during disasters and a roadmap with guidelines on how to improve communication effectiveness during emergencies. Helping organizations and agencies maintain public trust, manage limited resources, and limit harm and disruption is critical. Understanding the crucial role media can play during disasters and working symbiotically with the media are key success factors in disaster response. Similarly, well-planned and well-executed crisis communication interventions, conceptualized within a continuous communication lifecycle, are central pieces of effective disaster preparedness and response systems. Communities worldwide thus need to invest in communication as a core element of their readiness to respond to crises now and in the future.

References

1. UNISDR. Economic losses, poverty and disasters: 1998–2017. 2018. https://www.unisdr.org/we/inform/publications/61119.
2. IFRC. What is a disaster. 2018. http://www.ifrc.org/en/what-we-do/disaster-management/about-disasters/what-is-a-disaster/.
3. Houston JB, Hawthorn J, Perreault M, Park E, Hode M, Halliwell M, McGowen S, Davis R, Vaid S, McElderry J, Griffith S. Social media and disasters: a functional framework for social media use in disaster planning, response and research. Disasters. 2014;39(1):1–22.
4. Shklovski, I., L. Palen and J. Sutton. Finding community through information and communication technology in disaster response. Paper presented at Computer Supported Cooperative Work 2008, San Diego, CA, 8–12 Nov 2008.
5. Jaeger PT, et al. Community response grids: e-government, social networks, and effective emergency management. Telecommun Policy. 2007;31(10–11):592–604.
6. Rene PL. The influence of social media on emergency management. PA TIMES Online. 2016. https://patimes.org/influence-social-media-emergency-management.
7. Witte K. Generating effective risk messages: how scary should your risk communication be? In: Burleson BR, editor. Communication yearbook (18). Thousand Oaks, CA: Sage; 1995. p. 229–54.
8. WHO. Definition of risk communication. 2018. May be retrieved at http://www.who.int/risk-communication/background/en/.
9. Coombs WT. Ongoing crisis communication. 4th ed. Thousand Oaks, CA: Sage; 2014.
10. CDC (Centers for Disease Control and Prevention). Crisis and emergency risk communication. US Department of Health and Human Services, CDC. 2014.
11. Reynolds B, Seeger M. Crisis and emergency risk communication. 2012th ed. Atlanta, GA: Centers for Disease Control and Prevention; 2012.
12. Seeger M. Best practices in crisis communication: an expert panel process. J Appl Commun Res. 2006;34(3):232–4.
13. Houston JB. Public disaster mental/behavioral health communication: intervention across disaster phases. J Emerg Manag. 2012;10(4):283–92.
14. Nair P. Role of media in disaster management. Mass Communicator, January–March 2010. 2010:36–40.
15. Maron DF. How social media is changing disaster response. Sci Am. 2013. 7 June 2013. https://www.scientificamerican.com/article/how-social-media-is-changing-disaster-response.

16. Mills A, Lee C, Rao HR. Web 2.0 emergency applications: how useful can Twitter be for emergency response? J Inform Priv Secur. 2009;5(3):3–26.
17. Karamanis T. The role of culture of culture and political institutions in media policy. Creskill, NJ: Hampton Press; 2003.

Triage and Transport of Casualties in the First Response Phase

7

Panagiotis V. Koukopoulos and Dionysios Koufoudakis

7.1 Scenario

Superfast XII has just arrived in Rhodes and the disembarking started. Suddenly, an explosion is heard from the cargo area, and the field is full of smoke. There are spots of fire everywhere. People running all over, passengers are ejected into the sea; bodies are spread on the disembarking area. Coast guard headquarters receive the message of the incidence.

What is your action plan? How many are injured? Is there a way to recognize the critically injured? Are there enough resources to deal with the critical patients? Who will approach the scene?

7.2 Introduction

The main challenge when dealing with a major incident is finding the best way to treat outnumbered casualties. According to its definition, always the casualties exceed the number of the responders and the duty of the incident officer is to prioritize their treatment. The need for a patient selection was recognized in early historical years.

7.2.1 History

Since the Trojan War, we have the first written reference on a draft priority system. Later on, during the Napoleon's wars we had the first essay on a systemic selection system that was called triage. The term «**Triage**» comes from the French verb

P. V. Koukopoulos (✉) · D. Koufoudakis
School of Medicine, National and Kapodistrian University of Athens-NKUA, Athens, Greece

© Springer Nature Switzerland AG 2021
E. Pikoulis, J. Doucet (eds.), *Emergency Medicine, Trauma and Disaster Management*, Hot Topics in Acute Care Surgery and Trauma,
https://doi.org/10.1007/978-3-030-34116-9_7

«trier» meaning "to select." It was first reported in the Napoleon wars by the doctor Dominique Jean Larrey.

7.2.2 Triage

Triage is a mandatory prioritizing system for any mass casualty incident—MCI.

MCI is any incident in which emergency medical services resources are overwhelmed by the number and severity of casualties [1–4]. This could be a natural disaster, like earthquakes, floods, volcanos, avalanches, forest fires, blizzards, etc. Or it could be man-made, like industrial, transport, or even an epidemic incident. Nowadays, military, terrorism, and all the kinds of warfare are a potential MCI for every country. All the emergency services worldwide now recognize the need for triage training in order to command and control a massive incident [5].

It is axiom that the only way to deal with such an emergency is to use a prioritizing system for the patients. In normal urban circumstances, the philosophy of emergency medicine is to provide the best possible care for each casualty [6]. This is not possible in a massive event. A system to select the patients that you need the most is the cornerstone for a "successful" management in mass casualties.

Triage systems provide a simple and fast algorithm to recognize the life-threatening injuries and deal for most of them urgently. The quickest way to do this is by performing a gross selection of those who can wait for more than 4 h before they receive any care. All the modern systems do that as their first action. At most of the times this would cover the 65% of all involved victims. Then selecting those who should be treated urgently and those who can wait 2–4 h becomes easier. All systems use a numeric and a color code which is the same (Fig. 7.1). The letter "P" stand for priority and letter "T" stands for treatment, according to different systems.

Fig. 7.1 Classification of injured

P	T	Description	Colour
1	1	Immediate	Red
2	2	Urgent	Yellow
3	3	Delayed	Green
1 hold	4	Expectant	Blue
Dead	Dead	Dead	White/Black

Triage is a dynamic process over time and it should be repeated regularly. It is also escalating according to the facilities taking place or the available resources. There is the draft selection done in the field (the first response phase) which is simple and fast, and done preferably by low -level health professionals or firemen. Then at the Casualty Collection Point (First Aid Station), there is a more detailed triage done by higher level professionals, more accurate but it takes more time.

After the initial treatment, the priority might change to better or worse, and a new selection is made for transportation. And then, when arriving to hospital, new and more sophisticated selection system is performed in the emergency department. For those who need surgical interventions, an upgraded selection system chooses who goes first in the operating theater, and after that who goes first in the intensive care unit. So, triage is an ongoing and evolving process in order to treat the correct patient at the correct time and with the appropriate means.

In modern emergency and disaster medicine, this system evolved in a well-organized and evidence-based system, helping the responders to take difficult decisions: which patient, with what injuries, should be treated in a specific time-frame, and then transported to the right health facility, by the right transportation mean.

7.2.3 Interventions in the First Response Phase

First responders have the ultimate responsibility of choosing who gets help and how. This is a very hard decision and must be made in the split of a second. Following a validated algorithm is very helpful and makes the triage a very fast and, almost, an accurate process.

Medical interventions in the first response phase are limited. This is because of the low availability in health professionals and resources. Those accepted by the most validated triage systems worldwide are: basic airway maneuvers, turning the casualty in recovery position and stopping the life-threating hemorrhage [7]. If none of those help, then the casualty is considered dead. A rather new system, the SALT, encourages professionals to make more, like providing rescue breaths to pediatric casualties, chest decompression, and providing antidotes, which is more time-consuming and requests more resources.

The main goal in all systems is avoiding waste of recourses on casualties with low probability of survival. There are more similarities in between them, but those we could highlight are:

- Triage is a dynamic process
- Stop, look, listen and think
- No more than 30 s on each patient for the initial triaging
- Common color coding (red-yellow-green)
- Do more for the most

7.3   Triage Systems

- Available prehospital triage systems
- Triage labeling
- Choosing the best system
- Moving casualties during the first response phase
- Human recourses management
- Supporting the staff

There are a few triage systems around the world with variabilities according to local needs and clinical governance [8]. All of them have their strong points and their pitfalls, but deep inside, they all follow the same principles [9]. Decision is based according to the prevalence of dying within minutes, hours, or days. This is mostly orientated by the CABCDE steps. The treatment facilities are another factor affecting the triage system. Prehospital environment is certainly different than the A & E of a hospital, the operating room, or the ICU. So, it is the decision-making system we should follow according to where we are and the recourses available. Moving from prehospital toward the more sophisticated recourses (ICU, OR), the triage system is more detailed and more accurate.

We will take you through the most popular systems used for prehospital triage worldwide. It is true that although they have some differences, if used at the same patient, they all give the same result. Yet, there is not enough evidence to support any of them, so the system used is chosen by the local or national health authorities [10].

7.3.1   START—Simple Treatment and Rapid Transport

Triage **START**—Simple Treatment and Rapid Transport system (Fig. 7.3)—was established in the United states in 1983 [9], from the Newport Beach Fire Department, in order to categorize treatment of the casualties in a major incident. Nowadays, it is used for triaging adults in most of the States and European Countries. It is considered a simple and a fast procedure [11], requiring 30–45 s per patient, based on the mnemonic **30–2–Can do** (Fig. 7.2). Again, it follows the ABCDE rule and the only intervention allowed is the airway opening, and controlling the life-threatening bleeding.

Initial assessment is based on guiding the walking wounded into a controlled area. This is the easy way to separate the third category MINOR that can be treated

Respirations:	Is the patient's respiratory rate over or under 30?	30
Perfusion:	Is capillary refill over or under 2 seconds?	2
Mental status:	Is the patient able to follow simple commands?	Can Do

Fig. 7.2 30–2–Can do—mnemonic

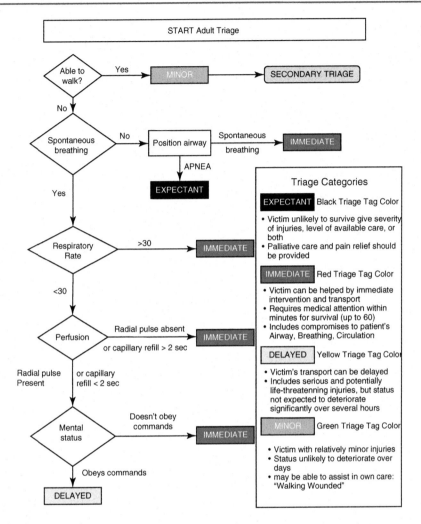

Fig. 7.3 START—triage system

by basic first aid, or even assist in treating other casualties. Statistically this covers the 50–60% of the injured (Fig. 7.3).

Next step is assessing breathing of the remaining casualties. If a casualty is not breathing, we open the airway and reassess. If still not breathing, he is categorized as EXPECTANT. CPR is contraindicated in MCI. Limited time and recourses will end up in low-quality resuscitation and an increase in reversible deaths.

If he starts breathing, he is prioritized IMMEDIATE. Next step is to check respiratory rate. If the rate is above 30, the casualty is an IMMEDIATE. If less than 30, we proceed in checking capillary refill time, with major bleeding control at the same time. If it is increased (more than 2 s), the casualty is an IMMEDIATE. We then check if he obeys simple orders. We ask him to move arms or legs, or squeeze our hand. If he obeys, then he is a DELAYDED; if not, he is an IMMEDIATE.

Triage is the key to success in a major incident. If the first responder is engaged in treatment and delays, precious time will be lost. Continuous reassessing is the cornerstone of the procedure, and labeling is very important to state the job is done.

According to START triage system tags label include:

- MINOR injuries: Any injuries can be treated with first aid

- DELAYDED injuries: Injuries required medical treatment, but not life threatening

- IMMEDIATE injuries: Life threatening injuries

- EXPECTANT injuries: Morgue/dead

7.3.2   Jump START Pediatric

Dealing with pediatric casualties during an MCI is stressful for all of us. Empathy for the juniors, vital signs differences, and the challenging communication are proved to stress the rescuers significantly. This is why JUMP START Pediatric is so significant (Fig. 7.4). Classifying tiny patients, having in mind all those differences, and performing the first life-saving interventions are done in a systematic way. Of course, there are always children with a body image of an adult, regardless the age. Treating them as children or adults is the first responder's call.

First described in Miami (1995), at the Florida Children's Hospital by Dr. Lou Romig [12], and Published in 2001 [13], but not validated by that time [14], this system is the most frequently used in pediatric patients all over the United States.

As the START, patients are categorized through three simple steps, starting with those who can walk and should be guided to a designated area. That way you have your MINOR category that can be treated with basic first aid.

Then we proceed by checking the airway. For those who are not able to breath, we perform simple maneuvers to open the airway. If they start breathing, they are IMMEDIATE. If they are still not breathing, we check for pulse. If no pulse is present, they are EXPECTANT. If there is a pulse, we give five rescue breaths. If still not breathing, then it is an EXPECTANT. If he starts breathing, he is an IMMEDIATE.

You see that giving rescue breaths is the main difference from the adult's START, following the cardiac arrest algorithm for children. But still, CPR is not indicated for the same reasons, as always mentioned.

Then we go on by counting the respiratory rate. Normal to those ages, it is between 15–45 bpm. If they have a rate outside those limits, it is an IMMEDIATE. If breathing is normal, we perform an AVPU neurological estimation. If they are in A or V, they are DELAYDED; if on P or U, they are IMMEDIATE.

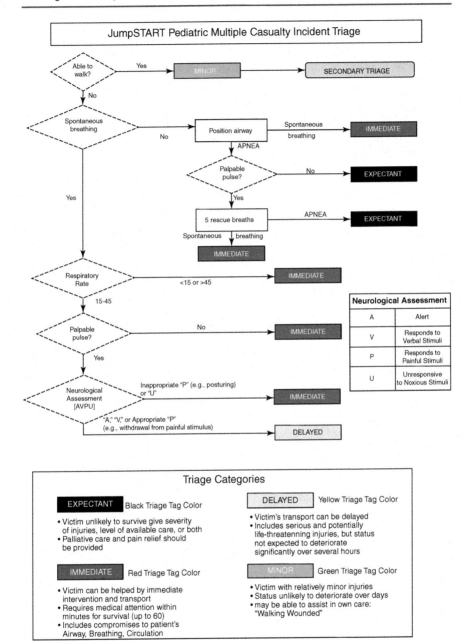

Fig. 7.4 Jump START system

According to Jump START Pediatric triage system tags label include:

- MINOR injuries: Any injuries can be treated with first aid

- DELAYDED injuries: Injuries required medical treatment, but not life threatening

- IMMEDIATE injuries: Life threatening injuries

- EXPECTANT injuries: Morgue/dead

7.3.3   Triage Sieve

Triage sieve is used in the United Kingdom and the commonwealth (Fig. 7.5). It is a rather modern system coming from simplifying the START system. The main benefit is that within the ambulance systems of the United Kingdom, the fire service and all the other emergency services are universal. They all get the same training, including the Armed Forces, and run national joined exercises giving a unique common language. The other important aspect is that it is a flexible system that can change immediately according to the national needs in very short time. It is based, of course, at the same ABCDE principles, but it was the first to adapt the catastrophic bleeding first step almost immediately after the 7–7 terrorist strike in London. This was the first triage system to introduce the CABCDE, giving priority in dealing with major bleeding.

The first step is to treat the catastrophic (life-threatening) hemorrhage by applying pressure dressings or tourniquet, and that immediately makes them priority 1 (red).

Then remove the walking casualties, or the uninjured, by asking them to help themselves and others away from the incident scene, pointing them an area to sit and wait (priority 3-green).

Then, walking among the casualties check if they are breathing. If they are not, you perform a jaw thrust and reassess. If they start breathe and are unconscious, they are priority 2 (yellow). If they are still not breathing, they are dead. If someone is breathing, you count their breathing rate for 10 s. If they have less than 10 or more than 30 breaths per min, they are priority 1. If they RR is between normal rates, then we assess the heart rate or the capillary refill. If they have more than 120beats per min, or CR > 2 s, they are priority 1. If they have less than 120 bpm or CR less than 2 s, they are priority 2.

The triage SIEVE categories are:

- P 3 injuries: Any injuries can be treated with first aid

- P 2 injuries: Injuries required medical treatment, but not life threatening

- P 1 injuries: Life threatening injuries.

- DEAD injuries: Morgue/dead.

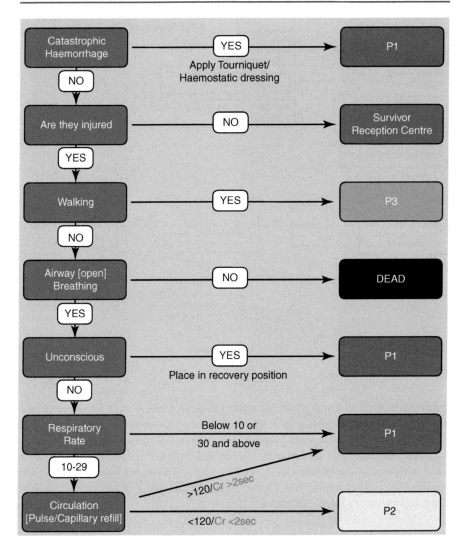

Fig. 7.5 SIEVE triage system

7.3.4 SALT—Sort, Assess, Lifesaving Interventions, Treatment and Transport

The SALT system [15] is a modern improved way to perform triage (Fig. 7.6). It was created in an effort to have a common system in the whole United States [9, 16].

Triage is performed in three levels. In the first level, we perform a draft estimation according the victim's movements. Those who walk are priority 3 and they will be taken care as last. Those who move their arm are 2, and they will be treated after we treat the first group. Those who do not move at all or have life-threatening

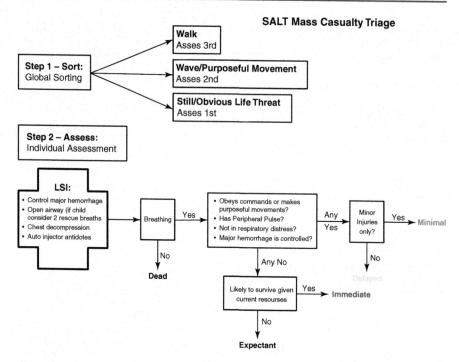

Fig. 7.6 SALT triage system

injuries are category 1 and need to be treated first. This step gives a rough idea to the rescuers so they can organize their actions. This way, those with minor injuries will be guided away from the scene giving space to the responders to work.

In the second level, we proceed to a tailored approach in recognizing those in need for life-saving interventions (LSI). At this point, when the other systems count respirations and heart rate, SALT only worries if they exist or not. If not, we perform any necessary interventions, as:

- Control of catastrophic bleeding
- Airway opening
- Two rescue breaths in non-breathing children
- Chest decompression
- Providing antidotes

At the last level, after opening the airway we check if the casualty is breathing. If not, he is DEAD. If he is breathing, then we check (a) if he obeys in simple commands, (b) if there is peripheral pulse, (c) if there is NO respiratory distress, and (d) if the catastrophic external bleeding is controlled. If all the above are a YES, and he has minor injuries, then the casualty is categorized as MINOR. If there are no minor injuries, he is a DELAYDED. If we have a NO in any of the above, we check if he can survive according to the recourses. If not, he is an EXPECTANT; if we can save him, he is an IMMEDIATE.

In general, SALT is a more active triage system, but needs to be done by trained health professionals, able to perform the LSI, and it is supposed to take as much time as any other system. The EXPECTANT category added is used to pick up those who have a low survival rate in the given circumstances.

The SALT categories are:

- MINOR injuries: Any injuries can be treated with first aid
- DELAYDED injuries: Injuries required medical treatment, but not life threatening.
- IMMEDIATE injuries: Life threatening injuries.
- EXPECTANT–DEAD injuries: Morgue/dead.

7.3.5   Triage Labeling

There are a few methods to state the triage category for patients [17]. They all follow the colored system and their role is to:

- Indicate the priority of the casualty
- Indicate that triage has been done
- Be the first form of the patient's record
- Be understood by all personnel involved in medical assessment and treatment

There are special cards (Figs. 7.7 and 7.8) with some common characteristics:

- They are waterproof, or they are in a plastic cover
- Easily identified

Fig. 7.7 Triage card

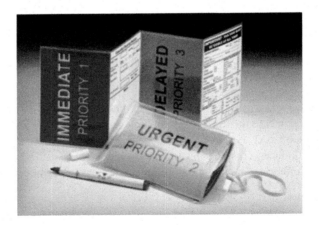

Fig. 7.8 Triage cards

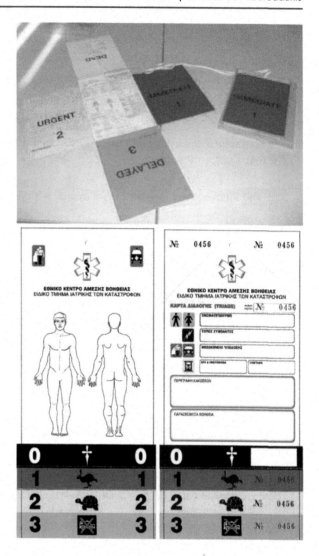

- Have a sticky area (or Velcro) to stay on the patient
- They have some space to write the timings and the vital signs, and of course the name of the casualty
- They can be easily changed when priority changes (foldable or cross-like)

It is not important which one your service uses, as long as you understand the way they work, which is always pretty straight forward.

In case the triage cards are not available, you can always use any alternative, as soon as everybody understands what it stands for. For example, colored sticky tape, cloth pegs, or you can write the priority number with a marker (or a lipstick) on their forehead. Anything is acceptable as long as we all understand it.

7.3.6 Comparing the Available Triage Systems

Literature review cannot prove the superiority of any of the available systems. It is true that there is a lack of scientific evidence about the effects of validated prehospital triage systems. We understand that running randomized or perspective trials is practically impossible, and even if they were not, the statistical difference could not be significant since mass casualties (thankfully) is not an everyday issue. The lack of evidence in the superiority of a system does not mean they do not work. All of them have the same principles, and if they are used to the same patient, the priority ends up the same. Choosing one of them has to do with local governance and training traditions. Sometimes it can be an "ego" issue between systems, like the UK and USA EMS services that historically they tend to agree that they disagree, but in the end they are doing the same thing. Judging from the results, all of them work and the services that they use can work effectively in those adverse situations.

So, which one should we choose? [10, 16, 18–20] We have the feeling that each one of them is efficient. Choose the simpler one that is closer to local training habits and can be reproduced between different areas and different emergency services. Since Fire Service and Ambulance Service need to work side by side, it is mandatory to have a common system to achieve a smooth patient flow. It would be ideal if a pan European system was adopted, when dreamers can wish for a universal triage system, even though we all know this is not going to happen.

7.3.7 Moving Casualties During the First Response Phase

The primary transportation happens when enough hands are available, to move patients from the incident scene to the Casualty Station (or First Aid, or Medical Station), the safe spot where medical staff can provide life-saving interventions, before getting victims to the hospital.

Transferring priority is based on the triage already done on scene. So, it is essential that all moving personnel can identify the triage labeling. This is important mostly when untrained volunteers are involved in the process.

The other main issue is that during this initial moving, spine control is not necessary since it wastes equipment and personnel on a hypothetical risk. Moving should be done by one or two rescuers using handling techniques with minimum equipment. There are some techniques well established, but sometimes according to the circumstances we need to improvise and use any method we can make off or modify one of the already tried, using your imagination.

We will report the most common, but one can find numerous online since transporting a patient could be as inventive as a KAMA SUTRA textbook.

7.3.8 One Rescuer

1. Drag from clothes

   We drag patients' clothes from the shoulder region, keeping his head between our two forearms. And alternative could be dragging him from his belt or vest or his trousers, according to access limitations (Fig. 7.9).
2. Fireman's method
   - Apply our feet against the victim's feet.
   - We drag his arms while we are bending our knees.
   - We kneel to the floor and let his weight drop over our shoulders.
   - We slowly stand up keeping our weight center on a wide base by spreading our legs slightly (Fig. 7.10).
3. Supporting the casualty

   A casualty that can walk is supported by the rescuer having his arm over his shoulder (Fig. 7.11).
4. Rautek maneuver

   The rescuer has his arms under the casualty's armpits and grabs one of his arm, walking backward (Fig. 7.12).

7.3.9 Two Rescuers

1. Supporting

   Two rescuers support the victim to walk by holding him under his arms (Fig. 7.13).
2. Carrying

   The first rescuer encircles the victim's chest by placing his arms under his armpits, and the second is holding the legs (Fig. 7.14).

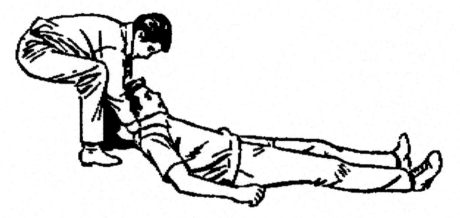

Fig. 7.9 Drag from clothes manoeuver

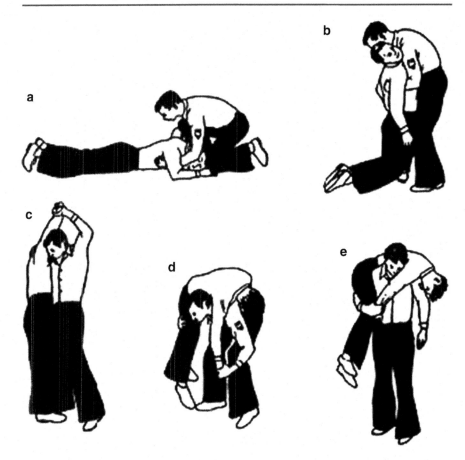

Fig. 7.10 Fireman's method

7.3.10 Using Special Equipment

Special equipment like trolleys, scoop-stretchers, army stretchers, baskets, etc., may be available. These require that there is enough manpower to use them properly, most unlikely in a mass casualty incidence, and it will be discussed in another chapter of this textbook.

7.3.11 Casualty Clearing Station—Casualty Collection Point

With the above methods, victims will be collected in a pre-specified area where they can receive medical treatment. Gathering all patients to a dedicated and protected area has the benefit of keeping the medical personnel and equipment in a space in order to treat more than one patient at the same time.

Choosing the most appropriate location and the characteristics that this should comply with will be further discussed in the appropriate chapter.

Fig. 7.11 Supporting the casualty

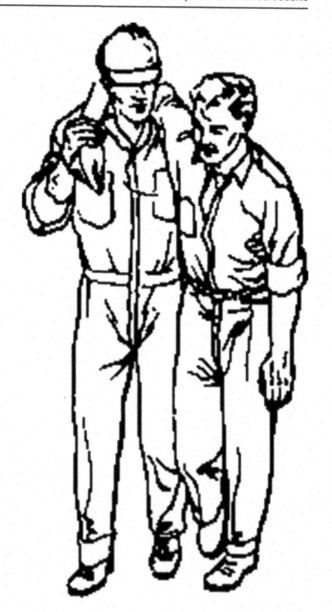

7.3.12 Human Recourses Management

During the MCI, one should not forget the staff. Working in such an incident is very hard, physically and emotionally. Remember that staff should have short breaks, something to eat and plenty of water to drink. In organized systems, a job-allocated person would be responsible for the staff welfare, but in most early stages, this should be your responsibility as well. Make sure that they take a break because tiredness can cause accidents and you do not need more accidents.

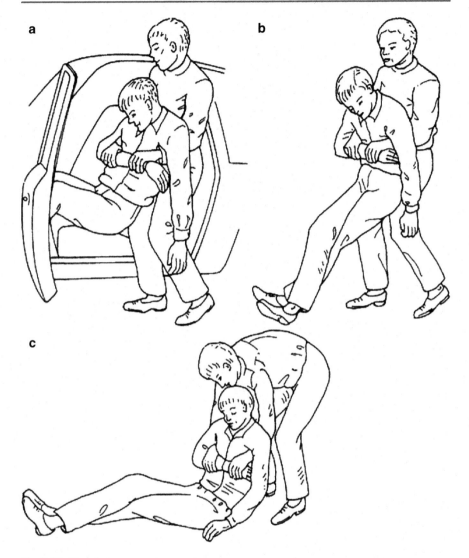

Fig. 7.12 Rautek maneuver

7.3.13 Supporting the Staff

When the incident comes to an end, you should make sure that all the involved personnel are safe. For this reason it is essential to keep a record of the people on site. This is also very important when urgent evacuation is needed due to a safe issue (e.g., fire).

The moment the last casualty is gone to the hospital, equipment should be collected and the rescuers should have a drink and an opportunity to get debriefed. Your focus now should be on saving the lives of your rescuers. Let

Fig. 7.13 Two rescuers maneuver, supporting

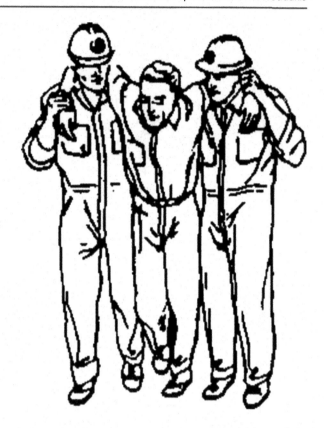

them express their grief and try to encourage their strong points; how many have been saved, not how many have been lost. Try to relieve their pain and save them from some nightmares.

7.4 Summary

The selection of the patients who need urgent medical interventions is the only way to save as many lives as possible, when the resources are limited. It is true that health professionals recognize the necessity of hard decisions in a split of a second. And it is indeed the only incident that may haunt our lives forever. No matter how hard you try, no matter how trained you are, you can't save them all, you never save enough, and you have to live with it.

Continuous education and training [2, 7, 10, 18, 21, 22] is mandatory to prepare ourselves for MCI. Triage is a fast and dynamic process with sometimes an unpredictable outcome. The first responder actions are very crucial for the successful control of such incidents, and training is the only way to get there.

Fig. 7.14 Two rescuers maneuver, carrying

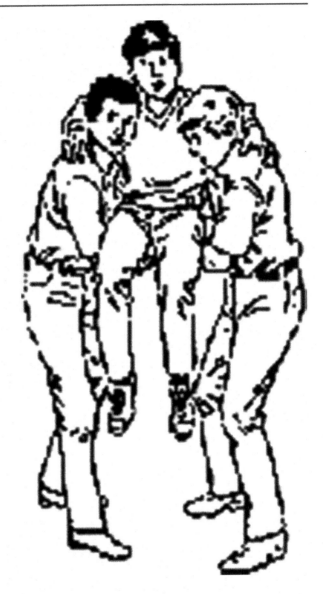

7.5   Scenario Continued

Triaging is the first step in getting in order such a chaos. "Do the best for most" is the main moto, and this will orientate the use of facilities and resources appropriately. That statement creates the need of establishing a reliable and fast method to categorize the casualties and prioritize our treatment.

Your first action as a first responder is to communicate with control and give them a detailed report on the incident. This will activate the system of response. The next step is to pick up a casualty gathering spot, safe and easy to access. Then ask all the walking wounded to exit the scene and guide them to the casualty station. Then triage should start. Until more help arrives, you should not try to treat any casualty. Triage them, tag them, and wait for help. The aim of this chapter is to present the available systems in prehospital care in most parts of the world. Training and having a common system within services will improve our performance in such incidents.

References

1. NAEMT. All hazards disaster response, course manual. Burlington, MA: Jones & Bartlett Learning; 2018.
2. Lewis AM, Sordo S, Weireter LJ, Price MA, Cancio L, Jonas RB, Dent DL, Muir MT, Aydelotte JD. Mass casualty incident management preparedness: a survey of the American College of Surgeons Committee on trauma. Am Surg. 2016;82(12):1227–31.
3. Stohler SA, Jacobs LM, Gabram SG. Roles of a helicopter emergency medical service in mass casualty incidents. J Air Med Transp. 1991;10(1):7–13.
4. Lidal IB, Holte HH, Vist GE. Triage systems for pre-hospital emergency medical services—a systematic review. Scand J Trauma Resusc Emerg Med. 2013;21:28. https://doi.org/10.118 6/1757-7241-21-28.
5. Billittier AJ, Lerner EB, Moscati RM, Young G. Triage, transportation, and destination decisions by out-of-hospital emergency care providers. Prehosp Disaster Med. 1998;13(2–4):22–7.
6. Ramesh AC, Kumar S. Triage, transportation, and destination decisions by out of hospital emergency care providers. J Pharm Bioallied Sci. 2010;2(3):239–47. https://doi.org/10.4103/0975-7406.68506.
7. Biddinger PD, Baggish A, Harrington L, et al. Be prepared—the Boston Marathon and mass-casualty events. 2013. https://www.nejm.org/doi/full/10.1056/NEJMp1305480.
8. Russo RM, Galante JM, Jacoby RC, Shatz DV. Mass casualty disasters: who should run the show? J Emerg Med. 2015;48(6):685–92. https://doi.org/10.1016/j.jemermed.2014.12.069. Epub 2015 Mar 30.
9. NAEMT. Pre hospital trauma life support. 8th ed. Burlington, MA: Jones & Bartlett Learning; 2016.
10. Jenkins JL, ML MC, Sauer LM, Green GB, Stuart S, Thomas TL, Hsu EB. Mass-casualty triage: time for an evidence-based approach. Prehosp Disaster Med. 2008;23(1):3–8.
11. Curran-Sills G, Franc JM. A pilot study examining the speed and accuracy of triage for simulated disaster patients in an emergency department setting: comparison of a computerized version of Canadian Triage Acuity Scale (CTAS) and Simple Triage And Rapid Treatment (START) methods. CJEM. 2017;19(5):364–71. https://doi.org/10.1017/cem.2016.386. Epub 2016 Oct 28.
12. Romig LE. Pediatric triage, a system to JumpSTART your triage of young patients at MCIs. JEMS. 2002;27(7):52–8, 60–3.
13. Wallis LA, Carley S. Comparison of paediatric major incident primary triage tools. Emerg Med J. 2006;23(6):475–8.
14. Sanddal TL, Loyacono T, Sanddal ND. Effect of JumpSTART trainng on immediate and short-term pediatric triage performance. Pediatr Emerg Care. 2004;20:749–53.
15. Silvestri S, Field A, Mangalat N, et al. Comparison of START and SALT triage methodologies to reference standard definitions and to a field mass casualty simulation. Am J Disaster Med. 2017;12(1):27–33. https://doi.org/10.5055/ajdm.2017.0255.
16. Lidal IB, Holte HH, Gundersen MW. Triage systems for Emergency Medical Services—prehospital and at hospital admission. https://www.ncbi.nlm.nih.gov/pubmed/29320102.

17. Rådestad M, Lennquist Montán K, Rüter A, Castrén M, Svensson L, Gryth D, Fossum B. Attitudes towards and experience of the use of triage tags in major incidents: a mixed method study. Prehosp Disaster Med. 2016;31(4):376–85. https://doi.org/10.1017/S1049023X16000480. Epub 2016 May 23.
18. Ryan K, George D, Liu J, Mitchell P, Nelson K, Kue R. The use of Field triage in disaster and mass casualty incidents: a survey of current practices by EMS personnel. Prehosp Emerg Care. 2018;22(4):520–6. https://doi.org/10.1080/10903127.2017.1419323. Epub 2018 Feb 9.
19. Lee CW, McLeod SL, Van Aarsen K, Klingel M, Franc JM, Peddle MB. First responder accuracy using SALT during mass-casualty incident simulation. Prehosp Disaster Med. 2016;31(2):150–4. https://doi.org/10.1017/S1049023X16000091. Epub 2016 Feb 9.
20. Streckbein S, Kohlmann T, Luxen J, Birkholz T, Prückner S. Triage protocols for mass casualty incidents: An overview 30 years after START. Unfallchirurg. 2016;119(8):620–31. https://doi.org/10.1007/s00113-014-2717-x.
21. Glow SD, Colucci V, Allington DR, Noonan CW, Hall EC. Managing multiple-casualty incidents: a rural medical preparedness training assessment. Prehosp Disaster Med. 2013;28(4):334–41. https://doi.org/10.1017/S1049023X13000423. Epub 2013 Apr 18.
22. Dittmar MS, Wolf P, Bigalke M, Graf BM, Birkholz T. Primary mass casualty incident triage: evidence for the benefit of yearly brief re-training from a simulation study. Scand J Trauma Resusc Emerg Med. 2018;26(1):35. https://doi.org/10.1186/s13049-018-0501-6.

Medical Evacuation of Emergency Affected Persons

8

Kenan Yusif-zade

8.1 Medical-Evacuation Measures: Concept and Essence

Medical evacuation is an integral part of medical-evacuation activities.

Medical evacuation means removal (withdrawal) of those affected from the lesion site, and their transportation until the stages of medical evacuation for timely medical treatment. Medical evacuation is a forced measure since it is impossible (there are no conditions) to organize comprehensive care and treatment in the area of mass sanitary losses.

Medical rescue of persons affected and their evacuation from impact zones are arranged through a phased treatment and evacuation process [1–4].

The medical evacuation phase requires public health care facilities to be deployed on routes of medical evacuation for reception, triage, specific aid to persons affected, and (when necessary) their preparation for further evacuation.

Currently, affected people undergo a 2-phase treatment and evacuation prior to being brought to destination.

The first phase of medical evacuation meant for premedical and first aid is unleashed in medical institutions, medical emergency stations that survived in a disaster area and are deployed by first aid teams, paramedics, and doctor-nurse teams that arrived in the disaster area from nearest health facilities, as well as in medical stations of military units drawn for rescue operations.

The second phase of medical evacuation is unleashed in medical facilities existing and operating outside the disaster area, and also in additionally deployed medical facilities for extensive medical support, both quality and specialty to treat

K. Yusif-zade (✉)
Military Medical Division, State Border Service, Baku, Azerbaijan

© Springer Nature Switzerland AG 2021
E. Pikoulis, J. Doucet (eds.), *Emergency Medicine, Trauma and Disaster Management*, Hot Topics in Acute Care Surgery and Trauma,
https://doi.org/10.1007/978-3-030-34116-9_8

affected people all the way through.Different transportation facilities are used to evacuate affected patients.

In peacetime and wartime, in case of emergency, medical and unadapted vehicles tend to be one of the primary means of evacuation across a "disaster area - nearest medical facilities" link [5, 6]. If necessary, air transport can be used for evacuation to specialized centers in the region or country. As sanitary evacuation and adapted transport will always be insufficient, and unadapted transport means have to be used to evacuate especially badly injured patients, it is necessary to comply strictly with the requirements of evacuation and transport triage.

The most difficult thing regarding organization and techniques in the emergency zones is to evacuate (remove, withdraw) those affected by the debris and seat of fire. If it is impossible to reach the affected by vehicles, they will be pulled out on stretchers by improvised tools (boards, etc.) to the point of possible loading on transport (by relay-race method).

Pickup points are chosen as close as possible to the sites of destruction, out of contamination and fire zones. In order to provide treatment of the casualties in the places of their concentration, ambulance staff and rescue parties are sent till the arrival of emergency teams and other units. First aid, evacuation and transport triage and arrangement of the loading platform are provided in these places.Evacuation by all types of vehicles is prohibited in the following cases [1, 7]:

– 2nd and 3rd-degree shock
– irretrievable loss of blood,
– terminal state,
– wounds and injuries of the skull and brain followed by loss of corneal and papillary reflexes, brain compression syndrome, meningoencephalitis, ongoing liquorrhea,
– post-tracheostomy (prior to establishment of sustainable external respiration),
– open eye injury potentially threatened by loss of membranes, bleeding or threat thereof, signs of endophthalmitis, sharp intraocular pressure caused by burnt eyeballs,
– severe respiratory failure, pleural empyema, and a septic state with breast wounds,
– diffuse peritonitis, intra-abdominal abscesses, acute intestinal failure, and threat or eventration signs of internal organs,
– suppurative urinary stasis, septic state in case of injuries of urogenital sphere,
– acute purulent-septic complications of wounds in case of injuries of long bones, pelvic bones, and large joints,
– anaerobic infection and tetanus,
– thrombosis of major vessels, state after ligation of external and common carotid artery (before removal of sutures),
– fat embolism and pulmonary embolism,
– acute hepatorenal failure,
– combined radiation injuries with irradiation equal to or above the dose of 6 g.

8.2   Main Triage Features

When in an emergency, 25–30% of affected patients need urgent medical measures appearing to be most efficient in the first hours after trauma. There is a severe need to choose—the priority should be given to the worst injured patients with chances to survive [8, 9].

Triage is a method of splitting injured people into groups according to the urgency of need of homogeneous medical and evacuation activities, depending on the medical indication and specific situation.

Triage includes prompt medical assistance and rational evacuation of injured people.

Triage is characterized by

– concreteness,
– succession,
– continuity.

Triage starts in casualty collecting points, continues across medical evacuation right up to all functional divisions. The triage scope is based on tasks assigned to functional divisions, a stage of medical evacuation, in the whole, and environmental context.

Types of triage. Depending on objectives set on stages of medical evacuation, there are two types of triage: in-point and evacuation transport.

In-point triage will assign injured people to groups according to the severity level of injury, a potential danger for the environment, to determine the need for the medical intervention and its priority and to assign a functional division (medical facility) of an evacuation phase (EP) in order to arrange medical intervention.

Evacuation Transport triage will split injured people into uniform groups to set evacuation priority and type of transportation (vehicle, air, etc.), will determine the position of the injured on evacuation means (lying, sitting), and identify a destination. Sensitive factors: condition, the severity level of injured, localization, character, and severity of the injury. These must be addressed through diagnosis, forecast, condition, and outcome; otherwise, it is impossible to deliver adequate triage.

Triage is based on three key features:

– Danger to others
– Medical indications
– Evacuation indications
– *Danger to others* determines the degree of need of sanitary and special treatment, isolation of affected patients.Therefore, affected persons are divided into the following groups:
– in need of special (sanitary) treatment (partial or total),
– subject to temporary isolation (in infectious and psycho-neurological medical isolation facilities),
– not in need of special sanitary treatment,

– *Therapeutic indication*—the degree of patients' need of medical care, priority and place (medical division) of its provision.
– According to the extent of need of medical care in appropriate divisions during evacuation phases, affected people are divided into those:
– in need of emergency medical assistance
– not in need of medical assistance (assistance may be postponed)
– with traumas incompatible with life and in need of symptomatic aid to relieve pain

Evacuation sign—necessity, the order of evacuation, transport mode, and the position of the affected in the transport. Based on these features, the affected persons are divided into groups:

– subject to evacuation outside the hearth, taking into account the evacuation destination, priority, method of evacuation (lying, sitting) and the mode of transport,
– subject to staying in a given medical institution (non-transportable, depending on the severity of their state) temporarily or until the outcome,
– subject to returning to a place of residence (resettlement) or short-term delay in the medical stage for medical observation,
– Particular attention is paid to the identification of those affected dangerous to others and in need of urgent medical care.
– The optimum composition of the triage team for the affected on stretchers: a doctor, a paramedic (a medical assistant), two nurses, two registering clerks. For the walking affected (patients), the triage team is composed of a doctor, a nurse and a registering clerk (Fig. 8.1).

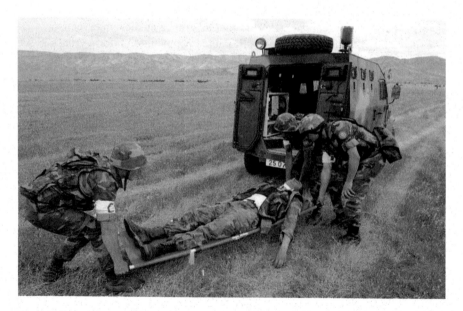

Fig. 8.1 Triage team

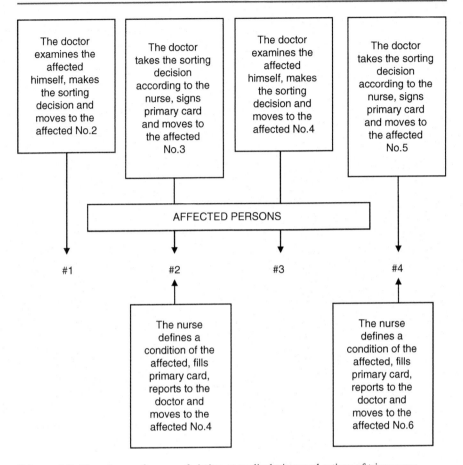

Scheme 8.1 The scheme of survey of victims at medical triage and actions of triage crew

The sequence of practical medical triage is as follows: a nurse, a paramedic—first a doctor identifies the affected (patients) who are dangerous to others. Afterwards, those affected in need of medical care and according to the urgency are identified by means of a brief inspection (external bleeding, asphyxia, convulsive state, and childbirth) and thus performing a "selective" triage (Scheme 8.1).

The priority is given to children and women in childbirth. After that, the medical staff moves to a consistent ("conveyer") examination of the affected (patients): a doctor, a nurse, and a registering clerk are with one of the patients, while a paramedic (a nurse), a nurse, and a registering clerk are with the other one. Having taken a triage decision for the first affected person, the doctor moves to the next one and receives information over the state of the affected person from a paramedic (a nurse) and, if necessary, completes the survey with personal information. After triage decision regarding the second affected person, the doctor moves to the third one. A paramedic with a registering clerk examines the fourth patient and fills in the medical documentation [3, 10].

The results of the medical triage are registered in the primary health card (Form 100), medical history (Fig. 8.2).

a

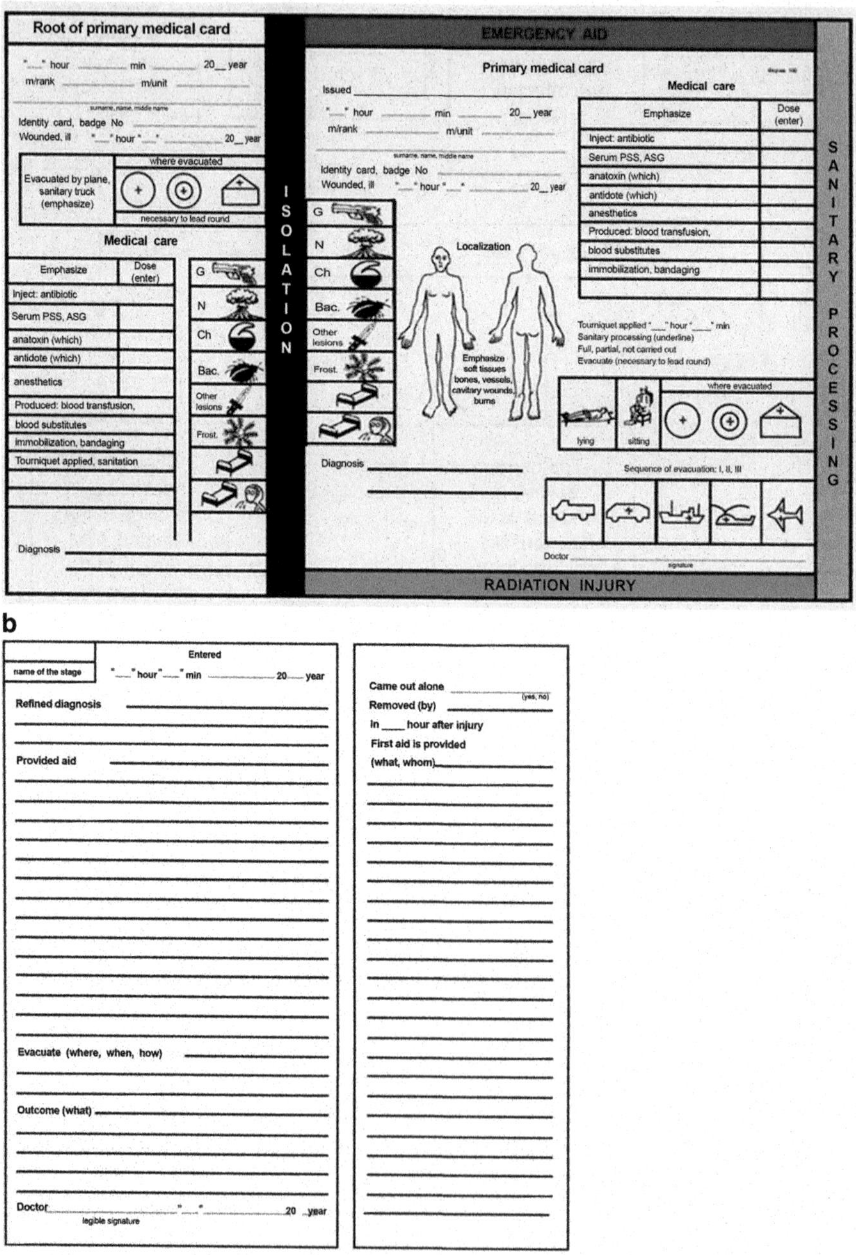

b

Fig. 8.2 Primary medical card: front side (**a**); reverse side (**b**)

Primary Medical Card (Form #100 in Azerbaijan) is a document of personal medical records, designed to ensure succession and consistency to provide medical assistance to the wounded, affected, and sick in advanced stages of medical evacuation. A completed medical card has a legal significance—it indicates the fact of injury (disease) and grants an affected person (patient) with the right to be evacuated to the rear.

At the stage of medical evacuation, where first medical aid is provided to the wounded, injured, or sick person for the first time, a front side of the primary medical card and its counterfoil are filled in.

A registration clerk completes the passport part of the card and its countercard; he circles the numbers of the assigned measures of medical care under the doctor's dictation and enters additional activities in free lines. The numbers of assignments are transferred to the counterfoil of the card. The marks of the performance of the medical prescriptions are marked by underlining the names of the corresponding medical measure in the card. Afterwards, the counterfoil is cut off the card and is left at this stage to produce a regular report on the health service. The completed card is signed by the doctor, stamped by the division and together with the evacuated patient (affected or sick) is sent for the next stage of the medical evacuation. At that, the medical card is attached to the bandage of the injured person, or is put in the left pocket of his overclothes.

While completing the front side of the card, the necessary data is recorded in the space provided. To indicate the type of sanitary losses, there are symbolic figures on the front side of the card and its counterfoil. To identify the nature and location of the injury, human silhouettes are used on the front side of the card.

In case of application of the tourniquet on the limb, hours and minutes of application are indicated. A mark of performance or non-performance of the special treatment is made. The nature of the injury is underlined, the location of injuries, burns, damages of bones and blood vessels are encircled. The order, mode of transport, and directions for the evacuation of the injured person (patient) are marked in a similar way.

Colored strips on the edges of the card are designed in order to signal the next stage of the medical evacuation to the doctor of the triage team concerning the performance of the urgent measures, which are necessary for the wounded (patient):

Red strips left in the cases, when an injured (patient) is in need of emergency medical care. If there is no necessity of urgent medical care, then the bar is cut off when the card is being completed. *Yellow strip* means the necessity of the sanitary treatment.

Black strip indicates the necessity of isolation of the wounded (patient) due to the infectious disease, reactive state, affection by the biological weapons.

Blue strip means the necessity to conduct special activities when affected by the penetrating radiation; the indications of the individual dosimeter are recorded here as well.

If an injured (patient) is in need of several medical measures at the same time, two or more colorful strips can be left on the card.

The health care activities are recorded in the section "medical aid" on the front side of the card. It is necessary to record all necessary volume of medical care for the given stage of the medical evacuation. The records should be specific, clear, indicating the dosage of medication, the multiplicity and methods of their introduction.

Four triage groups in wartime and *five groups in peacetime* are distinguished as a result of triage (triage) (Scheme 8.2).

First triage group—severely injured people with the lesion incompatible with life and writhing in agony are in need of symptomatic aid; prognosis is unfavorable, they are not subject to evacuation.

Second triage group—affected with severe lesion and in need of emergency medical care; however, the prognosis may be favorable, the medical care is given to the affected persons falling under this group in the first place at this stage.

Third triage group—those with severe and moderate lesion, which do not pose an immediate threat to life. They are given medical care in the second turn, or may be delayed until the beginning of the next stage.

Fourth triage group—those who have injuries of moderate severity. Prognosis is favorable, medical assistance is provided at the next stage.

In emergency situation during peacetime, the fifth group stands out of the fourth group—those that have minor injuries, not requiring medical assistance at this stage, they are sent to the outpatient treatment.

Hospital medical institutions providing qualified and specialized medical treatment for the majority of the affected (patients) represent the second final stage of medical evacuation. This determines a particular medical triage. They consist of the distribution of the affected to the corresponding groups.

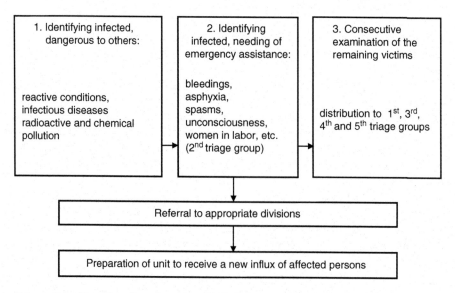

Scheme 8.2 Algorithm of carrying out medical triage

The affected (patients) in the receiving-triage department are divided into the following groups (after distinguishing of the affected and sick persons, in need of sanitary treatment and isolation):

- Those who require urgent medical care are sent to the appropriate functional units—a dressing ward, operating room, anaerobic, anti-shock and intensive therapy room.
- Those with removed bandage that require triage are sent to the dressing room.
- Those who require X-ray to confirm the diagnosis are sent to the X-ray unit.
- All other affected persons and patients (including those who require to be sent in the second turn to the dressing and operating rooms) are distributed according to the specialized hospital departments.

To perform medical triage in each stage of medical evacuation, specifically designed triage evacuation is deployed. As a rule, their composition includes:

- triage station,
- triage platform,
- reception and triage tent (tents, wards, units),
- evacuation tent (tents, wards, units),
- In all cases, medical triage should start with the allocation of the affected group, representing danger to others. This function is usually performed by the triage station, assigning "dangerous for others" to the isolation wards and platform (unit) of special treatment.
- The rest wounded and sick are sent to perform triage on the triage platform and triage tent (Fig. 8.3).

8.3   Types of Medical Care (Identification, Place of Performance, Optimal Timeliness to Render Its Various Types, Attracted Forces and Means)

Type of medical care is a combination of therapeutic and preventive activities, established for a certain stage of evacuation.

The following types of care are distinguished in the system of staged treatment of the affected and patients with their evacuation according to the assignment: first aid, predoctor care, first medical assistance, qualified medical assistance, and specialized medical assistance [5, 11–13].

First aid is a set of simple medical activities provided on the spot as a self and mutual aid by the sanitary helpers (in wartime), personnel of rescue formations, search-and-rescue services (in peacetime) with the use of basic and available tools. The optimal term is up to 30 minutes upon the receipt of the lesion [14, 15].

The purpose of the first aid is to halt the exposure of the damaging factor, elimination of the life-threatening events, and prevention of dangerous complications.

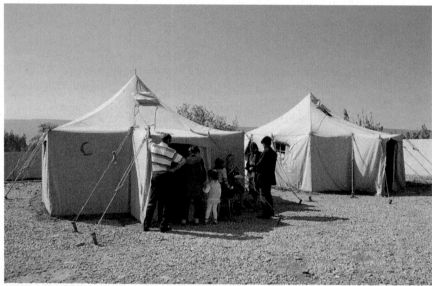

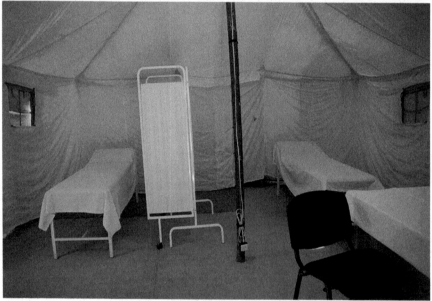

Fig. 8.3 Deployment of the field hospital (North Border in Azerbaijan)

Predoctor care is a paramedical personnel of the deployed units (usually in peacetime), *with the purpose to prevent life-threatening disorders.* Optimal term is 1–2 h. Authorized equipment is used for the predoctor care.

First medical assistance is provided by general practitioners in the Medical Detachment (MD), Mobile Medical Detachment (MMD) (in wartime) and by doctors of medical and nursing teams, working at the assembly point of the affected or deployed units of the medical assistance (in peacetime), *with the purpose of* elimination of the consequences of life-threatening lesion, prevention of the development of complications (shock, wound infection), preparations for further evacuation. The optimal term is 4–6 h (Fig. 8.4).

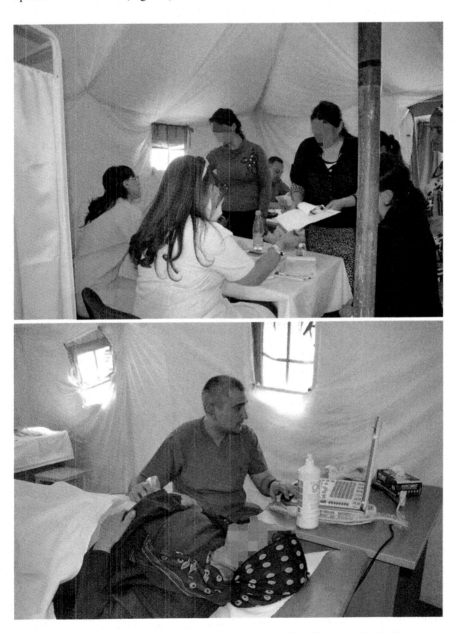

Fig. 8.4 Medical staff during active work in a field hospital. (North Border in Azerbaijan)

Qualified medical assistance is performed by doctors-surgeons and therapists in mobile formations, multidisciplinary medical institutions, already existing or additionally deployed (both in peacetime and wartime). It is *intended* to eliminate effects of life-threatening injuries and diseases (Fig. 8.5). The optimal term is 6–12 h.

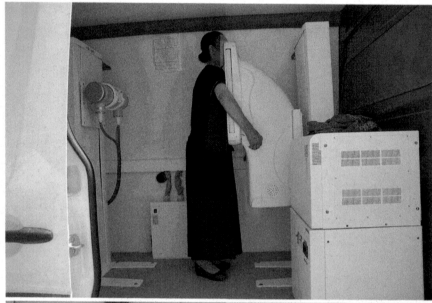

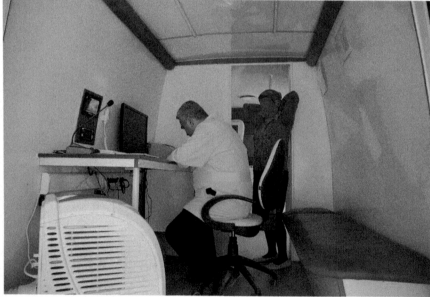

Fig. 8.5 Mobile formation. X-Ray Unit

Specialized medical assistance represents the highest form of medical care and is exhaustive in its nature. It is provided by the appropriate specialists with the necessary equipment, specially designed for the purpose of medical institutions no later than the day after the lesion [16].

The experience of elimination of many emergency situations strongly suggests that the list of activities of a particular type of medical care in real situation may be reduced or expanded. Nevertheless, the following requirements should be implemented during all options of the volume of medical aid:

- measures to eliminate life-threatening events have to be taken while rendering any medical assistance,
- measures to prevent severe complications,
- measures to provide transportation without any significant complications.

8.4   Volume of Medical Assistance

The volume of medical assistance means the "number" of activities conducted at the stages of the medical evacuation depending on the situation [17].

The content of the first aid depends on the nature of lesion [10, 16].

Both in peacetime and wartime, the following activities are included in the list of first aid in case of traumatic injuries:

- withdrawal of the affected from the debris and destroyed shelters,
- restoration of the patency of the upper respiratory tract,
- artificial ventilation,
- external cardiac massage,
- temporary arrest of bleeding with all available means,
- adjustment of sterile dressings on the wound and burnt surfaces,
- transport immobilization,
- assistance in provision of the physiologically advantageous position for the affected,
- adjustment of occlusive dressing in case of open pneumothorax,
- introduction of anesthetics, etc.

The list of measures in case of burns also includes extinguishing of the burning clothes.

In the hearths with the release of emergency hazardous substances (EHS) or with the application of the chemical weapons by the enemy, the first aid should be provided in the shortest terms (in the first minutes of lesion) and includes [18]:

- use of personal protective gear,
- provision of antidotes, sorbents, and gastric lavage without a probe,
- performance of partial sanitization of the open parts of the body,
- rapid evacuation from the hearth.

When there are radiation accidents and in case of the use of nuclear weapons, the first aid includes [19]

- performance of measures to stop the inflow of radioactive substances into the body (through air, water, food),
- rapid evacuation outside the territory contaminated with radioactive substances,
- use of means that arrest the primary reaction on irradiation, radio protectors, medication to protect thyroid,
- partial sanitization of the open parts of the body, the removal of radioactive substances from the clothes, shoes, etc.

When mass outbreaks of infectious diseases in the heart of bacteriological (biological) infection, the first aid includes

- use of available and authorized means of protection,
- active detection and isolation of patients and people suspected in infectious diseases,
- performance of emergency nonspecific prevention,
- complete and partial special (sanitary) treatment.

Predoctor care includes

- verification if the bandages are adjusted appropriately and if necessary, fix the adjusted bandages, tourniquet, immobilization,
- adjustment of aseptic dressings, tourniquet,
- adjustment of standard splint under the bad immobilization or its absence.

The elimination of asphyxia (cleaning of the mouth and throat, if necessary introduction of artificial airway, oxygen inhalation, mechanical ventilation of lungs):

- introduction of anesthetics,
- re-introduction of the antidotes according to the indications,
- performance of additional partial sanitary treatment (in case of necessity),
- simple measures against shock (warming at low temperatures, giving hot tea, introduction of anesthetics, cardiovascular means and medicaments that stimulate respiration).

First medical assistance. The total volume of the medical assistance consists of the measures that are held based on the urgency and activities, performance of which can be delayed.
Urgent measures are prescribed under the life-threatening conditions. They include:

- elimination of asphyxia (aspiration of mucus and blood from the upper respiratory tracts, introduction of airway, ligation of tongue, excision or suturing of the

hanging flaps of the soft palate and lateral sections of the pharynx, tracheostomy according to indications, mechanical ventilation of lungs, application of occlusive dressings under the open and pneumothorax, centesis of the pleural cavity or thoracentesis under stressed one),
- arrest of the impaired hemorrhage (suturing or ligation of the vessel in the wound, application of hemostat or tight tamponade of the wound, control of the tourniquet and if necessary, its secondary application),
- limb amputation (its segments) hanging on the flap,
- arrangement of anti-shock measures (blood transfusions and blood substitutes, procaine block, introduction of anesthetics and cardiovascular medicaments),
- catheterization or capillary puncture of the bladder under the damage of urethra,
- partial sanitary processing and change of clothes,
- introduction of antibiotics, anticonvulsants, bronchodilators, and antiemetic drugs,
- gastric lavage with the help of the probe in case of contact with toxic substances in the stomach,
- decompressive craniotomy (in wartime),
- degassing of the wound under its infection with persistent TS (toxic substances),
- application of antitoxic serum in case of poisoning by bacterial toxins and nonspecific prevention in case of affection by the biological weapon, etc.

The group of measures of the first medical assistance that *may be delayed* include:

- elimination of flaws of the first medical and predoctor care (readjustment of bandages and immobilization),
- introduction of tetanus toxoid and antibiotics,
- procaine block in case of limb injuries without signs of shock,
- prescription of various symptomatic drugs in situations that are not life-threatening for the affected.

Reduction of the first medical aid is performed at the expense of non-implementation of measures of the second group.
Measures of qualified medical assistance are divided into two groups:

- urgent,
- measures that can be delayed.

Urgent measures of qualified surgical aid involve

- final hemostasis,
- elimination of asphyxia and establishment of sustainable respiration,
- complex therapy of acute blood loss, shock, traumatic toxicosis,
- treatment of anaerobic infections,

- surgical debridement and suturing of the wounds in case of open pneumothorax, thoracocentesis in case of valvular pneumothorax,
- laparotomy in case of penetrating wounds and closed abdominal trauma with damage of internal organs, in case of closed injury of the bladder and rectum,
- amputation in case of extremity avulsion and massive destruction of limbs,
- decompressive craniotomy,
- surgical treatment of long bone fractures with extensive destruction of the soft tissues,
- necrotomy in case of circular burns of the chest and extremities accompanied by the disturbance of respiration and blood circulation,

Urgent measures of qualified therapeutic assistance include

- introduction of antidotes and anti-botulinum serum,
- complex therapy of cardiovascular insufficiency, cardiac arrhythmias, acute respiratory failure,
- treatment of toxic pulmonary edema,
- introduction of analgesic, desensitizing means, anticonvulsants, antiemetic means, and bronchodilators,
- complex therapy of acute renal failure,
- use of tranquilizers and antipsychotic drugs in case of acute reactive states and others,

Measures, the late implementation of which can lead to serious complications relate *to the second group of qualified surgical assistance*:

- adjustment of suprapubic fistula in case of urethra's injury and unnatural anus in case of intraperitoneal damage of the rectum,
- surgical treatment of wounds in case of long bone fractures (without extensive damage of soft issues),
- necrotomy in case of circular burns of the chest and extremities that do not cause failures in respiration and blood circulation,
- amputation in case of ischemic necrosis of a limb,
- primary surgical treatment of wounds that are contaminated with the radioactive substances (RS), chemical agents (CA),
- restoration of patency of the main arteries,

As well as measures, the delay of which under the application of antibiotics, *will not necessarily lead to complications*:

- primary surgical treatment of injuries of the soft tissues,
- primary surgical treatment of the burns,
- laminar suturing in case of the seamed injuries of face,
- ligature teeth binding in case of mandibular fractures, and others,

- *The second group of qualified therapeutic assistance* (the performance of which can be rejected under unfavorable conditions) include:
- introduction of antibiotics, sulfonamides with the purpose of prevention,
- treatment with vitamins,
- hemotransfusion with the aim of substitution,
- use of symptomatic means,
- physiotherapy, etc.

Specialized medical assistance represents the highest form of health care.

The following types of the specialized medical assistance in the specialized hospitals are as follows:

Specialized surgical	Assistance	Neuro-surgical	Ophthalmic
Otorhinolaryngological, dental, radiological, and other	Urological	Psycho-neurological	Toxicological

References

1. Musayev A. Mülki Müdafiə Tibbi xidmətinin təşkili. Dərslik. Bakı, 2011, 165 səh. (*Azerbaijani Lang*).
2. Ocaqov H.O.. Mülki müdafiə. Dərs vəsaiti. B.: Maarif, 1997, 144 s. (*Azerbaijani Lang*).
3. Харина М.В. Медицинская служба гражданской обороны. Учебно-методическое пособие. 2007, 100 с. (*Russian Lang*).
4. Medical management of chemical casualties handbook. 3rd ed. Aberdeen Proving Ground, MD: USAMRICO; 2000.
5. Cone DC, Schmidt TA, Mann NC, Brown L. Developing research criteria to define medical necessity in emergency medical services. Prehosp Emerg Care. 2004;8(2):116–25.
6. Martinez R. New vision for the role of emergency medical services. Ann Emerg Med. 1998;32(5):594–9.
7. Ocaqov H.O.. Fövqəladə halların nəticələrinin aradan qaldırılması. Ali məktəblər üçün dərslik. Bakı: Təhsil, 2009, 441 səh. (*Azerbaijani Lang*).
8. Бобов С.А., Юртушкин В.И. Чрезвычайные ситуации: защита населения и территорий. Учебное пособие. М., 2000. (*Russian Lang*).
9. Japanese Red Cross Society, Japan: Earthquake and Tsunami 24 Month Report Glide no. EQ-2011-000028-JPN 26 July 2013.
10. Боровко И.Р., Жогальский И.Я, Фролов Н.А. Основы гражданской обороны и службы экстренной медицинской помощи: Курс лекций. Мн.: БГМУ, 2005, 99 с. (*Russian Lang*).
11. A Journal of Civil-Military Disaster Management and Humanitarian Relief Collaborations. 2013–14, vol VI.
12. Analysis of Emergency Medical Systems Across the World. An interactive qualifying project submitted to the Faculty of the Worcester Polytechnic Institute. MIRAD Laboratory, 2013.
13. Razzak JA, Kellermann AL. Emergency medical care in developing countries: is it worthwhile? Bull World Health Organ. 2002;80:900–5.
14. Emergency safety and first aid handbook.
15. Improve the safety of your workers by training them in first aid CPR AED. American Heart Association. 2011.
16. Yusif-zada KY. Semi-public hospital management. The optimal integration of state funded and private healthcare services under a single hospital management. Germany: LAP LAMBERT Academic Publishing; 2016. 66p

17. Managing health for field operations in oil and gas activities. A guide for managers and supervisors in the oil and gas industry. OGP Report Number 343. 2011.
18. Ghazanfari T, Fagizadeh S, Aragizadeh H. Sardasht-Iran cohort study of chemical warfare victims: design and methods. Arch Iranian Med. 2009;12(1):5–14.
19. Ocaqov H.O.. Fövqəladə hallarda həyat fəaliyyətinin təhlukəsizliyi. Ali məktəblər üçün dərslik. Bakı: Casıoglu, 2010, 387 səh. (*Azerbaijani Lang*).

Ultrasound in Disasters and Austere Environments

9

Jay Doucet

9.1 Introduction

Natural disasters and some man-made mass casualty events can produce enough injured patients to overwhelm local health care systems and create loss of healthcare infrastructure, including imaging resources. They may also require healthcare to be provided in austere, resource-limited environments. Current healthcare in high-income nations is extensively based on advanced medical imaging. Organisation for Economic Co-operation and Development (OECD) 2018 data indicates that from 100 to 271 CT scans per 1000 inhabitants were performed in US and EU countries [1]. In the surge of patients occurring during loss of utilities and nonavailability of advanced medical imaging, there may be a critical lack of image-based clinical decision-making support. This will be a severe challenge for trauma care providers. A method to screen and diagnose trauma and non-trauma conditions that is rapid enough to deal with a large patient surge is ultrasound.

The characteristics of recently released ultrasound devices—lightweight, battery powered, handheld devices that use wireless, cloud-based image storage, can have considerable utility in disasters and austere environments. However, adequate preparation and training are required for successful deployment.

J. Doucet (✉)
Division of Trauma, Surgical Critical Care, Burns and Acute Care Surgery, Department of Surgery, University of California San Diego Health, San Diego, CA, USA
e-mail: jdoucet@ucsd.edu

© Springer Nature Switzerland AG 2021
E. Pikoulis, J. Doucet (eds.), *Emergency Medicine, Trauma and Disaster Management*, Hot Topics in Acute Care Surgery and Trauma,
https://doi.org/10.1007/978-3-030-34116-9_9

9.2   POCUS Training

Bedside ultrasonography by a non-fulltime sonographer clinician, also called Point of Care Ultrasonography (POCUS) has become a common part of the practice of trauma and acute care surgery [2]. Ultrasound facilitates diagnosis and increases the safety of procedures. Medical students in the US are now being taught ultrasonography skills in their junior years of medical school. Residencies and fellowships are increasingly adopting ultrasound curricula. The quality of ultrasound equipment and images are improving, ease of use is better and cost of equipment has decreased. Some newer devices are provided with integrated training modules for physicians.

The operator-dependent nature of the FAST exam and need for experience has led to a recognition that formal ultrasound curricula must be offered in medical school, residencies and fellowships. Facility with ultrasound is now required by Residency Review Committees' Milestones requirements for several specialties in the US. In 2017, new guidelines, including didactic education and a specified number of proctored examinations were provided in the US by the Surgical Critical Care Program Directors Society (SCCPDS), who train trauma surgeons and surgical intensivists in the US [3].

Training and credentialing in POCUS is available to all physicians. The American Medical Association has asserted that ultrasound imaging is not the exclusive property of any specialty, but that hospital medical staffs should determine requirements for privileging. These requirements should be based upon the physician's training for the use of ultrasound technology and strongly recommends that these criteria are in accordance with recommended training and education standards developed by each physician's respective specialty [4].

There is no single prescribed credential in POCUS that is universally accepted. Indeed, there is controversy whether external agencies should play a role versus using hospital-based training, required postgraduate training or continuing medical education (CME) courses alone. While an external credential for a specific clinical skill might demonstrate commitment to excellence and validation of training, there is no evidence that an external POCUS credential enhances patient safety. Indeed, in low and middle-income nations and in resource-limited environments, a requirement for an external credential could actually be a barrier to wider adoption of a critical patient care skill.

For those physicians who did not receive sufficient training in residency to be skilled in ultrasound, excellent resources are available on-line from sites such as pocus.org, sdms.org, aseuniversity.org and other sites. Finding a mentor who can observe your technique and review your examinations is also very helpful. There are also live CME-type POCUS ultrasound courses held in many countries, but these can be very expensive, and can only provide an introduction. If a physician is using POCUS to enhance decision-making or procedures, they should participate in a quality assurance (QA) program to allow ultrasound-facile peers to review complications and outcomes associated with POCUS use. Logs should be kept of POCUS exams to maintain privileges and enable QA processes.

9.3   POCUS Equipment

A revolution in wireless technology and microprocessors has also affected ultrasound devices. It is now possible to purchase a US FDA-approved ultrasound machine that performs most typical imaging modes, uses a robust semiconductor chip sound emitter, has digital image processing, connects to "cloud" storage via the provider's mobile phone and costs less than US$2000, not including annual subscriptions (~US$400) (Fig. 9.1). Pocket-sized ultrasound machines are decreasing in cost and will be carried by increasing numbers of providers. Ignoring the capabilities of this imaging modality will soon be impossible for trauma and acute care surgeons.

The small size of the newest handheld probes such as the Butterfly iQ, General Electric (GE) VScan or Philips Lumify simplifies their use in austere environments, they literally can be kept in a pocket. In the case of the Butterfly iQ, an Apple iOS device such as an iPhone or iPad is needed for visualization, while the Lumify needs an Android-based tablet. These devices could be easily taken on board aircraft or vehicles and brought to the billions of the world's population who lack good access to medical imaging. Battery life of these devices is typically 120 min, meaning some thought must be made for how these devices will be recharged between uses in resource-limited devices. Additional power sources, such as battery banks or solar chargers that provide mains power or USB power to charge the device and any visualization devices such as tablets should be also be acquired for use in disasters.

The current devices use Wi-Fi wireless connections to upload stored images. In the case of the GE VScan or Phillips Lumify, these can provide DICOM standard images for archiving in a hospital PACS system. The Butterfly iQ requires a separately-charged subscription to upload images to a cloud-based server system via Wi-Fi. If many images are to be stored and Wi-Fi with an internet connection is not available, images may be stored temporarily on the Android tablet or iOS device. In the case of

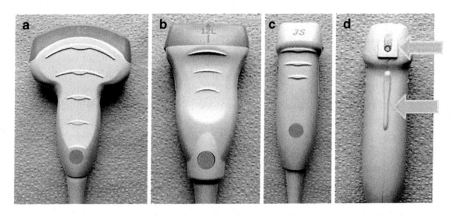

Fig. 9.1 Typical ultrasound probes. (**a**) Convex low frequency transducer—used in abdominal exams, (**b**) linear high frequency transducer—used in vascular and pleural exams, (**c**) phased array low frequency transducer specifically designed for cardiac imaging/echocardiography, (**d**) showing the transducer orientation index marker. Note the ridge on the probe housing and the LED

the Butterfly iQ being used in low resource environments, individual images taken are typically between 500 KB and 1 MB, and videos are 1–2 MB per second of recording. 16 GB of free space on a typical Apple iPhone or iPad would hold thousands of images and videos prior to internet connection. The Butterfly iQ does have to connect to the internet every 30 days for firmware updates and to check for recalls [5].

9.4   Conventional POCUS Studies

9.4.1   FAST

In 1996, "Focused *Abdominal* Sonography for Trauma" or FAST was described by Rozycki et al. The exam was "focused"—looking for free fluid only—to simplify the test and to make it faster [6]. However, within a year in the name of the exam had already changed to the "Focused *Assessment* with Sonography for Trauma" due to the realization that thoracic structures such as the heart, pericardium and pleura could also be evaluated [7]. FAST is useful not just in trauma patients, but can be adapted for the assessment of other acute surgical patients as well.

The purpose of the FAST examination is to determine the presence of pathologic intra-abdominal, intrapleural, or intraperitoneal free fluid, which has a distinctive hypoechoic or anechoic (that is, black) appearance on the screen [8]. About the only absolute contraindication to doing the FAST exam is when it delays performing a definitive operative procedure.

Ultrasound offers several advantages in the evaluation of the acute surgical patient. It is rapid and can be done at the bedside. It is noninvasive and does not require the use of radiation. It can be performed quickly, including in the middle of a trauma or shock resuscitation or even during CPR. The test can be repeated as often as desired. This makes it very suitable for the acute patient in shock, where the American College of Surgeons Advanced Trauma Life Support (ATLS) "Primary Survey Adjuncts" of FAST, Chest X-ray, and Pelvis X-ray can quickly locate the site of a large intracavitary hemorrhage and hematoma [9].

FAST ultrasound of the abdomen does have some significant limitations, the most significant is its lack of sensitivity, typically less than 75%. There are other tests that are more sensitive such as the CT scan of the abdomen, which is very sensitive and specific, or the diagnostic peritoneal lavage, which is exquisitely sensitive and not very specific. Sensitivities as low as 42% have been reported with FAST. However, that may not matter when FAST is employed by surgeons using an appropriate trauma or ICU algorithm. The low sensitivity of FAST is complemented by a good selectivity which means that a positive test is likely true and the negative test simply means more evaluation is necessary.

The FAST exam has been continually improved since the original four quadrant exam. The eFAST (enhanced FAST) means the addition of pleural views, which can detect a pneumothorax more rapidly and with greater sensitivity than a chest X-ray [10, 11] The thoracic views improve the utility of eFAST, even though it shares the relative lack of sensitivity of the traditional FAST abdominal exam compared to the CT scanner.

In patients in whom there is a doubt regarding the presence of pericardial effusion or tamponade, the FAST exam of the pericardium is invaluable and can be life-saving.

Some centers have improved the sensitivity of trauma ultrasonography by actually doing extra views and examining the organs, instead of just looking for fluid as done in FAST. At our Level I Trauma Center, we have previously demonstrated that a combination of a comprehensive negative screening ultrasonography (US) and negative clinical observation for 12–24 h, in the setting of blunt abdominal trauma, virtually excludes missed abdominal injury [12]. We call this complete examination CUST—Complete Ultrasonography for Trauma. Other advantages of CUST are the significant reduction in hospital charges as well as a large reduction in radiation exposure in trauma patients. Surgeon-selected blunt abdominal trauma screening with the CUST protocol appears to have similar outcomes as CTAP. While the initial CUST sensitivity was 76% in 19,128 patients, when combined with serial examination and selective CT scanning, the false negative rate was 0.29% with a NPV of 99% [13].

There are conditions in which a negative FAST cannot be accepted as definitive and a CT Scan should be performed.

A negative FAST examination should not be accepted as definitive if:

- it is of poor quality,
- it is a case of seat belt mark injury,
- it is a case of penetrating torso trauma,
- the patient is very obese,
- there is hematuria,
- the patient has significant abdominal pain without other operative indications, or,
- spinal and/or pelvic fractures are suspected.

In such cases, the patient should undergo CT scanning if available, or undergo serial examinations with a high suspicion for need for operative intervention.

Immediate laparotomy or thoracotomy without performing a FAST exam might be considered in penetrating trauma, or in blunt trauma with conditions such as peritonitis or evisceration. However, this means that there will be no evaluation of the pleura or pericardium prior to the procedure. The exact trajectory of penetrating trauma might not be immediately known at laparotomy. The presence of an occult pneumothorax might be missed and manifest only after intubation and anesthesia. Missed tamponade can be a lethal error, and can occur in both penetrating and blunt trauma.

Serial abdominal examination without FAST means that the opportunity to conduct repeat FAST exams is lost. Repeat FAST examinations increase the test's sensitivity and can indicate the need for CT or operation before peritonitis or abdominal pain manifests [14].

A limitation of FAST is that results are operator-dependent. Less experienced operators are less sensitive to detecting fluid—in one study about 10% of residents and attendings could detect 400 ml of intraperitoneal fluid, 85% could detect 850 ml and 97% could detect 1000 ml (Figs. 9.2 and 9.3) [15].

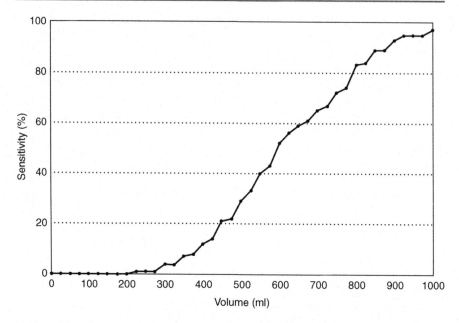

Fig. 9.2 Sensitivity of FAST to intraperitoneal fluid volume—EM attendings and residents

Fig. 9.3 Hand held, multimode, semiconductor chip ultrasound transducer, connects to iOS mobile phone, uses cloud storage, costs less than US$2000

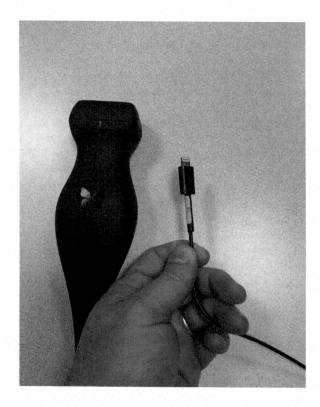

The principal probe positions for the FAST examination are shown at Fig. 9.4 along with typically appearances of hemoperitoneum and pericardial fluid (Fig. 9.5). eFAST adds pleural and parasternal windows as well.

9.4.2   Specific Abdominal Organs

The acute care surgeon, after mastering the FAST examination can expand their skills into an ultrasound repertoire that could include abdominal aortic aneurysm (AAA), gallbladder/hepatobiliary, spleen and appendix/intestinal examinations. Each new area requires additional training and a sufficient caseload to maintain proficiency. Most of these exams are not extremely time critical, with the possible exception of the AAA examination in a hypotensive patient. In most medical centers a skilled sonographic technician routinely performs these examinations. However these are also within the ability of an interested acute surgeon-sonographer.

Fig. 9.4 Solid ovals are probe locations for FAST abdominal ultrasound— Morrison's pouch (hepatorenal fossa), the splenorenal fossa (SR), the subcostal area (S), and the pelvis (P). Dashed circles are typical additional windows for eFAST— pleura (PL) and parasternal (P)

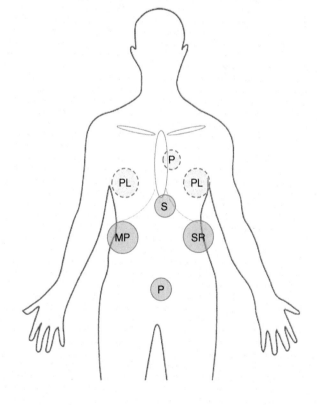

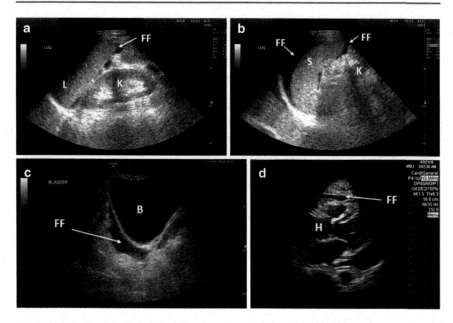

Fig. 9.5 (a–c) Example FAST images with hemoperitoneum—(**a**) Morrison's pouch (hepatorenal fossa), (**b**) splenorenal fossa, (**c**) pelvis with bladder, (**d**) FAST Subcostal SLAX view with large pericardial effusion. FF marks areas of free fluid. *L* liver, *S* spleen, *K* kidney, *B* bladder, *H* heart

9.5   Cardiac Ultrasound

The differential diagnosis and management of shock states are frequent challenges to the acute surgeon. Clinical examination is notoriously unreliable. Invasive monitoring techniques such as central venous pressure and pulmonary artery pressure catheters have fallen out of favor in many cases due to concerns for increased complications and difficulty of interpretation. These will also be difficult or impossible to manage in resource-limited settings. The latest addition to the FAST examination is the use of ultrasound to guide resuscitation of the acute surgical patient with shock. The intravascular volume status of the trauma patient has been estimated by the inferior vena cava (IVC) diameter and collapsibility as well as by ventricular filling [16]. More than 20 studies have been published describing the use of cardiac ultrasonography for resuscitation [2].

Bedside limited echocardiography has the advantages of being noninvasive, rapid, and being performed by the acute surgeons who will make immediate decisions on definitive management. Right and left ventricular function, intravascular volume and tamponade physiology can be rapidly identified. The Focus Assessed Transthoracic Echocardiography (FATE) examination was first described in 1989 in Denmark as a rapid way to assess shock states in critical care patients [17]. Similarly, the Focused Cardiac UltraSonography (FoCUS) examination was recommended by the American Society of Echocardiography (ASE) in 2014 for non-cardiologist clinicians to obtain rapid cardiac assessments [18]. The purpose of these exams is not to replace formal echocardiography, which can detect subtle and sophisticated findings such in as chronic valvular disease, but instead to make a shortened echocardiographic assessment of the current physiologic state, rule in or out critical diagnoses and guide resuscitative efforts.

Limited echocardiography is a step up in training complexity from the FAST examination. The target is moving, the useable sonographic windows are smaller and there is a greater demand on psychomotor skills to place the probe in the exact position to obtain the desired view. In trauma patients, typically less than 50% of the cardiac echocardiographic windows are useable due to subcutaneous air, pneumothoraces, edema, wounds, dressings, spinal precautions, and difficulty in positioning the patient [19]. Another training issue is that ultrasound machines switching from abdominal to cardiac modes by convention usually reverse the image, causing the index mark on the screen to shift from top left to top right. However, acute surgeons and trainees have routinely mastered these skills and are rewarded by the ability to make rapid assessments of cardiac physiology and intravascular volume status in the shock state.

9.5.1 Performing a Limited Echocardiography

There are three typical probe locations on the thorax for limited cardiac echo—the subcostal area (S), the left parasternal area (P) and the apical area (A) (Fig. 9.6).

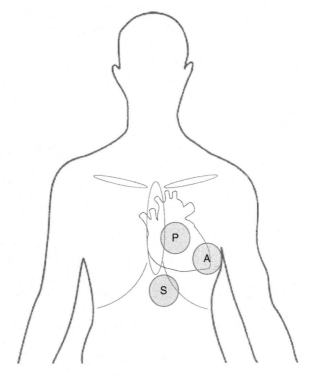

Fig. 9.6 Probe locations for point-of-care echocardiography—the subcostal area (S), the left parasternal area (P) and the apical area (A)

The subcostal location is included in the FAST examination and has two probe positions—subcostal long axis (SLAX) and subcostal short axis (SSAX) which give long axis and short axis views of the ventricles. A view of the inferior vena cava can also be obtained here (SIVC). The SLAX view requires placing probe below the xiphisternum, pointing the probe at the left acromion and rotating the probe on its long axis so that the index mark points away from the right shoulder, giving a long view of the ventricles (Fig. 9.7). The SLAX allows assessment of the left ventricle's performance. The SSAX view can then be obtained by continuing to point the probe at the left acromion while rotating the probe so that the index mark to pointing toward the patient's feet, giving a view across the ventricles (Fig. 9.8). This allows

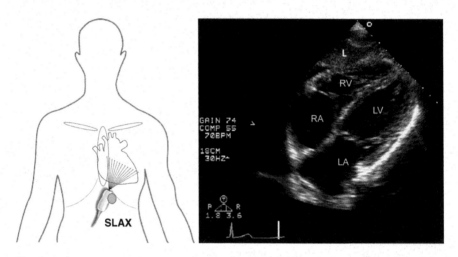

Fig. 9.7 The Subcostal Long Axis (SLAX) view—the index mark is to the patients left. *RV* right ventricle, *LV* left ventricle, *L* Liver. (From Adams D., Forsberg E. (2009) Conducting a cardiac ultrasound examination. In: Nihoyannopoulos P., Kisslo J. (eds) Echocardiography. Springer, London)

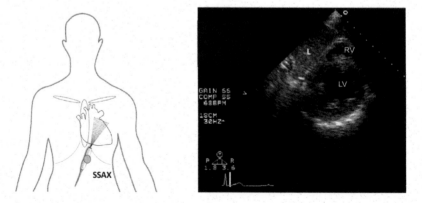

Fig. 9.8 The Subcostal Short Axis (SSAX) view—the index mark is to the patients feet. *RV* right ventricle, *LV* left ventricle, *L* Liver. (From Adams D., Forsberg E. (2009) Conducting a cardiac ultrasound examination. In: Nihoyannopoulos P., Kisslo J. (eds) Echocardiography. Springer, London)

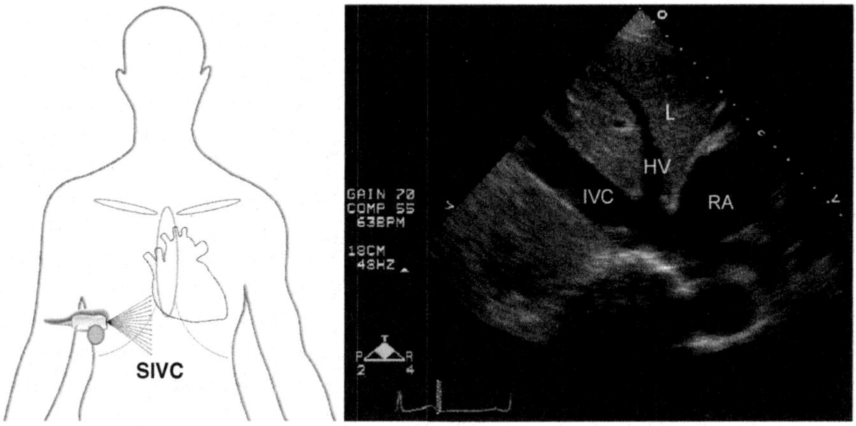

Fig. 9.9 The Subcostal IVC (SIVC) view—the index mark is towards the patients feet. *HV* hepatic vein, *IVC* inferior vena Cava, *RA* right atrium, *L* liver. (From Adams D., Forsberg E. (2009) Conducting a cardiac ultrasound examination. In: Nihoyannopoulos P., Kisslo J. (eds) Echocardiography. Springer, London)

assessment of the relative size of the left and right ventricle and comparison of performance of various areas of the left ventricle, as well as qualitative assessment of ejection fraction. The SIVC view is then obtained by pointing the probe in the subcostal area more medially to see the entry of the IVC into the inferior right atrium (Fig. 9.9). The SIVC allows assessment of intravascular volume status by IVC diameter.

If the IVC view cannot be obtained via the SIVC view due to interference from abdominal gas, incisions, dressings or subcutaneous air, it can also be assessed by placing the probe posteriorly at the right posterior costal margin in the posterior axillary line. This has the advantage of looking through the posterior liver anteriorly without the intestinal gas being interposed. Once the hepatorenal fossa (Morrison's pouch) is identified, the probe is tilted so that the IVC, near the center of the torso can be identified. In any view, the IVC diameter is typically assessed about 2–2–3 cm below the right atrial—IVC junction, in both transverse and longitudinal views [20].

The parasternal window offers the shortest distance to the heart, but is frequently affected by chest injury, dressings and pneumothoraces. The parasternal long axis (PLAX) view is obtained by placing the probe in about the fifth interspace just to the left of the sternum (Fig. 9.10). The probe is aligned so that the long axis of the probe head is aligned along a line from the right acromion to the left upper quadrant of the abdomen, with the index mark pointing away from the right shoulder, giving a long view of the ventricles, allowing assessment of left ventricle performance. The parasternal short axis (PSAX) view is obtained by rotating the probe 90° so that the long axis of the probe head is aligned along a line from the left acromion to the right upper quadrant of the abdomen, with the index mark pointing away from the left shoulder, giving a short view across the ventricles (Fig. 9.11). The probe can be tilted with a "fanning" motion to examine the ventricles from the tricuspid or mitral annulus to the chordae and to the apex of the heart.

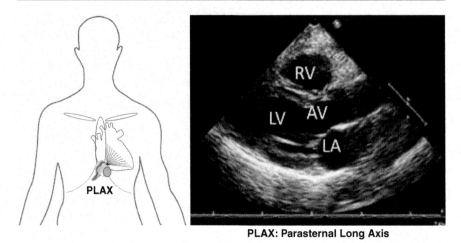

PLAX: Parasternal Long Axis

Fig. 9.10 The Parasternal Long Axis (PLAX) view—the index mark is to the patients left upper quadrant. *RV* right ventricle, *LV* left ventricle, *LA* left atrium, *AV* aortic valve. (From Walley, P.E., Walley, K.R., Goodgame, B. et al. A practical approach to goal-directed echocardiography in the critical care setting. Crit Care (2014) 18: 681. https://doi.org/10.1186/s13054-014-0681-z)

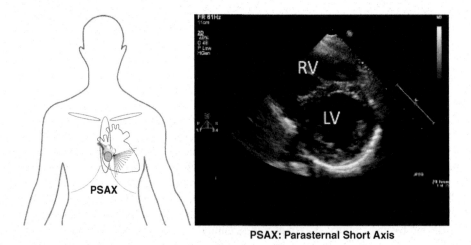

PSAX: Parasternal Short Axis

Fig. 9.11 The Parasternal Short Axis (PSAX) view—the index mark is to the patients right upper quadrant. *RV* right ventricle, *LV* left ventricle. (From Walley, P.E., Walley, K.R., Goodgame, B. et al. A practical approach to goal-directed echocardiography in the critical care setting. Crit Care (2014) 18: 681. https://doi.org/10.1186/s13054-014-0681-z)

The apical location is often unusable in critical patients as many patients must be positioned so that they are rolled onto their left side, allowing the apex of the heart to be more proximal to the chest wall. The apical 4 chamber view (A4CH) is obtained by placing the probe in about the fifth intercostal space in the midclavicular line pointing at the right acromion (Fig. 9.12). The index mark is pointed

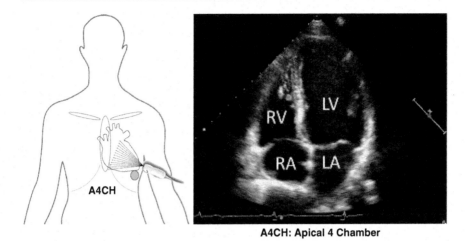

A4CH: Apical 4 Chamber

Fig. 9.12 The Apical 4 Chamber (A4CH) view—the index mark is to the patients right acromion. *RV* right ventricle, *LV* left ventricle, *RA* right atrium, *LA* left atrium. (From Walley, P.E., Walley, K.R., Goodgame, B. et al. A practical approach to goal-directed echocardiography in the critical care setting. Crit Care (2014) 18: 681. https://doi.org/10.1186/s13054-014-0681-z)

somewhat posteriorly. This will achieve a view of all four chambers of the heart as well as the intraventricular septum. Comparison of left and right ventricular size and function can be made as well as views of the tricuspid and mitral valves obtained. Septal motion can also be assessed. Allowing the probe position to slide slightly more anteriorly on the chest achieves the "five chamber" view where the aortic valve is also seen as well as the four ventricles.

9.5.2   Left Ventricle

A rapid qualitative assessment of left ventricular (LV) performance can be obtained from the above views. A stepwise assessment of the heart can be performed by first looking for obvious pathology such as tamponade, dilation or hypokinesis, next looking at ventricular size, wall thickness and filling and in systole and diastole and then looking at contractility in both left and right ventricles. The pleura should also be imaged bilaterally to identify pleural effusions or pneumothorax.

With a reasonable amount of practice, the acute surgeon can readily identify when LV ejection fraction is below 40–45% without need of formal measurements or calculations. A baseline bedside echocardiographic study in the acute ICU admission makes subsequent identification of acute versus chronic LV dysfunction easier. Global LV dysfunction can be seen in sepsis and septic shock, post-arrest states, stress cardiomyopathy, dilated cardiomyopathy, myocarditis and in chronic congestive heart failure. Generally the acute surgeon is looking for gross changes that will help explain a shock state. Subtle dysfunction such as diastolic heart failure is beyond the scope of the limited echocardiogram by the acute surgeon.

A special form of LV stress dysfunction can have a specific appearance—Takotsubo cardiomyopathy or "broken-heart syndrome" [21]. This can be triggered by physiologic or psychologic stress, usually in critically ill patients 50–80 years old. Women comprise 90% of cases. Classically, the base of LV is seen to have normal size and contractility while the apical segment is seen to balloon outwards in systole, giving the heart the shape of the Japanese octopus trap that provides the name of this condition.

Areas of localized LV hypokinesis may be caused by localized ischemia such as seen in acute coronary syndromes. The echocardiogram is more sensitive than EKG in detection of myocardial infarction in the postoperative patient, and can add sensitivity to troponin levels, which are already abnormal in 15–30% of non-cardiac surgery ICU patients. Although specific areas of the LV can be associated with particular coronary artery occlusions, this is beyond the scope of the usual acute surgeon echocardiographic examination—in suspected acute coronary syndromes cardiology consultation is warranted.

9.5.3   Right Ventricle and IVC

The right ventricle (RV) views should not be ignored as they can be significant in the shock state. The RV is harder to visualize due to its thinner wall. The normal RV wraps around a portion of the thicker walled circular LV as seen in the short axis PSAX or SSAX views. The interventricular septum normally bulges in a convex manner from the LV into the RV in both systole and diastole. In the healthy heart the stroke volume and ejection fraction are similar in the LV and RV, so the ventricular volumes should be equivalent, although each is shaped differently. As RV pressures increase such as in right heart failure, pulmonary embolism or pulmonary hypertension, the RV can be seen to enlarge and the septum increasingly flattens the side of the normally circular LV in the short axis views. As RV pressures increase further, the septum may begin to paradoxically bulge into the LV for a greater portion of the cardiac cycle.

Significant PE associated with shock is classically associated with a distended RV, flattened septum, under filled LV, and distended IVC. Echocardiography has a specificity of 81% and 94% and a positive predictive value of 71% and 86% for pulmonary emboli, however other sources of RV failure should be considered within the clinical context [22].

The IVC views should also be part of the cardiac ultrasound of the acute patient with a suspected shock state. Under normal conditions in healthy, spontaneously breathing, supine patients the IVC will nearly or completely collapse with inspiration and expand with expiration. Ultrasonographic assessment of the diameter of the inferior vena cava in expiration (IVCe) and in inspiration (IVCi) allows assessment of the collapsibility of the inferior vena cava (IVCe-IVCi) [23]. Another measurement of intravascular volume status is the IVC collapsibility index (IVC-CI). The IVC-CI is calculated using a standard formula IVC-CI = (IVCe) − (IVCi)/ (IVCe) × 100%, where IVCe is the maximum IVC diameter at expiration and IVCi is the minimum IVC diameter at inspiration [24]. Respiratory variation in IVC diameter has been found to be more pronounced in hypovolemia with abnormally low CVP being increasingly likely as IVC-CI approaches 100%. However there is not yet an exact cutoff value determined for IVC-CI for hypovolemia, although 75% has been suggested as the cutoff.

Similarly to central venous pressure measurements, techniques of IVC measurement have many of the same inaccuracies of CVP measurements. Positive pressure ventilation can invert the normal inspiratory-expiratory minimal and maximum size relationship, and high PEEP levels may reduce venous inflow to the chest and distend the IVC. Increased right atrial pressures are seen in right heart failure, valvular disease, and pulmonary hypertension and may cause increased IVC diameter that is not reflective of an increased volume status. However, these conditions would not be expected in most trauma or acute surgery admissions. Another issue with IVC diameter may be the effect of increased abdominal pressure such as seen in abdominal compartment syndrome causing narrowing of the IVC [25]. However, abdominal compartment syndrome is rarely present at admission in acute surgery patients, and when it is present at admission is usually accompanied by overt clinical signs that indicate immediate surgical intervention.

Following IVC diameters after initial therapeutic fluid challenge of the blunt trauma patient with hypotension may improve the utility of FAST in trauma patients. Yanagawa et al., in a study of 30 trauma patients presenting with shock (systolic BP < 90 mmHg) followed patients into two groups: a transient responder group ($n = 17$) in which shock recurred after an initial 2 L intravenous crystalloid fluid bolus in the emergency room and a responder group ($n = 13$) in which blood pressure remained stable [26]. IVC diameter predicted patients who would become hypotensive later despite equivalent fluid resuscitation. It also predicted those likely to need emergent hemostatic inventions such as laparotomy or angiography—the transient responder group contained a greater proportion of patients who underwent such procedures than the responder group (47.0% vs. 7.6%, $p < 0.05$).

In a American Association for Surgery of Trauma (AAST) multi-institutional trial of 144 major trauma patients, those with persistent IVC collapsibility on a second IVC measurement 60 min after admission compared with those who had increased IVC size, had significantly higher intravenous fluid requirements during the first 24 h of hospitalization (2503 ± 1751 mL vs. 1243 ± 1130 mL, $p = 0.003$) [27]. Those patients undergoing resuscitation can have repeated assessments by POCUS to assess the adequacy of resuscitation and need for further assessments.

9.5.4 Chest Injury—Pneumothorax

Rib fractures are common injuries in earthquakes and building collapses [28]. Rib fractures, sternal fractures, and pneumothorax can be detected by ultrasound [29]. Ultrasound can detect non-loculated pneumothorax more rapidly and more accurately that chest X-ray, although sensitivity can be affected by recent surgery, presence of a chest tube or subcutaneous air [10]. Specificity of a positive examination is excellent, and the size of the pneumothorax can be estimated in the supine patient, as the lung usually falls away from the anterior chest wall before the lateral chest wall. In this way, ultrasound can detect the presence of an "occult" pneumothorax that would not be visible on a supine chest X-ray. Either the phased-array or high-frequency linear probe can be used, although we prefer the higher resolution of the linear probe.

There are four ways ultrasound can be used to identify a pneumothorax:

1. Pleural sliding—the lung slides within the pleura during respirations and this sliding is evident by the sliding motion, especially of sonographic "B-lines," which appear as bright spots on the pleural surface with "ringdown" artifact, producing an appearance called "comet tails" (Fig. 9.13). There is no pleural sliding and no comet tails in locations where a pneumothorax is present.
2. M-mode—Using M-mode provides a time based graphical output of a single line over time. This can make pleural sliding more evident, with the normal exam with sliding producing an granular appearance below the ribs called the "Sandy beach" (Fig. 9.14) and where a pneumothorax without sliding generates an undifferentiated multilayered appearance called the "Stratosphere" sign (Fig. 9.15).
3. Lung point—This is a highly sensitive and specific sign of pneumothorax. As the probe is slid from the anterior portion of the chest where the pneumothorax is present to a more posterior and lateral position, the edge of the lung posterior to the pneumothorax that is just touching the chest wall may be seen. As the lung slides back and forth with respirations, periods of pleural sliding are interspersed with periods of no sliding. The edge of the lung is typically triangular in cross-section and so the name of Lung Point arises. Lung point may not be seen in large or tension pneumothoraces as no part of the lung may be found in contact with the chest wall.
4. Lung pulse—in some cases, there is little pleural sliding as respiratory movement may not be occurring in the portion of the lung under examination. This may occur during bronchial obstruction, apnea, contralateral mainstem intubation or near the heart. However, lung sliding can still be seen, only in small movements that correspond with the heart rate as the lung enlarges with every systole.

Fig. 9.13 Comet tails on pleural ultrasonography—normal—arrows indicate Comet tails

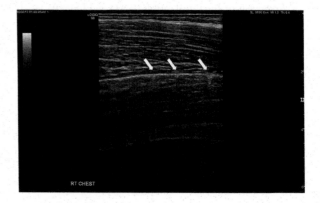

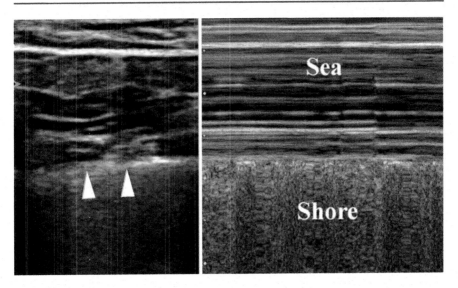

Fig. 9.14 Pleural ultrasonography—this is a split image with the left showing the 2D view of the pleural interface and the right side showing a normal M mode image showing the "Seashore" sign which is evidence of pleural sliding. (From Gillman LM, Ball CG, Panebianco N, Al-Kadi A, Kirkpatrick AW. Clinician performed resuscitative ultrasonography for the initial evaluation and resuscitation of trauma. Scandinavian Journal of Trauma, Resuscitation and Emergency Medicine. 2009;17:34. https://doi.org/10.1186/1757-7241-17-34)

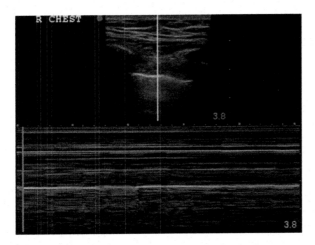

Fig. 9.15 Pleural ultrasonography—this is a split image with the top showing the 2D view of the pleural interface and the bottom showing an abnormal M Mode image showing the "Stratosphere sign" due to pneumothorax and no pleural sliding. (From Gillman LM, Ball CG, Panebianco N, Al-Kadi A, Kirkpatrick AW. Clinician performed resuscitative ultrasonography for the initial evaluation and resuscitation of trauma. *Scandinavian Journal of Trauma, Resuscitation and Emergency Medicine*. 2009;17:34. https://doi.org/10.1186/1757-7241-17-34)

9.5.5   Pleural Effusion, Atelectasis, and Pneumonia

In the same way the intra-abdominal fluid has a characteristic anechoic or black appearance on FAST examination, pleural effusions show as anechoic areas in the chest. These are usually best seen just above the diaphragm and posteriorly in the semi-recumbent patients. Ultrasound can differentiate between effusion and atelectasis or consolidation where the chest X-ray shows only basilar opacification of the lung field. Ultrasound can be superior to CT scanning in provide clues about the nature of the pleural fluid—featureless anechoic fluid is typically of a transudate, whereas exudates may have fibrinous strands that move with patient movement. Retained hemothorax will layer out into serous and cellular layers producing the "hematocrit sign". An empyema will often show areas of loculation. Assessment of pleural effusions over time in the ICU can help determine their progression, nature and potential for infection, indicating which should undergo drainage by thoracentesis.

Pneumonia with consolidation turns the normally air filled lung into a solid mass, and the lung takes on the ultrasonographic appearance of the liver. Lobar pneumonias can have quite sharp borders on ultrasound with the bright, consolidated lung adjacent to featureless normal lung lobes. Pulmonary edema increases the amount of interstitial lung water, making the "B-lines" of the lung more prominent and increasing the number of comet tails that are visible.

9.6   Useful Ultrasound Studies in Disaster and Resource-Limited Environments

9.6.1   Triage

In a high-income nation, trauma and critical acute surgery patients will typically have conventional X-rays and CT scans performed routinely at admission, such as recommended by the ATLS program [30]. In disasters and resource-limited settings, plain radiography and CT scanning may unavailable or severely limited in availability. Routine X-rays can also slow triage efforts. According to the U.S. Centers of Disease Control triage prediction tool, a single X-ray technician performing the ATLS-recommended chest, pelvis and other plain X-rays requires a mean of 10 min per patient. This would limit the flow of major trauma victims to six patients per hour per X-ray technician and X-ray machine [31]. This would be intolerably slow in many mass trauma situations.

POCUS can be used a screening tool by trauma providers at the bedside during the Initial Assessment to reduce reliance on immediate conventional radiology and CT scanning. Pneumothorax, hemothorax and shock states can be readily screened and identified. Stable patients with negative POCUS exams can forgo immediate scanning, freeing available X-ray technicians and CT scanners for more critical patients.

One of the first descriptions of POCUS in a natural disaster was following the 6.9 magnitude earthquake in Armenia in December 1988. This event caused over 25,000 deaths and approximately 150,000 injuries in area of about 700,000 people. The capital city, Yerevan was relatively unaffected, and its 1000 beds major hospital was the main medical facility for casualty victims. The only CT scanner in Yerevan was dedicated to managing head-trauma cases. Two triage areas, each with an ultra-sound machine, were created in the lobby of the hospital. Six physicians staffed the two rooms on a rotating basis and performed ultrasound examinations on as many trauma victims as time permitted. In a 72-h period, 750 patients came through the hospital. Four hundred of these patients received 530 ultrasound examinations either in the triage rooms or the emergency ward. 304 of the 503 exams were considered negative, and 96 (about 20%) demonstrated some form of pathology. Sixteen patients underwent operative intervention, usually laparotomy, based solely on clinical examination and ultrasound findings. There were four false negative cases (less than 1%) among the 530 studies performed, which illustrates the usual limitations in sensitivity of POCUS in trauma: one patient was found to have a ruptured kidney on laparotomy; another, a retroperitoneal hematoma; the third had a subcapsular hematoma of the spleen; and one obese patient had a massive hemothorax [32].

POCUS also has been shown to have a role in man-made events such as terrorist bombings and conflicts. FAST examinations were performed prehospital responders and hospital personnel after the 2004 Madrid train bombing and the 2005 London Underground bombing [33, 34]. Ultrasound was also successfully used for evaluation during explosive mass casualty incidents in a battlefield hospital in Iraq and equips even the smallest surgical teams in NATO forces [35].

9.6.2 PEA and CPR

Prolonged resuscitative efforts for trauma and acute patients under cardiac arrest during disaster and limited-resource scenarios are usually futile and incompatible with the adoption of a population-based standard of care. There is evidence that performance of limited echocardiography during PEA and CPR can be useful [36]. Four immediately significant conditions can be identified from the SLAX view, even while CPR is in progress. Cardiac standstill, with no visible cardiac motion, is associated with no meaningful survival in blunt trauma patients undergoing CPR for cardiac arrest, and is considered justification for suspension of resuscitative efforts, including no resuscitative thoracotomy [37]. Cardiac tamponade, identified as a pericardial effusion with RV or right atrial collapse with tamponade physiology requires pericardiotomy for surgical causes with pericardial clot and pericardiocentesis for medically caused non-clotting effusions. An empty heart points to severe hypovolemia. Massive pulmonary embolism is associated with RV distension, septal flattening, and small LV size.

9.6.3 Airway

Confirmation of successful intubation is routinely performed for all emergency intubations.. However, no technique used for confirmation of endotracheal tube (ETT) placement has been proven to be 100% accurate. Most physicians use a combination of auscultation, direct laryngoscopy, and end-tidal carbon dioxide detection to confirm ETT placement. However, in resource-limited, austere environments, end-tidal carbon dioxide and other intubation indicators may not be available.

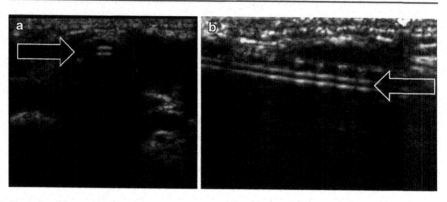

Fig. 9.16 Endotracheal tube in the proper position, as seen through the cricothyroid membrane in the transverse (**a**) and the longitudinal (**b**) views. (From Galicinao, J. et al. Pediatrics 2007;120:1297–1303)

Ultrasound has been used to confirm successful placement of the ETT after intubation, this is performed by scanning through the cricothyroid membrane with the linear probe and along the trachea. The ETT is visible as a double bright line (Fig. 9.16). A study of 99 children aged 1–17 years, revealed that the ETT was detected in all 99 patients by using bedside ultrasonography. Two views were required to show the ETT. In three cases, the colorimetric carbon dioxide detector gave negative or equivocal results but the ultrasound showed the ETT was correctly placed [38].

9.6.4 Crush Injury

Following large earthquakes, crush injury and crush syndrome may occur in thousands of extracted patients [39, 40]. Crush injury is defined as the result of physical trauma from prolonged compression of the torso, limb(s), or other parts of the body. The resulting injuries to soft tissues, muscles, and nerves can be due to the primary direct effect of the trauma or ischemia related to compression. In addition to possible direct muscle or organ injury, after release of the compressive force, severe crush injury results in swelling in the affected areas, with possible muscle necrosis and neurologic dysfunction. Crush injury can also be due to a secondary injury from subsequent compartment syndrome.

Crush syndrome is defined as the systemic manifestations resulting from crush injury, which can result in organ dysfunction predominantly acute kidney injury (AKI), but multisystem organ injury can also occur), or death. The manifestations of crush syndrome are the systemic consequences of muscle injury, specifically rhabdomyolysis, which commonly result in AKI [41, 42].

Following a 7.6 magnitude earthquake in Turkey in 1999, a study of the prognostic utility of renal Doppler ultrasound in determining the need for hemodialysis from crush injuries was performed. Out of 5302 patients admitted to regional hospitals, 639 had renal complications due to crush injuries, and 477 required hemodialysis after developing acute renal failure. Renal ultrasound in particular was used to gauge whether victims needed additional intravenous fluid resuscitation, urine alkalization and intravenous mannitol. Doppler flow to the kidneys was measured to calculate the renal resistive index, which was found to correlate well with the presence of oliguria and anuria and the need for hemodialysis. It was concluded that this measurement may be predictive for recovery from acute renal failure resulting from crush injury [43]. Similar utility for renal Doppler ultrasound was found after earthquakes in Haiti and Kashmir [44, 45].

9.6.5 Fractures

POCUS can be used to identify fractures, especially when the bone is largely subcutaneous such as in the hand, upper and lower extremities [46–48]. Fracture reduction guidance has been described for long bong fractures in children and in distal radial fractures and metacarpal fractures in adults [49–51]. Conventional X-ray has a low sensitivity for rib fractures, ultrasound has been suggested as being superior, but the quality of studies to date is poor [52].

9.6.6 Traumatic Brain Injury

Except in infants, where transfontanellar ultrasound of traumatic brain injury (TBI) can be sometimes be performed, ultrasound does not yet have a routine role in the evaluation of brain injury [53]. However there are investigations ongoing for the use of ultrasound in TBI.

Optic Nerve Sheath Diameter (ONSD) has been suggested as a potential noninvasive measure of the intracranial pressure (ICP). This would be very useful in environments where invasive ICP monitoring is unavailable or impractical. The exam is done using a linear probe and high-frequency setting. The measurement is taken of the diameter of the optic nerve sheath at the back of the eye, 3 mm behind the globe using an electronic caliper along the axis of the optic nerve. A meta-analysis of seven prospective studies of ONSD in with 320 patients with elevated ICP noted wide confidence intervals and significant heterogeneity in the studies. Transcranial Doppler has also been evaluated for noninvasive ICP assessment in three studies, with variable results. Both of these techniques are still considered investigational and should not yet be used to direct clinical management of TBI [54].

9.7 Conclusion

POCUS makes it possible to identify abdominal and thoracic injuries rapidly and efficiently, can guide procedural interventions and can hasten triage. The ability to utilize POCUS in conditions where conventional X-ray and CT imaging are unavailable further increases its utility. As physicians and allied providers become more facile with POCUS, and as POCUS machines become smaller, durable and more capable, POCUS will be an indispensable and integral component of disaster response and the provision of care in austere environments.

References

1. OECD. Health at a glance 2019. 2019.
2. Ferrada P. Image-based resuscitation of the hypotensive patient with cardiac ultrasound: an evidence-based review. J Trauma Acute Care Surg. 2016;80(3):511–8.
3. (SCCPDS) SCCPDS. Point of care ultrasound program for surgical critical care fellows. 2017. http://sccpds.org/scc-program-directors/ultrasound-curriculum/.
4. Association AM. Privileging for ultrasound imaging H-230.960. 2010. Cited 2019 30 Dec 2019.
5. Butterfly Networks. Use without internet. 2019. https://support.butterflynetwork.com/hc/en-us/articles/360030750152-Use-Without-Internet.
6. Rozycki GS, Ochsner MG, Schmidt JA, Frankel HL, Davis TP, Wang D, Champion HR. A prospective study of surgeon-performed ultrasound as the primary adjuvant modality for injured patient assessment. J Trauma. 1995;39(3):492–8; discussion 498–500.
7. Lichtenstein DA. Lung ultrasound in the critically ill. Ann Intensive Care. 2014;4(1):1.
8. Rozycki GS, Ochsner MG, Jaffin JH, Champion HR. Prospective evaluation of surgeons' use of ultrasound in the evaluation of trauma patients. J Trauma. 1993;34(4):516–26; discussion 26–7.
9. Subcommittee A, American College of Surgeons' Committee on T. International Awg. Advanced trauma life support (ATLS(R)): the ninth edition. J Trauma Acute Care Surg. 2013;74(5):1363–6.
10. Soult MC, Weireter LJ, Britt RC, Collins JN, Novosel TJ, Reed SF, Britt LD. Can routine trauma bay chest X-ray be bypassed with an extended focused assessment with sonography for trauma examination? Am Surg. 2015;81(4):336–40.
11. Hamada SR, Delhaye N, Kerever S, Harrois A, Duranteau J. Integrating eFAST in the initial management of stable trauma patients: the end of plain film radiography. Ann Intensive Care. 2016;6(1):62.
12. Brown MA, Casola G, Sirlin CB, Hoyt DB. Importance of evaluating organ parenchyma during screening abdominal ultrasonography after blunt trauma. J Ultrasound Med. 2001;20(6):577–83; quiz 85.
13. Dehqanzada ZA, Meisinger Q, Doucet J, Smith A, Casola G, Coimbra R. Complete ultrasonography of trauma in screening blunt abdominal trauma patients is equivalent to computed tomographic scanning while reducing radiation exposure and cost. J Trauma Acute Care Surg. 2015;79(2):199–205.
14. Blackbourne LH, Soffer D, McKenney M, Amortegui J, Schulman CI, Crookes B, Habib F, Benjamin R, Lopez PP, Namias N, et al. Secondary ultrasound examination increases the sensitivity of the FAST exam in blunt trauma. J Trauma. 2004;57(5):934–8.
15. Branney SW, Wolfe RE, Moore EE, Albert NP, Heinig M, Mestek M, Eule J. Quantitative sensitivity of ultrasound in detecting free intraperitoneal fluid. J Trauma. 1995;39(2):375–80.
16. Ratnasekera A, Ferrada P. Ultrasonographic-guided resuscitation of the surgical patient. JAMA Surg. 2018;153(1):77–8.
17. Jensen MB, Sloth E, Larsen KM, Schmidt MB. Transthoracic echocardiography for cardiopulmonary monitoring in intensive care. Eur J Anaesthesiol. 2004;21(9):700–7.
18. Via G, Hussain A, Wells M, Reardon R, ElBarbary M, Noble VE, Tsung JW, Neskovic AN, Price S, Oren-Grinberg A, et al. International evidence-based recommendations for focused cardiac ultrasound. J Am Soc Echocardiogr. 2014;27(7):683.e1–e33.

19. Gunst M, Sperry J, Ghaemmaghami V, O'Keeffe T, Friese R, Frankel H. Bedside echocardiographic assessment for trauma/critical care: the BEAT exam. J Am Coll Surg. 2008;207(3):e1–3.
20. Finnerty NM, Panchal AR, Boulger C, Vira A, Bischof JJ, Amick C, Way DP, Bahner DP. Inferior vena cava measurement with ultrasound: what is the best view and best mode? West J Emerg Med. 2017;18(3):496–501.
21. Izumo M, Akashi YJ. Role of echocardiography for takotsubo cardiomyopathy: clinical and prognostic implications. Cardiovasc Diagn Ther. 2018;8(1):90–100.
22. Hernandez C, Shuler K, Hannan H, Sonyika C, Likourezos A, Marshall J. C.A.U.S.E.: cardiac arrest ultra-sound exam—a better approach to managing patients in primary non-arrhythmogenic cardiac arrest. Resuscitation. 2008;76(2):198–206.
23. Barbier C, Loubieres Y, Schmit C, Hayon J, Ricome JL, Jardin F, Vieillard-Baron A. Respiratory changes in inferior vena cava diameter are helpful in predicting fluid responsiveness in ventilated septic patients. Intensive Care Med. 2004;30(9):1740–6.
24. Ciozda W, Kedan I, Kehl DW, Zimmer R, Khandwalla R, Kimchi A. The efficacy of sonographic measurement of inferior vena cava diameter as an estimate of central venous pressure. Cardiovasc Ultrasound. 2016;14(1):33.
25. Bauman Z, Coba V, Gassner M, Amponsah D, Gallien J, Blyden D, Killu K. Inferior vena cava collapsibility loses correlation with internal jugular vein collapsibility during increased thoracic or intra-abdominal pressure. J Ultrasound. 2015;18(4):343–8.
26. Yanagawa Y, Sakamoto T, Okada Y. Hypovolemic shock evaluated by sonographic measurement of the inferior vena cava during resuscitation in trauma patients. J Trauma. 2007;63(6):1245–8; discussion 8.
27. Doucet JJ, Ferrada P, Murthi S, Nirula R, Edwards S, Cantrell E, Han J, Haase D, Singleton A, Birkas Y, et al. Ultrasonographic inferior vena cava diameter response to trauma resuscitation after 1 hour predicts 24-hour fluid requirement. J Trauma Acute Care Surg. 2020;88(1):70–9.
28. Sirmali M, Turut H, Topcu S, Gulhan E, Yazici U, Kaya S, Tastepe I. A comprehensive analysis of traumatic rib fractures: morbidity, mortality and management. Eur J Cardiothorac Surg. 2003;24(1):133–8.
29. Rainer TH, Griffith JF, Lam E, Lam PK, Metreweli C. Comparison of thoracic ultrasound, clinical acumen, and radiography in patients with minor chest injury. J Trauma. 2004;56(6):1211–3.
30. Henry SM. Advanced trauma life support course student manual. 10th ed. American College of Surgeons: Chicago, IL; 2018.
31. Trauma ACoSCo. Disaster management and emergency preparedness course manual. 2nd ed. Chicago, IL: American College of Surgeons; 2017.
32. Sarkisian AE, Khondkarian RA, Amirbekian NM, Bagdasarian NB, Khojayan RL, Oganesian YT. Sonographic screening of mass casualties for abdominal and renal injuries following the 1988 Armenian earthquake. J Trauma. 1991;31(2):247–50.
33. Turegano-Fuentes F, Caba-Doussoux P, Jover-Navalon JM, Martin-Perez E, Fernandez-Luengas D, Diez-Valladares L, Perez-Diaz D, Yuste-Garcia P, Guadalajara Labajo H, Rios-Blanco R, et al. Injury patterns from major urban terrorist bombings in trains: the Madrid experience. World J Surg. 2008;32(6):1168–75.
34. Aylwin CJ, Konig TC, Brennan NW, Shirley PJ, Davies G, Walsh MS, Brohi K. Reduction in critical mortality in urban mass casualty incidents: analysis of triage, surge, and resource use after the London bombings on July 7, 2005. Lancet. 2006;368(9554):2219–25.
35. Raja AS, Propper BW, Vandenberg SL, Matchette MW, Rasmussen TE, Johannigman JA, Davidson SB. Imaging utilization during explosive multiple casualty incidents. J Trauma. 2010;68(6):1421–4.
36. Breitkreutz R, Price S, Steiger HV, Seeger FH, Ilper H, Ackermann H, Rudolph M, Uddin S, Weigand MA, Muller E, et al. Focused echocardiographic evaluation in life support and peri-resuscitation of emergency patients: a prospective trial. Resuscitation. 2010;81(11):1527–33.
37. Inaba K, Chouliaras K, Zakaluzny S, Swadron S, Mailhot T, Seif D, Teixeira P, Sivrikoz E, Ives C, Barmparas G, et al. FAST ultrasound examination as a predictor of outcomes after resuscitative thoracotomy: a prospective evaluation. Ann Surg. 2015;262(3):512–8; discussion 6–8.

38. Galicinao J, Bush AJ, Godambe SA. Use of bedside ultrasonography for endotracheal tube placement in pediatric patients: a feasibility study. Pediatrics. 2007;120(6):1297–303.
39. Oda J, Tanaka H, Yoshioka T, Iwai A, Yamamura H, Ishikawa K, Matsuoka T, Kuwagata Y, Hiraide A, Shimazu T, et al. Analysis of 372 patients with crush syndrome caused by the Hanshin-Awaji earthquake. J Trauma. 1997;42(3):470–5; discussion 5–6.
40. Bartels SA, VanRooyen MJ. Medical complications associated with earthquakes. Lancet. 2012;379(9817):748–57.
41. Sever MS, Vanholder R, Disasters RoIWGoRftMoCViM. Recommendation for the management of crush victims in mass disasters. Nephrol Dial Transplant. 2012;27(Suppl 1):i1–67.
42. Godat LN, Doucet J. In: Bulger E, editor. Severe crush injury in adults. Waltham, MA: UpToDate; 2019.
43. Keven K, Ates K, Yagmurlu B, Nergizoglu G, Kutlay S, Aras S, Ozcan H, Duman N. Renal Doppler ultrasonographic findings in earthquake victims with crush injury. J Ultrasound Med. 2001;20(6):675–9.
44. Vanholder R, van der Tol A, De Smet M, Hoste E, Koc M, Hussain A, Khan S, Sever MS. Earthquakes and crush syndrome casualties: lessons learned from the Kashmir disaster. Kidney Int. 2007;71(1):17–23.
45. Vanholder R, Gibney N, Luyckx VA, Sever MS, Renal Disaster Relief Task F. Renal Disaster Relief Task Force in Haiti earthquake. Lancet. 2010;375(9721):1162–3.
46. Kocaoglu S, Ozhasenekler A, Icme F, Pamukcu Gunaydin G, Sener A, Gokhan S. The role of ultrasonography in the diagnosis of metacarpal fractures. Am J Emerg Med. 2016;34(9):1868–71.
47. Tayal VS, Antoniazzi J, Pariyadath M, Norton HJ. Prospective use of ultrasound imaging to detect bony hand injuries in adults. J Ultrasound Med. 2007;26(9):1143–8.
48. Champagne N, Eadie L, Regan L, Wilson P. The effectiveness of ultrasound in the detection of fractures in adults with suspected upper or lower limb injury: a systematic review and subgroup meta-analysis. BMC Emerg Med. 2019;19(1):17.
49. Patel DD, Blumberg SM, Crain EF. The utility of bedside ultrasonography in identifying fractures and guiding fracture reduction in children. Pediatr Emerg Care. 2009;25(4):221–5.
50. Shen S, Wang X, Fu Z. Value of ultrasound-guided closed reduction and minimally invasive fixation in the treatment of metacarpal fractures. J Ultrasound Med. 2019;38(10):2659–66.
51. Bozkurt O, Ersel M, Karbek Akarca F, Yalcinli S, Midik S, Kucuk L. The diagnostic accuracy of ultrasonography in determining the reduction success of distal radius fractures. Turk J Emerg Med. 2018;18(3):111–8.
52. Battle C, Hayward S, Eggert S, Evans PA. Comparison of the use of lung ultrasound and chest radiography in the diagnosis of rib fractures: a systematic review. Emerg Med J. 2019;36(3):185–90.
53. Trenchs V, Curcoy AI, Castillo M, Badosa J, Luaces C, Pou J, Navarro R. Minor head trauma and linear skull fracture in infants: cranial ultrasound or computed tomography? Eur J Emerg Med. 2009;16(3):150–2.
54. Robba C, Santori G, Czosnyka M, Corradi F, Bragazzi N, Padayachy L, Taccone FS, Citerio G. Optic nerve sheath diameter measured sonographically as non-invasive estimator of intracranial pressure: a systematic review and meta-analysis. Intensive Care Med. 2018;44(8):1284–94.

Part II

Hospital Response

Basics of Hospital Response

10

Christos Christou

> *Functioning Plans of Response: Goals and Structure, Functions of Critical Importance for the Capacity of the Hospital, The Content of the Disaster Plan, What Every Staff Member Should Know, The Alert Process, Decision About the Level of Alert, Coordination and Command, Communication with the Command on Regional Level, Communication with the Command on National Level, Preparing the Hospital, Receiving Casualties, Registration of Patients, Hospital Information Center and Management of Media)*
>
> *If you fail to plan, you are planning to fail!*
>
> —Benjamin Franklin

10.1 Objective

The purpose of this chapter is to identify the basic principles of disaster planning and emergency preparedness of a health care facility/ hospital. The readers will get familiar with

- Functioning plans of response: goals and structure, functions of critical importance for the capacity of the hospital.
- The content of the disaster plan and what every staff member should know.
- The alert process, decision about the level of alert.
- Coordination and command, communication with the command on regional level, communication with the command on national level.

C. Christou (✉)
Department of Greece, Medecins Sans Frontieres (MSF), Athens, Greece
e-mail: christos.christou@athens.msf.org

© Springer Nature Switzerland AG 2021
E. Pikoulis, J. Doucet (eds.), *Emergency Medicine, Trauma and Disaster Management*, Hot Topics in Acute Care Surgery and Trauma,
https://doi.org/10.1007/978-3-030-34116-9_10

- Preparing the hospital, receiving casualties, registration of patients, hospital information center.
- Management of media.

10.2 Structure

Text with a scenario of emergency preparedness plan for a mass casualty incident in a small health structure.

10.3 Introduction

No definition of emergency incident/disaster is universally accepted. According to the Emergency Management Accreditation Program [1], a disaster is any severe or prolonged emergency which threatens life, property, environment, and/or critical systems; an emergency is any incident or set of incidents, natural or human caused, which require responsive actions to protect life, property, environment, and/or critical systems. Therefore, an emergency management program is the system that provides for management and coordination of prevention, mitigation, preparedness, response, and recovery activities for all hazards [2]. The system encompasses all organizations, agencies, departments, and individuals having responsibilities for these activities. In other words, any event that requires special planning to ensure capacity and capability for the provision of appropriate medical care to the attendees without adversely affecting medical care in the host community could be considered as emergency/disaster incident.

By the ATLS definition, a mass casualty incident (MCI) is a disaster, in which patient care resources are overwhelmed and cannot immediately be supplemented. Whenever a hospital or a health care facility is confronted by a situation where it has to provide care to a large number of patients in limited time, which is beyond its normal capacity, constitutes a disaster for the said hospital [3]. In others words when the resources of the hospitals (infrastructure, trained manpower, and organization) are overwhelmed beyond its normal capacity and additional contingency measure are required to control the event, the hospital can be said to be in a disaster situation [4]. This implies that a same event may have a disaster potential for a smaller hospital and not so for a bigger one. Therefore, disaster for a hospital is "a temporary lack of resources which is caused due to sudden influx of unexpected patient load." [5]

10.3.1 Why Planning?

Hospitals that are not prepared to respond effectively to public health emergencies, may risk increased morbidity and mortality of casualties, reduced ability to protect their own staff and facilities and a prolonged recovery phase resulting in financial losses and negative publicity within the community. Developing a community-wide emergency preparedness program for domestic preparedness requires that health care representatives collaborate with their public safety and emergency preparedness agencies to develop a clear appreciation for each other's capabilities and limitations.

The main objective of a hospital emergency/disaster plan is to optimally prepare the staff and institutional resources of the hospital for effective performance in different disaster situations. The hospital disaster plans should address not only the mass casualties which may result from a mass casualty incident (MCI) that has occurred away from the hospital, but should also address the situation where the hospital itself has been affected by a disaster [6]. Thus, a hospital disaster plan could be divided into two categories:

Internal Disaster Plan: It could be any event inside the hospital or on campus endangering patients or staff, creating a need for evacuation or relocation. Additionally, it may be any situation where additional staffing is needed. Examples of internal disasters are fire, explosion, flooding, or earthquake [7].

External Disaster Plan: It consists of any disaster outside the hospital (natural or man-made) requiring the activation of the emergency management plan, e.g., hurricane, plane crash, chemical spill, and mass casualty incident [8].

In case of incidents affecting the hospital itself, the further goals of the plan would be to protect life, environment, and property inside the hospital from any further damage [9]:

- By implementing the preparedness measures.
- By appropriate actions of the staff who have to know their tasks in such a situation.
- By soliciting help from outside in an optimal way.
- By re-establishing as quickly as possible an orderly situation in the hospital, enabling a return to normal work conditions.

In case of MCI away from the hospital (not affecting the hospital), the further goals of the disaster plan should be to control a large number of patients and manage the resulting problems in an organized manner [10]:

- By enhancing the capacities of admission and treatment.
- By treating the patients based on the rules of individual management, despite there being a greater number of patients.
- By ensuring proper ongoing treatment for all patients who were already present in the hospital.
- By smooth handling of all additional tasks caused by such an incident.
- By providing medications, medical consultation, infusions, dressing material, and any other necessary medical equipment.

10.3.2 How to Plan?

The following strategies are invaluable aids for revising a hospital's disaster poli-
cies/plans or upgrading to a comprehensive emergency preparedness plan:

- Review and, where needed, enhance and incorporate existing contingency or
  disaster plans as much as possible. It is not necessary to completely rewrite exist-
  ing plans to conform to the emergency management plan format, but all aspects
  of the existing emergency management plan need to be critically reviewed.
- Build layered protection by developing plans to defend both mission-critical sys-
  tems and mission-critical operations. Some key elements of this planning include:
  – Communications during emergencies.
  – Managing resources and assets.
  – Managing safety and security.
  – Defining and managing staff roles and responsibilities.
  – Managing utilities.
  – Managing patient clinical and support activities.
- The emergency management plan should use a common framework that incorpo-
  rates four separate process components: mitigation, preparedness, response, and
  recovery (well known as the life cycle).
- Those responsible for developing the plan need to involve community emer-
  gency management planners as well as public safety and public health providers
  to assure that the hospital's plan coincides and integrates with those in the
  community.
- All emergency management plans should be evaluated through regular exercises,
  and when necessary, revisions should be incorporated. Staff knowledge and competency fades with time, and hazards and vulnerabilities may change.

10.4   The Life Cycle

There are four main key aspects for the emergency management planning:mitigation,
preparedness, response, and recovery (Fig. 10.1).

When developing a comprehensive emergency management plan to address an
emergency incident/disaster, it is imperative that those responsible for the planning
understand these four key aspects. The first step to employing these aspects successfully is to understand how these terms are defined in relation to the principles of
emergency management planning for health care organizations (Fig. 10.2).

1. *Prevention (Mitigation)*
   Mitigation is defined as the activities an organization undertakes in order to
   lessen the severity and impact a potential emergency incident/disaster may have

Fig. 10.1 The life cycle

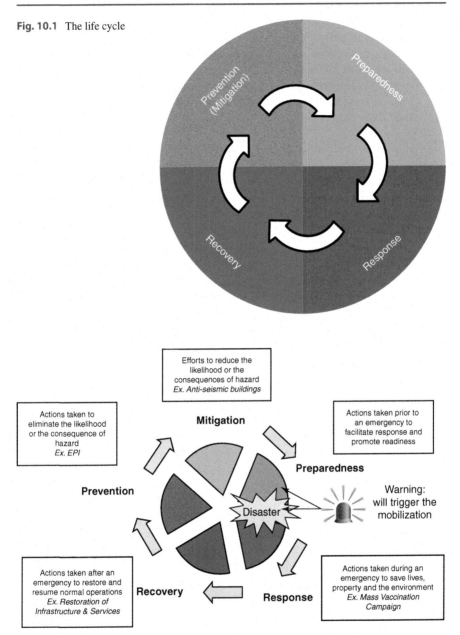

Fig. 10.2 The four key aspects (prevention/mitigation, preparedness, response, and recovery) to address a disaster

on its operations. Those responsible for implementing the emergency management plan must address mitigation from two perspectives:

- Mitigation activities are employed prior to an emergency incident/disaster that will eliminate or decrease the potential of vital system failures.
- Mitigation activities undertaken during an emergency incident/disaster to reduce the effects of the disaster that were not adequately alleviated by pre-event mitigation efforts.

2. *Preparedness*

Preparedness is defined as the aggregate of all measures and policies taken by those responsible for the development and implementation of the emergency management plan before the event occurs, which in turn provides programs designed to minimize loss of life and damage, to organize and facilitate effective rescue and relief, and to rehabilitate after disaster. Preparedness includes warning systems, sheltering in place, evacuation plans, energy management strategies, and disaster drills and exercises. Contingency and response plans are included in the steps of preparedness. As preparedness increases, the ability of a hospital and a community to absorb the event and mitigate the impact (damage) is augmented as a dependent variable of the level of preparedness. Preparedness addresses educating and training the organization and its management as well as the public. This aspect of emergency preparedness includes knowledge of plans, training of personnel, and stockpiling of supplies, as well as ensuring that needed funds and other resources are available.

3. *Response*

Response refers to actual emergency management. Response involves treating victims, reducing secondary impact to the organization, and controlling the negative effects of an emergency incident/disaster. The hospital must have an all hazards response plan to provide the foundation for organization readiness and to address the hospital's overall readiness. Each department needs to determine their responsibilities and how their response activities support and align with the hospital's all hazards response plan.

4. *Recovery*

Recovery consists of four key elements: finance, staffing, service, and communication. These are incorporated into the formulation of strategies and action plans and then implemented to address the primary and secondary effects resulting from the emergency incident/disaster.

- Primary effects are those that are a direct result of the event.
- Secondary effects are those that result from the primary effects or from the responses to the event.

Although described as acute, some effects may be ongoing and stretch over long periods of time (i.e., famine, drought, epidemics, complex human emergencies). These effects are functions of the vulnerability of the population and the environment and the human responses to the impact of the event.

The hospital emergency planning can be divided into three phases: the pre-disaster, the disaster, and the post-disaster phase.

10.4.1 Pre-disaster Phase

The primary aim of the district medical authorities during the pre-disaster phase would be to critically asses the available medical resources within the district and share them with other neighboring districts. In other words, the networking of the various medical resources and hospitals should be the main aim of the district medical authorities in the pre-disaster phase. The networking should not only be of facilities but of transport vehicles like ambulances, blood banks, CT scan, etc.

Emphasis should also be laid down on the organizational and functional aspects of such a medical networking.

(a) Planning: Most of the assessment and planning is done in the pre-disaster phase; the hospital plans are formulated and then discussed in a suitable forum for approval.
(b) The disaster manual: The hospital disaster plan should be written down in a document form and copies of the same should be available in all the areas of the hospital.
(c) Staff education and training: It is very important for the staff to know about and get trained in using the hospital disaster/emergency manual. Regular staff training by suitable drills should be undertaken in this phase.

10.4.1.1   Hospital Disaster Management Committee

The Hospital Disaster Management or Emergency Preparedness Committee is a multidisciplinary group representing key departments whose input is essential to planning and development of policies and procedures related to hospital and community emergency preparedness. Formation of a disaster/emergency committee is the first step for making a disaster plan for the hospital. Most of the hospitals already have such hospital management committees; therefore, an emergency/disaster management committee can be carved out from such already existing committees. The members of the disaster management committee should be from following basic facilities of the hospital administration:

- The director/head of the facility/hospital.
- Member/members from hospital management board.
- The chiefs/heads of various clinical departments supporting the emergency service,; e.g., acute and emergency services, orthopedics, general surgery, medicine, neurosurgery (if present), cardio-thoracic surgery (if present), anesthesia.
- The chiefs/heads of various ancillary departments, e.g., radio-diagnosis, transfusion medicine/ blood bank, laboratory services/pathology, forensic medicine.
- The chief nursing matron.
- The finance department.
- The stores and supplies department.
- The hospital engineering department.
- The public relation and liaison office.
- The chief of security of the hospital.

- The sanitation department.
- Hospital kitchen/dietary services.
- The social welfare department (if present).
- Hospital unions.

10.4.1.2 Central Command Structure (Incident Command System)

In order to ensure effective control and avoid duplication of action, there should be a unified command system which should be based on the individual hospital hierarchical chain. The advantages of ICS are many: it has predictable chain of management; flexible organization charts allowing flexible response to specific emergencies; prioritized response checklists; accountability of position function; improved documentation; a common language to promote communications and facilitate outside assistance; cost-effective emergency planning within the hospital.

Although this sort of chain of command is ideal to avoid chaos in emergency situations, it is seen that there is a strong opposition to formation of any such hierarchical command system by the physicians and hospital personnel. Nevertheless, all doctors including the administrator should emphasize that such a command system would come into effect only at the time of mass casualty incident and would close down on withdrawal of disaster alert. Therefore, all hospital personnel including doctors should respect the command hierarchy during emergencies and disasters.

Any command system may be used by the hospital but the most important rule is to make an organizational chart. Each position on the chart should be function based and not position or individual based. An individual can be assigned more than one position on the chart, so a person might have to perform multiple tasks until additional support comes. Also the titles used in a disaster/emergency plan are carried by functions and not individual people/designation (Fig. 10.3).

10.4.1.3 Action Cards

Action sheets or job cards are basis of a successful disaster/emergency management plan. These sheets should be made for each and every position in the organizational chart of the command system. The job cards should be detailed, stored safely (in disaster manual), color coded, and laminated.

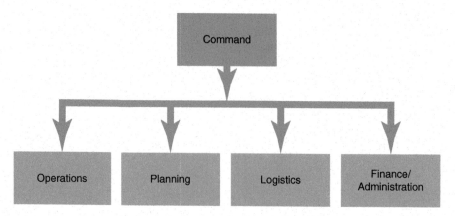

Fig. 10.3 Basic incident command diagram. Each position on the chart should be function based

10.4.1.4   Plan Activation of Different Areas of Hospital

The areas which should find a mention in a hospital emergency plan are:

- Command center.
- Communications office/paging/hotline area/telephone exchange.
- Security office.
- Reception and triage area.
- Decontamination area (if needed).
- Minor treatment areas.
- Acute care area (emergency department).
- Definitive care areas (OTs, wards).
- Intensive treatment area and activation of high dependency units.
- Mortuary.
- Holding area for relatives/non-injured.
- Area for holding media briefings.
- Area for holding patients in case a part of the hospital is evacuated.

1. All these areas should be mapped on the outlay map of the hospital. The normal capacities of the existing areas should be mentioned on these maps.
2. Disaster beds/how to increase bed capacity in emergencies.
3. The newly arriving patients would require admission for definitive treatment; therefore, plans should be there to increase the bed capacity when needed. This can be achieved by the following actions:
   - Discharge elective cases.
   - Discharge stable recovering patients. Stop admitting non-emergency patients.
   - Convert waiting/non-patient care areas into makeshift wards.

10.4.1.5   Planning of Public Information and Liaison (Crisis and Emergency Risk Communication)

We live in the age of mass and multimedia. Every news and information source will seek access to the latest and most up-to-date information. In most cases there is absence of clear and credible information. This leads to media speculations and increases the stress and pressure of the incident, especially on hospital and its staffs. Communicating in disaster situations has become increasingly difficult for responding organizations and hospital representatives. The organization's credibility and the credibility of the spokespersons who deliver messages is of critical importance as it can build the necessary trust and prevent confusion in public opinion.

The disaster committee should designate one person from the hospital for regular media/press briefing. One of the areas in the hospital should be designated as media room where media persons can be accommodated for controlled access to information. Media always gets its information—the better way is the controlled one.

In order to communicate successfully in a crisis, one must be fast, accurate, honest, credible, consistent, and empathetic. In every crisis, there is a right message that needs to be shared at the right time.

Speed of response, avoiding errors during the crisis response, and asking for forgiveness when mistakes occur greatly contribute to building and maintaining trust. Expressing empathy in a crisis situation is not a luxury but a necessity and everyone involved as a spokesperson must be prepared to express and repeat empathy sincerely toward the community and those affected by the incident. In addition, he must show competence and expertise by remaining honest and open.

During a crisis, people may experience a multitude of feelings and a wide range of emotions like fear, anxiety, confusion, hopelessness, helplessness, uncertainty, or panic. Many of these psychological barriers, which could interfere with the cooperation and response from the public, can be mitigated through the work of an experienced spokesperson with an empathetic and honest health risk communication style. In other words, the right spokesperson at the right time with the right message can save lives.

The following communication principles should be incorporated into messages:

- Acknowledge fears.
- Express wishes, show empathy.
- Give people things to do.
- Acknowledge the shared misery.
- Give anticipatory guidance.

If spokespersons acknowledge the risk, its severity and complexity and acknowledge fears, they can then ask people to bear the risk during the emergency and work toward solutions together. Some of the common pitfalls and communication failures that inhibit operational success are:

- Mixed messages from multiple experts through multiple sources with lack of absolute agreement.
- Late released information that may leave space to others to fill the gap by an opportunistic and fraudulent response.
- Paternalistic attitudes that do not treat public like intelligent adults.
- Countering rumors or myths in real time may serve to spread them.

The WHO checklist recommended actions are:

- Appoint a public information spokesperson to coordinate hospital communication with the public, the media, and health authorities.
- Designate a space for press conferences (outside the immediate proximity of the emergency department, triage/waiting areas, and the command center).
- Draft brief key massages for target audiences (e.g., patients, staff, public) in preparation for the most likely disaster scenarios.
- Ensure that all communications to the public, media, staff (in general), and health authorities are approved by the incident commander or ICG.
- Establish streamlined mechanisms of information exchange between hospital administration, department/unit heads, and facility staff.
- Brief hospital staff on their roles and responsibilities within the incident action plan.

- Establish mechanisms for the appropriate and timely collection, processing, and reporting of information to supervisory stakeholders (e.g., the government, health authorities), and through them to neighboring hospitals, private practitioners, and pre-hospital networks.
- Ensure that all decisions related to patient prioritization (e.g., adapted admission and discharge criteria, triage methods, infection prevention, and control measures) are communicated to all relevant staff and stakeholders.
- Ensure the availability of reliable and sustainable primary and back-up communication systems (e.g., satellite phones, mobile devices, landlines, Internet connections, pagers, two-way radios, unlisted numbers), as well as access to an updated contact list.

10.4.1.6 Planning for Security of Hospitals in Emergency Situation

During emergency situation, the hospital is the focus of not only the patients being brought in but a lot of other persons including relatives, by-standers, media, etc. They more often than not block the entrance and other areas hampering the smooth functioning of the hospital. It is therefore recommended that all hospitals should have some security arrangements even in non-disaster phases. The hospital security should be operational at a very early stage of disaster. Some of the duties recommended by WHO are:

- Appoint a hospital security team responsible for all hospital safety and security activities.
- Prioritize security needs in collaboration with the hospital ICG. Identify areas where increased vulnerability is anticipated (e.g., entry/exits, food/water access points, pharmaceutical stockpiles).
- Ensure the early control of facility access point(s), triage site(s), and other areas of patient flow, traffic, and parking. Limit visitor access as appropriate.
- Establish a reliable mode of identifying authorized hospital personnel, patients, and visitors.
- Provide a mechanism for escorting emergency medical personnel and their families to patient care areas.
- Ensure that security measures required for safe and efficient hospital evacuation are clearly defined.
- Ensure that the rules for engagement in crowd control are clearly defined.
- Solicit frequent input from the hospital security team with a view to identifying potential safety and security challenges and constraints, including gaps in the management of hazardous materials and the prevention and control of infection.
- Identify information insecurity risks. Implement procedures to ensure the secure collection, storage, and reporting of confidential information.
- Define the threshold and procedures for integrating local law enforcement and military in-hospital security operations.
- Establish an area for radioactive, biological, and chemical decontamination and isolation.

10.4.1.7 Transportation

Transportation (to and from the site or other hospitals) is necessary in emergency situation mainly to bring the patients from the site of mass casualty incident to the hospital. Transport is also required to transfer patients to other hospitals if the facilities at the hospital in question are overwhelmed or are unable to perform its functions due to internal damage.

10.4.1.8 Stores Planning

It is recommended that adequate stores of linen, medical items, surgical items should be kept separately in the Emergency/Casualty and should be marked as the "Disaster Store." The activation of this store is done only after the disaster has been notified by the appropriate authorities. As immediate measures, the buffer stocks earmarked for the Casualty/Emergency Services should be utilized till the fresh stocks are replenished from main hospital stores/disaster stores. Any requirements to the operational areas/treatment areas are conveyed to the command center. WHO recommendations are:

- Develop and maintain an updated inventory of all equipment, supplies and pharmaceuticals; establish a shortage-alert mechanism.
- Estimate the consumption of essential supplies and pharmaceuticals (e.g., amount used per week) using the most likely disaster.
- Consult with authorities to ensure the continuous provision of essential medications and supplies (e.g., those available from institutional and central stockpiles and through emergency agreements with local suppliers and national and international aid agencies).
- Assess the quality of contingency items prior to purchase; request quality certification if available.
- Establish contingency agreements (e.g., memoranda of understanding, mutual aid agreements) with vendors to ensure the procurement and prompt delivery of equipment, supplies, and other resources in times of shortage.
- Identify physical space within the hospital for the storage and stockpiling of additional supplies, taking ease of access, security, temperature, ventilation, light exposure, and humidity level into consideration. Ensure an uninterrupted cold chain for essential items requiring refrigeration.
- Stockpile essential supplies and pharmaceuticals in accordance with national guidelines. Ensure the timely use of stockpiled items to avoid loss due to expiration.
- Define the hospital pharmacy's role in providing pharmaceuticals to patients being treated at home or at alternative treatment sites.
- Ensure that a mechanism exists for the prompt maintenance and repair of equipment required for essential services. Postpone all non-essential services when necessary.
- Coordinate a contingency transportation strategy with pre-hospital networks and transportation services to ensure continuous patient transferal.

10.4.1.9 Human Resources Planning

Medical Staff: In addition to the members of clinical staff, para and preclinical disciplines (if present in the facility) should render their services in managing the casualties. Duty roster for standby staffs should be available. The nursing matron should be able to prepare a list of nursing staffs who may be made available at a short notice. The nursing personnel officer should be also able to mobilize additional nursing staffs from non-critical areas.

Other Staff: Duty roster (including those on standby duty) of all ancillary medical services (e.g., radiology, laboratory, blood bank) and also other hospital services (house-keeping, sanitation, stores, pharmacy, kitchen, etc.) should be available with the duty officer/hospital administrator.

Volunteers: The role which volunteers will assume in the course of a disaster should be predetermined, rehearsed, coordinated, and supervised by the regular senior staff of the health facility.

Reserved Staff: In cases of large-scale disaster, the recommendations are made for community participation and reserve staff concept.

Preparedness will be enhanced by the development of a community-wide concept of "reserve staff" identifying physicians, nurses, and hospital workers who are retired, have changed careers to work outside of healthcare services, or now work in areas other than direct patient care (e.g., risk management, utilization review). While developing the list of candidates for a community-wide "reserve staff" will require limited resources, the reserve staff concept will only be viable if adequate funds are available to regularly train and update the reserves so that they can immediately step into roles in the hospital which allow regular hospital staffs to focus on incident casualties.

Hospital preparedness can be increased if state medical councils, working through the State Medical Services, develop procedures allowing physicians licensed in one system of medicine to practice in another under defined emergency conditions.

Recommended actions as per WHO checklist are:

- Update the hospital staff contact list.
- Estimate and continuously monitor staff absenteeism.
- Establish a clear staff sick-leave policy, including contingencies for ill or injured family members or dependents of staff.
- Identify the minimum needs in terms of health-care workers and other hospital staff to ensure the operational sufficiency of a given hospital department.
- Establish a contingency plan for the provision of food, water, and living space for hospital personnel.
- Prioritize staffing requirements and distribute personnel accordingly.
- Recruit and train additional staff (e.g., retired staff, reserve military personnel, university affiliates/students, and volunteers) according to the anticipated need.
- Address liability, insurance, and temporary licensing issues relating to additional staff and volunteers who may be required to work in areas outside the scope of their training or for which they have no license.

- Establish a system of rapidly providing health-care workers (e.g., voluntary medical personnel) with necessary credentials in an emergency situation, in accordance with hospital and health authority policy.
- Cross-train health-care providers in high-demand services (e.g., emergency, surgical, and intensive care units).
- Provide training and exercises in areas of potential increased clinical demand, including emergency and intensive care, to ensure adequate staff capacity and competency.
- Identify domestic support measures (e.g., travel, child care, care for ill or disabled family members) to enable staff flexibility for shift reassignment and longer working hours.
- Ensure adequate shift rotation and self-care for clinical staff to support morale and reduce medical error.
- Ensure the availability of multidisciplinary psychosocial support teams that include social workers, counsellors, interpreters, and clergy for the families of staff and patients.
- Ensure that staffs dealing with epidemic-prone respiratory illness are provided with the appropriate vaccinations, in accordance with national policy and guidelines of the health authority.

10.4.1.10 Financial Planning

An important aspect of any management plan is the financial management. It is recommended that the disaster plans are made in close association with the financial advisors of the hospital/institution. This will make them more cost-effective and avoid unnecessary and repeated expenditure. Financial planning includes (but is not limited to) purchasing, procurement, patient tracking, insurance, document security, building safety, building repair, and inventory/supplies. These responsibilities need to be assessed and carried out by those individuals who are responsible for job actions under the finance branch of the incident command system.

10.4.1.11 Operations Planning

The incident commander after notification of the hospital disaster activates and alerts the in-charges of different important areas of the hospital. The in-charges of various facilities in turn notify and alert the staff (medical/nursing/others staff) working in these areas to immediately reach the area and carry out their functions. The in-charges also call up the reserved staff which is not on duty to be ready in case they are needed.

Reception and Triage Area: Triage is the term used to describe the process of sorting out casualties and prioritizing care. Historically, triage has been used within multiple military conflicts [11]. Civilian emergency medical services and hospital emergency departments who use the process show increased evidence of improved outcomes. Decreasing time to treat those in need of immediate care has been shown to increase survival rates. The triage process may be used for both injured and ill patients [12]. Acuity levels may change in three ways for patients from the initial assigned level, during their reassessments, and through the care process:

 – Improvement in status.
 – Decline in status.
 – Stable status.

Despite the large number of triage systems extant throughout the world, most have several features in common. A majority of these systems use a "walking filter" to identify quickly less severely injured patients and remove from the immediate disaster zone. START (Simple Triage and Rapid Treatment) (Fig. 10.4) and JumpSTART (for triaging children younger than 8 years of age) (Fig. 10.5) are considered to be the standard triage methods, mostly used by pre-hospital EMS and disaster volunteers. They are also appropriate for use by hospitals with a large group of patient arrivals as a tool to quickly identify those in most need of immediate care [13]. The goal is to quickly identify the red casualties among the total injured group.

START Triage

Walking wounded are directed to go to treatment area. (All are triaged as Green.)

Those unable to walk are assessed by the "RPM" method:

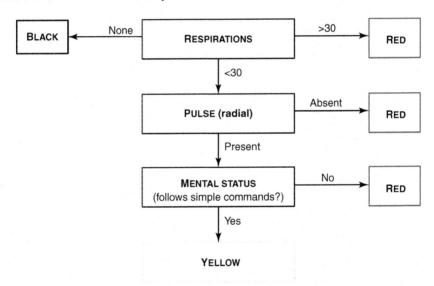

Important:
Once any RED criteria are met, tag patient and MOVE ON!
Triage is sorting, not treatment. Only 2 interventions may made during triage:
   1) Open/clear airway.
   2) Apply direct pressure to major bleeding sites.
Patients will be reassessed at treatment area(s).

Fig. 10.4 START card as a "walking filter" to identify quickly less severely injured patients and remove them from the immediate disaster zone

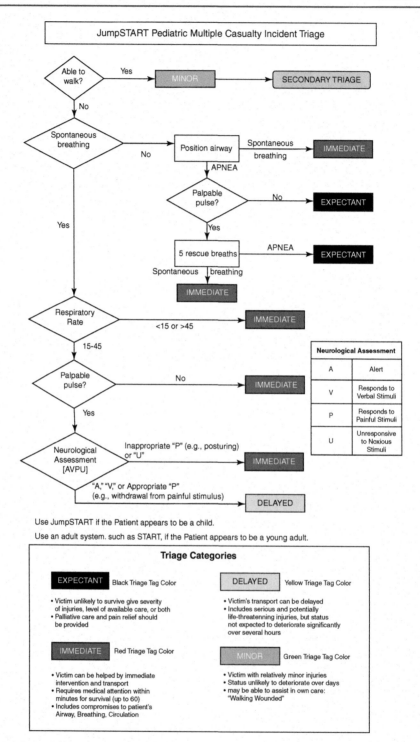

Fig. 10.5 JumpSTART card for triaging children younger than 8 years of age

To accomplish this:

- All ambulatory casualties are moved away from the rest of the injured and are given a green (minor care) designation. This process removes the largest group in most disasters and makes it much easier to identify the more severely injured patients. Stating a simple phrase like "If you can hear the sound of my voice, come over here (point to the location)." A bullhorn or other voice amplification device, and gestures to point to those who are ambulatory, may help to guide them toward a staging area.
- A rapid screening of each remaining person on the scene may be conducted with less than 1 min spent per casualty. The parameters used for screening include: respiratory status (R), perfusion (P), and mental status (M).
- Only the simplest of interventions are given, such as opening an airway or directing a bystander to apply direct pressure to external bleeding.

Reassessment helps direct resources to those who would benefit the most. For example, persons who have no medical needs but are psychological casualties may be directed to a support center for care instead of an emergency department. A primary goal of triage is to decongest emergency departments allowing them to care for the highest acuity level patients. Triage methods assist responders in identifying alternate care sites for green-tagged persons who are in need of minor treatment and likely to be ambulatory.

Reassessment conducted periodically after the initial sorting may validate that an appropriate triage level is identified. Reassessment also attempts to avoid under-triaging (assigning a less serious acuity which could lead to a higher potential risk of mortality or disability) or over-triaging (assigning a higher acuity level which could lead to patients using treatment space that others need).

The triage area is the first area of contact between hospital personnel and the incoming patients. This area should be manned by:

- Registration officer on the registration desk.
- Triage doctors/nurses.
- Adequate number of doctors in the emergency room/casualty.
- Adequate number of stretchers/trolley bearers.
- Hospital attendants. The initial registration and triage should be done in this area.
- Triage criteria for disasters and the patients will be color coded according to the kind of treatment they deserve (Fig. 10.6).
  - ONE—immediate resuscitation (**RED**).
  - TWO—potentially Life-threatening injuries (**YELLOW**).
  - THREE—walking wounded (**GREEN**).
  - FOUR—dead (**BLACK**).
  - An additional color (**BLUE**) can be applied for palliative care patients.

Decontamination Area (Nuclear, Biological, or Chemical Disasters): Hospital emergency operation plans should include information related to decontamination

Color	Acuity	Need for Treatment	Comments
RED	Emergent	Immediate	Threat to life, limb, or organ
YELLOW	Urgent	Delayed	Significant injury or illness but can tolerate a delay in care
GREEN	Non-Urgent	Minimal / Non-urgent	Can safely wait for treatment
BLACK	Expired or Expected	No treatment; Expectant: Treat if resources are available	Consider transport and care for expectant patients after initial "Reds" are cleared, if resources exist and it does not delay care for Yellows. FEMORS offers guidelines on palliative care.

Fig. 10.6 Patients will be color coded according to the kind of treatment they deserve. An additional color (BLUE) can be applied for palliative care patients

and how it is going to be performed, as necessary. This may include any of the following:

- A process for communicating with and directing patients to a decontamination area(s).
- Communications protocols to be used by team members within decontamination area(s) and between other units.
- Processes for activation/de-activation of the team.
- Specific triggers and/or scenarios where decontamination would be appropriate.
- Location of primary and alternative decontamination areas.
- Set-up, designation of space, and operational procedures for each space.
- Segregation and decontamination of prioritized contaminated individuals and their belongings.
- The segregation of contaminated vehicles, equipment, and supplies.
- A process for human and material resource staging and demobilization/reconstitution.
- A plan for staging and rehabilitation of decontamination team staff
- These measures support proper decontamination procedures and processes which helps to ensure everyone's (patient and staff member) safety is taken seriously.

Acute Care Area (Emergency Department), Definitive Care areas (Operation Theatres, Wards), *Intensive Treatment Area Activation* (HDU/ICU), *Treatment Areas*: Hospital planning has traditionally anticipated the number of casualties to be treated as potentially up to 20% of the total licensed bed capacity of the hospital. This number does not necessarily indicate an increase of in-patient admissions and hospitals should determine what is a realistic number based on surge capability and capacity (staff, space, and equipment and supplies).

Clinical treatment for casualties may be provided in a traditional or non-traditional area. Hospital planning should include information detailing how a surge of patients is going to be accommodated. A mass casualty incident (MCI) may result in both higher and lower numbers of patient arrivals, varied acuity levels, and varying pediatric casualties, depending on the type of disaster scenario.

The staffs, mainly nursing staffs and hospital attendants who are familiar with first aid, splinting, and dressings, can be sent to the minor treatment areas, thus saving the medical staffs for more intensive and resuscitation areas.

Typically, only 10% of the red-tagged emergent casualties from a conventional MCI require stat, emergency, life-saving (resuscitative) surgery [14]. A significant number of casualties may require one or more surgical interventions during their hospital stay. Hospitals may consider bundling procedures per casualty to reduce anesthesia time, increase the operation room availability, and shorten the recovery process for patients. This coordinated approach to surgical care has been used by the military and may be called "parallel operating." The type of operations expected to be performed may include:

- Life-saving operations (hemorrhage control, craniotomy).
- Open fractures.
- Penetrating eye injuries.
- Neurological surgery (urgent).
- Chest surgery.
- Oral/maxillary/facial surgery.
- Burns.

Holding Area for Relatives/Non-Injured: A hospital staff member will stay with the family members. (Social services will be assigned here after reporting to the command center and other personnel assigned as needed). A list of the visitors' names in association with the patient they are inquiring about should be kept. Volunteers may be needed to escort visitors within the facility.

10.4.1.12 Essential Ancillary Services
- *Laboratory Services*: The department head or designee will call in their own personnel as needed after reporting to command center. He/she will call personnel from nearby hospitals and clinics as necessary and will have arrangements made to obtain additional blood, equipment, and supplies from area agencies.
- *Radiology Services Department*: the head of designee will call any or all personnel needed, will arrange for extra supplies to be brought in if needed, and will coordinate the flow of work and delegation of work areas. Other members of the radiology staff will perform all x-ray exams/CT scans/Ultrasounds, etc., as needed and assigned.
- *Blood Bank*: The need for blood products is often overestimated but during a disaster blood and blood product usage may rise above normal levels. The resurgent use of tourniquets and newer products such as bandages with hemostatic

properties may be able to control blood loss. Consultation with the hospital laboratory, local blood bank, and materials management may identify the availability of blood, blood products, and other supplies improving patient outcomes. Emergency operating plans may want to consider including the level of blood supply needed based on current information related to appropriate transfusion criteria, blood availability, and other measures that conserve blood or prevent blood loss.

- *Mortuary Services (Care for the dead)*: Mortuary should be situated away from the main entrance of the hospital. It should be adequately staffed with senior forensic specialist/any designee appointed for that purpose [15]. Patients pronounced dead on arrival (DOA) should be tagged with a disaster tag and body should be sent to mortuary. The emergency department should also notify about all deaths to the command control room. Bodies should be stored in the alternate morgue area if the capacity of mortuary to store bodies is overwhelmed. Mortuary personnel will remain with bodies until removed by mortuary in-charger. After bodies have been identified, the information will be filed on the disaster tag and medical records notified as to the identification of the patient. The bodies may be removed via a separate gate of the hospital with the knowledge of the mortuary in-charge [16]. A complete record of all bodies must be maintained along with the name of the agency removing them (police, fire department, hearse, etc.).
- *Sanitation Services*: Adequate sanitation services within and around the hospital should be ensured by the hospital administration.
- *Hospital Laundry and Sterile Supply*: The hospital administration should ensure adequate supply of clean hospital linen, sterile dressing, and sterile supply of instruments to the essential areas of the hospital.

10.4.2 Disaster Phase

The district medical authorities should play a leading role in medical treatment of victims once the disaster strike. The chief district medical officer/equivalent position should take the role of incident commander and should set up a medical command structure which would work in tandem with the district administrative authorities. [17, 18] The steps are as following:

(a) Phase of activation—alert and notification of emergency.
(b) Activation of the chain of command in the hospital.
(c) Operational phase. This is the phase in which the actual tackling of mass casualties is performed according to the disaster/emergency plan.
(d) Phase of deactivation. This is a crucial phase of the hospital emergency plan when the administration/command of the hospital is satisfied that the influx of mass casualty victims is not continuing to overwhelm the hospital facilities.

10.4.3 Post-disaster Phase

Once the incident commander and the leaders of respective areas are convinced that there will be no more casualties who will come to the hospital, they would take a decision to deactivate the plan and resume the normal functioning of the hospital. This is an important phase of disaster planning where the activities of the disaster/emergency phase are discussed and the inadequacies are noted for future improvements [19]. The deactivation should not be too early (premature) or too late. Once the decision is taken, it is very difficult to reactivate the plan within a short period of time.

The WHO recommended actions are as follows:

- Appoint a disaster recovery officer responsible for overseeing hospital recovery operations.
- Determine essential criteria and processes for incident demobilization and system recovery.
- In case of damage to a hospital building, ensure that a comprehensive structural integrity and safety assessment is performed.
- If evacuation is required, determine the time and resources needed to complete repairs and replacements before the facility can be reopened.
- Organize a team of hospital staff to carry out a post-action hospital inventory assessment; team members should include staff familiar with the location and inventory of equipment and supplies. Consider including equipment vendors to assess the status of sophisticated equipment that may need to be repaired or replaced.
- Provide a post-action report to hospital administration, emergency managers and appropriate stakeholders that includes an incident summary, a response assessment, and an expenses report.
- Organize professionally conducted debriefing for staff within 24–72 h after the occurrence of the emergency incident to assist with coping and recovery, provide access to mental health resources and improve work performance.
- Establish a post-disaster employee recovery assistance program according to staff needs, including, for example, counselling and family support services.
- Show appropriate recognition of the services provided by staff, volunteers, external personnel and donors during disaster response and recovery.

Debriefing: Importance of debriefing exercises as a part of planning cannot be stressed further. Debriefing is a process in which the Disaster Committee sits down after the disaster has been deactivated and tries to figure out how things went. It can be best described as a critical self-review of one hospital's own performance during a disaster. [20, 21] What went right is taken cognizance of and what went wrong is further incorporated into the disaster plans. This is arguably the most time-consuming part of a major incident. It will include action reports, follow-up, debrief, and even preparation for inquests. The process may take months to years and lessons learned in individual cases should be disseminated throughout the medical community to improve on responses when other major incidents inevitably occur.

Glossary

Compound (Combination) Disaster Disasters are not always limited to a single hazard. Sometimes two or more completely independent disasters occur at the same time—an earthquake strike during a flood, for instance. More commonly, however, one disaster triggers a secondary hazard. Some secondary hazards only occur as result of a primary hazard, such as a tsunami (from earthquakes), while others can occur either because of or independent of other disasters. Compound disasters, which can occur either sequentially or simultaneously with one or more disasters, have a tendency to exacerbate consequences, and increase victims' issues [25].

Coping Capacity The ability of people, organizations, and systems, using available skills and resources, to face and manage adverse conditions, emergencies, or disasters.

Disaster A serious disruption of the functioning of a community or a society involving widespread human, material, economic, or environmental losses and impacts, which exceeds the ability of the affected community or society to cope using its own resources. Disasters are often described as a result of the combination of: the exposure to a hazard; the conditions of vulnerability that are present; and insufficient capacity or measures to reduce or cope with the potential negative consequences [22].Disaster impacts may include loss of life, injury, disease, and other negative effects on human physical, mental, and social well-being, together with damage to property, destruction of assets, loss of services, social and economic disruption, and environmental degradation.

Early Warning System The set of capacities needed to generate and disseminate timely and meaningful warning information to enable individuals, communities, and organizations threatened by a hazard to prepare and to act appropriately and in sufficient time to reduce the possibility of harm or loss.

Emergency Preparedness Plan versus Contingency Plan Contingency planning means making a plan to respond to a potential crisis or emergency. This includes developing scenarios *(anticipating the crisis)*, determining the objectives of the organization in these situations, and defining what will be needed to reach those objectives [23]. Contingency planning is one tool of emergency preparedness, but it is not emergency preparedness itself. Emergency preparedness consists of all activities taken in anticipation of a crisis to expedite effective emergency response. This includes contingency planning, but is not limited to it: it also covers stockpiling, the creation and management of stand-by capacities, and training staff and partners in emergency response.

Emergency A crisis or emergency is a threatening condition that requires urgent action. Effective emergency action can avoid the escalation of an event into a disaster.

Hazards A dangerous phenomenon, substance, human activity, or condition that may cause loss of life, injury or other health impacts, property damage, loss of livelihoods and services, social and economic disruption, or environmental damage.

Risk Risk is the likelihood of an event occurring multiplied by the negative consequence of that event, were it to occur. Risk = Likelihood x Negative Consequence Likelihood is expressed either as a probability (e.g., 0.15; 50%) or as a frequency (e.g., 1 in 1,000,000; 5 times per year). Consequences are a measure of the effect of the hazard on people or property.

Vulnerability Vulnerability is a measure of the propensity of an object, area, individual, group, community, country, or other entity to incur the consequences of a hazard. This measurement results from a combination of physical, social, economic, and environmental factors or processes. Resilience, the opposite of vulnerability, is a measure of propensity to avoid loss [24].

References

1. Emergency Management Program Guidebook. Emergency Management Strategic Healthcare Group (EMSHG) emergency management academy, Washington, DC. St. Louis, MO: VHA Centre for Engineering & Occupational Safety and Health. https://www.emap.org/index.php/root/for-programs/23-2013-emergency-management-standard/file.
2. Carlin E, et al. Foundations in community resilience and the national preparedness system. In: Strengthening the disaster resilience of the Academic Biomedical Research Community: protecting the nation's investment. USA: National Academies Press; 2017.
3. Born CT, et al. Disasters and mass casualties: II. Explosive, biologic, chemical, and nuclear agents. J Am Acad Orthop Surg. 2007;15(8):461–73.
4. Nekoie-Moghadam M, et al. Tools and checklists used for the evaluation of hospital disaster preparedness: a systematic review. Disaster Med Public Health Prep. 2016;10(5):781–8.
5. Ullah S, et al. Challenges of hospital preparedness in disasters in Balochistan. Pak J Public Health. 2017;7(1):30–7.
6. Born CT, et al. Disasters and mass casualties: II. Explosive, biologic, chemical, and nuclear agents. J Am Acad Orthop Surg. 2007;15(8):461–73.
7. Lewis CP, Aghababian RV. Disaster planning. Part I: Overview of hospital and emergency department planning for internal and external disasters. Emerg Med Clin. 1996;14(2):439–52.
8. Department of Homeland Security. Homeland security presidential directive/HSPD-21: public health and medical preparedness. Washington, DC: Department of Homeland Security; 2007.
9. World Health Organization, et al. Mass casualty management systems: strategies and guidelines for building health sector capacity. 2007.
10. Manley WG, et al. Realities of disaster preparedness in rural hospitals. Disaster Manag Response. 2006;4(3):80–7.
11. Iserson KV, Moskop JC. Triage in medicine. Part I: Concept, history, and types. Ann Emerg Med. 2007;49(3):275–81.
12. Schultz CH, Koenig KL, Noji EK. A medical disaster response to reduce immediate mortality after an earthquake. N Engl J Med. 1996;334(7):438–44.

13. Ngabirano, Annet Alenyo. A comparison between differently skilled pre-hospital emergency care providers in major incident triage in South Africa. PhD thesis. Stellenbosch: Stellenbosch University; 2018.
14. Lynn M, et al. Management of conventional mass casualty incidents: ten commandments for hospital planning. J Burn Care Res. 2006;27(5):649–58.
15. Brassil KE, Zillman MA. Design for a hospital mortuary. Pathology. 1993;25(4):333–7.
16. Morgan O, Tidball-Binz M, van Alphen D. Management of dead bodies after disasters: a field manual for first responders. Pan American Health Organization (PAHO). 2006.
17. Guidelines for Hospital Emergency Preparedness Planning, Government of India, National Disaster Management Division Ministry of Home Affairs. http://asdma.gov.in/pdf/publication/undp/guidelines_hospital_emergency.pdf.
18. Lincoln EW, Khetarpal S, Strecker-McGraw MK. EMS, incident command. In: StatPearls [Internet]. Treasure Island, FL: StatPearls Publishing; 2019.
19. Tekin E, et al. Evacuation of hospitals during disaster, establishment of a field hospital, and communication. Eurasian J Med. 2017;49(2):137.
20. Cohen RE. Mental health services in disasters: Instructor's guide. Pan American Health Organization (PAHO). 2000.
21. Wilson JP, Friedman MJ, Lindy JD, editors. Treating psychological trauma and PTSD. New York: Guilford Press; 2012.
22. Watson SK, Rudge JW, Coker R. Health systems' "surge capacity": state of the art and priorities for future research. Milbank Q. 2013;91(1):78–122.
23. Choularton R. Contingency planning and humanitarian action: A review of practice. Humanitarian Practice Network. 2007. Chapters 2–3.
24. Coppola DP. Introduction to international disaster management. Amsterdam: Elsevier; 2006. Chapter 1.
25. Nelson SA. Natural disasters & assessing hazards and risk. Research Paper for Tulane University. 2014, p 20.

The Art of Triage

11

Ari Leppäniemi

11.1 Definition of Triage

The standard definition of triage is "the sorting of and allocation of treatment to patients and especially battle and disaster victims according to a system of priorities designed to maximize the number of survivors." In real mass casualty situations, the principle of triage is to identify and transfer (after life-saving initial interventions in the field) those patients among the initial survivors that have a reasonable chance of meaningful survival if their injuries are treated rapidly and effectively.

11.2 Principles of Triage

A large number of casualties, limited resources on the scene, and the critical time factor typical to a mass casualty incident preclude a thorough evaluation and definitive treatment of individual injured patients according to accepted practices. Therefore, the standard goal of providing the greatest good for each individual patient must change in mass casualty setting to "the greatest good for the greatest number." The main instrument to achieve this is the application of sorting out patients according to the severity of their injuries, or triage, and assigning those who are the most seriously injured to receiving priority care.

Depending on the circumstances, up to 20% of mass casualty victims die on the scene (immediate deaths). Of those surviving the immediate insult (immediate survivors), about 10–20% are severely injured. Delay in the treatment of this patient group increases mortality and disability, and many need surgery and intensive care.

A. Leppäniemi (✉)
Emergency Surgery, Abdominal Center, Meilahti Hospital, University of Helsinki,
Helsinki, Finland
e-mail: ari.leppaniemi@hus.fi

© Springer Nature Switzerland AG 2021   147
E. Pikoulis, J. Doucet (eds.), *Emergency Medicine, Trauma and Disaster
Management*, Hot Topics in Acute Care Surgery and Trauma,
https://doi.org/10.1007/978-3-030-34116-9_11

However, about 60–80% of immediate survivors have minor and nonfatal injuries, some of them not even requiring hospital admission. In these instances, efficiency of care can be degraded by *overtriage* (proportion of survivors assigned to immediate care, hospitalization, or evacuation who are not critically injured).

The main aim of any mass casualty plan is to facilitate the selection and timely treatment of the severely injured patients. Because the resources in mass casualties are almost always stretched to the limit, the basic principles of triage should be implemented. From the trauma care perspective, it has been emphasized that successful coping with a mass casualty does not mean streamlining the flow of 80 casualties, but rather providing high-quality trauma care to very few but critical (and salvageable) patients.

A useful tool to assess the overall performance of the health care system in mass casualties is to calculate the *Critical Mortality Rate* (CMR) of immediate survivors, i.e., the proportion of deaths out of the total of severely injured but initially surviving patients (Injury Severity Score > 15). It has been shown that CMR is directly proportional to the overtriage percentage.

11.3   Selection of Triage Site and Assigning Key Duties

The medical commander in the field, after consultation with the overall incident commander in the field, should select the triage sites. The site should be safe and secured, placed on a dry and possibly sheltered area, upwind from the incident, and close to the evacuation route for the ambulances with a one-way traffic direction.

After assigning the leaders of the initial three key responsibilities (primary triage, secondary triage and treatment, and evacuation) with appropriate teams, and establishing communication with the overall regional medical commander who has the knowledge of the current situation and capabilities of each hospital in the region, the field medical commander directs and supervises the organized field triage process. It also includes the establishment of a place for deceased victims, separate from the treatment areas.

11.4   Categories of Triage

The initial sorting of the victims by the primary triage officer is based on the ability of the victims to walk and follow orders (Fig. 11.1). Directing the "walking wounded" to another site for appropriate evaluation and treatment separates them from the more severely injured who are collected to the main secondary triage point to be evaluated by the secondary triage and treatment officer. Overtriage can be reduced by focusing on physiologic and anatomic criteria rather than on injury mechanism in selecting patients for transport to trauma centers, and this can be achieved without increasing *undertriage* (not detecting patients with severe injuries, delaying their transfer or sending them to an inappropriate facility).

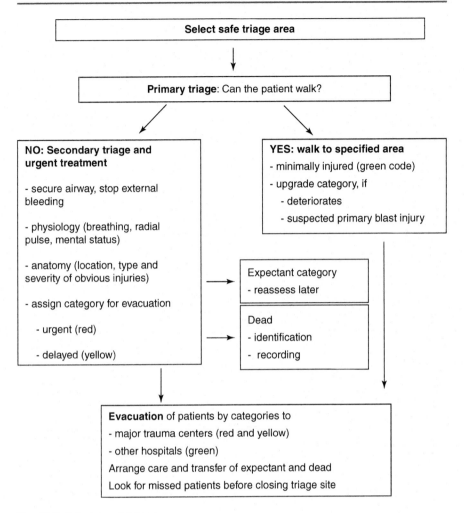

Fig. 11.1 Principles of field triage

Table 11.1 Field triage categories and commonly used color codes	Immediate (red)
	Delayed (yellow)
	Minimal (green)
	Expectant (violet)
	Dead (black)

Patients with severe injuries are first evaluated, sorted out, and treated by the secondary triage officer for immediately life-threatening problems (airway and breathing, external bleeding) and assigned a category for evacuation (Table 11.1). It should be noted that triage is a dynamic process and the condition of the patient can change, either because of the immediate life-threatening problem has been solved (by establishing a secure airway or stopping external bleeding, for example) or because the deterioration of a patient with an unrecognized severe injury, such as internal bleeding from a pelvic fracture, for example. The triage category should reflect the urgency of evacuation to get the patient to the hospital for definitive treatment, not the initial condition.

11.5 Transfer

Patients who need immediate evacuation (red code) should be transported first to the nearest appropriate medical facility that has the capability to deal with the suspected injuries. Typical injuries include conditions that might have been treated in the field initially but need subsequent definitive surgical treatment, such as airway compromise, open chest wounds, tension pneumothorax and major external hemorrhage, or conditions that cannot be treated in the field such as hypotension caused by cavitary bleeding, intermediate burns, or unconscious patients with focal signs. The receiving hospital is usually the major trauma center in the area, but under some circumstances it might be the hospital with special expertise, such as a burn unit, cardiothoracic surgery, or neurosurgery. If possible, no hospital should receive more than five severely injured patients during the first hour.

The delayed category (yellow code) includes patient who need definitive treatment that often includes surgery, such as hemodynamically stable patients with penetrating abdominal wounds, extremity vascular injuries, unconscious patients without airway compromise or lateralizing signs, pelvic, spinal, or extremity fractures, or major soft tissue wounds. They should be transported after the immediate category patients following the same stratification according to the potential injuries as the immediate category patients.

The minimally injured patients (green code) should be equally divided among the lower echelon or more distant hospitals in the area using mass transportation means, such as buses, if possible. The actual updated capacity situation of the receiving hospitals should be taken into account, and the field medical commander can obtain this information from the overall medical commander (usually located in the major trauma center) and pass that on to the evacuation officer.

The expectant category (violet code) refers to patients who are alive but with unsurvivable injuries or patients with such severe injuries that their rapid evacuation would unlikely lead to survival and might divert the limited resources away from patients with potentially more survivable injuries. Examples for this type of injuries include severe head injuries with open skull fractures and unconsciousness, extensive deep burns, and imminent cardiac arrest with major torso trauma. This category is the most difficult to assign patients to and requires the necessary mindset and medical competence from the triage officer. These patients should be segregated from the others at least in the initial phase, and kept comfortable and monitored for any improvement in their condition that may warrant care later in the evolution of the incident response.

Dead victims (black code) should be segregated from all others to decrease the possibility of resource-utilizing treatment efforts, and to facilitate later identification and communication of their outcome to families.

11.6 Record Keeping

One important aspect of triage is record keeping that prevents losing track of casualties and allowing a post-event analysis of triage decisions, casualty management, and casualty outcomes, from which important decisions can be derived to improve performance in future events. Most likely in the future it will be possible to track mass casualties utilizing the existing databases and creating a unique mass casualty code to be added to the patient codes.

11.7 Summary

The essence of triage is to identify the critically injured victims rapidly and reliably, intervene in the immediately life-threatening but treatable problems (airway, external bleeding), and evacuate the patients as soon as possible to the most appropriate hospital. Utilizing a unified EMS system and a regional agreement of multiple hospitals within reasonable distances and stratified according to their trauma management capacity and resources, a rational plan can be developed to ensure that the most critically injured patients are sent directly to the right hospitals without overwhelming these hospitals with minor injuries. Avoiding overtriage and not exceeding the surge capacity of the major trauma hospitals are the most efficient ways of decreasing the critical mortality rate, the hallmark of the efficiency of the medical response to a mass casualty incident.

Acknowledgments This chapter is partially based on the chapter "EMS and Pre-Hospital Issues", by Ari Leppäniemi. In: Shmuel C. Shapira, Jeffrey S. Hammond, Leonard A. Cole (eds) Essentials of Terror Medicine, Springer New York, 2009 (with permission).

Bibliography

1. Avidan V, Hersch M, Spira RM, Einav S, Goldberg S, Schecter W. Civilian hospital response to a mass casualty event: the role of the intensive care unit. J Trauma. 2007;62:1234–9.
2. Einav S, Feigenberg Z, Weissman C, et al. Evacuation priorities in mass casualty terror-related events. Implications for contingency planning. Ann Surg. 2004;239:304–10.
3. Epley E. Regional medical disaster planning: an integrated approach to ESF-8 planning. J Trauma. 2007;62:596.
4. Frykberg ER. Medical management of disasters and mass casualties from terrorist bombings: how can we cope? J Trauma. 2002;53:201–12.
5. Frykberg ER. Triage: principles and practice. Scand J Surg. 2005;94:272–8.
6. Garthe E, Mango N. A method for tracking mass casualty or terrorism incidents in existing databases. J Trauma. 2002;53:793–5.

7. Hammond J. Mass casualty incidents: planning implications for trauma care. Scand J Surg. 2005;94:267–71.
8. Hirshberg A. Multiple casualty incidents. Lessons from the front line. Ann Surg. 2004;239:322–4.
9. Hirshberg A, Scott BG, Granchi T, Wall MJ Jr, Mattox KL, Stein M. How does casualty load affect trauma care in urban bombing incidents? A quantitative analysis. J Trauma. 2005;58:686–95.
10. Kluger Y, Kashuk J, Mayo A. Terror bombing – mechanisms, consequences and implications. Scand J Surg. 2004;93:11–4.
11. Lockey DJ, MacKenzie R, Redhead J, et al. London bombings July 2005: the immediate pre-hospital medical response. Resuscitation. 2005;66:ix–xii.
12. Peral Gutierrez de Ceballos J, Turegano Fuentes F, Perez Diaz D, Sanz Sanchez M, Martin Llorente C, Guerrero Sanz JE. Casualties treated at the closes hospital in the Madrid, March 11, terrorist bombings. Crit Care Med. 2005;33:S107–12.
13. Torkki M, Koljonen V, Sillanpää K, et al. Triage in bomb disaster with 166 casualties. Eur J Trauma. 2006;32:374–80.

Injuries and Scoring Systems

12

Gennaro Perrone, Elena Bonati, Antonio Tarasconi,
Harishine K. Abongwa, and Fausto Catena

12.1 Trauma Score Evolution

In recent decades, there has been a change in the management of conflict between different states. There has been a change in the management of the conflict compared to the collective imagination. Metropolitan cities have become battlefields due to increasing adverse events such as terrorist attacks, bioterrorism, etc. It must also be borne in mind that man has gone wildly into dangerous places and this behavior associated with natural disasters has led to real disasters. This socioeconomic evolution made it necessary to adapt hospitals and their resources. New scientific concepts have been introduced in order to increasingly standardize certain behaviors during adverse events. This has resulted in an ever faster response in patient care [1].

In the medical field, the concept of "disaster" has taken hold, understood as an accident or an event in which the needs of patients exceed the resources necessary for their treatment [2]. Emergency planning has made it possible to improve the efficiency of the health system in responding to the problems that arise from it. Usually the response to catastrophic events is negatively conditioned by the discrepancy between requests, capabilities, and organizational structures available.

Disaster management teams are critical to the mass casualty incident response given the complexity of today's disaster threats. Current disaster planning and response emphasizes the need for an all-hazards approach. Flexibility and mobility are the key assets required of all disaster management teams. Medical providers must respond to both these challenges if they are to be successful disaster team members.

G. Perrone · A. Tarasconi · H. K. Abongwa · F. Catena (✉)
Department of Emergency Surgery, Maggiore Hospital, Parma, Italy

E. Bonati
General Surgical Clinic, Maggiore Hospital, Parma, Italy

© Springer Nature Switzerland AG 2021
E. Pikoulis, J. Doucet (eds.), *Emergency Medicine, Trauma and Disaster Management*, Hot Topics in Acute Care Surgery and Trauma,
https://doi.org/10.1007/978-3-030-34116-9_12

The variety of events to which we are exposed does not make it possible to predict the place, the characteristics, and the moment in which a disaster will occur. For this reason, today we tend to use multi-risk approaches based on a single and common initial response to the emergency with subsequent treatment routes based on the type of disaster that has occurred. The goal is to do the best possible for the greatest number of victims.

The aforementioned adverse events generate unique demands for the medical community [3]. In particular, surgeons must be better educated in disaster management. Triage changes according to the various situations; disasters require a completely different approach to assessment and assistance that often goes beyond one's ethics and training. An ability is required to adapt and apply fundamental principles of disaster management universally to any mass incidents caused by people or nature. Organizational tools such as the incident control system and the hospital incident control system contribute to a quick and coordinated response to specific situations. This problem in recent years has been the focus of discussions that led to the formation of international emergency response teams able to provide medical, surgical, and intensive care services in hostile environments throughout the world.

Hospitals must undertake all activities aimed at identifying potential risks, training staff, and being aware of their resources. These activities are based on an emergency plan that must be simple and flexible, periodically reviewed, and which must provide for the continuous training of the personnel in charge.

The American College of Surgeons Committee on Trauma (ASCOT) commissioned the Major Trauma Outcome Study (MTOS) in 1982 to pool data on injured patients and to develop and test survival probability norms based on injury severity scores [4]. The MTOS data was collected retrospectively with four countries participating: the United States, Canada, the United Kingdom, and Australia. Many injury severity measures were developed to support epidemiological research and performance evaluation; examples include abbreviated injury scale (AIS), injury severity score (ISS), and new injury severity scores (NISS), a severity categorization of trauma, and International Classification for Diseases-9 ISS (ICISS).

The ever-growing need to establish a common language regarding traumas has led over time to the introduction of two types of injury dictionaries: one specific for trauma and one non-specific. The first category includes the Abbreviated Injury Scale (AIS) classification system, while the nonspecific classification system is based on the disease classification method (ICD) [5]. This formulation arose from the need for a precise description of the injuries of an accident and the damage associated with it in order to obtain uniform epidemiological, clinical, and evaluative data. This need for uniformity has taken hold since the end of the 1960s, a period in which the work of the Baltimore group led by Dr. Becker goes back.

Determining the extent of the injuries for a patient, both subjectively and objectively, is fundamental since this leads to the financing of healthcare, patient triage and epidemiology, and research. The injury severity score (ISS) was probably the severity parameter of the most used injury since its initial development. Although the ISS has a number of recognized mathematical, administrative, and clinical limits, its importance in monitoring and assessing trauma has led to the ISS being considered the "gold standard" in assessing the severity of trauma. In the AIS system, the assignment of severity measures is based on consensus among groups of experts; it is therefore a subjective classification system. At the level of clinical outcome, a trauma can be described according to two fundamental dimensions which are the anatomical aspect and the physiological consequences.

In 1993, Osler tried to schematize the main variables that influence the outcome, focusing on the relationship between anatomical injury, physiological damage, and previous health status [6]. The outcome measure of greater use is the probability of survival (or death). The physiological consequences of the trauma can be measured by appropriate scales, such as that of the revised trauma score (RTS). The assessment of the physiological damage is based on the ISS, while with regard to the state of health a proxy variant is inserted as the age of the patient because the seniority of the subject is an important indicator of the state of health.

The abbreviated injury scale (AIS) system arose from the need to standardize the lesions according to a classification by establishing a gravity scale [7]. The American Association for the Advancement of the Automotive Medicine (AAAM) through the formation of a Committee for the Graduation of Injuries contributed to the drafting of the first version of the AIS published in 1971 in a pioneering work by Dettaven. The initial version identified 73 types of traumas that instead became 1300 in the most recent version. AIS is based on an anatomical basis and consists of six characters for each diagnosed lesion. The combination of the aforesaid characters makes it possible to identify the various levels of the anatomical part involved in the lesion taking into account the region of the affected body, the type of structure involved (both the specific anatomical structure and the lesion level), generating a score. The lesions are then also classified according to an ordinal gravity scale ranging from 1 to 6 (maximum degree of severity). It should be emphasized that this is not a system of systemic assessment of the traumatized, but takes into consideration only the severity of the individual lesions and therefore does not provide an overall assessment of the severity of the traumatized because it does not even take into account the summing effects of the various injuries. This system is expensive both in terms of information requirements and requires a coding of the injuries that requires highly qualified personnel. To overcome these obstacles and in the attempt to obtain an automated coding, a system for the conversion of ICD 9-CM codes into MAIS or ISS scores was developed.

To solve the problem of the overall assessment of the severity of a polytraumatized initial reference was made to the MSS score (MAIS), that is, to the index of the patient's most serious injury. However, the problem arose of having to pass to an objective measurement and to analyze the correlation between AIS scores and mortality. A demonstration of the non-linearity of the relationship between AIS and probability of death was given by Becker in 1974 with a study of 2128 traumatized patients admitted to eight Baltimore hospitals, in which he developed the ISS system.

From this study, it emerged that the mortality rate increased more than proportionally to the severity score and that the secondary lesions also had effects on mortality. Individual injuries that are not fatal can have a significant effect on mortality when combined with others.

Given these data, it has been proven over the years to obtain non-linear equations which are as close as possible to actual results.

The Becker study found that the mortality rate increased disproportionately with respect to the assigned severity score. Secondary lesions, which were singularly not fatal, in this study had a significant effect if added together. It also emerged that the influence on mortality of a number of associated lesions of more than three was not relevant. The following algorithm was proposed: ISS: MAIS region 1+ MAIS region 2+ MAIS region 3. Region MAIS refers to the most severe lesion of a body region. The ISS score is expressed on an ordinal scale ranging from 0 to 75. It has become a universally accepted method for evaluating trauma while undergoing various adaptations imposed by the evolution of knowledge.

Given the short faults of the ISS system, in the early nineties a severity score of the ICD-9 injury (ICISS) was introduced [8], defined as the product of all the survival risk ratios for the traumatic codes ICD-9 of a patient. ICISS is a much better survival predictor than ISS in injured patients. Using the ICD-9 lexicon can avoid the need for AIS coding. Subsequently, we tried to perform a similar revision based on ISS data using the AIS vocabulary. In fact, the lexicon used to divide the "landscape" of injury into individual injuries may be of little importance.

Although the ISS is widely used for the assessment of trauma, it has some limitations, as it considers only the most serious damage in a single part of the body and does not measure other minor injuries in the same body region; therefore, the new accident severity score (NISS) was developed to exceed the ISS limits; it considers severe injuries in different areas of the body regardless of the region of the affected body [9]. The severity score of the injury was initially introduced to estimate the mortality of patients with trauma; however, other applications for the ISS have been demonstrated in several studies.

The NISS is a better choice for case mix control in trauma research than the ISS for predicting intensive care unit admission and length of hospital stay [10]. This data from the Canadian study by Lavoie is in contrast with the previous Saeedi's study which does not evince this superiority.

As we could initially describe, physiological damage is a determining part of the outcome of a trauma. Over the years it has been tried to develop appropriate indicators of this damage, some of which are specific to the trauma. One of these is the revised trauma score (RTS) which is obtained by linearly combining three different physiological indicators: Glasgow coma scale (GCS), systolic pressure (SP), and respiratory rate (RR) [11, 12]. These parameters are designed to measure the state of consciousness of the individual and the cardiocirculatory and respiratory function at the systemic level. This index is expressed on a continuous scale ranging from 0 representing the absence of vital signs to 7.84 which is the reference value for normal vital signs. These results are obtained with the following formula: RTS = 0.9368 GCS + 0.7326 PS + 0.2908 RF. Figure 12.1 shows a precompiled model used in our region (Fig. 12.1). The RTS is a well-established predictor of mortality in trauma populations, but there is a lack of definitive evidence supporting its use as a primary triage tool and as a predictor of outcomes other than mortality.

The flaw of this index is that the calculation is too complicated for easy use in emergency departments. Many times it is developed by parmedici so it may not have high reliability. The respiratory rate (RR), one of the parameters used for its calculation, is less reliable than other factors because it is influenced by the patient's age, injury mechanism, and mechanical ventilation. The RTS Triage (T-RTS) is

	Cognome	
SERVIZIO SANITARIO REGIONALE EMILIA-ROMAGNA	Nome	Barcode
	Data di nascita	
Logo Azienda	N° CCI/Nosologico	

SCALA RTS (Revised Trauma Score di Champion)

	Descrizione	Punteggio
Glasgow coma scale (GCS)	13-15	4
	9-12	3
	6-8	2
	4-5	1
	3	0
PA sistolica	>89	4
	76-89	3
	50-75	2
	1-49	1
	0	0
Frequenza respiratoria	10-29	4
	>29	3
	6-9	2
	1-5	1
	0	0
	Totale	

Punteggio	rischio
≤ 9/10	Trauma severo

DATA.............................. Ora.............................. FIRMA..............................

Fig. 12.1 An Italian regional example of revised trauma score of Champion

based on the same risk intervals and RTS variables and is easier to use, but nevertheless has the same problems as RTS. T-RTS is currently used by ambulance personnel to choose the most appropriate hospital facilities based on the severity of trauma. Moreover, it is an independent predictor of mortality in hospital.

T-RTS is currently used by ambulance personnel to select the most appropriate hospital facilities based on the severity of the trauma. Furthermore, it is an independent predictor of hospital mortality. From the literature it emerges that in severe traumatized patients, pre-hospital changes of T-RTS are also an independent predictor of mortality and are very useful for establishing prognosis.

So far we have discussed the systems for assessing the severity of traumas of an objective or subjective nature, expressed through specific indices or scales, and the validity of these indicators in terms of the predictive capacity of the outcome was discussed [13]. The relationship between gravity indicator, ISS type, and outcome measure, such as the mortality rate, was investigated. The severity level of the trauma expressed by an outcome measure is expressed by TRISS (TRauma score, Injury Severity Score), which combines the ISS as an anatomical lesion measure, the RTS for the physiological damage, and age as a proxy of the patient's general health status (physiological reserve). The idea behind this indicator is that the simultaneous use of health measures based on different aspects of the description of the lesion allows a greater accuracy in the prediction of the outcome with respect to each measure considered individually. Champion has linked, in his relationship, a link between the probability of survival and the indicators previously mentioned.

Currently the calculation formula of the TRISS is $SP = 1/(1 + e - b)$ where ps = probability of survival, $b = B0 + b1$ (RTS) $+ b2$ (ISS) $+ b3$ (age). In this formula, the regression coefficients originate from the MTOS study [4]. As can be seen from the above formula, we start from anatomical and physiological measures of severity of the trauma, to estimate the functional relationship with the probability of survival in a study population, and then use it as a measure of the overall severity of the trauma.

The probability of survival was used to observe the different levels of severity of a pathology even without being related to measures of functional and anatomic damage. Rutledge et al. [14] used diagnoses and procedures codified according to the ICD-9-CM system for classification of diseases and by grading them by gravity according to the lethality rate (DRR: death risk ratio) relative to each ICD-9 code calculated on a sample of 10,000 patients by dividing the number of deaths observed for each category by the total number of patients in the category. In this work a diagnosis pattern and procedures are defined for each type of patient, each with a probability of death, which identifies the specific type of patient and determines the probability of survival. Patterns and related DRRs are applied to any other patient population for considered trauma. The approach behind this process is of the typical type and is based on the idea that the mortality rate for a traumatic disease is stable. Therefore the lethality rate can be extrapolated to another population.

This model, the ICD-9-based illness severity score (ICISS), was developed from the Agency for Health Care Policy Research's Health Care Utilization Project database and is used to predict hospital survival, hospital length of stay, and hospital charges of injured patients admitted to University of North Carolina Hospitals. ICISS expressed the severity of a patient's trauma as a product of the survival probability calculated for each diagnosis, encoded according to the ICD-9-CM system, based on the observed survival rate in a sufficiently large patient population. This system has proved statistically significant with respect to the predictive capacity of the probability of survival, hence the severity of the diseases, and is universally applicable to all types of pathologies, both traumatic and non-traumatic.

However, among studies published after 2003, the Trauma Mortality Prediction Model based on ICD-9 codes (TMPM-9) demonstrated superior discriminative ability than ICISS using the product of traditional survival proportions. Several methods for predicting mortality after trauma were examined [15]. Two classifications are used to provide a taxonomy for diseases, including injuries. The ICD-9 is the classification system for administrative data in the United States. AIS has been developed for the characterization of lesions only. The trauma mortality prediction model (TMPM) is based on empirical assessments of severity for each lesion in the ICD-9 and AIS lexicons. Every chance of mortality (POD) is estimated from the five worst injuries per patient. The TMPM.ado command allows users to efficiently apply TMPM to fundamental ICD-9 or AIS data sets. The command makes use of model-mediated regression coefficients (MARCs) that assign empirically derived gravity measurements for each of the 1322 AIS codes and 1579 ICD-9 hazard codes. The risk codes are grouped into a set of regression coefficients. A logical model is generated to calculate the probability of death. This model is also applied to the ICD-10. The basic idea of the development of TMPM was to adapt a probit model with death as a result with 1000 possible lesions as binary predictors starting from a cohort extrapolated from the National Trauma Data Bank (NTDB). The design matrix was 1000 variables long and 1,000,000 cases. The sum of the data set provided a rich mosaic of lesions with the survival of the associated patient. Two separate probit models were created using the lesions described in the coding system. The first model used as possible lesions as binary predictors and death as a binary outcome and a second model was based on the severity indicators of the body region. The empirical gravity of the injury to the injury was estimated by taking a weighted average of the two regression models. TMPM-ICD10 provides better discrimination and calibration than the ISS and can be computed without recourse to AIS coding the TMPM-ICD10 should replace the ISS as the standard measure of overall injury severity for data coded in the ICD-10-CM lexicon.

Other registries and datasets using ISS >15 as an inclusion criterion may exclude a substantial body of data relating to significantly morbid trauma patients [16].

GCS, ISS, TRISS, and RTS are the most commonly used injury measures; however, some attempts have been made to develop new injury measures. Examples include exponential injury severity score (EISS), Ganga Hospital score for lower limb fractures, tangent injury severity score (TISS), and some novel biomarkers such as lactate and serum acetylcholinesterase. Other scores that were not traditionally used in injury or trauma research such as McLaughlin, Modified Rankin, South African Triage Score, Modified Early Warning System, and Rwanda mortality prediction model have also been used for the prediction of mortality in trauma populations.

The basic deficit is a more objective indicator of physiological stress after trauma than the vital signs that make up the RTS score. A model of prediction of trauma survival based on the basic deficit was developed [model of deficit severity score and basic lesion (BISS)], in which the RTS was replaced by the basic deficit as a measure of the physiological imbalance.

The BISS model, a trauma model based on the basic survival prediction deficit, has shown equivalent performance to those of TRISS and ASCOT [17] and can offer a more simplified calculation method and a more objective evaluation. Replacing ISS with NISS can greatly improve model accuracy, but further confirmation is needed because there are not many studies on this data in the literature.

TRISS can be employed for different purposes, that is, preliminary outcome-based evaluation (PRE) and definitive outcome-based evaluation (DEF) [18]. TRISS is a method which is now the most extensively used for the outcome evaluation of trauma. Even so, it still has some shortcomings; e.g., trauma cannot be given the weights that should be given, and the section of age is too simple. ASCOT is also a physiologic and anatomic combined method for the evaluation of injury severity and outcome. To some extent, this method obviates the shortcomings of TRISS in the calculation of probability of survival (Ps) with injury severity score (ISS). Therefore, ASCOT is considered to be superior to TRISS in the evaluation of Ps.

The scientific community is still looking for a model of forecasting the best mortality in the general traumatic population [19]. Ideal future models should be developed and/or validated using an appropriate sample size with sufficient events for the predictor variable, use multiple imputation patterns to correct missing values, use the continuous variant of the predictor if available, and incorporate all different types of predictors readily available (i.e., physiological variables, anatomical variables, cause/mechanism of the lesion, and demographic variables). Furthermore, while mortality rates are decreasing, it is important to develop models that provide physical, cognitive, or quality of life to measure the quality of care. Injuries and their physiological response are complex mechanisms, and the outcome of injuries is frequently affected by a number of factors ranging from age and pre-existing conditions of the patient to biochemical response of the body. It is difficult to account for all factors in a single model or severity measure; therefore, the use of non-injury-specific measures such as APACHE II, SOFAS, and SAPS has gained traction in trauma research.

12.2 Trauma Registry Utility

Trauma registries are an essential part of trauma quality improvement programs aimed at decreasing morbidity and mortality in high-income countries [20, 21]. In low- and middle-income countries (LMICs), where the burden of injury is disproportionately high, hospitals have faced challenges in adapting trauma registry models implemented in high-income countries. Many LMICs face unique challenges to implementation that must be overcome to create sustainable trauma databases.

The implementation and development of an emergency medical services (EMS) system is varied among LMICs. Many LMICs lack an organized EMS system with most ambulances used purely for transport and not as an emergency care vehicle. Financial issues are the most common problems faced by LMICs with support from developed countries a necessity.

The literature on pediatric trauma epidemiology in LMICs is limited. The injuries seen in these trauma admissions also differed significantly between LMICs and high-income countries (HICs). Most of the current scoring systems have been created for HICs and therefore are not optimal for LMICs. The Kampala trauma score assessed in a LMIC was useful in injury monitoring and resource evaluation in limited settings. This is a way to improve the experience of associated pediatric patients. Kampala trauma score (KTS) [22] is a simplified composite of the RTS and the ISS and closely resembles the TRISS method. The validity of the KTS was demonstrated when compared with RTS and ISS alone, or compared with the TRISS method. The KTS has proven reliable when used in trauma registries in Uganda, both in urban and rural settings.

The KTS score is a severity instrument designed to differentiate severe injuries from non-severe injuries [23]. However, the outcomes it predicts, mortality and prolonged hospitalization, are often not as frequently involved and vary less widely for non-severe injuries. Also, the relationship between patient outcomes and injury severity is neither linear not binary in its nature, making the use of cut-offs difficult. If the KTS score categorizes patients as "severe," a more effective application of clinical interventions can be applied to those who will gain the most. In the trauma registry, at its "best cut-off" (70.9% sensitivity, 77.9% specificity) the KTS will still mislabel 29% of the patients who will go on to die. Therefore, the KTS is more difficult to utilize for individual patient triage as opposed to its potential usage to determine, for example, resource allocation on a population-wide basis. The use of this score in the various studies used is not able to determine a limit point to differentiate patients from severe to non-severe patients in order to allow a tailor-made treatment. Until further applied research is undertaken, the utility of KTS as a triage tool is limited. However, it will continue to be used effectively for population-based approaches for the assessment, evaluation, and research of health care needs.

12.3 Pediatric Scores

The pediatric trauma score (PTS) was devised specifically for the triage of pediatric trauma patients [24]. PTS is based on the assignment of a score ranging from +2 to −1 (0 excluded) of the following parameters: weight in kg, arterial pressure expressed in mmHg, mental state, evaluation of the airways, bone fractures, and open wounds. Researchers, policymakers, and directors of medical centers should take steps toward implementing precise patient evaluation and preventive programs, in order to improve the quality of services and care. The GCS, PTS, and ISS can be used to predict mortality with statistical significance in child patients with trauma.

The pediatric BIG score [25] is a reliable mortality prediction score for children with traumatic injuries; it uses international normalization ratio (INR), base excess (BE), and Glasgow coma scale (GCS) values that can be measured within a few minutes of sampling, so it can be readily applied in the Pediatric Emergency Department, but it cannot be applied on patients with chronic diseases that affect INR, BE, or GCS.

12.4   Conclusions

There are still many shady areas regarding the various types of scores. The implementation of research at a global level, also thanks to free magazines, and the current awareness of the scientific community about mutual collaboration will certainly lead to improvements regarding the treatment of various types of trauma. Currently the development of the ICD-10, for example, should begin to improve the performance of traumatized patients and the first large-scale results are now at the door.

References

1. Strous RD, Gold A. Ethical lessons learned and to be learned from mass casualty events by terrorism. Curr Opin Anaesthesiol. 2019;32(2):174–8. https://doi.org/10.1097/ACO.0000000000000684. PMID: 30817391.
2. Briggs SM. Disaster management teams. Curr Opin Crit Care. 2005;11(6):585–9.
3. Born CT, Briggs SM, Ciraulo DL, Frykberg ER, Hammond JS, Hirshberg A, Lhowe DW, O'Neill PA. Disasters and mass casualties: I. General principles of response and management. J Am Acad Orthop Surg. 2007;15(7):388–96.
4. Champion HR, Copes WS, Sacco WJ, Lawnick MM, Keast SL, Bain LW Jr, Flanagan ME, Frey CF. The Major Trauma Outcome Study: establishing national norms for trauma care. J Trauma. 1990;30(11):1356–65. PMID: 2231804.
5. Baker SP, O'Neill B, Haddon W, et al. The Injury Severity Score: a method for describing patients with multiple injuries and evaluating emergency care. J Trauma. 1974;14:187–96.
6. Osler T. Injury severity scoring: perspectives in development and future directions. Am J Surg. 1993;165(2A Suppl):43S–51S. PMID: 843899.
7. Gennarelli & Wodzin. CMAAS (Committee on Medical Aspects of Automotive Safety). Rating the severity of tissue damage: I. The abbreviated scale. JAMA. 1971;215:277–80.
8. Osler T, Rutledge R, Deis J, Bedrick E. ICISS: an international classification of disease-9 based injury severity score. J Trauma. 1996;41(3):380–6; discussion 386–8.
9. Salehi O, Dezfuli SAT, Namazi SS, Khalili MD, Saeedi M. A new injury severity score for predicting the length of hospital stay in multiple trauma patients. Trauma Mon. 2016;21(1):e20349.
10. Lavoie A, Moore L, LeSage N, Liberman M, Sampalis JS. The injury severity score or the New Injury Severity Score for predicting intensive care unit admission and hospital length of stay? Injury. 2005;36(4):477–83.
11. Gabbe BJ, Cameron PA, Finch CF. Is the revised trauma score still useful? ANZ J Surg. 2003;73(11):944–8.
12. Lichtveld RA, Spijkers AT, Hoogendoorn JM, Panhuizen IF, van der Werken C. Triage revised trauma score change between first assessment and arrival at the hospital to predict mortality. Int J Emerg Med. 2008;1(1):21–6. https://doi.org/10.1007/s12245-008-0013-7.
13. Champion HR, Sacco WJ, Carnazzo AJ, Copes W, Fouty WJ. Trauma score. Crit Care Med. 1981;9(9):672–6.
14. Rutledge R, Fakhry S, Baker C, Oller D. Injury severity grading in trauma patients: a simplified technique based upon ICD-9 coding. J Trauma. 1993;35(4):497–506; discussion 506–7.
15. Osler T, Glance LG, Cook A, Buzas JS, Hosmer DW. A trauma mortality prediction model based on the ICD-10-CM lexicon: TMPM-ICD10. J Trauma Acute Care Surg. 2019;86(5):891–5. https://doi.org/10.1097/TA.0000000000002194.
16. Palmer C. Major trauma and the injury severity score – where should we set the bar? Annu Proc Assoc Adv Automot Med. 2007;51:13–29. PMCID: PMC3217501. PMID: 18184482.

17. Lam SW, Lingsma HF, van Beeck EF, Leenen LP. Validation of a base deficit-based trauma prediction model and comparison with TRISS and ASCOT. Eur J Trauma Emerg Surg. 2016;42(5):627–33.
18. Zhu P, Jiang J. Employment of trauma and injury severity score and a severity characterization of trauma in the outcome evaluation of trauma care and their research advances. Chin Med J (Engl). 1998;111(2):169–73.
19. Mehmood A, Hung YW, He H, Ali S, Bachani AM. Performance of injury severity measures in trauma research: a literature review and validation analysis of studies from low-income and middle-income countries. BMJ Open. 2019;9(1):e023161.
20. Bommakanti K, Feldhaus I, Motwani G, Dicker RA, Juillard C. Trauma registry implementation in low- and middle-income countries: challenges and opportunities. J Surg Res. 2018;223:72–86. https://doi.org/10.1016/j.jss.2017.09.039.
21. Suryanto, Plummer V, Boyle M. EMS systems in lower-middle income countries: a literature review. Prehosp Disaster Med. 2017;32(1):64–70.
22. Macleod JBA, Kobusingye O, Frost C, Lett R. Kampala Trauma Score (KTS): is it a new triage tool? East Cent Afr J Surg. 2006;12(1):74–82.
23. Bradshaw CJ, Bandi AS, Muktar Z, Hasan MA, Chowdhury TK, Banu T, Hailemariam M, Ngu F, Croaker D, Bankolé R, Sholadoye T, Olaomi O, Ameh E, Di Cesare A, Leva E, Ringo Y, Abdur-Rahman L, Salama R, Elhalaby E, Perera H, Parsons C, Cleeve S, Numanoglu A, Van As S, Sharma S, Lakhoo K. International study of the epidemiology of paediatric trauma: PAPSA research study. World J Surg. 2018;42(6):1885–94. https://doi.org/10.1007/s00268-017-4396-6.
24. Furnival RA, Schunk JE. ABCs of scoring systems for pediatric trauma. Pediatr Emerg Care. 1999;15(3):215–23.
25. El-Gamasy MAE-A, Elezz AAEBA, Basuni ASM, Elrazek MESAA. Pediatric trauma BIG score: predicting mortality in polytraumatized pediatric patients. Indian J Crit Care Med. 2016;20(11):640–6.

Wound Care Management, Non-penetrating Injuries, and Wounds Penetrating into Body Cavities

Nelson Olim

13.1 Penetrating Trauma

Penetrating wounds are injuries that result from tissue penetration by a foreign material. Most commonly these injuries are caused by weapons that can be further classified into low-energy (knifes and hand-energized missiles); medium-energy (handguns, pistols, and revolvers), and high-energy weapons (military or hunting rifles). Injuries by projectiles propelled by the energy of a blast explosion (also called secondary blast injuries) will be covered in a different chapter, but according to the size of the projectile, the energy of the blast and the distance traveled, they usually fall under the medium- or high-energy categories.

13.1.1 Stab Wounds

Stab wounds to the chest and abdomen often cause life-threatening injuries as both cavities contain vital organs and major blood vessels that can be disrupted. Life or limb-threatening injuries can also result from stab wounds to other anatomical locations if neuro-vascular structures are affected. Because the energy transfer is done along a tract, the size and shape of the blade, as well as the exact anatomical location, play an important role in the outcome of these wounds. As a rule of thumb, damage is only inflicted to local tissues along the path, or paths, of the blade. Surrounding tissues that do not directly contact the blade are usually unaffected. This being said, one should not assume that blades always produce straight paths, as movements of the victim and the perpetrator may create multiple injuries in the cavities despite the existence of one single entry point.

N. Olim (✉)
World Health Organization, Geneva, Switzerland

© Springer Nature Switzerland AG 2021
E. Pikoulis, J. Doucet (eds.), *Emergency Medicine, Trauma and Disaster Management*, Hot Topics in Acute Care Surgery and Trauma, https://doi.org/10.1007/978-3-030-34116-9_13

13.1.2 Gunshot Wounds (GSW)

Gunshot wounds are becoming increasingly common all around the world. Conflict, violence, and criminality coupled with flexible legislation that allows easy access to military rifles in some countries have been producing some of the most devastating injuries seen in civilian settings.

The original size of the entry and exit wounds per se do not give enough information on the path of the bullet or the damage produced, as this is dependent on many other factors. Entry wounds can be larger than the exit wounds and small-entry/small-exit wounds may conceal damage caused by the large temporary cavity that was formed in between.

Small Arms
Small arms are hand-held small caliber firearms with less than 20 mm bore size. Under the tag "Small Arms," we mainly find revolvers, pistols, rifles, carbines, assault rifles, submachine guns, and light machine guns.

Ammunition Terms
A typical cartridge contains a case (with a primer and different amounts of gunpowder) and a bullet (the projectile). Most bullets used nowadays have a lead or steel core. This core is then either fully jacketed with a harder material like a copper alloy (FMJ bullets) or semi-jacketed (SJ), leaving the tip of the core exposed (soft point/hollow point bullets).

Energy Transfer
When gunpowder ignites, expanding gas is generated. The more gunpowder, the more gas is generated. Bigger cartridges like the ones used in assault rifles have much more gunpowder than smaller cartridges used in revolvers and pistols (handguns). The extreme pressure generated by the expanding gas propels the bullet out of the case and through the weapon's barrel into the air at a certain speed. On impact, all the energy left on the bullet is transferred to the human body causing the injury.

Kinetic energy (E_k) of the bullet (muzzle energy) is calculated (in J) using the formula

$$E_k = \frac{1}{2}mv^2$$

where m is the mass of the bullet (in Kg) and v is velocity of the bullet (in m/s). The bullet of a typical 9 mm Luger cartridge used by many police forces has an average of 470 J. An AK47 Kalashnikov rifle's bullet has an average of 3000 J.

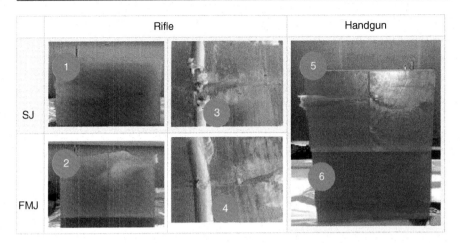

Fig. 13.1 FMJ bullets (2, 4, 6) vs SJ bullets (1, 3, 5)

13.1.3 Patterns of Injury

The pattern of injury is mainly determined by the type of bullet (FMJ vs SJ) and by the energy still left upon impact (handgun vs rifle). The bullets on image 1 (SJ) and 2 (FMJ) had exactly the same energy, but the energy was deposited at different depths (Fig. 13.1):

- Rifle FMJ bullets penetrate deeper (2,4) before they start tumbling to create a temporary cavity.
- Handgun FMJ bullets (6) do not create temporary cavities.
- SJ bullets (1,3,5) deform or expand on impact, depositing most of the energy in the first centimeters after penetration. SJ bullets are used for hunting and by some police departments, but are prohibited for use in war by the 1899 Hague Convention.

13.2 Hemorrhage

Noncompressible hemorrhage is the immediate major concern following penetrating trauma to the chest or abdomen, even in the absence of obvious external exsanguination. Some injuries will inevitably lead to death almost instantly. If we consider that on an average 70 kg man, an estimated 5000 ml of blood flows through the aorta every minute, and that volume amounts for the whole blood volume, then we can easily infer that a complete disruption of the aorta will lead to death in less than a minute. Complete disruptions of other smaller arteries would imply different timings as, for example, the 600 ml/min flow rate of the superior mesenteric artery or the 450 ml/min flow rate of a renal artery. Fortunately, not every penetrating injury disrupts a major blood conduct but rather a series of smaller arterial and venous vessels, and numerous capillaries.

During hemorrhage, the natural physiological response will focus on preserving blood pressure as the circulating volume is progressively lost, and this is mainly achieved through peripheral vasoconstriction. However, the buffering capacity of the system is limited and the potential for inadequate cardiac output leading to inadequate organ perfusion is high even if the blood pressure remains within the normal range. This is particularly true when we are facing a massive hemorrhage, defined by one or more of the following criteria:

- Loss of more than total blood volume within 24 h (around 70 ml/kg, >5000 ml in a 70 kg adult)
- 50% of total blood volume loss in less than 3 h
- Bleeding in excess of 150 ml/min
- Bleeding which leads to a systolic blood pressure of less than 90 mmHg or a heart rate of more than 110 beats per minute

13.2.1 Shock

Hypoxia due to inadequate tissue perfusion is called shock, and until otherwise proven, in patients with penetrating injuries to the chest or abdomen this is due to hypovolemia secondary to hemorrhage.

Shock can also be classified into different classes according to the volume of blood loss and the resulting abnormalities identified in some physiological parameters (i.e., pulse rate, blood pressure, and mental status) (Table 13.1).

Patients presenting with tachycardia, hypotension, and visible blood loss are easily identified as being in shock, however, trauma patients may be shocked even if presenting with normal blood pressure and pulse rate. Thus, in trauma patients with penetrating injures, adequate cardiac output cannot be inferred from blood pressure. A relationship between the two only happens when blood loss is critical or rapid.

Table 13.1 Shock classifications

	Class I	Class II	Class III	Class IV
Blood loss (ml)	Up to 750	750–1500	1500–2000	>2000
Blood loss (% of volume)	Up to 15%	15–30%	30–40%	>40%
Pulse rate	<100	>100	>120	>140
Blood pressure	Normal	Normal	Decreased	Decreased
Mental status	Normal to slightly anxious	Slightly anxious, restless	Anxious, confused	Confused, lethargic

13.2.2 The Trauma Triad of Death

Massive and ongoing blood loss inevitably leads to tissue hypoperfusion. This means that there is less oxygen being delivered to the cells. Less oxygen delivery makes the individual cells shift into anaerobic metabolism. The problem with anaerobic metabolism is that it produces lactic acid as an end product (leading to lactic acidosis), and is less efficient in terms of ATP production. Less ATP being produced, means less ATP is available for heat production, thus further contributing to hypothermia (temperature ≤ 35 °C) (Fig. 13.2).

Lactic acidosis will further impair myocardial contractility, contributing to reduced tissue perfusion. Hypothermia, on the other hand, is further aggravated by the adrenergic stimulation vasoconstriction that attempts to keep the blood pressure within acceptable values.

The clotting cascade enzymes and platelets only operate within a narrow temperature range; thus, hypothermia together with the vigorous immunologic response (cytokines) both contribute to the establishment of a trauma-induced coagulophaty. Furthermore, hypoperfusion together with tissue injury results in hyperfibrinolysis and activation of the protein C pathway, leading to fibrinogen depletion and systemic anticoagulation also called trauma-induced coagulophaty (TIC) by some authors.

Hypothermia is one of the most important physiological predictors for early and late mortality in trauma patients, and coagulopathy, independent of hypothermia but strongly correlated with acidosis and ISS, is also associated with increased mortality in trauma patients. Some studies suggest an overall in hospital mortality rate of 47.8% for those patients arriving at the emergency department presenting with the

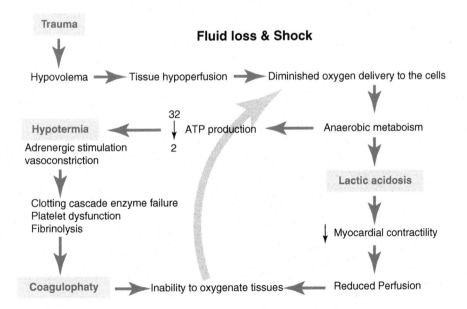

Fig. 13.2 Fluid loss and shock scheme

full triad: coagulopathy (international normalized ratio (INR) >1.5), hypothermia (temperature <35 °C), and acidosis (pH <7.2).

13.3 Damage Control Concepts

Damage control can be seen as a principle, a concept, and a philosophy. The founding pillars of damage control have been imported from naval military experience, where in the aftermath of a battle-damaged ship, all internal resources are mobilized in order to limit the extension of the damages and keep the ship afloat with a functional steer. In practical terms, all the actions taken during this emergency situation aim at: temporarily stop the flooding, extinguish the fires, and keep the propellers running.

The extrapolation of these naval damage control principles into penetrating trauma thus requires a set of measures aiming to stop the bleeding, limit contamination and soilage, and preserve blood flow to vital organs. The most important goal is to keep the patient alive at all costs, and ideally this process should begin at the point of injury.

13.3.1 Damage Control Resuscitation

Although the initial management of every single trauma patient starts with the traditional "ABCDE" or "(C)ABCDE" approach (which prioritizes catastrophic blleding), the modern approach to trauma management includes a series of clinical interventions known as damage control resuscitation which also target the complications of major hemorrhage (coagulophaty, hypothermia, and acidosis).

Hemodinamically unstable patients should be simultaneously assessed and resuscitated. The goal is to have normal perfusion restored, thus recovering from shock. However, it has been demonstrated that in trauma patients with penetrating injuries presenting with active bleeding, attempts to restore perfusion, before adequate hemostasis is achieved, are counterproductive. Damage control resuscitation thus relies on three basic principles:

- Hemorrhage control (preserving circulating volume and minimizing blood loss)
- Permissive hypotension/hypovolemia (keeping systolic blood pressure around 80–90 mmHg in order to avoid "popping the clots")
- Early empiric use of red blood cells and clotting products (thus limiting fluids that may dilute coagulation proteins) and consequently preventing and treating trauma induced coagulopaty

The single most important step in the management of the severely injured patient is to arrest bleeding and restore blood volume. Still, fluids should be judiciously used and prioritized according to their availability, knowing that the most effective resuscitation fluid is the patient's own blood. In order of preference, the following should be used:

- Fresh warm whole blood (better than stored whole blood)
- Plasma (1) + red blood cells (1) + platelets (1)
- Plasma (1) + red blood cells (1)
- Plasma or red blood cells
- Warm colloids (HES)
- Warm crystalloids (Plasmalyte A; better than Ringer lactate, better than normal saline)

When homeostasis has been achieved, definitive resuscitation to restore organ perfusion is initiated, and although this strategy clearly sacrifices perfusion for homeostasis (prioritizing TIC), several studies have demonstrated that it is associated with a decrease in mortality and reduced duration of stay in intensive care and hospital.

Certain procedures like tourniquets and splints, as well as some adjuncts like tranexamic acid or topical hemostatic agents (combat gauze), or some interventions such as resuscitative endovascular balloon occlusion of the aorta, may all play a role until definitive surgical or radiological hemorrhage control is achieved.

Having this in consideration, during the initial "ABCDE" or "(C)ABCDE" approach, the initial resuscitation end points are:

- Radial pulse present.
- Systolic blood pressure around 80–90 mmHg.
- Improved mental status.

13.3.2 Damage Control Surgery

Damage control surgery (DCS) is part of the damage control resuscitation (DCR) philosophy and sacrifices the completeness of the immediate surgical repair and restoration of anatomy in order to adequately address the combined physiological insult of trauma and subsequent surgery.

In practical terms, damage control surgery is done to treat the physiology and not the anatomy. Historically, the first time the term was used was in 1993 by Rotondo and colleagues. The initial description was of an abbreviated laparotomy followed by intensive resuscitation and later return to the operating theater for definitive repair, thus defining three damage control stages:

- DCS Stage 1
  - Hemorrhage control
  - Limit peritoneal contamination
  - Temporary abdominal closure
- DCS Stage 2
  - Hypothermia prevention and treatment
  - Correction of coagulopathy
  - Correction of acidosis

- DCS Stage 3 (no longer than 72 h from Stage 1)
  - Definitive surgery
  - Creation of ostomies, feeding access, fascial closure

Since then and in the past 25 years, the DCS concept has been broadly applied in different surgical fields including, orthopedic surgery, vascular surgery, neurosurgery, and plastic surgery. Additionally and more recently, two new stages were added in order to cover for the prehospital and early resuscitation phase (DCS Stage 0) and reconstructive surgery (DCS Stage 4).

Important to note that most trauma patients who present to an emergency department, even those with penetrating wounds, do not require a damage control approach. Only a few who are seriously injured, in shock, should require damage control resuscitation and damage control surgery, and these should be identified as early as possible.

13.4   Penetrating Abdominal Wounds

All patients should be initially managed using the traditional ABCDE/(C)ABCDE approach, and it is important to early identify patients who have an immediate indication for laparotomy. This patient population shall not undergo axial imaging, but rather be immediately transferred to the operating theatre.

Gunshot and stab wounds are always contaminated. All patients undergoing surgery should receive tetanus prophylaxis and antibiotic prophylaxis to deal with the eventual bacteremia produced by the manipulation of contaminated tissues.

Violation of the peritoneum occurs in between 20% and 80% of patients with penetrating trauma, and the peritoneum can accommodate nearly all of a patient's circulating blood volume.

Unlike blunt trauma, injuries to the stomach, duodenum, small intestine, and colon are common in penetrating trauma. The small intestine is actually the most common site of injury in both blunt and penetrating trauma.

Evisceration of bowel or omentum and bleeding from the wound are indications for surgical exploration, regardless of the patient hemodynamic status. All abdominal gunshot wounds require exploration but anterior abdominal stab wounds are best managed following the "Western Trauma Association algorithm for local wound exploration and abdominal stab wounds" (Fig. 13.3).

13.4.1 Damage Control Laparotomy

For the selected subset of unstable patients requiring immediate laparotomy, the whole team should be aware of the surgical goals (and resist the temptation to embark into definitive repairs):

- Hemorrhage control
- Limiting peritoneal contamination
- Temporary abdominal closure

Fig. 13.3 D/C—discharge;
Cbc—complete blood count

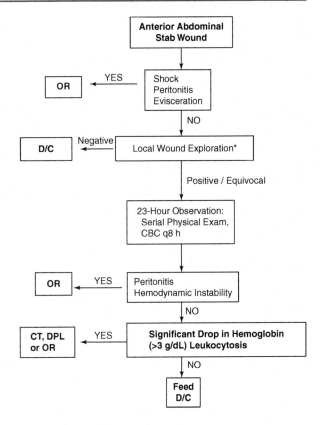

Hemorrhage control: As soon as entering the abdomen, vascular control of the abdominal hemorrhage should be paired with packing of all four quadrants. Vascular control can be achieved either by direct digital pressure applied to the abdominal aorta or through performing an initial left anterior lateral thoracotomy for proximal aortic control before the laparotomy. The later technique is currently subject to debate as some authors suggest that the physiologic cost of this thoracotomy is greater than direct control or endovascular occlusion techniques. Whatever the choice of technique, this initial maneuvers usually improve cardiac and cerebral perfusion, thus contributing to the overall resuscitation process.

Bleeding from solid organs should be controlled by either direct compression or removal of the organ. In the case of splenic bleeding, the damage control approach favors immediate splenectomy instead of time-consuming splenorrhapies. For a massive liver hemorrhage, the initial approach can follow the sequence "Push, Pringle, Pack," thus buying some time for further decisions to be taken.

Lateral expanding hematomas of the retroperitoneum are best approached laterally to medially through a Mattox maneuver (left-medial visceral rotation) or through a Cattel–Braasch maneuver (right-medial visceral rotation). In both cases if the kidney is identified as the source of injury, a quick palpation of a normal kidney on the contra-lateral renal fossa will give you the peace of mind to proceed with the nephrectomy.

Shunting is probably one of the best options when leading with a major vascular injury, but even major truncal arteries and veins may have to be ligated if no other option is available on the table. Vascular repair at DCS Stage 1, should only be attempted if time permits and in agreement with the anesthetist.

Limiting peritoneal contamination: Although hollow viscus injuries do not often contribute to hemodynamic instability, they are associated with significant morbidity and mortality.

Stool and other enteric content should be washed out. Ongoing leakage from non-circumferential holes in the bowel can be easily and quickly repaired with 3-0 or 2-0 silk sutures, whether major leaks should not undergo any attempt for anastomosis and should be addressed with linear stapling devices, umbilical tapes, skin staplers, or abdominal clamps that will remain in place until DCS Stage 3.

Injuries to the pancreas and duodenum are particularly challenging. Duodenal injuries should be simply debrided and closed. In the damage control situation, the addition of nasogastric decompression will be enough, and considerations of pyloric exclusion can be taken at DCS Stage 3. Pancreatic injuries in this setting are better managed by closed suction drainage or a combination of closed suction drainage and resection, which is the case of distal injuries with ductal involvement who will benefit from a distal pancreatectomy with splenectomy plus close suction drainage. Attempting a pancreaticoduodenectomy in a damage control setting defies the whole concept of Damage Control surgery.

Temporary abdominal closure: Primary fascial closure is not an option under damage control mode and it is important to recognize that the role for an open abdomen (OA) is not exclusive to the damage control population. OA has been an effective treatment for abdominal catastrophes in traumatic and general surgery. Damage control surgery, severe abdominal infection, planned second look operation, and prevention of abdominal compartment syndrome are all indications for temporary closures. Intra-abdominal hypertension (IAH) and abdominal compartment syndrome (ACS) have been increasingly recognized as contributing factors for mortality.

Historically, abdominal packing, Bogota bags, and towel clip skin closure have been used as temporary means to achieve temporary closures. Currently the most commonly used techniques derive from the initial vacuum pack technique described by Barker et al. In summary, a perforated polyethylene sheet is placed over the intraperitoneal viscera and beneath the peritoneum of the anterior and lateral abdominal wall. Then, a layer consisting of compressible material, such as sterile surgical gauzes, applied over the polyethylene sheet. Two silicone drains positioned between the gauzes and connected to an aspiration source at -20 cm H_2O. A plastic polyester drape to cover the skin surrounding the wound.

Today, different and more efficient, pre-assembled commercial systems are available to provide negative pressure therapy, sub-atmospheric pressure or vacuum sealing techniques. The underlying principle is the same as the Barker system, and availability of resources will probably dictate the method of choice.

13.5   Penetrating Chest Wounds

Penetrating chest injuries account for 12% of all trauma-penetrating injuries, yet thoracic injuries account for up to 25% of early trauma related deaths, second only to head and neck injuries.

Paradoxically, however, thoracic trauma can uniquely benefit from bedside procedures like tube thoracotomy, emergency airway creation and emergency department thoracotomy, to alleviate the immediate threat of mortality and allow further definitive treatment.

All patients should be initially managed using the traditional ABCDE/(C)ABCDE approach, and, as in abdominal trauma, it is important to early identify patients who have an immediate indication for thoracotomy.

13.5.1 Damage Control Thoracotomy

The principles of thoracic damage control are the same as abdominal damage control: DCS Step 1 to stop the hemorrhage and limit contamination, DSC Step 2 at the ICU unit in an effort to restore physiologic condition, and DSC Step 3 for definitive repair.

For an abbreviated thoracic operation, the patient should be positioned in the supine position with the arms extended out at 90° with a slight elevation under the left chest to increase exposure. In the event of a nonanticipated emergency laparotomy, this is the more convenient position.

For patients who present in extremis, an anterolateral incision is simpler and quicker than a midline sternotomy.

Once inside, three main actions can be taken: release of cardiac tamponade, compression of the supradiaphragmatic aorta, and packing of the chest for hemorrhage control.

If a pericardial tamponade is found and released (pericardium incision parallel to the frenic nerve), then one should focus on the control of the cardiac/great vessel bleeding. Digital pressure followed by a quick staple closure or simple suture will often work. For bigger defects, a bladder catheter can be inserted an inflated into the bleeding cavity to buy some time.

Vascular injuries should also be approached in a damage control manner: either lateral repair, shunt placement, or ligation.

Lung injuries are traditionally easier to solve from a technical perspective. In cases where the source of a significant hemorrhage is the lung, releasing of the inferior pulmonary ligament, followed by a twisting maneuver of the lung around its hilum will compress both the pulmonary veins and arteries. Alternatively, a pulmonary hilar clamp can be placed, with similar results.

Hemorrhage from through and through pulmonary parenchymal injuries are best managed by a technique called tractotomy, by which, using a surgical stapler or between clamps the "roof" of the tract/channel is opened, exposing the underlying bleeding vessels that can now be individually addressed.

Esophageal injuries are usually very challenging. In a damage control setting the best options to deal with esophageal injuries are: primary closure (reinforced with pericardium) with wide drainage, or wide drainage alone with two chest tubes together with a nasogastric tube placed at the level of injury.

Most upper airway injuries can be managed by passing an endotracheal tube past the site of injury.

A subset of patients presenting with penetrating chest trauma with witnessed previous cardiac activity which as seen been lost, or patients deteriorating rapidly prior to arrest of cardiac activity, are strong candidates for a bedside left anterolateral resuscitative thoracotomy. The primary aim is to release a cardiac tamponade, apply digital pressure to the descending aorta, or allow for internal cardiac massage. Additionally, this approach also allows for a quick lung twist (180° rotation of the lung) or a lung tractotomy with a surgical stapler, in order to temporary control pulmonary sources of bleeding. If needed the incision can be extended to the contralateral side over the fifth intercostal space, creating a clamshell thoracotomy and allowing for a total chest exposure. Even knowing that the survival rates in these cases are quite low (18–33%), these patients are almost always candidates for a subsequent thoracic damage control procedure.

It is debatable whether the chest can be definitively closed after a damage control operation. Some authors favor the vacuum sealing techniques, while others prefer the immediate traditional closure leaving the chest tubes in place. Whatever technique is used, it is important to remember that the goal is to achieve adequate perfusion and oxygenation while monitoring for any ongoing hemorrhage.

13.6   Wound Care

Entry and exit wounds, whether caused by bullets or knifes, require proper debridement. Unless strictly unavoidable, these wounds should not be part of the main surgical incision (laparotomy or thoracotomy) and should not be used to pass drains (abdominal or chest). Proper debridement of these wounds may however require a combination of incision (to extend the wound and expose deeper layers of subcutaneous fat, fascia and muscle) plus excision (the removal of all contaminated and necrotic tissue). As a rule of thumb, with very few exceptions, all wounds should be left open (covered by a dressing) for a period of 2–5 days, when safe delayed primary closure of the clean wound can then be achieved.

Head Injuries

14

Freiderikos Sotiriou, Panagiotis Papadopoulos-Manolarakis, Stefanos Korfias, and Andreas Pikoulis

Abbreviations

ASDH	Acute subdural hematoma
BBB	Blood brain barrier
CPP	Cerebral perfusion pressure
CSF	Cerebrospinal fluid
CT	Computed tomography
DAI	Diffuse axonal injury
DTI	Diffusion tensor imaging
DWI	Diffusion weighted imaging
E/R	Emergency room
EDH	Epidural hematoma
GCS	Glasgow Coma Scale
ICH	Intracerebral hematoma
ICP	Intracranial pressure
ICU	Intensive care unit
IPC	Intraparenchymal catheter
IVC	Intraventricular catheter

F. Sotiriou (✉)
Neurosurgical Clinic Athens Naval Hospital, Athens, Greece

P. Papadopoulos-Manolarakis
Neurosusrgical Department, General Hospital of Nikaia—Piraeus, Athens, Greece

S. Korfias
National & Kapodistrian University of Athens, Evangelismos Hospital, Athens, Greece

A. Pikoulis
University General Hospital "Attikon", National and Kapodistrian University of Athens, Athens, Greece

© Springer Nature Switzerland AG 2021
E. Pikoulis, J. Doucet (eds.), *Emergency Medicine, Trauma and Disaster Management*, Hot Topics in Acute Care Surgery and Trauma,
https://doi.org/10.1007/978-3-030-34116-9_14

IVH	Intraventricular hemorrhage
LOC	Loss of consciousness
PTV	Posttraumatic vasospasm
SAH	Subarachnoid hemorrhage
SDH	Subdural hematoma
TBI	Traumatic brain injury

14.1 Head Injuries

Traumatic brain injury (TBI) constitutes the main cause of death and long-term disability in young adults worldwide and its challenging management requires collaboration between many specialties. However, prevention strategies, such as seat belt combined with air bags, helmet use, or well-organized pre-hospital care, are the most effective means to limit the impact of closed TBI in "developed regions". Nowadays, this impact is particularly high and mortality rates are affected accordingly (from 4% to 8% for moderate TBI until 50% for severe TBI).

Neurotrauma is the most prevalent disorder with *two important factors* that affect the outcome:

1. The *primary brain injury*, when the initial impact and the transmission of its force causes an immediate damage or even shearing of long axons of neurons.
2. The *secondary brain injury* which refers to the subsequent neuronal damage due to pathophysiologic mechanisms such as intracranial hypertension, hypoxia, systemic hypotension, or posthemorrhagic hydrocephalus.

Thus, the neurosurgeon's involvement in the management of moderate or severe TBI, and therefore in prevention of *secondary brain damage*, is decisive and includes, in principle, methods like decompressive craniectomy or multimodality monitoring techniques supported by specially trained staff in neurological intensive care units (ICU).

Advances in understanding the neurobiology of TBI have shown that most of the secondary damage which was long thought to be fully established at the moment of impact is actually an evolving process that may be halted, reversed, or repaired by therapies.

14.2 Classification of Head Injury

Different approaches to classification of TBI exist.

From a *mechanistic aspect*, head injuries are distinguished in:

(a) Closed (the most common type)
(b) Penetrating [*missile* (e.g., due to bullets) and *nonmissile* (e.g., due to knives)]

(c) Crush
(d) Blast, which has recently been identified as a separate entity and is frequently caused by improvised explosive devices used during armed conflicts and terrorist activities

Regardless of the mechanism of head injury, its severity can be clinically classified assessing the patient's state of consciousness through the *Glasgow Coma Scale (GCS)* score (Table 14.1) [1]. There are, however, restrictions in the application of GCS in some patients who arrive at the emergency room (E/R) sluggish because of cardiovascular shock, sedation, or other similar causes. In these cases, for example, a precise clinical evaluation cannot be performed until the shock or the drugs metabolism is overcome. Similar challenges are faced during intensive care unit (ICU) management because many intracranial pressure (ICP)-lowering therapies render patients heavily sedated, paralyzed, or both. In addition, intubation or craniofacial injuries which involve orbits can interfere verbal or eye response respectively.

Evaluating the initial GCS, TBI can be classified as [1]:

(a) Mild (GCS 13–15)
(b) Moderate (GCS 9–12)
(c) Severe (GCS 3–8)

Table 14.1 The Glasgow Coma Scale Score

Neurological response[a]	Points
Best eye response (E)	
Open spontaneously	4
Open to verbal command	3
Open to pain	2
No eye opening	1
Best verbal response (V)	
Oriented	5
Confused	4
Inappropriate words	3
Incomprehensible sounds	2
No verbal response	1
Best motor response (M)	
Obeys commands	6
Localizing response to pain	5
Withdrawal from pain	4
Abnormal flexion to pain/decorticate posturing	3
Extensor response to pain/decerebrate posturing	2
No motor response	1
Minimum score (E + V + M)	*3*
Maximum score	*15*

Modified after Teasdale and Jennett [1]
[a]The GCS is determined by adding the scores of the best neurological responses in each of three categories

Furthermore, two subcategories are:

(d) Minimal [GCS 15, no loss of consciousness (LOC) or amnesia]
(e) Critical (GCS 3–4)

Another classification of TBI based on initial brain computed tomography (CT) scan refers to *anatomical injury patterns*:

(a) Focal (contusions or intracranial hematomas)
(b) Diffuse

and could be used to evaluate patients at high risk of delayed deterioration due to secondary brain injury and therefore with poor clinical outcome. The indications for initial brain CT scan to determine the severity of a head injury are briefly summarized in Table 14.2.

In 1991, Marshall score [2], and later an alternative version known as Rotterdam score (Table 14.3) [3], was introduced to predict the outcome of TBI.

Table 14.2 Indications for initial brain CT scan

Indications for initial brain CT scan: (*Remember*: LOC, PTA, VOM, RF, FND, P.A.D.D.)
1. GCS ≤14/15 or progressive headache or deterioration
2. Loss of consciousness (LOC)
3. Posttraumatic amnesia (PTA)
4. Vomiting ≥2 episodes (VOM)
5. Risk factors (RF) as anticoagulation or/and antiplatelet therapy
6. Focal neurological deficit (FND)
7. Psychiatric patient, alcohol, drugs, dementia (P.A.D.D.)
8. Any sign of basal fracture (raccoon eyes, battle sign, CSF rhinorrhea/otorrhea)

Table 14.3 Rotterdam score

Initial brain CT findings (Mneumonic: "S.E.B.AH.")	Points
Midline brain shift (S)	
0–5 mm	0
>5 mm	1
Epidural space lesion (E)	
Yes	0
No	1
Basal cisterns (B)	
Normal	0
Compressed	1
Absent	2
Traumatic IVH or SAH (AH)	
No	0
Yes	1
Minimum score (S + E + B + AH)	*0*
Maximum score	*5*

Modified from Maas et al. [3]
CT computed tomography, *IVH* intraventricular hemorrhage, *SAH* subarachnoid hemorrhage

This grading system substantially correlates the findings of the initial CT scan (e.g., traumatic intraventricular or subarachnoid hemorrhage, midline brain shift, basal cisterns, or brainstem compression) with the clinical course and eventually the outcome of the patient [4].

Specifically, 6 months mortality in adults with TBI increases with the score as follows: 0% for score 1, 7% for score 2, 16% for score 3, 26% for score 4, and 53% for score 5 [3].

14.2.1 Focal Brain Injury

Focal brain injuries typically refer to (1) *contusions* and (2) *traumatic intracranial hematomas.*

14.2.1.1 Brain Contusions

This entity represents hemorrhagic areas, under the pia matter (supial), owing to rupture of small vessels and extravasation or blood into parenchyma. The frontal and temporal poles are most often involved because of close contact with bony surfaces of the cranial base and vault (Fig. 14.1). Occasionally, these focal hemorrhagic regions can produce remarkable mass effect due to their progression to an intra-cerebral hematoma (traumatic-ICH) with the concomitant surrounding edema.

A classification of contusions based on anatomical and mechanical criteria is usually suggested:

1. *Fracture contusions*, due to direct contact injuries under a skull fracture.
2. *Coup contusions*, directly under the site of impact without concomitant skull fracture.
3. *Contre-coup contusions*, in regions distant to but not always opposite the impact.
4. *Gliding contusions,* representing bilateral focal hemorrhages into the gray and the underlying white matter of the parasagittal brain tissue, owing to rotational forces.

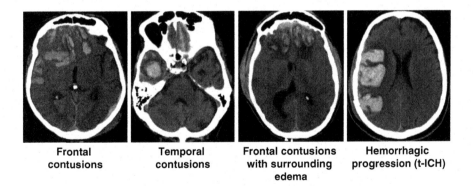

| Frontal contusions | Temporal contusions | Frontal contusions with surrounding edema | Hemorrhagic progression (t-ICH) |

Fig. 14.1 Brain contusions. CT images from different patients

5. *Intermediary contusions,* as punctuate hemorrhages in deep cerebral structures (basal ganglia with adjacent thalamus and hypothalamus, corpus callosum, brainstem).
6. *Herniation contusions,* in brain tissue near the tentorial edge or near the foramen magnum. The types of brain herniation are schematically represented in Fig. 14.2.

Herniation produces brain injury along free edges of dural reflections and dysfunction in blood supply or white matter pathways, followed by the corresponding clinical symptoms in each case. More specifically, in the case of subfalcine herniation, compression of the pericallosal arteries by the herniated cingulated gyrus could cause leg weakness. A tentorial herniation may result in ptosis, ipsilateral mydriasis, contralateral hemiparesis, and decreased level of consciousness because of compression of the oculomotor nerve and the posterior cerebral artery by the

Fig. 14.2 Schematic representation of the types of brain herniation. (1) Subfalcine/cingulate: under the edge of falx cerebri. (2) Tentorial/uncal: over the tentorial edge. (3) Transtentorial/central: through the tentorial notches. (4) Transcalvarial: swollen brain tissue through dural and skull defects. (5) Tonsilar: through the foramen magnum

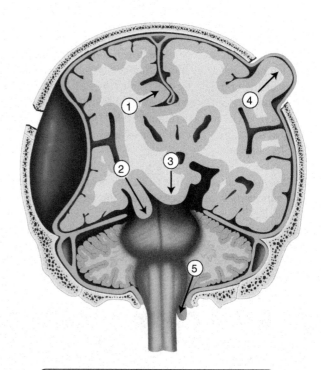

1. Subfalcine/Cingulate: under the edge of falx cerebri
2. Tentorial/Uncal: over the tentorial edge
3. Transtentorial/Central: through the tentorial notches
4. Transcalvarial: swollen brain tissue through dural and skull defects
5. Tonsilar: through the foramen magnum

herniated medial edge of the uncus. In massive herniation, the cerebral peduncle on the opposite side to the hernia may be indented by the tentorium, producing a Kernohan's notch and a false localizing and paradoxical ipsilateral hemiparesis. The most dramatic type of herniation, central herniation, could result in coma with respiratory and cardiovascular (bradycardia and hypertension) irregularity because of the downward compression of the brainstem and the perforating branches of the basilar artery that finally cause its ischemia. In the case of tonsilar herniation, the compression of the medulla by the herniated cerebral tonsils through the foramen magnum causes apnea.

The indications for surgical treatment of traumatic intracerebral hematomas (t-ICH) and/or hemorrhagic contusions are summarized as follows [5]:

(a) In cases with persistent elevated intracranial pressure (ICP) (see below)
(b) T-ICH volume* >50 cm^3
(c) Initial GCS 6–8 and frontal or temporal t-ICH volume >20 cm^3 on brain CT-scan, with midline shift ≥0.5 cm or/and compressed basal cisterns
(d) Neurological deterioration due to hemorrhagic progression of contusions (signs of mass effect—imminent herniation)

*The estimation of T-ICH volume is based on the ellipsoid volume equation as described by Kothari et al. [6] [$ABC/2$, A = maximum length (in cm), B = width perpendicular to A on the same head CT slice, and C = the number of slices multiplied by the slice thickness].

14.2.1.2 Traumatic Intracranial Hematoma

This entity refers to any posttraumatic hemorrhagic lesion developed into the skull and it is divided, according to the location of the bleeding in relation to the meninges, into three types: (1) epidural, (2) subdural, and (3) intracerebral (t-ICH, see above). Traumatic intracranial hematoma causes a progressive mass effect, usually detected on the initial CT brain scan, which is responsible for the delayed neurological deterioration and requires surgical evacuation as soon as possible.

Epidural Hematoma (EDH)

EDH develops between the dura mater and the skull and the bleeding source is arterial in most of the cases because of laceration of middle meningeal artery by fracture at the pterion [7]. However, the remainder of cases are due to bleeding from a skull fracture or a vein sinus. Incidence: 1–2% of head injury admissions [8], commonly in young adults (rare in <2 years and >60 years).

Classification of EDH according to its radiographic progression:

- *type I* (1st day—acute and hyperacute, associated with "swirl" fresh arterial blood)
- *type II* (2nd–4th day—subacute)
- *type III* (7th–20th day—chronic, hemorrhagic elements of different time)

Clinical presentation (the classic triad):

- Initial posttraumatic loss of consciousness
- Transient complete recovery ("lucid interval")
- Sudden neurological impairment with rapid deterioration (obtundation, ipsilateral pupillary dilatation, and contralateral hemiparesis, followed by *Cushing triad* due to brainstem compression: (1) respiratory disturbances and (2) arterial hypertension with (3) bradycardia, and finally death).

However, this typical presentation occurs only in a limited rate of patients with EDH (<10–27%) [9]. Other symptoms or findings could be: headache, seizure, vomiting. Although the severity of these symptoms is affected by the hematoma size, the postoperative prognosis remains excellent for patients with a "pure EDH" (without associated contusions or other hemorrhagic lesions) if there are no delays in diagnosis and subsequent treatment. The indications for surgical evacuation of EDHs are summarized as follows [10]:

(a) GCS <9 and anisocoria as soon as possible
(b) Volume >30 cm³, *regardless of GCS*
(c) Thickness >15 mm (Fig. 14.3)
(d) Midline shift >5 mm (Fig. 14.3)

Fig. 14.3 Acute epidural hematoma in axial CT

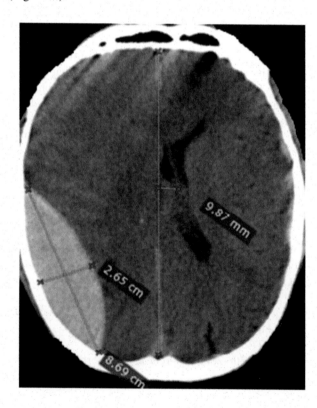

(e) Establishment of focal neurological deficit
(f) Position: EDH of the middle or posterior cranial fossa needs more "flexible" criteria for surgery.

Subdural Hematoma (SDH)

SDHs constitute bleeding collections between the arachnoid and the dura mater (subdural space) and occur either due to tearing of bridging veins (Fig. 14.4) that drain part of cortical blood directly into superior sagittal sinus or as a result of bleeding from superficial brain contusions.

Classification of SDHs:

Clinically, an acute SDH (a) becomes evident within 3 days of injury, subacute (b) between 3 and 21 days, and chronic (c) if more than 21 days pass between injury and clinical presentation (Table 14.4 and Fig. 14.5).

Acute Subdural Hematoma (ASDH)

This entity, commonly associated with underlying brain injury, account for about 60% of all SDHs. The majority of ASDHs occur after rupture of cortical veins by two distinct pathologies:

- *First type*: Accumulation around brain contusion (extension of cortical bleeding over the arachnoid membrane). This complex of SDH and damaged-necrotic brain is termed "*burst lobe*" and is more common in the temporal lobe. In this type the underlying primary brain injury is usually severe.
- *Second type*: Stretching and tearing of bridging veins owing to inertial forces causes a low-pressure venous bleeding into the subdural space followed by

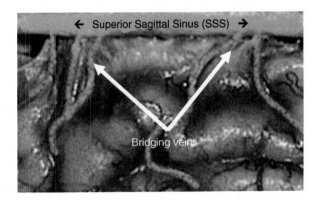

Fig. 14.4 Schematic representation of cortical veins

Table 14.4 Subdural hematoma classification and changes on CT with time

Type	Days	Consistency	CT appearance
Acute	0–2	Clotted blood	Hyperdense
Subacute	2–14	Clotted and fluid blood	Isodense
Chronic	>14	Fluid blood	Hypodense

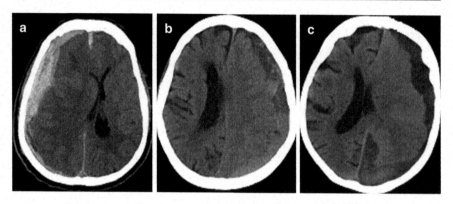

Fig. 14.5 Appearance of each type (**a–c**) of subdural hematoma in axial CTs

secondary brain damage because of the progressive mass effect, the venous out-flow obstruction, and finally the local cerebral ischemia. However, in some rare cases of rapture of a cortical artery, an even more rapid neurological deterioration is observed.

The severity of initial impact damage is occasionally much higher in ASDH than in EDH because of the associated underlying brain injury following subdural hematomas. Without early surgical evacuation of clot (within 4 h), much more in cases of "non-pure" ASDH (with concomitant contusions, t-SAH, DAI), the prognosis is extremely poor because the mass effect and intracranial hypertension affect the cerebral blood flow, causing further cerebral ischemia (secondary brain damage). The indications for surgical treatment of ASDHs are summarized as follows [11]:

(a) Every ASDH with a midline shift >0.5 cm *or* thickness >1 cm, regardless of GCS
(b) ICP monitoring in all comatose patients (GCS <9) with an ASDH and surgical evacuation if ICP exceeds 20 mmHg
(c) ASDH with midline shift <0.5 cm *or* thickness <1 cm should undergo evacuation if GCS drops by ≥2 points from injury to admission and/or if the pupils become asymmetric or fixed and dilated.

14.2.2 Diffuse Brain Injury

Diffuse brain injury is the most common type of TBI and includes a wide range of clinical entities, from concussions to the persistent posttraumatic coma.

14.2.2.1 Concussion
Concussion, as a result of rotational acceleration/deceleration head injury without mechanical contact, is the mildest type of diffuse brain injury; and patients usually experience an impermanent loss of consciousness (LOC). Although previously

thought harmless, concussion is now considered as a brain damage and repeated episodes can occasionally cause a significant impairment of neurological status.

Although the pathophysiology of this entity is not clearly understood, the usually immediate return to the normal state of alertness suggests that the LOC is a result of transient disturbances in the function of diencephalon or brainstem. Whereas brain CT-scan and GCS levels may be normal, signs of cytotoxic cerebral edema can be observed in the diffusion tensor imaging (DTI).

14.2.2.2   Diffuse Axonal Injury (DAI)

DAI occurs after severe rotational or angular acceleration and deceleration that can be caused by shear forces to axons. Therefore, DAI is the main reason for severely impaired TBI patients even if significant cerebral contusions or intracranial hematomas are lacking. Minimal or mild DAIs can be a result of acceleration/deceleration forces in the sagittal or oblique plane, whereas severe DAIs result after the corresponding lateral or coronal forces. The histological characteristics of DAI include axonal disconnection and swelling associated with punctuate ("strich") hemorrhages in eloquent areas that undergo maximal acceleration forces during head injury (peri-ventricular white matter and adjacent structures, such as corpus callosum, fornix, internal capsule, hypothalamus, basal nuclei, and superior cerebellar peduncles).

14.2.2.3   Traumatic Subarachnoid Hemorrhage (T-SAH)— Posttraumatic Vasospasm (PTV)

Traumatic SAH, as a result of rupture of the superficial cortical vessels into the subarachnoid spaces due to the initial impact, remains a common brain CT-scan sign associated with severe (33–60% of all cases) TBI [12–14]. This entity can be followed by posttraumatic vasospasm (PTV), a serious secondary brain damage that usually causes permanent neurological deficits and corresponds to a poor outcome. PTV typically develops between approximately first and fifth day after TBI and it can last from 12 h to 30 days [15], involving both posterior and anterior circulation arteries. The major differences between aneurysmal and traumatic SAH involve distribution and time course. Specifically, t-SAH has a different distribution, mainly involving inter-hemispheric, cortical convexity, and supratentorial spaces. Secondly, vasospasm following aneurysmal SAH occurs and resolves later on serial CT than PTV.

14.2.2.4   Intraventricular Hemorrhage (IVH)

Between all the patients with severe TBI, about 25% will develop hemorrhage into the brain's ventricular system. This entity, typically occurring after a powerful head injury, is usually accompanied by punctuate hemorrhages in adjacent deep cerebral structures, such as basal ganglia and hypothalamus. Post-hemorrhagic communicating hydrocephalus, due to cerebrospinal fluid (CSF) malabsorption at the level of arachnoid granulations, is more likely to occur after traumatic IVH than acute obstructive hydrocephalus.

14.3 Management of Severe Head Injury

14.3.1 Pre-hospital Management

A well-organized pre-hospital management composed of experienced and well-trained rescuers and medical staff is crucial to prevent secondary brain injury. Since most treatment strategies aim to prevent its disastrous consequences, rapid correction of hypoxemia and hypotension, the two most important predictors for mortality, is recommended [16].

First of all, intubate any patient with a GCS score ≤8 (after immobilization of cervical spine) and give controlled ventilation with continuous monitoring of oxygenation by pulse oximetry. Management is similar in TBI patients with significant impairment or deterioration of neurological status, accompanied even by seizures and respiratory, or severe craniofacial and other thoracoabdominal injuries.

The guidelines for the step-by-step pre-hospital management outlined by the Brain Trauma Foundation are as follows [16]:

- *Assessment phase*:
  - Continuous oxygen saturation and blood pressure monitoring to prevent hypoxemia (<90% O_2 saturation) and hypotension (<90 mmHg systolic blood pressure), respectively.
  - Estimate the severity of TBI by assessing the GCS score after securing airway, breathing, and circulation and before administering sedatives or paralytics.
  - Record bilateral pupillary size and reflex after patient stabilization. Note any evidence of orbital trauma.
- *Treatment phase*:
  - Establish airway in severe TBI, inability to maintain airway or hypoxemia with supplemental oxygen.
  - Avoid hypoxemia (SpO_2 <90%) and maintain normocapnia (PCO_2: 35–40 mmHg).
  - Use isotonic fluids to treat hypotensive patients.
  - In a normoventilated, well-oxygenated, and normotensive patient with clinical signs of cerebral herniation (dilated unreactive or asymmetric pupils, extensor posturing or no motor response, decrease in GCS score by more than 2 points from prior best score), hyperventilation (20 breaths/min in adult, 25 in child and 30 in infant) can be used as a temporary measure until hospitalization.

14.3.2 E/R Management

The first-line management of the TBI patient (Diagram 14.1), just like the multi-injured patient, follows a sequential flow according to Advanced Trauma Life Support (ATLS) guidelines of the American College of Surgeons (ACS), known as the *primary survey* or "ABCDEs" [17].

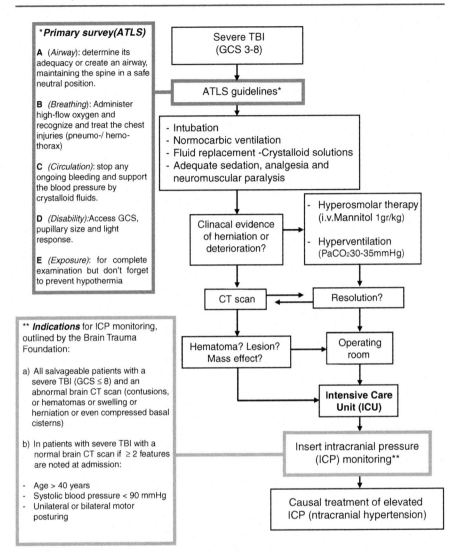

Primary survey(ATLS)

A *(Airway)*: determine its adequacy or create an airway, maintaining the spine in a safe neutral position.

B *(Breathing)*: Administer high-flow oxygen and recognize and treat the chest injuries (pneumo-/ hemo-thorax)

C *(Circulation)*: stop any ongoing bleeding and support the blood pressure by crystalloid fluids.

D *(Disability)*:Access GCS, pupillary size and light response.

E *(Exposure)*: for complete examination but don't forget to prevent hypothermia

Indications for ICP monitoring, outlined by the Brain Trauma Foundation:

a) All salvageable patients with a severe TBI (GCS ≤ 8) and an abnormal brain CT scan (contusions, or hematomas or swelling or herniation or even compressed basal cisterns)

b) In patients with severe TBI with a normal brain CT scan if ≥ 2 features are noted at admission:

- Age > 40 years
- Systolic blood pressure < 90 mmHg
- Unilateral or bilateral motor posturing

Severe TBI (GCS 3-8)

ATLS guidelines*

- Intubation
- Normocarbic ventilation
- Fluid replacement -Crystalloid solutions
- Adequate sedation, analgesia and neuromuscular paralysis

Clinacal evidence of herniation or deterioration?

- Hyperosmolar therapy (i.v.Mannitol 1gr/kg)
- Hyperventilation (PaCO₂30-35mmHg)

CT scan → Resolution?

Hematoma? Lesion? Mass effect? → Operating room

Intensive Care Unit (ICU)

Insert intracranial pressure (ICP) monitoring**

Causal treatment of elevated ICP (ntracranial hypertension)

Diagram 14.1 Initial management in severe TBI. (Modified from Aarabi et al. [17])

General guidelines for urgent neurosurgical consultation during the primary or secondary survey include: open depressed skull fracture, open head injury with visible brain tissue, lateralizing neurological signs (unilateral third cranial nerve palsy, decerebrate or decorticate posturing, hemiparesis, or hemiplegia), any alteration of GCS, and abnormal head CT findings.

14.3.2.1 Initial Management of Severe Head Injury Outlined by the Brain Trauma Foundation

Clinical presentation of raised ICP, such as impaired level of consciousness, headache, vomiting, or nausea, could not be evaluated in comatose patients. Thus, in ICU we use ICP monitoring techniques to prevent the catastrophic consequences of secondary brain injury as a result of raised ICP due to diffuse brain swelling or the extra volumes of intracranial hematomas or contusions.

14.3.2.2   ICP Values

1. Normal-resting ICP is <10 mmHg
2. Sustained ICP >20 mmHg is typically abnormal
3. ICP 20–40 mmHg → moderate intracranial hypertension
4. ICP >40 mmHg → severe, usually life-threatening intracranial hypertension

Although some CT signs, such as compression or even absence of basal cisterns and midline shift, are predictive of brain swelling and intracranial hypertension, an increased value of ICP could occur without these findings. It is also observed that the number and duration of raised ICP episodes significantly correlates with worse functional outcome and death after TBI. The recent guidelines [18] for TBI management recommend *treating ICP > 20 mmHg (recommendation level II)* or using clinical and CT signs in addition to the range of ICP values to decide the appropriate treatment (*recommendation level III*).

14.3.2.3   Techniques of ICP Monitoring

1. *Intraventricular* catheter (IVC): Its tip is preferably positioned into the right frontal horn of the lateral ventricle and is connected to an external pressure transducer via fluid-filled tubing [19].

Advantages of this method:	*Disadvantages of this method*:
(1) Relief of elevated ICP by CSF drainage	(1) Risk for ventriculitis and intracranial hemorrhage
(2) Most accurate	(2) Difficult to insert in "slit ventricles"
(3) Lower cost	

2. *Intraparenchymal* catheter (IPC): effective and similar to IVC, but more expensive.
3. *Extracerebral* catheters (epidural, subdural, or subarachnoid): less accurate types of monitoring.

Routine catheter exchange or/and systemic prophylactic antibiotics are not recommended in the recent TBI guidelines.

14.3.2.4   Duration of ICP Monitoring

Withdrawal of catheter when ICP values remain normal for 48–72 h.

Attention: Don't remove the catheter too early, because a secondary rise in ICP values is observed between third and tenth day after TBI in about one-third of patients with intracranial hypertension due to the delayed development of entities such as intracranial hematomas, PTV, posttraumatic hydrocephalus, or even cardiovascular reasons.

The surgical steps for ICP catheter placement are discussed in Fig. 14.6.

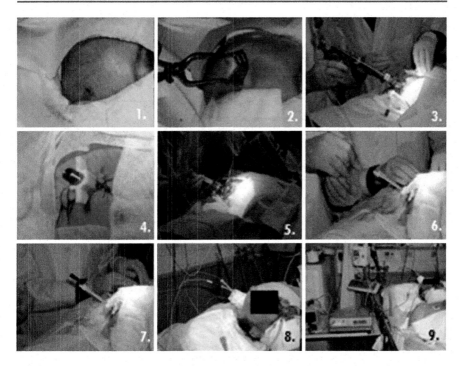

Fig. 14.6 Images showing the step-by-step placement of an ICP catheter in the ICU. First of all, find and mark Kocher's point (roughly 11 cm behind the nasion and on the mid-papillary line laterally) and then inject local anesthetic with lidocaine. Skin incision is made centered on Kocher's point and a self-retaining retractor is placed (1–2), Burr hole using a hand drill (3), bolt placement and fixation (4–5), catheters insertion (6–7), connection and ICP activation (8–9)

Table 14.5 Causes of traumatic intracranial hypertension

*Keep in mind: Traumatic intracranial hypertension, may be due any of the following *reversible* causes:

1. Brain swelling (*see below*)
2. Traumatically induced lesions (SDH, EDH, t-ICH, depressed skull fracture, tension pneumocephalus)
3. Posttraumatic hydrocephalus (obstruction of CSF circulation or absorption)
4. Sustained posttraumatic seizures (status epilepticus)
5. Hypoventilation (causing hypercarbia → vasodilatation)
6. Systemic hypertension (HTN)
7. Venous sinus thrombosis
8. Increased muscle tone and valsalva maneuver as a result of agitation or posturing
9. Hyperemia (possibly due to vasomotor paralysis—loss of cerebral autoregulation)

14.3.3 ICU Management

Management of severe TBI aims to prevent secondary brain injury by optimizing cerebral perfusion pressure (CPP), brain tissue oxygenation, and generally avoiding the devastating effects of increased intracranial pressure (Table 14.5). There is good

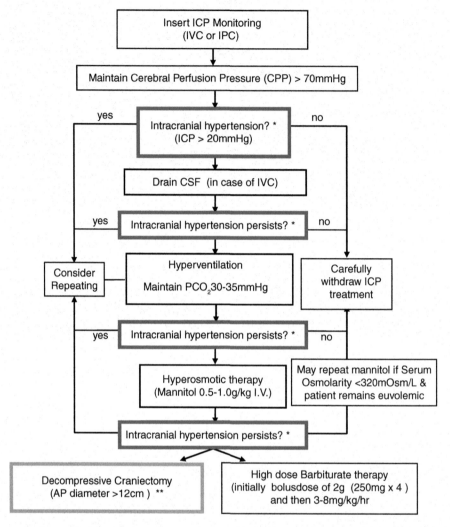

Diagram 14.2 Management of severe TBI in ICU (Modified from Bratton et al. [16] and Aarabi et al. [17])

evidence that a standardized treatment protocol system leads to improved outcome after TBI [20, 21]. An example of such an algorithm is shown in Diagram 14.2.

**Decompressive craniectomy*:

For real brain decompression (Fig. 14.7), the bone flap diameter should be 12 cm or more with a reverse C-shaped dural opening (86 ml additional volume for lateral craniectomy).

Thus, causal treatment of elevated ICP at any time is demanded [22].

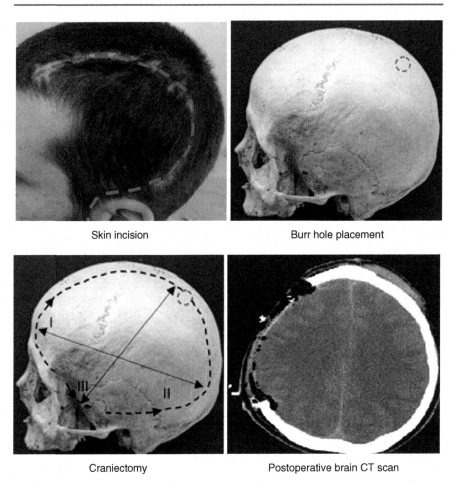

Skin incision   Burr hole placement

Craniectomy   Postoperative brain CT scan

Fig. 14.7 Decompressive lateral (left) craniectomy

14.4   Brain Swelling in Head Injury

Some degree of brain swelling is present in most TBIs and may be an important contributor the raised ICP. Three main patterns of brain swelling (Diagram 14.3) follow head injury:

1. Swelling around cerebral contusions and intracerebral hemorrhages
   Called "penumbra," a combination of vascular damage leading to BBB disruption and vasogenic edema and ischemic damage resulting in cytotoxic (intracellular) swelling. Osmotic edema may also contribute because of the high osmolality of the central necrotic areas of contusions.
2. Diffuse swelling of one cerebral hemisphere

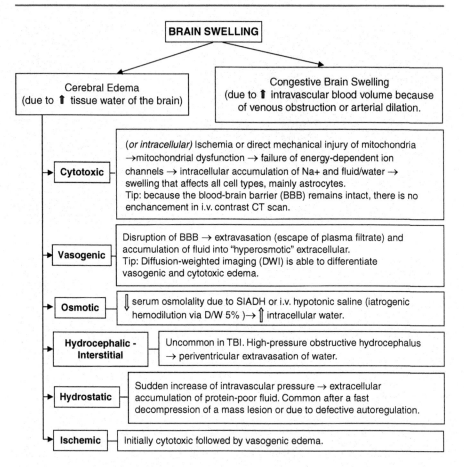

Diagram 14.3 Types of brain swelling from a pathophysiological point of view

Diffuse swelling of one cerebral hemisphere unrelated to contusion, intracerebral hemorrhage, or infarction may be associated with an ipsilateral ASDH but may also occur with larger epidural hematomas or as an isolated event.

3. Diffuse cerebral swelling of the entire brain

The reported incidence of diffuse brain swelling (Fig. 14.8) following head trauma on head CT scanning varies from 5% to 40%. Diffuse cerebral swelling occurs more frequently in children than in adults and may occur rapidly. A particularly severe catastrophic fatal form without obvious evidence of contusions or hemorrhages on neuroimaging occurs in young children. The pathogenesis of this progressive diffuse swelling unresponsive to treatment is poorly understood.

14.5   Conclusion

The primary goals of trauma resuscitation *are preventing hypoxia and hypotension, maintaining low normocarbia*, rapidly assessing *and decompressing mass lesions*, and *controlling ICP*. When possible, emergency medical technicians should begin

Fig. 14.8 Diffuse brain swelling in axial CT

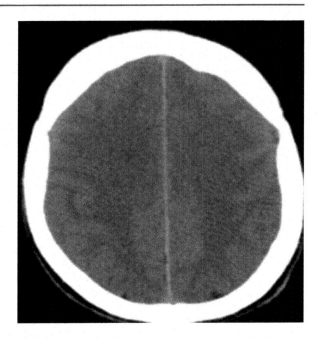

these actions in the prehospital setting. In the emergency department, the traumatologist and neurosurgeon must develop an organized approach to evaluating and treating these patients. Although some have found that life-saving decompression performed by trained general surgeons can be effective, a limited number of studies by non-neurosurgeons performing neurosurgical procedures suggest that outcome is improved if these procedures are performed by a neurosurgeon and further indicate that there is normally enough time to transfer these patients to a facility with specialists. In some very isolated communities, particularly where it is difficult to obtain neurosurgical trauma coverage, there may be an increasing role played by acute care surgeons.

References

1. Teasdale G, Jennett B. Assessment of coma and impaired consciousness. A practical scale. Lancet. 1974;2:81–4.
2. Marshall LF, Marshall SB, Klauber MR, van Berkum Clark M, Eisenberg HM, Jane JA, Luerssen TG, Marmarou A, Foulkes MA. A new classification of head injury based on computerized tomography. J Neurosurg. 1991;75:S14–20.
3. Maas AI, Hukkelhoven CW, Marshall LF, Steyerberg EW. Prediction of outcome in traumatic brain injury with computed tomographic characteristics: a comparison between the computed tomographic classification and combinations of computed tomographic predictors. Neurosurgery. 2005;57:1173–82.
4. Cowie R. Neurosurgery: principles and practice. Ann R Coll Surg Engl. 2006;88:244.
5. Bullock MR, Chesnut R, Ghajar J, Gordon D, Hartl R, Newell DW, Servadei F, Walters BC, Wilberger J. Surgical management of traumatic parenchymal lesions. Neurosurgery. 2006a;58:S2-25–46.
6. Kothari RU, Brott T, Broderick JP, Barsan WG, Sauerbeck LR, Zuccarello M, Khoury J. The ABCs of measuring intracerebral hemorrhage volumes. Stroke. 1996;27:1304–5.

7. Zee CS, Go JL. CT of head trauma. Neuroimaging Clin N Am. 1998;8:525–39.
8. Freytag E. Autopsy findings in head injuries from blunt forces. Statistical evaluation of 1,367 cases. Arch Pathol. 1963;75:402–13.
9. McKissock W, Taylor J, Bloom W, Till K. Extradural haematoma: observations on 125 cases. Lancet. 1960;276:167–72.
10. Bullock, M. R., Chesnut, R., Ghajar, J., Gordon, D., Hartl, R., Newell, D. W., Servadei, F., Walters, B. C. & Wilberger, J. E. 2006b. Surgical management of acute epidural hematomas. Neurosurgery, 58, S7–15; discussion Si–iv.
11. Bullock MR, Chesnut R, Ghajar J, Gordon D, Hartl R, Newell DW, Servadei F, Walters BC, Wilberger JE. Surgical management of acute subdural hematomas. Neurosurgery. 2006c;58:S2-16–24.
12. Bullock R, Golek J, Blake G. Traumatic intracerebral hematoma—which patients should undergo surgical evacuation? CT scan features and ICP monitoring as a basis for decision making. Surg Neurol. 1989;32:181–7.
13. Mattioli C, Beretta L, Gerevini S, Veglia F, Citerio G, Cormio M, Stocchetti N. Traumatic subarachnoid hemorrhage on the computerized tomography scan obtained at admission: a multicenter assessment of the accuracy of diagnosis and the potential impact on patient outcome. J Neurosurg. 2003;98:37–42.
14. Morris GF, Bullock R, Marshall SB, Marmarou A, Maas A, Marshall LF. Failure of the competitive N-methyl-D-aspartate antagonist Selfotel (CGS 19755) in the treatment of severe head injury: results of two phase III clinical trials. The Selfotel Investigators. J Neurosurg. 1999;91:737–43.
15. Armonda RA, Bell RS, Vo AH, Ling G, Degraba TJ, Crandall B, Ecklund J, Campbell WW. Wartime traumatic cerebral vasospasm: recent review of combat casualties. Neurosurgery. 2006;59:1215–25; discussion 1225.
16. Bratton S, Chesnut R, Ghajar J, McConnell Hammond F, Harris O, Hartl R, Manley G, Nemecek A, Newell D, Rosenthal G. Brain trauma foundation; American Association of Neurological Surgeons; Congress of Neurological Surgeons; Joint Section on Neurotrauma and Critical Care, AANS/CNS. Guidelines for the management of severe traumatic brain injury. J Neurotrauma. 2007a;24:S59–64.
17. Aarabi B, Mehta R, Eisenberg HM. Management of severe head injury. In: Moore AJ, Newell DW, editors. Neurosurgery: principles and practice. London: Springer London; 2005.
18. Bratton SL, Chestnut RM, Ghajar J, McConnell Hammond FF, Harris OA, Hartl R, Manley GT, Nemecek A, Newell DW, Rosenthal G, Schouten J, Shutter L, Timmons SD, Ullman JS, Videtta W, Wilberger JE, Wright DW. Guidelines for the management of severe traumatic brain injury. VIII. Intracranial pressure thresholds. J Neurotrauma. 2007c;24(Suppl 1):S55–8.
19. Bratton SL, Chestnut RM, Ghajar J, McConnell Hammond FF, Harris OA, Hartl R, Manley GT, Nemecek A, Newell DW, Rosenthal G, Schouten J, Shutter L, Timmons SD, Ullman JS, Videtta W, Wilberger JE, Wright DW. Guidelines for the management of severe traumatic brain injury: VII. Intracranial pressure monitoring technology. J Neurotrauma. 2007b;24(Suppl 1):S45–54.
20. Elf K, Nilsson P, Enblad P. Outcome after traumatic brain injury improved by an organized secondary insult program and standardized neurointensive care. Crit Care Med. 2002;30:2129–34.
21. Patel HC, Menon DK, Tebbs S, Hawker R, Hutchinson PJ, Kirkpatrick PJ. Specialist neurocritical care and outcome from head injury. Intensive Care Med. 2002;28:547–53.
22. Stocchetti N, Maas AI. Traumatic intracranial hypertension. N Engl J Med. 2014;370:2121–30.

Eye and Maxillofacial Injuries

15

Marilita M. Moschos

15.1 "Eye Injuries and Maxillofacial Injuries"

Maxillofacial fractures have been associated with severe morbidity, disfigurement, financial cost, as well as vision-threatening ocular injuries. The prevalence of ocular injuries, which complicate such fractures, ranges between 2.7% and 94% [1–3]. A facial fracture, especially localized at upper face and forehead, makes the presence of ocular injuries 6.7 times more frequent [2, 4]. Moreover, fractures that involve the posterior third of the orbit are associated with worse visual acuity compared to that of the anterior two-thirds of the orbit [5]. According to the literature, ocular injuries are more probable in patients with mild (41.2%) or moderate (59.5%) orbital trauma compared to those with a severe one [6]. The main causes of such fractures are road traffic accidents (64% of all cases), which usually involve motorcycles, bicycles, and heavy vehicles, followed by accidental fall and inter-personal violence related to alcohol consumption. Sports injuries are also implicated in maxillofacial fractures [4, 7, 8].

Ocular trauma, induced due to maxillofacial fractures, has been correlated to age (lower risk in children under 12 years old), sex (male dominance), pattern, and position of maxillofacial fractures and etiology of damage [4]. They are estimated to be 7% of all body injuries and 10–15% of eye diseases [9]. The consequent impairment of vision usually affects occupational and social functions. Vision loss and blindness is apparent in 0.32–10.8% of facial fractures [10, 11].

The major mechanisms of visual impairment involve direct injury to the globe, direct or indirect damage on optic nerve, systemic perfusion disturbances, and loss of eye integrity [11, 12]. Subsequent to the management of life-threatening

M. M. Moschos (✉)
Ophthalmology, National and Kapodistrian University of Athens and in the General Hospital of Athens "Gennimatas", Athens, Greece

problems, a complete ocular examination is mandatory. The latter should include visual acuity measurements (if the patient's general health permits this), tests of pupillary reactions and ocular movements, evaluation of globe integrity, and fundus examination.

The disturbances on patients' emotional and financial status, the impairment in quality of their life, and the consequent socioeconomic problems explain the importance of both effective treatment and prolepsis [9, 13, 14]. The collaboration of multiple specialties, including ophthalmology, otolaryngology, neurology, plastic surgery, trauma surgery, and oral surgery, are needed to evaluate and treat patients with maxillofacial fractures [6, 15]. The former would be facilitated by a standardized classification, such as Birmingham eye trauma terminology system (BETTS) (Fig. 15.1). The definitions of ocular injuries are presented below:

1. Closed injury is commonly due to blunt trauma, leaving the corneo-scleral wall of the globe intact.
2. Contusion is a closed injury due to blunt trauma and the damage can be present at the site of impact or at a distant site.
3. Lamellar laceration is a partial-thickness wound caused by a sharp object.
4. Open injury involves a full-thickness wound of the corneo-scleral wall.
5. Rupture is a full-thickness wound caused by blunt trauma, observed at the weakest point of the globe (not always at the site of the impact).
6. Laceration involves a full-thickness wound caused by a sharp object at the site of the impact.
7. Penetration presents a single full-thickness injury, usually caused by a sharp object, without an exit wound. It may be associated with intraocular presence of a foreign body.
8. Perforation consists of two full-thickness wounds, being originated from the entry and the exit of a missile.

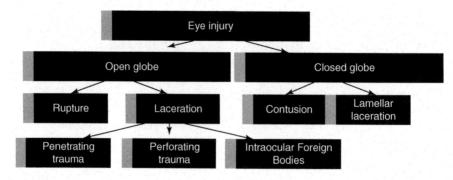

Fig. 15.1 The Birmingham eye trauma terminology system (BETTS)

15.2   Closed-Globe Ocular Injuries

The most common cause of closed trauma is the blunt one, which results in antero-posterior compression, expansion in the equatorial plane, posterior displacement of the lens–iris diaphragm, rupture of ocular tissues, and severe increase in intraocular pressure. Although a blow-out fracture of the orbit (typically inferiorly into the maxillary sinus) usually protects the globe, 30 per cent of the cases present ruptured globe combined with orbital fracture [13]. Hypahema and retinal detachment seem to be the most common manifestations of the anterior and posterior segment, respectively. The prognosis for visual acuity has been related to retinal and choroid lesions, along with optic nerve damage. The latter involves avulsion of the optic nerve, traumatic optic neuropathy, and optic atrophy [16].

The main causes of blunt ocular trauma are squash balls, elastic luggage straps, and champagne corks. Golf-related ocular injuries account for 1.5–5.6% of sports-induced ocular trauma [17, 18]. The incidence of sports-related ocular trauma in children is estimated to be 11–18% of cases. The most common sports related to such trauma are cycling, football, tennis, trampolining, fishing, and swimming. Children between 10–14 years old and boys are at high risk, due to the competitive nature of activities [19]. Although sports are a main cause of ocular damage among children, the most injuries seem to take place within the house (48% of all cases) [20]. Education and use of eye protection during sports are mandatory for preventing such accidents, which are implicated in 50% of uniocular blindness in children [19, 20]. High explosive and fragmentation power are the main cause of war-related ocular injuries. Closed-globe injuries are less common (20–43% of cases) than the open-globe ones (29.6–80% of cases), exhibiting better anatomical and visual outcome and treatment is mandatory [21, 22].

15.2.1 Anterior Segment

Corneal abrasion is a default of the epithelium, which is diagnosed with fluorescein staining under blue light vision (Figs. 15.2 and 15.3). The symptoms include impaired vision, pain, photophobia, tearing, and foreign body sensation. Visual acuity is severely diminished, if the trauma is extended over the papillary area. The treatment involves an antibiotic ointment and topical cycloplegia. The former lubricates the eye surface and protects the trauma from any secondary infection, whereas the latter reduces the pain. The use of pressure patching does not seem beneficial anymore, because it does not promote healing or improve rest symptoms [11–13]. *Acute corneal edema* is subsequent to focal or diffuse dysfunction of corneal epithelium, usually associated with folds in Descement membrane and stromal thickening. The latter recesses spontaneously [23–25].

Hyphema characterizes the hemorrhage into the anterior chamber, coming from iris or ciliary body (Fig. 15.4). Red blood cells form an inferior fluid level, which

Fig. 15.2 Corneal
abrasion observed with
fluorescein staining

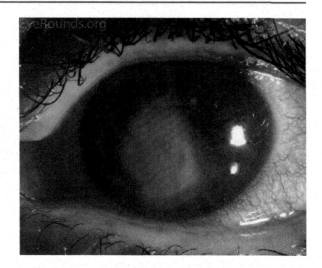

Fig. 15.3 Corneal
abrasion stained with
fluorescein under cobalt
blue light

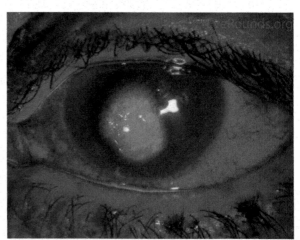

Fig. 15.4 Traumatic
hyphaema with inferior
level of blood in
anterior chamber

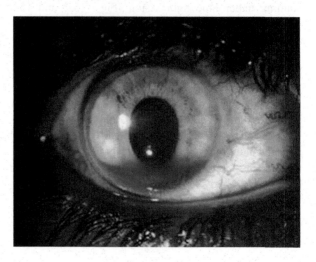

must be measured and evaluated. The lysis and retraction of the fibrin clot, which is present in the bleeding vessel, are implicated in rebleeding. The latter occurs within 2–5 days post-traumatically, varying in incidence. The consequent complications involve glaucoma, iridocorneal angle recession, iridodialysis, optic atrophy, amblyopia, corneal blood staining (when the hyphaema is prolonged), optic atrophy, and peripheral anterior synechia [13, 26]. Reading disability related to accommodative impairment, greater than 2.5 dioptres, has also been observed in post-traumatic hyphema [27].

The initial management includes bed rest with 30° head elevation for 4 days to prevent rebleeding, discontinuation of electives anticoagulants, topical mydriatics, and steroids for 2 weeks. Atropine and steroids are installed daily to prevent further hemorrhage and treat associated uveitis. The prevalence of secondary hemorrhage can be reduced by the administration of systemic antifibrinolytic agents, including E-aminocaproic and tranexamic acid, which is 8–10 times more potent than the former. Tranexamic acid prevents plasminogen and plasmin from fibrin binding, minimizing the chances for clot lysis. The common dose is 25 mg/kg three times a day, whereas the possible side effects involve muscle cramps conjunctival suffusion, nasal congestion, headache, rash, pruritus, dyspnea, cardiac arrhythmias, systemic hypotension, and gastrointestinal disturbances. Recently, the topical administration of 5% solution of tranexamic acid has been suggested as treatment for traumatic hyphaema [13, 26]. The incidence of raised intraocular pressure is estimated to be 30% of cases, due to angle damage. Glaucoma medications are used to lower the increased pressure [13]. The elevation of intraocular pressure in the fellow eye, related to neuronal control between the two eyes, has also been reported [28]. Intracameral injection of tissue plasminogen activator (tPA) has also been associated with lower incidence of secondary hemorrhage, decrease in intraocular pressure, and diminish of complications [29]. Surgical wash-out of the anterior chamber is rarely used.

Pupil damage leads to miosis, which can be accompanied by pigmen deposits on the anterior lens capsule (Vossius ring), or mydriasis, usually permanent due to trauma to the iris sphincter. The latter are developed as pupillary tears iridocorneal angle recession and trabecular meshwork damage, which are associated with secondary glaucoma (7–9% of cases), as it has been already referred. Annually, follow-up is demanded. The dehiscence of the iris root from the ciliary body is another possible lesion, which is known as *iridodialysis*. Patients suffer from uniocular diplopia, unless the lesion is covered by the upper lid. The "D" formation of the pupil is common and the treatment is surgical [13]. The traumatic detachment of the ciliary body from the sclera spur is called *cyclodialysis*. The symptoms include hypotony, shallow anterior chamber, abnormal architecture of anterior segment, cataract, retinal and choroidal folds, hypotony maculopathy, and decreased visual acuity. The diagnosis is based on gonioscopy, anterior segment ultrasound biomicroscopy (UBM) (Fig. 15.5), and optical coherence tomography (OCT). Conservative treatment involves administration of topical atropine for 6–8 weeks, which leads to resolution. The surgical option combines cyclopexy, phacoemulsification, and transcleral Cionni ring [30, 31].

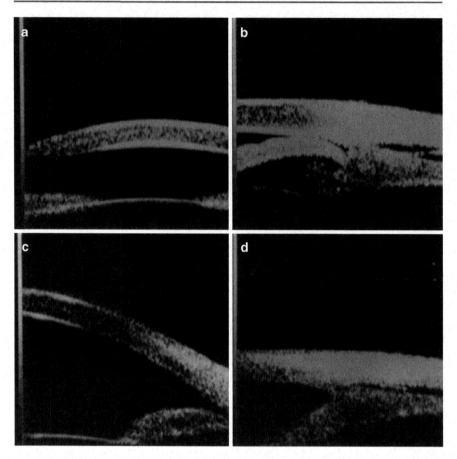

Fig. 15.5. UBM of an eye with cyclodialysis. (**a**) The anterior chamber is shallow 1 day after blunt ocular injury. (**b**) Ciliary effusion with anterior rotation, thickening of the ciliary processes, and iris bombe are noted. After 7 days, (**c**) a deeper anterior chamber and (**d**) partial resolution of the subciliary fluid are noted

Cataract is developed due to damage of the lens fibers and capsule, resulting in aqueous humor input and opacification. The presentation of opacifications along the anterior lens capsule form the Vossius ring, whereas a flower-shaped formation occurs within the posterior capsule. The treatment is surgical. *Subluxation* occurs when the zonular support is disturbed and the lens is dislocated into the anterior or posterior (when the lens capsule is intact) chamber (Fig. 15.6). Clinical findings include iridodonesis (tremble on ocular movements), uniocular diplopia, and lenticular astigmatism. The location of the lens can be restored with mydriasis, supine position of the patient and corneal indentation [13].

Fig. 15.6 Traumatic lens dislocation

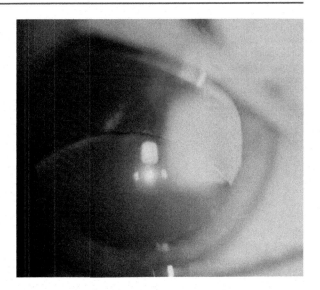

15.2.2 Vitreoretinal and Optic Nerve Damages

The presence of *vitreous hemorrhage* due to closed-globe trauma has been associated with severe pathologies of anterior segment, including hyphema, traumatic cataract, and lens dislocation, as well as posterior segment damages. The latter usually involve retinal tears and detachment, proliferative vitreoretinopathy (PVR), submacular hemorrhage, whereas macular hole, choroidal rapture, retinal dialysis, and vessels occlusion are less common complications. Early vitrectomy is indicated to prevent poor visual outcome, related to posterior segment pathologies [32]. When vitreous hemorrhage is developed with subarachnoid or subdural bleeding is known as Terson's syndrome. The prognosis is usually good and the visual acuity is rehabilitated, when the intraocular hemorrhage has been absorbed.

Berlin's edema or commotion retina is a frequent pathology subsequent to closed globe blunt ocular trauma. The transmission of trust wave to the retina is probably responsible for severe vision loss and the development of the macular whitening thickening, which can be accompanied by retinal hemorrhages [33]. Prognosis is related to the severity and location of lesions; if the latter are situated in the retinal periphery, they are not usually diagnosed. Spontaneous recession can also occur [34].Vision loss has been associated with damage or necrosis of photoreceptors [35]. Not treatment is effective. The development of peripheral retinal cracks needs to be treated with laser or cryopexy [36]. *Choroidal ruptures* can be occurred after severe trauma, which are located as yellowish crescent-shaped lesions (Fig. 15.7). They can be direct, situated anteriorly at the site of the impact and parallel to the ora serrata, or indirect, which are located at the opposite site [34, 37, 38]. If the situation is complicated with choroidal neovascularization can lead to exudative maculopathy [39].

Fig. 15.7 Choroidal macular rupture, complicated with secondary epiretinal membrane formation (arrows) and retinal traction (arrowheads)

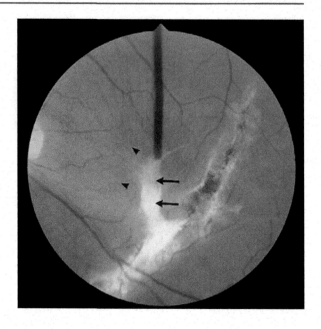

Optic neuropathy can be subsequent to blunt or penetrating orbital trauma due to direct damage from sharp objects (hemorrhage or compression) or transmission wave. The visual prognosis is poor, associated with optic nerve atrophy [40].

15.3 Open-Globe Ocular Injuries

Open-globe injuries are the leading cause of visual loss for working individuals and children. The prevalence among adolescents is estimated to be around 19.8% whereas pediatric patients account for 8–14% of all cases [41–44]. The prognosis of penetrating injuries has been associated with advanced age, poor initial visual acuity, severity of trauma and development of vitreous hemorrhage, retinal detachment, or PVR [9, 44]. The latter is sequel of retinal detachment and exhibits high prevalence after trauma, accessing the 43%, 21%, 15%, and 11% of cases in perforation, rupture, penetration, and presence of intraocular foreign body, respectively [44].

Scleral lacerations can be developed anterior or posterior. The former have been associated with iridociliary prolapse and vitreous incarceration, which can lead to fibrous proliferation and consequent retinal detachment. The rehabilitation of uveal tissue and vitreous are mandatory for the management of such trauma. Posterior sclera lacerations have poorer prognosis, compared to anterior ones, and are complicated with retinal breaks.

The severity and management of *corneal open injuries* depend on the extent of the wound as well as the involvement of iris or lens. Small wounds, which leave intact the anterior chamber, can be spontaneously healed or using a soft contact lens. Larger corneal traumas, combined with shallow or flat anterior chamber, are treated with sutures. Iris prolapsed is managed with abscission, whereas phacoemulsification is needed in case of lenticular trauma. The prevalence of *intraocular pressure elevation or traumatic glaucoma* after open-globe injury is estimated to be 32.4% and 11%, respectively. Such complications have been related to trabecular meshwork damage, hyphema, lenticular damage, iris inflammation, peripheral anterior synechiae, vitreous hemorrhage, and topical steroid administration [45]. A wound size larger than 6 mm has been correlated to post-traumatic elevation of intraocular pressure [46].

Optic nerve avulsion is a rare sequel of extreme rotation or anterior displacement of the globe. It is related to entrance of an object between the glob and the orbit. There is no treatment and the prognosis depends on the severity of avulsion (partial or complete). *Isolated third nerve palsy* due to penetrating trauma has also been reported. Complete recession of subsequent anisocoria, ptosis, and binocular diplopia was noted [47].

Intraocular foreign bodies appear increased incidence among open-globe injuries, estimated to be 18 PVR 41% of all cases [48–50]. The vast majority of them remain in the posterior segment of the eye [51]. Organic materials are less tolerated then the inorganic ones, including glass, stone, and plastic. However, iron, copper, and lead should urgently be removed due to their toxicity [52, 53]. The entrance of the foreign bodies is usually through the cornea (65%), while sclera (25%) and limbus (10%) are less frequent points of penetration [54]. They are usually detected in the posterior segment (58–88%), but they can also be found in anterior chamber (10–15%) and lens (2–8%) [50]. Their complications are related to their direct effect or can be sequel to chemical reactions of metals, such iron and copper. *Siderosis bulbi* characterizes the consequences of iron deposition, involving iris eterochromia, mydriasis, lens opacification, glaucoma, and retinal pigmentary lesions [55, 56]. Chalcosis, which is consequence of copper presence in the globe, may be apparent as Kayser-Fleischer ring in the cornea (depositions within the Descement membrane), refractile particles in the anterior chamber or iris, or even as a sunflower cataract [57]. The diagnosis is based on detailed history, ophthalmological examination, and imaging with plain X-ray computed tomography (CT), ultrasonography, B-scan, and magnetic resonance imaging (MRI) [51, 58, 59].

Early removal predicts the visual outcome, which has been also associated with the size of the foreign body (poor vision if it is over 3 mm) and the ocular lesions [60]. Vision-threatening complications include endophthalmitis (2.1–17%), retinal detachment, PVR, and sympathetic ophthalmia [51, 60]. Increasing pain after injury stabilization, progressive visual loss, hypopyon, vitritis, lid edema, conjunctival and corneal edema, fibrous papillary membranes, and loss of red reflex are signs of endophthalmitis [61–63]. The microorganisms implicated in endophthalmitis are mainly gram-positive, including coagulasenegative Staphylococci, which includes *Staphylococcus* epidermis, *Streptococcus* species, *Bacillus* species, and *Staphylococcus aureus*. However, gram-negative microbes and fungal can be also detected in post-traumatic endophthalmitis [61, 62, 64]. Intravenous antibiotics, culture of the wound, and surgical removal of the foreign body are indicated for the management of intraocular bodies. The prevalence of postoperative retinal detachment is estimated to be between 6% and 40%, whereas it has been associated to foreign bodies over 4 mm [51, 65]. Both retinal detachment and PVR seem to be dependent on the size of intraocular foreign body [51].

In conclusion, the visual prognosis of open-globe injuries depends on the type and extent of wound, early diagnosis and management, as well as postoperative follow-up. In addition, age, initial visual acuity, lens damage, hyphema, vitreous hemorrhage, retinal detachment, presence of relative afferent pupillary defect (RAPD) and type of intraocular foreign body play a role in the visual prognosis of injuries [66–69].

15.4   Ocular Manifestations Related to Maxillofacial Injuries

Periorbital bruise is a common sign of direct trauma, due to blood effusion via the subcutaneous tissue. Although the contusion remains for several weeks, no treatment is necessary. *Subconjunctival ecchymosis* and *conjunctival edema* (chemosis) are additional signs of such fractures (Fig. 15.8). Edema of upper eyelid can lead to *ptosis* (mechanic ptosis), which may be also sequel of traumatic nerve paresis. Mechanical entrapment or paresis of extraocular muscles can restrict ocular movements. In this case, the force duction test can discriminate mechanical causes of *diplopia* from neurogenic disorders. Diplopia is the most frequent clinical sign in patients with lateral wall fractures [3]. Inferior and posterior displacement of zygoma induces *enopthalmos*, whereas any medial dislocation may lead to *exopthalmos* [3, 8, 12]. The increase in inter-canthal distance (over 38.7 mm in men and over 37.5 mm in women) characterizes the *traumatic telecanthus*, related to disruption of medial canthal ligament [8]. *Le fort fractures* are manifested with panda facies and bilateral raccoon eyes, chemosis, battles sign (bruising over the mastoid process), ecchymosis of the maxillary vestibule, mobile maxilla and nasal bridge, palatal laceration, cerebrospinal fluid rhinorrhea, and otorrhoea. Plain X-rays and CT are needed for the diagnosis [70]. Proptosis is apparent in up to 3% of major trauma patients and is caused by herniated tissue, orbital edema, and retrobulbar hemorrhage [71].

Besides open- and closed-globe injuries, which have been already described, the main causes of vision loss in maxillofacial fractures include retrobulbar hemorrhage, traumatic optic neuropathy, loss of eyelid integrity, and chemical injury [12].

Retrobulbar hemorrhage is usually clinically diagnosed, based on decreased visual acuity, pain, ptosis, proptosis, RAPD, progressive ophthalmoplegia, eyelid

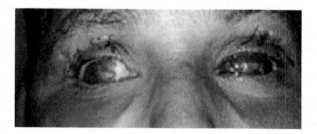

Fig. 15.8 Bilateral upper lid tear with circumorbital ecchymosis. Coexistent sub-conjunctival haemorrhage on right eye and chemosis on left eye

and conjunctival edema, and increased intraocular pressure [12, 70–72]. Retinal lesions can include pulsations of the central retina artery and choroidal folds [71]. The trauma is usually located at orbitozygomatic area. It is an emergency, given that irreversible damage can occur, if ischemia lasts over 60 min [12]. The management includes immediate surgical decompression along with the intravenous administration of mannitol (200 ml of solution 20% or 1 g/kg), acetazolamide (250–500 mg), and dexamethasone (4 mg/kg bolus and 2 mg/kg six hourly for 24 h). The medical treatment should be started before surgery and continued until the globe pressure is rehabilitated [12, 70, 71].

Traumatic optic neuropathy accounts for 0.5–6% of closed head injuries. Stretching, contusion, or shearing of the optic nerve are the main causes of such damage, inducing inflammatory and neurological mediators. The latter result in vasospasm and vaso-occlusion, edema and necrosis, mechanisms which interpret the permanent visual loss in 50% of the cases. Normal eye with reduced visual acuity and RAPD are signs of optic nerve damage, whereas CT can contribute to diagnosis [2, 12]. The immediate administration of intravenous methylprednisolone is indicated to eliminate edema and inflammation. The loading dose is 30 mg/kg over 30 min, followed by 15 mg/kg 6 hourly over 2 days and then an oral dose of 80 mg (progressive reduction 20 mg every 3 days) [12].

Chemical injuries are diagnosed in 10% of ocular trauma and are caused by substances exhibiting different pH from the ocular one (ocular pH = 7.4). The majority of chemicals are alkalis, which penetrate lipid membranes and result in greater lesions than acids. Necrosis of ocular surface is developed, when conjunctival endothelium and cornea are abrupted. The presence of ischemia in more than three quarters of the limbal induces visual loss, corneal scarring and vascularization, cataract, flaucoma, and uveitis. Visual rehabilitation can be achieved by limbal stem cell and corneal transplantation [12].

Traumatic globe avulsion characterizes the dislocation of the globe out of its normal anatomical position [73]. It is an extremely rare condition, followed by severe trauma to the head or orbit, which are complicated with multiple facial and orbital fractures [73, 74]. Avulsion of the globe (avulsio bulbi) can be classified as a single avulsion of the optic nerve (avulsio incompleta) or combined with disruption of the extraocular muscles (avulsio completa), which may cause total luxation of the ocular bulbus [74]. They are observed after traffic accidents, firearm projectiles, or during sports accidents. Three possible mechanisms of traumatic globe avulsion have been described: (1) anterior propulsion of the globe caused by the entrance of an elongated object into the medial orbit; (2) anterior luxation of the globe induced by a wedge-shaped object; and (3) optic nerve direct transection by a penetrating object [75, 76]. Traumatic globe dislocation into the paranasal sinuses is an extremely rare condition, reported in the literature (24 cases), present in patients mostly involved in traffic accidents (42% of the cases). Among paranasal sinuses, the maxillary one was the most affected (87.5%), followed by ethmoid sinus (12.5%) [77].

The anatomic restoration of the orbit and globe is mandatory, although primary enucleation has also been suggested. The latter is used to avoid sympathetic opthalmia, which develops in 3–5% of all penetrating trauma. It is caused when the uveal pigment of the disrupted globe enters into contact with the immune system, resulting in immunological reaction against the contralateral eye [74]. The enucleation technique involves the isolation of all extraocular muscles, cleaning and debridement of the orbit, cultures taking and fitting of an orbital implant [75]. However, repositioning of the globe is related to cosmetic and psychological benefits for the patients, while favoring children's facial bone development [74]. Overall, the anatomic restoration of the orbit and globe is necessary for the protection of optic nerve and visual rehabilitation. Direct traction of the globe is the surgical technique used in the majority of the cases (50% of the cases), but manual repositioning of the globe via trans-maxillary approach has also been applied (21% of the cases). The main materials used for the reconstruction of orbital wall are titanium mesh, silicone sheets, porous polyethylene, and autogenous bone [77]. Titanium meshes are most popular due to their properties, which include small thickness, easy fitting to the orbital wall, long-term maintenance of its shape, and resistance to corrosion, whereas they can be sterilized [3].

15.5 Conclusions

The increased traffic accidents and sports injuries, associated with modern lifestyle, reflect the significance of maxillofacial fractures. The latter have indisputably severe physical, physiological, and socio-economic implications. Vision loss and blindness, which is apparent in 0.32–10.8% of facial fractures, definitely impair occupational and social functions. The collaboration of multiple specialties, including ophthalmology, otolaryngology, neurology, plastic surgery, trauma surgery, and oral surgery, is needed to evaluate and treat such patients. As soon life-threatening problems have been managed, a complete ocular examination is mandatory. The latter should include visual acuity measurements (if the patient's general health permits this), tests of pupillary reactions and ocular movements, evaluation of globe integrity, and fundus examination. Imaging techniques are also necessary. Ophthalmologists and maxillofacial surgeons should cooperate to restore orbital wall and treat ocular injuries. Immediate treatment can protect the globe from permanent lesions and improve the visual prognosis.

References

1. Patil SG, Kotwal IA, Joshi U, Allurkar S, Thakur N, Aftab A. Ophthalmological evaluation by a maxillofacial surgeon and an ophthalmologist in assessing the damage to the orbital contents in midfacial fractures: a prospective study. J Maxillofac Oral Surg. 2016;15(3):328–35. PubMed PMID: 27752202; PubMed Central PMCID: PMC5048320.
2. Jamal BT, Pfahler SM, Lane KA, Bilyk JR, Pribitkin EA, Diecidue RJ, Taub DI. Ophthalmic injuries in patients with zygomaticomaxillary complex fractures requiring surgical repair. J Oral Maxillofac Surg. 2009;67(5):986–9. https://doi.org/10.1016/j.joms.2008.12.035. PubMed PMID: 19375007.

3. Sales PHDH, Rocha SSD, Rodrigues PHC, Cetira Filho EL, Silva LF, Mello MJR. Surgical treatment of posttraumatic ophthalmoplegia through the reconstruction of the lateral orbital wall. J Craniofac Surg. 2017;28(5):e444–6. https://doi.org/10.1097/SCS.0000000000003634. PubMed PMID: 28538072.
4. Zhou HH, Liu Q, Yang RT, Li Z, Li ZB. Ocular trauma in patients with maxillofacial fractures. J Craniofac Surg. 2014;25(2):519–23. https://doi.org/10.1097/SCS.0000000000000683. PubMed PMID: 24561369.
5. Tsai HH, Jeng SF, Lin TS, Kueh NS, Hsieh CH. Predictive value of computed tomography in visual outcomes in indirect traumatic optic neuropathy complicated with periorbital facial bone fractures. Clin Neurol Neurosurg. 2005;107:200–6.
6. Kreidl KO, Kim DY, Mansour SE. Prevalence of significant intraocular sequelae in blunt orbital trauma. Am J Emerg Med. 2003;21:525–8.
7. Septa D, Newaskar VP, Agrawal D, Tibra S. Etiology, incidence and patterns of mid face fractures and associated ocular injuries. J Maxillofac Oral Surg. 2014;13(2):115–9. https://doi.org/10.1007/s12663-012-0452-9. PubMed PMID: 24822001; PubMed Central PMCID: PMC4016399.
8. Rajkumar GC, Ashwin DP, Singh R, Prashanth R, Rudresh KB. Ocular injuries associated with midface fractures: a 5 year survey. J Maxillofac Oral Surg. 2015;14(4):925–9. https://doi.org/10.1007/s12663-015-0778-1. PubMed PMID: 26604465; PubMed Central PMCID: PMC4648769.
9. Yüksel H, Türkcü FM, Çınar Y, Cingü AK, Sahin A, Sahin M, Özkurt Z, Murat M, Çaça I. Etiology and prognosis of penetrating eye injuries in geriatric patients in the Southeastern region of Anatolia Turkey. Ulus Travma Acil Cerrahi Derg. 2014;20(4):253–7. https://doi.org/10.5505/tjtes.2014.71597. PubMed PMID: 25135019.
10. Magarakis M, Mundinger GS, Kelamis JA, Dorafshar AH, Bojovic B, Rodriguez ED. Ocular injury, visual impairment, and blindness associated with facial fractures: a systematic literature review. Plast Reconstr Surg. 2012;129(1):227–33. https://doi.org/10.1097/PRS.0b013e3182362a6d. Review. PubMed: 21915081.
11. Andrews BT, Jackson AS, Nazir N, Hromas A, Sokol JA, Thurston TE. Orbit fractures: identifying patient factors indicating high risk for ocular and periocular injury. Laryngoscope. 2016;126(Suppl 4):S5–11. https://doi.org/10.1002/lary.25805. PubMed PMID: 26690301.
12. Perry M, Dancey A, Mireskandari K, Oakley P, Davies S, Cameron M. Emergency care in facial trauma—a maxillofacial and ophthalmic perspective. Injury. 2005;36(8):875–96. Review. PubMed PMID: 16023907.
13. Scott R. The injured eye. Philos Trans R Soc Lond Ser B Biol Sci. 2011;366(1562):251–60. https://doi.org/10.1098/rstb.2010.0234. Review. PubMed PMID: 21149360; PubMed Central PMCID: PMC3013431.
14. Kuhn F, Morris R, Witherspoon CD, Heimann K, Jeffers JB, Treister G. A standardized classification of ocular trauma. Ophthalmology. 1996;103:240–3. https://doi.org/10.1007/BF00190717.
15. Kulkarni A, Chandrasala S, Nimbeni B, Vishnudas P, Dev A. An interesting case of penetrating craniofacial trauma involving a wooden stick. J Clin Diagn Res. 2016;10(4):ZD01–3. https://doi.org/10.7860/JCDR/2016/16916.7571. PubMed PMID: 27190963; PubMed Central PMCID: PMC4866261.
16. Feng K, Ma ZZ. Clinical features, anatomical and visual outcomes, and prognostic factors in closed globe injuries presenting with no light perception: Eye Injury Vitrectomy Study. Acta Ophthalmol. 2012;90(6):e493–4. https://doi.org/10.1111/j.1755-3768.2011.02325.x. PubMed PMID: 22151827.
17. Peate WF. Work-related eye injuries and illnesses. Am Fam Physician. 2007;75(7):1017–22. Review. PubMed PMID: 17427615.
18. Park SJ, Park KH, Heo JW, Woo SJ. Visual and anatomic outcomes of golf ball-related ocular injuries. Eye (Lond). 2014;28(3):312–7. https://doi.org/10.1038/eye.2013.283. PubMed PMID: 24384962; PubMed Central PMCID: PMC3965816.

19. Hoskin AK, Yardley AM, Hanman K, Lam G, Mackey DA. Sports-related eye and adnexal injuries in the Western Australian paediatric population. Acta Ophthalmol. 2016;94(6):e407–10. https://doi.org/10.1111/aos.12911. PubMed PMID: 26647756.
20. Kadappu S, Silveira S, Martin F. Aetiology and outcome of open and closed globe eye injuries in children. Clin Exp Ophthalmol. 2013;41(5):427–34. https://doi.org/10.1111/ceo.12034. PubMed PMID: 23145496.
21. Islam QU, Ishaq M, Yaqub A, Saeed MK. Functional and anatomical outcome in closed globe combat ocular injuries. J Pak Med Assoc. 2016;66(12):1582–6. PubMed PMID: 28179694.
22. Cockerham GC, Lemke S, Rice TA, Wang G, Glynn-Milley C, Zumhagen L, Cockerham KP. Closed-globe injuries of the ocular surface associated with combat blast exposure. Ophthalmology. 2014;121(11):2165–72. https://doi.org/10.1016/j.ophtha.2014.06.009. PubMed PMID: 25124272.
23. Lim CH, Turner A, Lim BX. Patching for corneal abrasion. Cochrane Database Syst Rev. 2016;7:CD004764. https://doi.org/10.1002/14651858.CD004764.pub3. Review. PubMed PMID: 27457359.
24. Campanile TM, St Clair DA, Benaim M. The evaluation of eye patching in the treatment of traumatic corneal epithelial defects. J Emerg Med. 1997;15(6):769–74. PubMed PMID: 9404791.
25. Kaiser PK. A comparison of pressure patching versus no patching for corneal abrasions due to trauma or foreign body removal. Corneal Abrasion Patching Study Group. Ophthalmology. 1995;102(12):1936–42. PubMed PMID: 9098299.
26. Jahadi Hosseini SH, Khalili MR, Motallebi M. Comparison between topical and oral tranexamic acid in management of traumatic hyphema. Iran J Med Sci. 2014;39(2 Suppl):178–83. PubMed PMID: 24753640; PubMed Central PMCID: PMC3993038.
27. Thériault FA, Pearce WG. Incidence of accommodative impairment following traumatic hyphema. Can J Ophthalmol. 1993;28(6):263–5. PubMed PMID: 8299050.
28. Anid G, Powell RG, Elkington AR. Postural response of intraocular pressure following traumatic hyphaema. Br J Ophthalmol. 1985;69(8):576–9. PubMed PMID:4016055; PubMed Central PMCID: PMC1040682.
29. Laatikainen L, Mattila J. The use of tissue plasminogen activator in post-traumatic total hyphaema. Graefes Arch Clin Exp Ophthalmol. 1996;234(1):67–8. PubMed PMID: 8750854.
30. Kluś A, Kosatka M, Kozera M, Rękas M. Surgical reconstruction of traumatic ciliary body dialysis: a case report. J Med Case Rep. 2017;11(1):22. https://doi.org/10.1186/s13256-016-1170-6. PubMed PMID: 28110637; PubMed Central PMCID: PMC5256542.
31. Chen HC, Chang SH, Chen SN, Ho JD. Ciliary effusion complicates blunt ocular trauma. Eye (Lond). 2003;17(7):835–6. PubMed PMID: 14528246.
32. Yeung L, Chen TL, Kuo YH, Chao AN, Wu WC, Chen KJ, Hwang YS, Chen Y, Lai CC. Severe vitreous hemorrhage associated with closed-globe injury. Graefes Arch Clin Exp Ophthalmol. 2006;244(1):52–7. Epub 2005 Jul 26. PubMed PMID: 16044322.
33. Flatter JA, Cooper RF, Dubow MJ, Pinhas A, Singh RS, Kapur R, Shah N, Walsh RD, Hong SH, Weinberg DV, Stepien KE, Wirostko WJ, Robison S, Dubra A, Rosen RB, Connor TB Jr, Carroll J. Outer retinal structure after closed-globe blunt ocular trauma. Retina. 2014;34(10):2133–46. https://doi.org/10.1097/IAE.0000000000000169. PubMed PMID: 24752010; PubMed Central PMCID: PMC4175068.
34. Gass JDM. Stereoscopic atlas of macular diseases: diagnosis and treatment. 4th ed. St. Louis: CV Mosby; 1997. p. 206–8. and 737–74.
35. Sipperley JO, Quigley HA, Gass DM. Traumatic retinopathy in primates. The explanation of commotio retinae. Arch Ophthalmol. 1978;96(12):2267–73. PubMed PMID: 718521.
36. Lean JS. Diagnosis and treatment of peripheral retinal lesions. In: Freeman WR, editor. Practical atlas of retinal disease and therapy. New York: Raven Press; 1993. p. 211–20.
37. Levin DB, Bell DK. Traumatic retinal hemorrhages with angioid streaks. Arch Ophthalmol. 1977;95(6):1072–3. PubMed PMID: 869751.
38. Baltatzis S, Ladas ID, Panagiotidis D, Theodossiadis GP. Multiple posttraumatic choroidal ruptures obscured by hemorrhage: imaging with indocyanine green angiography. Retina. 1997;17(4):352–4. PubMed PMID: 9279955.

39. Hart CD, Raistrick R. Indirect choroidal tears and late onset serosanguinous maculopathies. Graefes Arch Clin Exp Ophthalmol. 1982;218(4):206–10. PubMed PMID:7084698.
40. Nazir SA, Westfall CT, Chacko JG, Phillips PH, Stack BC Jr. Visual recovery after direct traumatic optic neuropathy. Am J Otolaryngol. 2010;31(3):193–4. https://doi.org/10.1016/j.amjoto.2008.11.015. PubMed PMID: 20015731.
41. Yüksel H, Türkcü FM, Ahin M, Cinar Y, Cingü AK, Ozkurt Z, Bez Y, Caça H. Vision-related quality of life in patients after ocular penetrating injuries. Arq Bras Oftalmol. 2014;77(2):95–8. PubMed PMID: 25076473.
42. Page RD, Gupta SK, Jenkins TL, Karcioglu ZA. Risk factors for poor outcomes in patients with open-globe injuries. Clin Ophthalmol. 2016;10:1461–6. https://doi.org/10.2147/OPTH.S108901. eCollection 2016. PubMed PMID: 27536059; PubMed Central PMCID: PMC4975575.
43. Malla G, Bhandari R, Gupta PP, Giri R. Penetrating orbit injury: challenge to emergency medicine. BMC Res Notes. 2013;6:493. https://doi.org/10.1186/1756-0500-6-493. PubMed PMID: 24283618; PubMed Central PMCID: PMC4222094.
44. Morescalchi F, Duse S, Gambicorti E, Romano MR, Costagliola C, Semeraro F. Proliferative vitreoretinopathy after eye injuries: an overexpression of growth factors and cytokines leading to a retinal keloid. Mediat Inflamm. 2013;2013:269787. https://doi.org/10.1155/2013/269787. Review. PubMed PMID: 24198445; PubMed Central PMCID: PMC3806231.
45. Bojikian KD, Stein AL, Slabaugh MA, Chen PP. Incidence and risk factors for traumatic intraocular pressure elevation and traumatic glaucoma after open-globe injury. Eye (Lond). 2015;29(12):1579–84. https://doi.org/10.1038/eye.2015.173. PubMed PMID: 26381097; PubMed Central PMCID: PMC5129804.
46. Acar U, Yıldız EH, Ergintürk Acar D, Altıparmak UE, Yalnız Akkaya Z, Burcu A, Unlü N. Posttraumatic intraocular pressure elevation and associated factors in patients with zone I open globe injuries. Ulus Travma Acil Cerrahi Derg. 2013;19(2):115–8. https://doi.org/10.5505/tjtes.2013.51437. PubMed PMID: 23599193.
47. Story C, Patterson M, McWilliams W, Markowitz BBA. Rare case of penetrating trauma resulting in isolated third nerve palsy. Neuroophthalmology. 2016;40(1):28–30. eCollection 2016 Feb. PubMed PMID: 27928379; PubMed Central PMCID: PMC5122935.
48. Patel SN, Langer PD, Zarbin MA, Bhagat N. Diagnostic value of clinical examination and radiographic imaging in identification of intraocular foreign bodies in open globe injury. Eur J Ophthalmol. 2012;22(2):259e68.
49. Yigit O. Foreign body traumas of the eye managed in an emergency department of a single-institution. Ulus Travma Acil Cerrahi Derg. 2012;18(1):75e9.
50. Zhang Y, Zhang M, Jiang C, Qiu HY. Intraocular foreign bodies in China: clinical characteristics, prognostic factors, and visual outcomes in 1,421 eyes. Am J Ophthalmol. 2011;152(1):66e73.e1.
51. Loporchio D, Mukkamala L, Gorukanti K, Zarbin M, Langer P, Bhagat N. Intraocular foreign bodies: a review. Surv Ophthalmol. 2016;61(5):582–96. https://doi.org/10.1016/j.survophthal.2016.03.005. Review. PubMed PMID: 26994871.
52. Fulcher TP, McNab AA, Sullivan TJ. Clinical features and management of intraorbital foreign bodies. Ophthalmology. 2002;109(3):494–500. https://doi.org/10.1016/S0161-6420(01)00982-4.
53. Garg SJ, Benson W, Fineman M, Bilyk JR. Bone from an orbital floor fracture causing an intraocular foreign body. Am J Ophthalmol. 2005;139(3):543–5. https://doi.org/10.1016/j.ajo.2004.08.054.
54. Rathod R, Mieler WF. An update on the management of intraocular foreign bodies. Retin Physician. 2011;8(3):52e5.
55. Tawara A. Transformation and cytotoxicity of iron in siderosis bulbi. Invest Ophthalmol Vis Sci. 1986;27(2):226e36.
56. Zhu L, Shen P, Lu H, et al. Ocular trauma score in siderosis bulbi with retained intraocular foreign body. Medicine (Baltimore). 2015;94(39):e1533.
57. Lit ES, Young LH. Anterior and posterior segment intraocular foreign bodies. Int Ophthalmol Clin. 2002;42(3):107e20.

58. Mete G, Turgut Y, Osman A, Gülşen U, Hakan A. Anterior segment intraocular metallic foreign body causing chronic hypopyon uveitis. J Ophthalmic Inflamm Infect. 2011;1(2):85–7. https://doi.org/10.1007/s12348-010-0011-9. PubMed PMID: 21484173; PubMed Central PMCID: PMC3102852.

59. Al-Mujaini A, Al-Senawi R, Ganesh A, Al-Zuhaibi S, Al-Dhuhli H. Intraorbital foreign body: clinical presentation, radiological appearance and management. Sultan Qaboos Univ Med J. 2008;8(1):69–74.

60. Nicoară SD, Irimescu I, Călinici T, Cristian C. Intraocular foreign bodies extracted by pars plana vitrectomy: clinical characteristics, management, outcomes and prognostic factors. BMC Ophthalmol. 2015;15:151. https://doi.org/10.1186/s12886-015-0128-6. PubMed PMID: 26526732; PubMed Central PMCID: PMC4631100.

61. Dehghani AR, Rezaei L, Salam H, Mohammadi Z, Mahboubi M. Post traumatic endophthalmitis: incidence and risk factors. Glob J Health Sci. 2014;6(6):68–72. https://doi.org/10.5539/gjhs.v6n6p68. PubMed PMID: 25363107; PubMed Central PMCID: PMC4825498.

62. Durand ML. Endophthalmitis. Clin Microbiol Infect. 2013;19(3):227–34. https://doi.org/10.1111/1469-0691.12118. Review. PubMed PMID: 23438028; PubMed Central PMCID: PMC3638360.

63. Kuhn F, Pieramici DJ. Endophthalmitis. In: Ferenc K, Pieramici D, editors. Ocular trauma: principles and practice. New York: Thieme; 2002. p. 293–300.

64. Chhabra S, Kunimoto DY, Kazi L, et al. Endophthalmitis after open globe injury: microbiologic spectrum and susceptibilities of isolates. Am J Ophthalmol. 2006;142(5):852–4.

65. El-Asrar AM, Al-Amro SA, Khan NM, Kangave D. Retinal detachment after posterior segment intraocular foreign body injuries. Int Ophthalmol. 1998;22(6):369–75.

66. Baban TA, Sammouh FK, ElBallouz HM, Warrak EL. Complete visual rehabilitation in a patient with no light perception after surgical management of a penetrating open-globe injury: a case report. Case Rep Ophthalmol. 2015;6(2):204–9. https://doi.org/10.1159/000434636. eCollection 2015 May–Aug. PubMed PMID: 26265906; PubMed Central PMCID: PMC4519596.

67. Agrawal R. Prognostic factors for final vision outcome in patients with open globe injuries. Indian J Ophthalmol. 2011;59(3):259–60. https://doi.org/10.4103/0301-4738.81030. PubMed PMID: 21586860; PubMed Central PMCID: PMC3120258.

68. Agrawal R, Ho SW, Teoh S. Pre-operative variables affecting final vision outcome with a critical review of ocular trauma classification for posterior open globe (zone III) injury. Indian J Ophthalmol. 2013;61(10):541–5. https://doi.org/10.4103/0301-4738.121066. PubMed PMID: 24212303; PubMed Central PMCID: PMC3853448.

69. Agrawal R, Rao G, Naigaonkar R, Ou X, Desai S. Prognostic factors for vision outcome after surgical repair of open globe injuries. Indian J Ophthalmol. 2011;59(6):465–70. https://doi.org/10.4103/0301-4738.86314. PubMed PMID: 22011491; PubMedCentral PMCID: PMC3214417.

70. Ceallaigh PO, Ekanaykaee K, Beirne CJ, Patton DW. Diagnosis and management of common maxillofacial injuries in the emergency department. Part 4: Orbital floor and midface fractures. Emerg Med J. 2007;24(4):292–3. Review. PubMed PMID: 17384387; PubMed Central PMCID: PMC2658241.

71. Tuckett JW, Lynham A, Lee GA, Perry M, Harrington U. Maxillofacial trauma in the emergency department: a review. Surgeon. 2014;12(2):106–14. https://doi.org/10.1016/j.surge.2013.07.001. Review. PubMed PMID: 23954483.

72. DeAngelis AF, Barrowman RA, Harrod R, Nastri AL. Review article: maxillofacial emergencies: maxillofacial trauma. Emerg Med Australas. 2014;26(6):530–7. https://doi.org/10.1111/1742-6723.12308. Review. PubMed PMID: 25292416.

73. Tunçbilek G, Işçi E. Traumatic evulsion of the globe: a very rare complication of maxillofacial trauma. J Craniofac Surg. 2008;19(2):313–5. https://doi.org/10.1097/SCS.0b013e318163e2db. Review.

74. de Santana Santos T, Vajgel A, Ribeiro CF, de Santana Júnior JR, Andrade Filho ES. Avulsion of globe following maxillofacial trauma. J Craniofac Surg. 2012;23(4):1097–100. https://doi.org/10.1097/SCS.0b013e318252d25c. PubMed PMID: 22777472.

75. Morris WR, Osborn FD, Fleming JC. Traumatic evulsion of the globe. Ophthal Plast Reconstr Surg. 2002;18:261–7.
76. Norazah AR, Akmal HZ, Hashima H, Vasantha T, Samsudin A. Globe avulsion secondary to maxillofacial trauma. Med J Malaysia. 2011;66(4):359–60. PubMed PMID: 22299558.
77. Amaral MB, Nery AC. Traumatic globe dislocation into the paranasal sinuses: literature review and treatment guidelines. J Craniomaxillofac Surg. 2016;44(5):642–7. https://doi.org/10.1016/j.jcms.2016.01.028. Review. PubMed PMID: 26948171.

Neck Injuries

16

Antonios Athanasiou

16.1 Introduction

Neck consists of multiple vital structures, with significant relationship to each other, in a very small space and without bony framework protection. As a result, any trauma patient with neck injury is considered to be an acute emergency. Neck injuries (NIs) can be blunt or penetrating and both are considered to have complex and challenging management. Even if the trauma patient has not major, superficial injuries, the clinicians must have high index of suspicious due to possible underlying injuries. Blunt NIs refer to injuries as a result of motor vehicle accidents, sport injuries, strangulation, or blows while penetrating NIs occur after stab or projectile injuries as well as penetrating debris. According to the literature, penetrating NIs represent approximately 10% of all trauma incidents [1]. Furthermore, the mortality rate of penetrating NIs is approximately 10% [2], which means that NIs require urgent attention not only by surgeons, but radiologists as well. This chapter will discuss the epidemiology, initial approach, and management of any neck injury.

16.2 Epidemiology

The two main mechanisms of NIs are penetrating and blunt NIs. Penetrating NIs in adults account for approximately 5–10% of all traumatic injuries while stab injuries from violent assault are the most common mechanism followed by gunshot wounds [3]. Stab injuries from Knife, glass razor, or blades have more predictable damage pathway, higher percentage of subclavian laceration, and lower proportion of spinal cord damage compared with projectile NIs. On the other hand, NIs caused by

A. Athanasiou (✉)
Department of Upper GI, Bariatric & Minimally Invasive Surgery, St. James University Hospital, Leeds, UK

© Springer Nature Switzerland AG 2021
E. Pikoulis, J. Doucet (eds.), *Emergency Medicine, Trauma and Disaster Management*, Hot Topics in Acute Care Surgery and Trauma,
https://doi.org/10.1007/978-3-030-34116-9_16

projectile, mainly handgun, shotgun and rifle, tend to create serious injuries and significantly increased mortality. The distance from the patient and the velocity of the projectile are crucial elements regarding the outcome of the injury. High-velocity weapons (for example AK 47s) cause more vascular and aerodigestive injuries [4]. Furthermore, weapons with high velocity (610–910 M/s) can cause NIs beyond the track of the bullet, the so-called cavitation phenomenon [5].

Penetrating NIs have been classified by the anatomical zones according to the level of injury (Fig. 16.1). Zone I is described as the area between the clavicles and the cricoid cartilage and includes the major thoracic vessels, proximal carotid and vertebral arteries, superior mediastinum, esophagus, lungs, trachea spinal cord, and thoracic duct. Zone II, between zones I and III, comprises the area between the inferior margin of the cricoid and the angle of the mandible. Structures within this zone include the jugular veins, vertebral and carotid arteries, trachea, esophagus, spinal cord, and larynx. Zone III extends from the angle of mandible and the base of the skull. The vertebral and carotid arteries, spinal cord, and pharynx are found in this zone [6].

The vast majority of penetrating NIs take place in zone II, mainly due to the density of vital structures; however, the surgical access and the proximal and distal vascular control are relatively easier compared with Zones I and III [7]. Zone I has the highest mortality rate after NIs, approximately 12%, mainly because of the severity of vessel injuries, the close proximity of mediastinal anatomical structures, and the difficult surgical access [8]. Arterial injury after penetrating NIs is reported to be 25%. Furthermore, carotid artery injury range from 6% to 17% [9].

Fig. 16.1 Zone classification of penetrating injuries to the neck

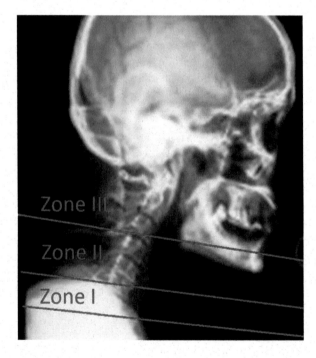

Exsanguination is considered to be the most frequent cause of death [8], while the mortality rate post laryngo-tracheal injuries is as high as 20% [10]. Last but not least, the mortality rate post pharyngo-esophageal trauma is reported to be 22% [11].

16.3 Prehospital Management

Patients with NIs can decompensate quickly and should be monitored very closely and transferred directly to a trauma center. Prehospital providers should minimize the time that they spent on scene. Movement of any impaled object should be avoided in the field. Following the main algorithm of Advanced Trauma Life Support (ATLS) is crucial due to the fact that it provides adequate initial management. This management includes possible advanced airway intervention such as cricothyroidotomy or endotracheal intubation, venous line placement and fluid infusion, cardiovascular monitoring, administration of medications, and diagnostic or therapeutic needle thoracostomy [12].

Airway management can be very difficult in trauma patient with NIs because direct trauma to the airway structures may require urgent airway protection. Endotracheal intubation can be the primary intervention for airway control while bag mask ventilation is an alternative option during transportation in hospital, when a definitive airway is not needed urgently. Nevertheless, bag mask ventilation may cause anatomical distortion if there is airway injury. The main clinical signs that suggest that patients with NIs need airway protection are subcutaneous neck emphysema, neck hematoma and active bleeding, hemoptysis, distorted neck anatomy, hoarseness, stridor, difficulty when swallowing secretions, dyspnea, and cyanosis [13]. Surgical airway (cricothyroidotomy) is generally indicated when orotracheal intubation is unsuccessful or when hemoptysis, obstruction above the larynx, edema, hematemesis, or severe neck or facial injury is present. Percutaneous needle transtracheal can also provide oxygen to trauma patients before establishing a definitive airway [14].

Cervical spine immobilization is strongly recommended only in the presence of clinical signs and symptoms that are associated with neurologic deficit, when the mechanism of the trauma is correlated with possible column or spinal injury and also when a physical examination cannot be completed accurately (unconscious patient) [15]. Penetrating neck trauma infrequently causes cervical spine injuries, especially after stab wounds. For this reason cervical spine immobilization should not hinder management, including airway visualization and protection. Rhee et al. showed in a retrospective study that the cervical spine injury is significantly dependent on the mechanism of injury following blunt and penetrating assault. More specifically, the incidence of cervical spine injury from gunshot wounds was 1.35% while the incidence from stab wounds was 0.12% [16].

16.4   Emergency Management

Patients with NIs should be inspected to identify any injury to platysma muscle. If this muscle is intact, then the wound is superficial and not penetrated. Platysma violation is by definition penetrating or deep neck injury and surgical consultation is recommended [17]. During the evaluation of patients with Nis, it is critical to check for hard and soft signs of penetrating injury (Table 16.1) [3]. Hemodynamically stable patients should be observed closely during the diagnostic studies because they may decompensate rapidly. The emergency clinician should focus on delayed occurrence of the hard signs of penetrating neck injury (Table 16.1), and the presentation of vascular, laryngo-tracheal, and pharyngo-esophageal injuries. Surgical review should always be obtained except if the platysma muscle has not been breached [17]. Asymtomatic patients with NIs should be monitored closely for at least 24 h.

Hemodynamically unstable patients must be resuscitated (ABCDE approach) and transferred to the theater immediately for definitive treatment. The lack of hard signs not always precludes underlying injuries such as pharyngo-esophageal injuries. For this reason, the management of these patients depends not only on the multidetector computed tomography with angiography (MDCT-A) findings but also on their physiological status [18].

16.5   Management of Vascular Injuries

Exsanguination is the most common cause of death due to penetrating neck injuries, representing approximately 50% of the mortality after NIs [3]. Patients with vascular injuries need urgent consultation by a vascular specialist. A variety of interventional and surgical treatments are available including stent placement or embolization, surgical ligation or primary vascular repair, and also revascularization. The latter offers the highest success rate after injuries to the carotid artery [19]. Surgical techniques for carotid repair include vein or polytetrafluoroethylene patch angioplasty and transverse arteriorrhaphy [20]. Cardiothoracic surgeon may be required for

Table 16.1 Hard vs soft signs of neck injury

Hard signs of vascular injury		
Vascular injury	Aerodigestive injury	Soft signs of injury
Expanding hematoma	Airway compromise and respiratory distress	Oropharyngeal blood
Shock with response to fluids		Dyspnea, dysphagia, dysphonia
Severe active hemorrhage	Massive hematemesis or hemoptysis	Hemoptysis, hematemesis
Cerebral ischemia	Air bubbling from a wound	Chest tube air leak
Absent or decreased radial pulse		Focal neurologic deficits
Vascular thrill or bruit		Subcutaneous or mediastinal air
Hemothorax more than 1 L		Non-expanding hematoma

vascular injuries in Zone I due to the fact that thoracotomy or sternotomy may be needed in order to achieve proximal control to vascular structures. For NIs with uncontrollable bleeding after external compression, Foley-catheter balloon for tamponade is recommended. This technique provides temporary bleeding control before definitive interventional and surgical treatment [21].

16.6 Management of Laryngotracheal Injuries

MDCT is the gold standard for the detection of laryngotracheal (LT) injuries in hemodynamically stable patients with NIs. MDCT has high sensitivity and specificity for detecting extraluminal air and cartilaginous fracture [22]. Moreover, bronchoscopy and panendoscopy are recommended for additional evaluation of laryngotracheal injuries prior to any surgical intervention [3]. Immediate repair of significant laryngotracheal injuries is crucial in order to avoid long-term complications including voice change, chronic pain, and strictures.

16.7 Management of Pharyngoesophageal Injuries

Cervical esophageal injuries are uncommon due to the anatomic position of the esophagus; however, the morbidity and mortality rate is high. These injuries are usually asymptomatic without clinical signs; however, hemoptysis, dysphagia, surgical emphysema, and hematemesis suggest the diagnosis. Patients with pharyngoesophageal injury need antibiotics and antifungal treatment, nil by mouth and nutritional support [23]. Patients who are unstable and demonstrating any of the "hard signs," mediastinitis or empyema due to esophageal leak, need surgical exploration. The patient with esophageal perforation post NIs need surgical debridement, primary repair of the injury, drainage, and feeding jejunostomy tube placement.

16.8 Conclusions and Recommendations

First of all, neck injuries, which penetrate the platysma, are considered to be penetrating neck injuries. Secondly, mortality seems to be highest within Zone 1 injuries concerning patients with NIs. Moreover, each and every patient with NIs is recommended to be transported immediately to the closest trauma unit due to the fact that he or she can decompensate very quickly. Furthermore, the airway of the patients with NIs who are suffering from any obvious distress (for example, severe hemorrhage, extensive neck wound, respiratory distress or shock) should be immediately stabilized. However, patients with NIs who were initially stable might still require airway protection, depending on either the projected course of their injury or some evidence of deterioration. A number of signs suggesting that the airway of the patients with NIs should be secured urgently include the following: hematoma or significant bleeding; subcutaneous emphysema; hemoptysis; bruit or thrill;

distorted neck anatomy; neurologic deficit; abnormal voice; and difficulty or pain when swallowing secretions.

Additionally, in most cases of patients with NIs, when necessary, a rapid sequence intubation (RSI) can be used in order to establish an airway. The RSI should be performed under fiberoptic or laryngoscopic visualization. Furthermore, due to the fact that the physical examination can miss significant esophageal and venous injuries despite identifying most arterial wounds, additional evaluation is necessary. In other words, additional evaluation is recommended for patients with NIs, which not only violates the platysma, but also it is connected with either signs of injury or signs seen on MDCT-A, which suggest injury.

Laryngotracheal injuries can cause respiratory distress, hemoptysis, anterior neck tenderness, stridor, subcutaneous air, odynophagia, or dysphonia. Pharyngo-esophageal injuries are not common, but connected with high morbidity and mortality. Clinicians should search for the referred injuries in patients with signs including blood in the saliva, dysphagia, subcutaneous air, and hematemesis. Penetrating neck injury NIs is possible to involve the central nervous system or the peripheral nervous system. According to the research, stable patients with NIs should be treated with selective operative management and newer protocols support a no-zone approach, which is stratified by the stability of the patient. However, the indications for mandatory surgical exploration, especially with Zone II injuries, are surrounded by controversy. The definite management of stable patients with NIs differentiates from institution to institution and local surgical practice.

Lateral neck radiograph demonstrates the anatomical zones according to the level of injury. Zone I is described as the area between the clavicles and the cricoid cartilage. Zone II comprises the area between the inferior margin of the cricoid and the angle of the mandible. Zone III extends from the angle of mandible and the base of the skull.

References

1. Vishwanatha B, Sagayaraj A, Huddar SG, Kumar P, Datta R. Penetrating neck injuries. Indian J Otolaryngol Head Neck Surg. 2007;59(3):221–4.
2. Saito N, Hito R, Burke PA, Sakai O. Imaging of penetrating injuries of the head and neck:current practice at a level I trauma center in the United States. Keio J Med. 2014;63(2):23–33.
3. Burgess CA, Dale OT, Almeyda R, Corbridge RJ. An evidence based review of the assessment and management of penetrating neck trauma. Clin Otolaryngol. 2012;37(1):44–52.
4. Penn-Barwell JG, Brown KV, Fries CA. High velocity gunshot injuries to the extremities: management on and off the battlefield. Curr Rev Musculoskelet Med. 2015;8(3):312–7.
5. Rahme R, Hamilton JF. Vertebral artery injuries in penetrating neck and cervical spine trauma. In: Neurotrauma management for the severely injured polytrauma patient. New York: Springer; 2017. p. 103–13.
6. McConnell DB. Management of penetrating trauma to the neck. Adv Surg. 1994;27:97–127.
7. Schroll R, Fontenot T, Lipcsey M, et al. Role of computed tomography angiography in the management of Zone II penetrating neck trauma in patients with clinical hard signs. J Trauma Acute Care Surg. 2015;79(6):943–50; discussion 950.

8. Rodriguez-Luna MR, Guarneros-Zarate JE, Hernandez-Mendez JR, Tueme-Izaguirre J, Noriega-Usi VM, Fenig-Rodriguez J. Defining Zone I of penetrating neck trauma: a surgical controversy in the light of clinical anatomy. J Trauma Acute Care Surg. 2016;80(4):670–3.
9. Demetriades D, Asensio JA, Velmahos G, Thal E. Complex problems in penetrating neck trauma. Surg Clin North Am. 1996;76(4):661–83.
10. Bryant AS, Cerfolio RJ. Esophageal trauma. Thorac Surg Clin. 2007;17(1):63–72.
11. Asensio JA, Berne J, Demetriades D, et al. Penetrating esophageal injuries: time interval of safety for preoperative evaluation-how long is safe? J Trauma Acute Care Surg. 1997;43(2):319–24.
12. Jain RK, Chakraborty P, Joshi P, Pradhan S, Kumari R. Penetrating neck injuries: from ER to OR. Indian J Otolaryngol Head Neck Surg. 2019;71(Suppl 1):352–7.
13. Walls RM, Brown CA, Bair AE, Pallin DJ. Emergency airway management: a multi-center report of 8937 emergency department intubations. J Emerg Med. 2011;41(4):347–54.
14. Koletsis E, Prokakis C, Baltayiannis N, Apostolakis E, Chatzimichalis A, Dougenis D. Surgical decision making in tracheobronchial injuries on the basis of clinical evidences and the injury's anatomical setting: a retrospective analysis. Injury. 2012;43(9):1437–41.
15. Tisherman SA, Bokhari F, Collier B, et al. Clinical practice guideline: penetrating zone II neck trauma. J Trauma Acute Care Surg. 2008;64(5):1392–405.
16. Rhee P, Kuncir EJ, Johnson L, et al. Cervical spine injury is highly dependent on the mechanism of injury following blunt and penetrating assault. J Trauma Acute Care Surg. 2006;61(5):1166–70.
17. Siau RT, Moore A, Ahmed T, Lee MS, Tostevin P. Management of penetrating neck injuries at a London Trauma Centre. Eur Arch Otorhinolaryngol. 2013;270(7):2123–8.
18. Osborn TM, Bell RB, Qaisi W, Long WB. Computed tomographic angiography as an aid to clinical decision making in the selective management of penetrating injuries to the neck: a reduction in the need for operative exploration. J Trauma Acute Care Surg. 2008;64(6):1466–71.
19. Scott WW, Sharp S, Figueroa SA, et al. Clinical and radiographic outcomes following traumatic Grade 1 and 2 carotid artery injuries: a 10-year retrospective analysis from a Level I trauma center. The Parkland Carotid and Vertebral Artery Injury Survey. J Neurosurg. 2015;122(5):1196–201.
20. Wehbe MR, Hoballah JJ. The management of penetrating neck injuries. In: Reconstructing the war injured patient. New York: Springer; 2017. p. 31–8.
21. Nowicki J, Stew B, Ooi E. Penetrating neck injuries: a guide to evaluation and management. Ann R Coll Surg Engl. 2017;100(1):6–11.
22. Bodanapally UK, Shanmuganathan K, Dreizin D, et al. Penetrating aerodigestive injuries in the neck: a proposed CT-aided modified selective management algorithm. Eur Radiol. 2016;26(7):2409–17.
23. Madiba TE, Muckart DJJ. Penetrating injuries to the cervical oesophagus: is routine exploration mandatory? Ann R Coll Surg Engl. 2003;85(3):162–6.

Thoracic Trauma

17

Christo Kole, Michail Vailas, Nikolaos Koliakos, and Dimitrios Schizas

17.1 Introduction

Thoracic trauma is one of the most common death-related injuries worldwide, accounting for 25% of trauma-associated deaths [1, 2]. More specifically, in the United Kingdom, it is responsible for 17,000 trauma deaths, 720,000 admissions, and over six million attendances to emergency departments annually [3]. Violence, falls, and motor vehicle accidents are reported as main causes of thoracic trauma [2], while blunt chest trauma incidence reaches 90% [4]. Severity of thoracic trauma varies from rib fractures, pneumothorax, lung contusion to thoracic vascular injury accounted for 49%, 20%, 12%, and 6% respectively [5]. Potentially life-threatening thoracic injuries such as aortic disruption, tracheobronchial disruption, esophageal disruption, myocardial contusion, and traumatic diaphragmatic rupture necessitate immediate surgical care and treatment [6].

Patient medical history may provide important information and clues concerning the severity of injury. Inspection and assessment of patient's chest movement and breathing pattern is of paramount importance during initial evaluation. Reduced thoracic movements or instability of the thoracic cage, signs of agony, severe pain, and discomfort during respiration may be apparent. Dyspnea, hemorrhagic shock, low cardiac output, and prominent intrathoracic bowel sounds indicating diaphragm rupture are several clinical signs that may be observed in cases of thoracic injuries [7]. Clinical examination of the thorax includes palpation which may reveal

C. Kole · M. Vailas · D. Schizas (✉)
First Department of Surgery, National and Kapodistrian University of Athens, Laikon General Hospital, Athens, Greece

N. Koliakos
Third Department of Surgery, National and Kapodistrian University of Athens, Attikon University Hospital, Athens, Greece

© Springer Nature Switzerland AG 2021
E. Pikoulis, J. Doucet (eds.), *Emergency Medicine, Trauma and Disaster Management*, Hot Topics in Acute Care Surgery and Trauma,
https://doi.org/10.1007/978-3-030-34116-9_17

localized tenderness and discomfort over the area of injury. Crackling and discomfort are associated with rib fractures and/or fractures of the costochondral junctions [8].

Therapeutic approach of thoracic trauma consists of three distinct levels of care. During the pre-hospital level [9], hemodynamic stabilization of the patient is a priority based on the ABCDE (Airway, Breathing, Circulation, Disability, Exposure) principles of advanced trauma life support (ATLS) [10], followed by detection and treatment or exclusion of immediately life-threatening injuries such as airway obstruction, tension pneumothorax, hemothorax, flail chest, cardiac tamponade [6]. In the emergency room level, thoracic fractures, pneumothorax, hemothorax, etc., may be confirmed by imaging techniques, chest X-ray, contrast-enhanced computed tomography (CT) scan [11]. Ultrasound examination is also considered valid in clinical entities such as cardiac tamponade, pneumothorax, and hemothorax [12–15]. Finally, during the third level of care, surgical intervention is essential for the management and definite treatment of thoracic injuries.

17.2   Thoracic Fractures

Thoracic fracture injuries include rib fractures, sternum fractures, and flail chest injury. Fractures may occur due to direct or indirect blunt trauma, falls, and aggressive cardiopulmonary resuscitation efforts [16]. Thoracic fractures cause severe pain and tenderness amplified by respiratory movements, deep breathing, or coughing, which eventually could lead to severe shortness of breath. Disorder of breathing mechanism due to trauma may be life threatening since it is often associated with respiratory disturbance, hypoventilation, hypoxia, and cyanosis [7]. Pneumonia in particular can be devastating, especially for elderly patients [17]. Penetrating trauma caused by fractured ribs may lead to lung and/or heart contusion, hemopneumothorax, cardiac tamponade, injuries which can progressively cause severe hypoxia [7]. Furthermore, prolonged ventilation, increased intensive care support, and hospital stay may have a negative impact on patient's recovery [17].

Flail chest injury occurs when several ribs are broken bilaterally. In trauma cases, this type of injury may be associated with sternal fractures. Sternal fracture is usually accompanied by myocardial contusion which is expressed with typical precordial pain and dyspnea [18]. Inspection of patient's chest reveals paradoxical movement during breathing accompanied by severe pain. This condition leads quickly to ventilation disorders since air flow is prevented from entering the lung parenchyma. Further examination of the injured patient is important as it may reveal head/neck and other organ-associated injuries. CT scan is considered the gold standard imaging tool used to evaluate thoracic fractures and associated complications [19].

Treatment in cases of the aforementioned injuries includes the use of analgesic drugs, proper treatment and management of other organ injuries, respiratory physiotherapy, and pulmonary toilet. Pain control in severe thoracic fractures is achieved by using oral/parenteral or intrapleural catheter analgesia (opiates, NSAIDS), intercostal nerve block [20] or a non-pharmacological technique, transcutaneous electrical nerve stimulation [21]. Chest wall stabilization may be performed using mechanical ventilation with positive end-expiratory pressure, while surgical treatment includes internal pneumatic stabilization of the chest wall [22]. Stabilization of rib fractures by intramedullary or Kirschner wires or management of sternal and rib fractures with the use of plates may be performed if necessary [23].

17.3 Lung Contusion

Lung contusion is usually the effect of blunt chest trauma involving injury of alveolar capillaries, resulting in accumulation of blood and other fluids within the alveolar capillaries. Impaired gas exchange due to fluid accumulation at alveolar level leads to low level of blood oxygen, hypoxia, and cyanosis [24, 25]. Clinically, patients are presented with dyspnea, tachypnea with decreased breath sounds, and reactive tachycardia, while laboratory blood analysis may reveal hypoxemia and hypercarbia [26]. Most lung contusions will not require any specific surgical treatment, except of supportive care, analgesia, ventilation, and maintenance of adequate blood oxygenation [27, 28].

17.4 Traumatic Pneumothorax

Pneumothorax is characterized by the presence of air inside the pleural space caused by penetrating injury of the chest and/or the lungs [29]. Injuries without exit wound usually are associated with rib fractures and may lead to the development of tension pneumothorax. On the other hand, open pneumothorax is caused by open chest trauma associated with penetrating injuries following insults from firearms, weapons, etc. Tension pneumothorax is a life-threatening condition which needs immediate diagnosis and treatment. Patients present with ipsilateral chest pain, severe dyspnea, and cough due to accumulation of air in pleural space that gradually increases, leading to lung collapse and shifting of the mediastinum away from the side of the pneumothorax [30]. Tachycardia, cyanosis, hypotension, distended jugular veins are also present, while air blood gas analysis shows hypoxia. If remained untreated, hypoxemia, metabolic acidosis, and decreased cardiac output lead to cardiac arrest and death [31].

Inspection findings include significant expansion of the affected hemithorax and trachea displacement away from the affected site, while clinical examination of the patient shows decreased or absent respiratory sounds and tympanism on the affected side. Chest X-ray and CT scan may confirm the presence of air in pleural space and organ displacements such as trachea and mediastinal structures shifting away from the side of pneumothorax, while ipsilateral diaphragm may be lowered due to decrease in trans-diaphragmatic pressures [30, 32].

As mentioned above, tension pneumothorax is a medical emergency. It requires immediate decompression by the insertion of an intercostal drain or wide bore catheter. Immediately chest decompression must be performed with a large-bore needle in the second or third intercostal space in the midclavicular line at the upper site of the rib. Following this, tension pneumothorax is converted to open pneumothorax, easier to treat. A chest tube placement must follow [33].

In the event of open pneumothorax, no valve mechanism exists; therefore it is less life threatening than tension pneumothorax. Initially, proper treatment of thoracic trauma is performed to avoid bacterial contamination of intrapleural space and/or mediastinum. Hermetization, sealing of the open wound, is required to prevent the development of tension pneumothorax [34]. Ultimately a thoracotomy tube is placed ipsilateral to the side of the wound, but at a different anatomic location than the wound using a small transverse incision just above rib to avoid vascular injury. After tube is introduced into the pleural space, incision is closed with interrupted skin sutures. Finally, tube is connected to underwater-seal drainage system [35] while needle aspiration is rarely applied for traumatic pneumothorax management [36].

17.5   Traumatic Hemothorax

Hemothorax is characterized by blood accumulation within the pleural space. This may be caused by penetrating or blunt trauma of the chest, diaphragm, or lungs. Hemothorax results in atelectasis of lungs, often leading to respiratory disorders. In cases of massive hemothorax, the mediastinum is shifted away from the side of the hemothorax. If blood is not drained, coagulated blood can produce a clotted hemothorax, empyema, and fibrothorax, resulting in prolonged disturbance of ventilation, leading to life-threatening conditions [37]. Furthermore, hemothorax may cause hypovolemic shock due to increased blood lost in the pleural space [38]. More than 1500 mL ($\geq$20 mL/kg) or 300–500 mL/h of blood loss is considered an indication for thoracotomy to manage the source of bleeding [7] (Table 17.1).

Table 17.1 Thoracic surgeon involvement due to the ATLS guidelines [4]	Recommended thoracic surgical intervention
	Penetrating chest trauma
	Blood loss: >1500 mL initially or >200 mL/h more than 2–4 h
	Important air-leakage over the chest tube
	Hemoptysis
	Massive subcutaneous emphysema
	Uncertain images on the chest X-ray or CT thorax
	Immediate thoracic surgical intervention
	Blood loss: >1500 mL initially or >200 mL/h more than 2–4 h
	Massive contusion-significant impairment of mechanical ventilation
	Endobronchial blood loss
	Tracheobronchial tree injury (Pneumothorax/Hemothorax)
	Injury of the heart or large vessels (blood loss/pericardial tamponade)

Patient with hemothorax may have the same clinical symptoms as patients suffering from pneumothorax, i.e., tachypnea, tachycardia, and cyanosis in advanced conditions. During physical examination however, percussion on the side of hemothorax shows dullness and decreased tactile fremitus of the lower lung fields, caused by pleural effusion in contrast to pneumothorax in which tympanism is apparent (see pneumothorax). Breathing murmurs may be decreased or absent depending on the amount of blood existing into the pleural space [38].

Hemothorax is confirmed by the presence of pleural fluid in chest X-ray (meniscus sign) and/or CT scan which may identify the presence of even small intrapleural collections of fluid, differentiating hydrothorax from hemothorax [39]. Furthermore, ultrasound may also be used in emergency situations [12]. Patients with thoracic trauma should be followed by radiography for at least 6 h after the initial injury in order to exclude potentially life-threatening developing hemothorax.

The stabilization of vital signs of the injured patient is imperative. Treatment of hemothorax consists of the evacuation of collected blood from the pleural space and re-expansion of lungs. Thoracic drainage may suffice in the management of hemothorax, without the need for a thoracotomy, if blood in the pleural space is not coagulated [40]. Surgical exploration by open thoracotomy is necessary if >1.500 mL of blood has accumulated during the last 24 h and/or an ongoing blood production of >200 mL of blood per hour is observed.

17.6 Cardiac Contusion

Cardiac contusion is usually injury of myocardium, caused by blunt chest trauma occurring by sudden decrease of body speed. Cardiac contusion may cause life-threatening arrhythmias and cardiac failure [41]; however non-specific ECG abnormalities are observed in such patients [42]. Such ECG changes may be also caused by non-cardiac factors including abnormal concentrations of electrolytes, hypoxia, anemia, and changes in vagal or sympathetic tone [18, 43–45]. Left ventricular injury can present with ST segment abnormalities or Q waves in case of extensive myocardial necrosis [42]. Damage and/or necrosis of myocardium may be diagnosed by the elevation of cardiac troponin I and T, which are highly sensitive markers [43, 46, 47]. Management of cardiac contusion in severely injured patients consists of hemodynamic stabilization and treatment of associated injuries. Surgical intervention is performed under general anesthesia [48]. Surgery is performed in case of significant effusion and tamponade, significant valvular heart disease, and LV dysfunction.

17.7 Cardiac Tamponade

Cardiac tamponade is an emergency situation that must be excluded or treated if diagnosed [6, 49]. It is caused by external compression of the heart and significant blood accumulation into the pericardial sac after blunt cardiac or intrapericardial aorta injury. Accumulation of blood increases intracardiac pressures leading to impediment of normal cardiac filling and reduction in cardiac output [50]. In case of rapid accumulation, 200 mL is sufficient to cause cardiac tamponade, increasing intrapericardial pressure to more than 15 mmHg and leading to compression of all cardiac chambers, decreased diastolic filling, and reduction of total venous return and cardiac output [51].

Patients may present with chest pain, tachypnea, dyspnea, cool extremities, and peripheral cyanosis. Physical examination will often reveal Beck's triad (hypotension, jugular venous distension and muted or distant heart sounds). Reactive sinus tachycardia presents in almost all patients with cardiac tamponade in order to maintain sufficient cardiac output. A narrow difference between systolic and diastolic blood pressure (normal pulse pressure is 30–40 mmHg), paradoxical pulse (i.e., a decline of 10 mmHg or more in systolic BP on inspiration), and distant (muffled) heart sounds may be present. Echocardiogram, two-dimensional and Doppler, is a sensitive and specific noninvasive test, which may identify the presence of pericardial effusion, determining its hemodynamic significance. Cardiac chamber collapse, dilated inferior vena cava, or respiratory variations in cardiac blood volumes and flow rates may occur. Electrocardiogram (ECG) may show electrical alterations (amplitude of QRS complexes varies), sinus tachycardia, and low-voltage recordings. However, chest radiography is not very sensitive in acute tamponade since cardiomegaly is usually absent and size of pericardium is relatively small [51, 52].

Therapeutically, little can be done in the pre-hospital setting other than the initial treatment of associated cardiogenic shock. Emergency thoracotomy to remove clots in the pericardium caused by a penetrating chest injury may be necessary in some cases. However, in most of the cases, pericardiocentesis is considered the sole tool for decompression of the cardiac tamponade in the emergency basis. Hospital care may include two strategies, pericardiocentesis or pericardial window [53]. Pericardiocentesis is performed using local anesthesia.

Pericardial puncture is performed using a needle insertion in the fifth or sixth left intercostal space near the sternum or through the costoxiphoid angle. The needle is advanced at 45° angle, 1–2 cm left of the costoxiphoid, and then up and backward toward the tip of the scapula until it reaches the pericardial sac.

Pericardial window is a surgical procedure in which part of the pericardial sac is removed, allowing the excess of fluid to drain, followed by sealing of the source of bleeding and repair of pericardium. There are two surgical options most commonly used: (1) the surgical (transthoracic or subxiphoid) pericardial window [54, 55] and (2) the video-thoracoscopic pericardial window [56, 57].

17.8 Mediastinal Organ Injury

Mediastinal organ injury consists of several entities such as esophageal injury, thoracic aorta injury, and tracheobronchial injury. Injuries may be caused by motor vehicle crash or penetrating trauma such as stab wounds or gunshot injuries. Mediastinal organ injuries are usually multiple injuries. Penetrating trauma of trachea may be accompanied by hemopneumothorax in 32% of the cases, with esophageal injuries in 11%, with major vascular injuries in 18%, with cardiac injuries in 5% of the cases, and intra-abdominal injuries in 18% of the cases, as well as aorta injury and pulmonary artery injuries [58].

17.9 Esophageal Injury

The esophagus is a muscular conduit, approximately 25 cm long divided into three main anatomical regions: cervical, thoracic, and intra-abdominal esophagus [59]. Esophageal injuries (Table 17.2) are caused by tear or lacerations of the wall of the esophagus, which subsequently lead to leakage of contents into the mediastinum [60, 61].

Patient with esophageal injuries are presented with chest or epigastric pain, which may reflect on shoulder tip. Other symptoms such as shock, cyanosis, dyspnea, tachypnea, cough, vomiting, hematemesis, dysphagia, and fever may be present [62–64]. Accumulation of air or fluid into the mediastinum or even pneumothorax may be a result of esophageal injury [65]. Another important diagnostic sign is subcutaneous emphysema in the neck.

Clinical evaluation is based on imaging techniques. Chest X-ray will reveal pleural effusion and/or pneumothorax on the side of the ruptured esophagus, while the presence of gastrografin extravasation will confirm the diagnosis and may locate the site of the rupture [63]. Computed tomography (CT) scan is useful to evaluate non-transmural esophageal perforations, which are not detected on esophagogram. Findings may include air and fluid around the injury of the esophagus or collection in the mediastinum; esophageal wall thickening; and radiographic evidence of inflamed mucosa. Finally, pleural effusions, pneumopericardium, and pneumoperitoneum may also occur [66].

Esophageal injury is accompanied by a high morbidity and mortality rate, if diagnosis and treatment are delayed. Treatment of esophageal trauma is mainly surgical. Primary repair involves the debridement of all affected tissues. Necrotic or devascularized tissue must be removed since their presence will endanger the repair. Moreover, esophageal trauma repair must be tension free, and mobilization of the esophagus should be minimal in order to maintain its blood supply [67–69]. Overzealous mobilization can render the anastomosis ischemic, resulting in

Table 17.2 Esophageal injury classification according to the American Association for the Surgery of Trauma (AAST) [66]	Grade I	Contusion/hematoma, partial thickness tear
	Grade II	Laceration less than 50%
	Grade III	Laceration more than 50%
	Grade IV	Less than 2 cm disruption of tissue or vasculature
	Grade V	More than 2 cm disruption of tissue or vasculature

postoperative leak. For cervical esophageal injuries, the sternocleidomastoid muscle can be used as a barrier between adjacent structures or to reinforce the repair. Due to its abundant blood supply and location, the sternocleidomastoid or platysma muscle can be used as a tissue flap [66]. In accompanying tracheobronchial injuries, the surgical management of the injury may be performed in two layers. Muscle with proper vascularization or tissue flap must be placed between the trachea and esophagus.

Diverting cervical esophagostomy should be performed in cases that primary repair is not possible [70]. Esophagectomy is performed rarely, only if the primary repair fails or cannot be performed after extensive damage. The most common surgical techniques used are transthoracic esophagectomies [71]. Transverse colonic interposition or a Roux-en-Y jejunal limb may be also used.

T-Tube diversion is used for smaller, distal injuries in patients who are not candidates for primary repair. T-tube is placed directly through the injury into the site of injury and kept on constant suction to encourage the formation of a controlled fistula. Once stable, the patient will need a gastrostomy tube for decompression and a feeding jejunostomy [72].

17.10 Tracheobronchial Injuries

Tracheobronchial injury is a life-threatening condition occurring in the area between the cricoid cartilage and the tracheal bifurcation [73] caused by blunt and/or penetrating trauma [74]. Tracheobronchial injury is linked with a high mortality rate due to associated asphyxia, whereas respiratory tract insufficiency may develop as a result of lack of injury recognition or incorrect management [75]. Main symptoms are respiratory distress and dyspnea [58, 76]. Clinical examination reveals stridor during auscultation, a sign of tracheal stenosis [77], while X-ray and CT scan may reveal emphysema, pneumomediastinum and/or pneumothorax, over-inflation of endotracheal tube cuff or displacement of endotracheal tube, mediastinal air, separation in the tracheal or bronchial air column, and respiratory tract deviation [78, 79].

In such cases, it is very important to secure airway since death may be caused within minutes induced by asphyxia [75]. Patients in distress and clinical suspicion of airway injury must be immediately intubated, while patients with penetrating cervical injury and air leakage are intubated directly through the tracheal lumen [76]. In case of a transected cervical trachea retracted into the mediastinum, location of the distal trachea is possible by palpation in front of the esophagus and it is followed by clamp holding and distal intubation by withdrawing it to the cervical wound [80].

Surgical treatment includes removal of necrotic tissue and debris, and an end-to-end anastomosis using absorbable sutures using healthy and well-vascularized tissues. In case of serious tracheobronchial damage, all devitalized tissues must be debrided preserving as much as viable airway tract is possible [81] (Table 17.1).

During post-operative period, pulmonary toilet is important to clear mucus and secretions from the airways. Ventilated patients should be treated with low airway pressure sufficient for oxygenation, and should be extubated as soon as possible.

Satisfactory healing should be assessed by bronchoscopy 7–10 days after tracheo-bronchial repair or prior to discharge [75].

17.11 Thoracic Aortic Injury

Thoracic aortic injury is another life-threatening condition accounting for 22% of blunt trauma [82, 83] or penetrating associated traumas [84].

Thoracic aorta is composed of the ascending aorta which is relatively mobile, aortic arch which is fixed, and descending aorta a second mobile aortic segment. Areas between these regions such as aortic isthmus, the transition zone between the mobile ascending aorta and the fixed descending aorta, the tethered site of the aorta at the ligamentum arteriosum and ascending aorta, just proximal to the origin of the brachiocephalic vessels, are possible sites of injury [85]. Depending on the location, thoracic aortic injury subsequently leads to leakage of contents into the surrounding mediastinum or into the pericardial sac leading to cardiac tamponade formation.

Patients usually are presented with severe chest and/or back pain, dyspnea, tachycardia, and cough. Moreover, patients may also present with voice hoarseness or vocal cord paralysis if there is damage of the left recurrent laryngeal nerve, which travels posterior to the distal aortic arch, loops around, and travels back staying in an anterior position from the aortic arch. Inspection of the patient may reveal bruising of the chest wall, while clinical examination presents a faint peripheral pulse palpation. Upper limb hypertension or normal upper limb pulses with decreased lower limb pulses (acute coarctation syndrome) may be also present. Systolic murmur can be heard during auscultation [86]. Widened mediastinum or left hemothorax, an abnormal aortic outline, opacification of the aortopulmonary window are findings in X-ray and CT scan indicative for this type of injury [86]. The gold standard method for the diagnosis is angiography or CT-angiography, which may reveal contrast extravasation outside the aorta [87, 88].

The initial treatment requires strict adherence to advanced trauma life support (ATLS) principles and hemodynamic stabilization of the patient. The assessment of other injuries will determine the subsequent management of thoracic aortic injury. The gold standard procedure for aortic injury treatment is endovascular stent placement [89]; however, such procedure is only available for injuries in which the external wall of the aorta is spared. Open surgery is performed in patients with significant left hemothorax, pseudocoarctation, or extensive mediastinal hematoma. Delay in aortic repair is associated with a high mortality; therefore, urgent and immediate repair through thoracotomy is necessary [90].

17.12 Ruptured Diaphragm

Diaphragm is a curved muscular structure which separates thoracic from abdominal cavity. Ruptured diaphragm represents less than 1% of traumatic injuries, usually associated with motor vehicle crashes, penetrating trauma, falls, and crush injuries

[91, 92]. Penetrating injury to the abdomen or chest from the level of T4 to T12 anteriorly and L3 posteriorly could lead to diaphragmatic injury [93]. 88–95% of diaphragmatic injuries occur on the left side [94], including spleen injury.

Apart from severe chest or abdominal pain, clinical features may vary based on the mechanism of injury. Ruptured diaphragm is usually associated with severe trauma including injuries of other surrounding thoracic organs, such as lungs, heart, or abdominal organs such as spleen, stomach, liver [95]. Patients with diaphragmatic injury may present with respiratory distress, dyspnea, orthopnea [96], and cough [97]. Severe herniation occurs when spleen is injured, whereas tachycardia and signs of intestinal obstruction or sepsis in the abdomen may be present [97]. Clinical examination shows absent or reduced breath sounds in the affected chest area. Bowel sounds may be present in case of bowel displacement into the thoracic cavity. Tympanic or dull sounds may be present during percussion in cases where intestines or liver migrate, respectively, in the thoracic cavity [95].

Chest X-ray has low sensitivity and specificity [97] since other injuries such as pulmonary contusion, hemothorax, or pneumothorax may be present, masking the injury on the X-ray film [98]. Chest X-ray findings may reveal the presence of air bubbles within the affected hemithorax. Mediastinum may appear shifted toward the other side, while the diaphragm may appear higher than normal due to the presence of stomach in the left hemithorax [95]. CT scan is considered as the gold standard technique since it offers a precise evaluation of the size and location of the diaphragmatic rapture [95, 99, 100].

Operative repair is required since a ruptured diaphragm cannot heal spontaneously. Stabilization of the A-airway, B-breathing, and C-circulation is always a priority. Surgical repair of ruptured diaphragm is usually performed through open abdominal approach involving primary or patch repair of the diaphragm. In case of delayed diagnosis, a thoracotomy or combined thoracic-abdominal approach is performed to avoid viscera and chest adhesions [101].

Laparoscopic or thoracoscopic approach may be used in less severe injuries including small diaphragmatic defects [102, 103]. In large defects, tension-free synthetic or biologic mesh repair is used. Biological meshes have lower rate of hernia recurrence, higher resistance to infections, and lower risk of displacement [104].

17.13 Conclusions

Most of the thoracic injuries may be life threatening. The complexity of thoracic trauma and associated respiratory failure increase the mortality rates of these injuries. Management should always follow the advanced trauma life support principles (Airway, Breathing, Circulation, Disability, Exposure), and rapid identification of life-threatening injuries such as airway obstruction, pneumothorax, hemothorax, cardiac tamponade is of paramount importance. Other thoracic injuries, such as aortic rupture, esophageal disruption, and myocardial contusion should not be missed as well, since they are linked with many fatalities.

Patient medical history can provide useful information regarding the type of injury, while inspection, clinical examination of the thorax, and imaging when necessary can aid the correct diagnosis and the proper therapeutic strategy (Table 17.3). Surgeon's involvement, as defined by the ATLS guidelines, is necessary during all three different levels of care: the pre-hospital setting, the emergency room, and the definite treatment of thoracic injuries in the operating room. Treatment depends on the nature of injury (Table 17.3) with the ultimate goal to establish normal gas exchange and normal hemodynamics, and prevent the development of long-term complications such as impairment of pulmonary function.

Table 17.3 Clinical features and management of thoracic trauma entities

Thoracic trauma entities	Clinical features	Diagnosis	CT-scanning and X-ray findings	Management
Thoracic fractures	Dyspnea, pain, hypoventilation, hypoxia, cyanosis, chest wall paradoxical movement	Pain in palpation	Thoracic and/or rib fractures	Pain control, mechanical ventilation with positive end-expiratory pressure, chest wall stabilization
Lung contusion	Reduced concentration of oxygen in arterial blood, hypoxia, cyanosis, dyspnea, tachypnea, tachycardia	Decreased breath sounds may be also present	No specific findings	Supportive care, ventilation, and maintenance of adequate blood oxygenation
Traumatic pneumothorax	Reduced hemithorax movement *on the side* of pneumothorax, tachycardia, hypotension, distended neck veins, ipsilateral chest pain, dyspnea, tachypnea cough, hypoxia, cyanosis	Decreased breath sounds, hyperresonance to percussion: *on the side* of pneumothorax	Shift of trachea *away* from the side of pneumothorax, air presence air in the pleural space thoracic cavity	*Medical emergency,* chest decompression with a needle (second or third intercostal space in the midclavicular line), followed by chest tube placement
Traumatic hemothorax	Reduced hemithorax movement *on the side* of hemothorax, tachypnea, tachycardia, hypotension, distended neck veins	Decreased or absence breath sounds, dullness to percussion, decreased tactile fremitus lower lung: *on the side* of pneumothorax	Shift of trachea *toward* the opposite side of hemothorax, presence of intrapleural collection of fluid	*Medical emergency,* evacuation of collected blood from the pleural space and re-expansion of lungs
Cardiac contusion	Chest pain, arrhythmias, cardiac failure	Increased cardiac troponin I and T		Hemodynamic stabilization and treatment of associated injuries

(continued)

Table 17.3 (continued)

Thoracic trauma entities	Clinical features	Diagnosis	CT-scanning and X-ray findings	Management
Cardiac tamponade	Chest pain, tachypnea, tachycardia dyspnea, cool extremities and cyanosis, Beck's triad (hypotension, jugular venous distension, muted, or distant heart sounds)	Narrow systolic-diastolic blood pressure, paradoxical pulses, distant heart sounds	Chest radiography-not very sensitive potential presence of pericardial effusion	*Medical emergency*, pericardiocentesis, emergency thoracotomy in case of clotting in the pericardium, pericardial window surgical procedure
Esophageal injury	Chest or epigastric pain with reflection on shoulder tip, dyspnea, tachypnea, cough, vomiting, hematemesis, dysphagia and fever		Pleural effusion and/or pneumothorax, pneumomediastinum leak of gastrografin, mediastinal air	Tension-free esophageal trauma repair, mobilization of the esophagus, sternocleidomastoid or platysma muscle can be used as a tissue flap, transthoracic esophagectomy, stomach mobilization or colonic interposition, and anastomosis end to end
Tracheobronchial injuries	Respiratory distress and dyspnea	Stridor	Emphysema, pneumomediastinum and/or pneumothorax. mediastinal air, separation in the tracheal or bronchial air column, respiratory tract deviation	*Medical emergency* Maintenance of an *adequate airway*, intubation if necessary. removal of necrotic tissue and debris, end-to-end anastomosis using absorbable sutures with healthy and proper vascularized tissues
Thoracic aortic injury	Severe chest and/or back pain, dyspnea, tachycardia, bruising of the anterior chest wall, hypotension and upper limb hypertension	Faint, but detectable peripheral pulse palpation. systolic murmur on the bottom of the heart	Widened mediastinum, massive left hemothorax, abnormal aortic outline, opacification of the aortopulmonary window, deviation of trachea to the right of midline and downward displacement of the left mainstem bronchus *CT angiography*: contrast outside the lumen of the aorta	*Medical emergency* ATLS principles and hemodynamic stabilization of the patient, endovascular placement of a covered stent

Table 17.3 (continued)

Thoracic trauma entities	Clinical features	Diagnosis	CT-scanning and X-ray findings	Management
Ruptured diaphragm	Chest/abdominal pain, dyspnea, orthopnea and coughing, tachycardia	No breath sounds *on affected side*, abdominal sounds, tympanic/dull sounds on percussion	Gas bubbles in the chest, mediastinal shift or lung/diaphragm displacement, stomach in left hemithorax	*Medical emergency* Stabilization of airway, breathing, and circulation Patch closure of the diaphragm or synthetic or biologic mesh repair

References

1. Bouzat P, et al. WITHDRAWN: chest trauma: first 48 hours management. Anaesth Crit Care Pain Med. 2017; https://doi.org/10.1016/j.accpm.2017.01.004.
2. Al-Koudmani I, Darwish B, Al-Kateb K, Taifour Y. Chest trauma experience over eleven-year period at al-mouassat university teaching hospital-Damascus: a retrospective review of 888 cases. J Cardiothorac Surg. 2012;7:35. https://doi.org/10.1186/1749-8090-7-35.
3. Blyth A. Thoracic trauma. BMJ. 2014;348:g1137. https://doi.org/10.1136/bmj.g1137.
4. Ludwig C, Koryllos A. Management of chest trauma. J Thorac Dis. 2017;9:S172–7. https://doi.org/10.21037/jtd.2017.03.52.
5. Kulshrestha P, Munshi I, Wait R. Profile of chest trauma in a level I trauma center. J Trauma. 2004;57:576–81.
6. Yamamoto L, Schroeder C, Morley D, Beliveau C. Thoracic trauma: the deadly dozen. Crit Care Nurs Q. 2005;28:22–40.
7. Richter T, Ragaller M. Ventilation in chest trauma. J Emerg Trauma Shock. 2011;4:251–9. https://doi.org/10.4103/0974-2700.82215.
8. Mayberry JC, Trunkey DD. The fractured rib in chest wall trauma. Chest Surg Clin N Am. 1997;7:239–61.
9. Waydhas C, Sauerland S. Pre-hospital pleural decompression and chest tube placement after blunt trauma: a systematic review. Resuscitation. 2007;72:11–25. https://doi.org/10.1016/j.resuscitation.2006.06.025.
10. Olgers TJ, Dijkstra RS, Drost-de Klerck AM, Ter Maaten JC. The ABCDE primary assessment in the emergency department in medically ill patients: an observational pilot study. Neth J Med. 2017;75:106–11.
11. Agladioglu K, et al. Chest X-rays in detecting injuries caused by blunt trauma. World J Emerg Med. 2016;7:55–8. https://doi.org/10.5847/wjem.j.1920-8642.2016.01.010.
12. Brooks A, Davies B, Smethhurst M, Connolly J. Emergency ultrasound in the acute assessment of haemothorax. Emerg Med J. 2004;21:44–6.
13. Chung MH, et al. The benefit of ultrasound in deciding between tube thoracostomy and observative management in hemothorax resulting from blunt chest trauma. World J Surg. 2018;42:2054–60. https://doi.org/10.1007/s00268-017-4417-5.
14. Dulchavsky SA, et al. Prospective evaluation of thoracic ultrasound in the detection of pneumothorax. J Trauma. 2001;50:201–5.
15. Ma O, Mateer JR. Trauma ultrasound examination versus chest radiography in the detection of hemothorax. Ann Emerg Med. 1997;29:312–5.
16. Calhoon JH, Grover FL, Trinkle JK. Chest trauma. Approach and management. Clin Chest Med. 1992;13:55–67.
17. Senekjian L, Nirula R. Rib fracture fixation: indications and outcomes. Crit Care Clin. 2017;33:153–65. https://doi.org/10.1016/j.ccc.2016.08.009.

18. Alborzi Z, et al. Diagnosing myocardial contusion after blunt chest trauma. J Tehran Heart Cent. 2016;11:49–54.
19. Talbot BS, et al. Traumatic rib injury: patterns, imaging pitfalls, complications, and treatment. Radiographics. 2017;37:628–51. https://doi.org/10.1148/rg.2017160100.
20. Hwang EG, Lee Y. Effectiveness of intercostal nerve block for management of pain in rib fracture patients. J Exerc Rehabil. 2014;10:241–4. https://doi.org/10.12965/jer.140137.
21. Oncel M, Sencan S, Yildiz H, Kurt N. Transcutaneous electrical nerve stimulation for pain management in patients with uncomplicated minor rib fractures. Eur J Cardiothorac Surg. 2002;22:13–7.
22. Benfield JR. Traumatic bronchial rupture and other major thoracic injuries. Ann Thorac Surg. 1990;50:523.
23. Ginsberg RJ, Kostin RF. 5. New approaches to the management of flail chest. Can Med Assoc J. 1977;116:613–5.
24. Hoff SJ, Shotts SD, Eddy VA, Morris JA Jr. Outcome of isolated pulmonary contusion in blunt trauma patients. Am Surg. 1994;60:138–42.
25. Miller DL, Mansour KA. Blunt traumatic lung injuries. Thorac Surg Clin. 2007;17:57–61, vi. https://doi.org/10.1016/j.thorsurg.2007.03.017.
26. Ganie FA, et al. Lung contusion: a clinico-pathological entity with unpredictable clinical course. Bull Emerg Trauma. 2013;1:7–16.
27. Sutyak JP, Wohltmann CD, Larson J. Pulmonary contusions and critical care management in thoracic trauma. Thorac Surg Clin. 2007;17:11–23, v. https://doi.org/10.1016/j.thorsurg.2007.02.001.
28. Moloney JT, Fowler SJ, Chang W. Anesthetic management of thoracic trauma. Curr Opin Anaesthesiol. 2008;21:41–6. https://doi.org/10.1097/ACO.0b013e3282f2aadc.
29. Porpodis K, et al. Pneumothorax and asthma. J Thorac Dis. 2014;6(Suppl 1):S152–61. https://doi.org/10.3978/j.issn.2072-1439.2014.03.05.
30. Sharma A, Jindal P. Principles of diagnosis and management of traumatic pneumothorax. J Emerg Trauma Shock. 2008;1:34–41. https://doi.org/10.4103/0974-2700.41789.
31. Barton ED, Rhee P, Hutton KC, Rosen P. The pathophysiology of tension pneumothorax in ventilated swine. J Emerg Med. 1997;15:147–53.
32. Zarogoulidis P, et al. Pneumothorax: from definition to diagnosis and treatment. J Thorac Dis. 2014;6:S372–6. https://doi.org/10.3978/j.issn.2072-1439.2014.09.24.
33. Baumann MH, Patel PB, Roney CW, Petrini MF. Comparison of function of commercially available pleural drainage units and catheters. Chest. 2003;123:1878–86.
34. Kotora JJ, Henao J, Littlejohn L, Kircher S. Vented chest seals for prevention of tension pneumothorax in a communicating pneumothorax. J Emerg Med. 2013;45:686–94.
35. Kwiatt M, et al. Thoracostomy tubes: a comprehensive review of complications and related topics. Int J Crit Illn Inj Sci. 2014;4:143–55.
36. Parlak M, Uil S, Van den Berg J. A prospective, randomised trial of pneumothorax therapy: manual aspiration versus conventional chest tube drainage. Respir Med. 2012;106:1600–5.
37. Tanaka H, et al. Surgical stabilization of internal pneumatic stabilization? A prospective randomized study of management of severe flail chest patients. J Trauma. 2002;52:727–32; discussion 732.
38. Broderick S, Hemothorax R. Etiology, diagnosis, and management. Thorac Surg Clin. 2013;23:89–96, vi–vii. https://doi.org/10.1016/j.thorsurg.2012.10.003.
39. Sinha P, Sarkar P. Late clotted haemothorax after blunt chest trauma. J Accid Emerg Med. 1998;15:189–91.
40. Boersma WG, Stigt JA, Smit HJ. Treatment of haemothorax. Respir Med. 2010;104:1583–7. https://doi.org/10.1016/j.rmed.2010.08.006.
41. Helling TS, Duke P, Beggs CW, Crouse LJ. A prospective evaluation of 68 patients suffering blunt chest trauma for evidence of cardiac injury. J Trauma. 1989;29:961–5; discussion 965–6.
42. Tenzer ML. The spectrum of myocardial contusion: a review. J Trauma. 1985;25:620–7.

43. Salim A, et al. Clinically significant blunt cardiac trauma: role of serum troponin levels combined with electrocardiographic findings. J Trauma. 2001;50:237–43.
44. Hiatt JR, Yeatman LA Jr, Child JS. The value of echocardiography in blunt chest trauma. J Trauma. 1988;28:914–22.
45. Garcia-Fernandez MA, et al. Role of transesophageal echocardiography in the assessment of patients with blunt chest trauma: correlation of echocardiographic findings with the electrocardiogram and creatine kinase monoclonal antibody measurements. Am Heart J. 1998;135:476–81.
46. Bertinchant JP, et al. Evaluation of incidence, clinical significance, and prognostic value of circulating cardiac troponin I and T elevation in hemodynamically stable patients with suspected myocardial contusion after blunt chest trauma. J Trauma. 2000;48:924–31.
47. Kaye P, O'Sullivan I. Myocardial contusion: emergency investigation and diagnosis. Emerg Med J. 2002;19:8–10.
48. End A, et al. Elective surgery for blunt cardiac trauma. J Trauma. 1994;37:798–802.
49. Spodick DH. Acute cardiac tamponade. N Engl J Med. 2003;349:684–90. https://doi.org/10.1056/NEJMra022643.
50. Appleton C, Gillam L, Koulogiannis K. Cardiac tamponade. Cardiol Clin. 2017;35:525–37. https://doi.org/10.1016/j.ccl.2017.07.006.
51. Richardson L. Cardiac tamponade. JAAPA. 2014;27:50–1. https://doi.org/10.1097/01.JAA.0000455653.42543.8a.
52. Agabegi SS, Agabegi ED. Chapter 1: Diseases of the cardiovascular system. In: Agabegi SS, Agabegi ED, editors. Step-up to medicine step-up. Philadelphia: Wolters Kluwer/Lippincott Williams & Wilkins; 2016. p. 39–40.
53. Moores DW, Dziuban SW Jr. Pericardial drainage procedures. Chest Surg Clin N Am. 1995;5:359–73.
54. Hommes M, Nicol AJ, van der Stok J, Kodde I, Navsaria PH. Subxiphoid pericardial window to exclude occult cardiac injury after penetrating thoracoabdominal trauma. Br J Surg. 2013;100:1454–8. https://doi.org/10.1002/bjs.9241.
55. Arom KV, Richardson JD, Webb G, Grover FL, Trinkle JK. Subxiphoid pericardial window in patients with suspected traumatic pericardial tamponade. Ann Thorac Surg. 1977;23:545–9.
56. Morales CH, Salinas CM, Henao CA, Patino PA, Munoz CM. Thoracoscopic pericardial window and penetrating cardiac trauma. J Trauma. 1997;42:273–5.
57. Mann GB, Nguyen H, Corbet J. Laparoscopic creation of pericardial window. Aust N Z J Surg. 1994;64:853–5.
58. Kelly JP, et al. Management of airway trauma: I: Tracheobronchial injuries. Ann Thorac Surg. 1985;40:551–5.
59. Abdullah I, Rosato EF. In: Roses RE, Paulson EC, Kanchwala SK, Morris JB, editors. Gowned and gloved surgery: Introduction to common procedures. Philadelphia: W.B. Saunders; 2009. p. 34–43.
60. Yamada T, Motomura Y, Hiraoka E, Miyagaki A, Sato J. Nasogastric tubes can cause intramural hematoma of the esophagus. Am J Case Rep. 2019;20:224–7. https://doi.org/10.12659/AJCR.914133.
61. Hagedorn KN, et al. Characterization of all-terrain vehicle-related chest injury patterns in children. Emerg Radiol. 2019;26:373. https://doi.org/10.1007/s10140-019-01679-y.
62. Attar S, et al. Esophageal perforation: a therapeutic challenge. Ann Thorac Surg. 1990;50:45–9; discussion 50–1.
63. Triggiani E, Belsey R. Oesophageal trauma: incidence, diagnosis, and management. Thorax. 1977;32:241–9.
64. Goldstein LA, Thompson WR. Esophageal perforations: a 15 year experience. Am J Surg. 1982;143:495–503.
65. Maniatis V, et al. Perforation of the alimentary tract: evaluation with computed tomography. Abdom Imaging. 2000;25:373–9.
66. Mubang RN, Stawicki SP. Esophageal trauma. Treasure Island, FL: StatPearls Publishing; 2019.

67. Jones WG 2nd, Ginsberg RJ. Esophageal perforation: a continuing challenge. Ann Thorac Surg. 1992;53:534–43.
68. Brewer LA 3rd, Carter R, Mulder GA, Stiles QR. Options in the management of perforations of the esophagus. Am J Surg. 1986;152:62–9.
69. Skinner DB, Little AG, DeMeester TR. Management of esophageal perforation. Am J Surg. 1980;139:760–4.
70. Rigberg DA, Centeno JM, Blinman TA, Towfigh S, McFadden DW. Two decades of cervical esophagostomy: indications and outcomes. Am Surg. 1998;64:939–41.
71. Flanagan JC, et al. Esophagectomy and gastric pull-through procedures: surgical techniques, imaging features, and potential complications. Radiographics. 2016;36:107–21. https://doi.org/10.1148/rg.2016150126.
72. Gill RC, Pal KMI, Mannan F, Bawa A, Fatimi SH. T-tube placement as a method for treating penetrating oesophageal injuries. Int J Surg Case Rep. 2016;28:255–7. https://doi.org/10.1016/j.ijscr.2015.12.025.
73. Welter S. Repair of tracheobronchial injuries. Thorac Surg Clin. 2014;24:41–50. https://doi.org/10.1016/j.thorsurg.2013.10.006.
74. Lee RB. Traumatic injury of the cervicothoracic trachea and major bronchi. Chest Surg Clin N Am. 1997;7:285–304.
75. Altinok T, Can A. Management of tracheobronchial injuries. Eurasian J Med. 2014;46:209–15. https://doi.org/10.5152/eajm.2014.42.
76. Rossbach MM, et al. Management of major tracheobronchial injuries: a 28-year experience. Ann Thorac Surg. 1998;65:182–6.
77. Symbas PN, Hatcher CR Jr, Vlasis SE. Bullet wounds of the trachea. J Thorac Cardiovasc Surg. 1982;83:235–8.
78. Lupetin AR. Computed tomographic evaluation of laryngotracheal trauma. Curr Probl Diagn Radiol. 1997;26:185–206.
79. Stark P. Imaging of tracheobronchial injuries. J Thorac Imaging. 1995;10:206–19.
80. Mathisen DJ, Grillo H. Laryngotracheal trauma. Ann Thorac Surg. 1987;43:254–62.
81. Mitchell JD, et al. Clinical experience with carinal resection. J Thorac Cardiovasc Surg. 1999;117:39–52; discussion 52–3.
82. Strassman G. Traumatic rupture of the aorta. Am Heart J. 1947;33:508–15.
83. Bertrand S, et al. Traumatic rupture of thoracic aorta in real-world motor vehicle crashes. Traffic Inj Prev. 2008;9:153–61. https://doi.org/10.1080/15389580701775777.
84. Pelletti G, et al. Traumatic fatal aortic rupture in motorcycle drivers. Forensic Sci Int. 2017;281:121–6. https://doi.org/10.1016/j.forsciint.2017.10.038.
85. McKnight JT, Meyer JA, Neville JF Jr. Nonpenetrating traumatic rupture of the thoracic aorta. Ann Surg. 1964;160:1069–72.
86. O'Conor CE. Diagnosing traumatic rupture of the thoracic aorta in the emergency department. Emerg Med J. 2004;21:414–9.
87. Beel T, Harwood AL. Traumatic rupture of the thoracic aorta. Ann Emerg Med. 1980;9:483–6.
88. Mokrane FZ, Revel-Mouroz P, Saint Lebes B, Rousseau H. Traumatic injuries of the thoracic aorta: the role of imaging in diagnosis and treatment. Diagn Interv Imaging. 2015;96:693–706. https://doi.org/10.1016/j.diii.2015.06.005.
89. Uzieblo M, et al. Endovascular repair of traumatic descending thoracic aortic disruptions: should endovascular therapy become the gold standard? Vasc Endovasc Surg. 2004;38:331–7. https://doi.org/10.1177/153857440403800404.
90. Oozawa S, Aoki A, Otsubo S, Miyajima Y, Ishimaru Y. [Nonpenetrating traumatic injury of the thoracic aorta and left subclavian artery; report of a case]. Kyobu Geka. 2005;58:573–5.
91. Corbellini C, Costa S, Canini T, Villa R, Contessini Avesani E. Diaphragmatic rupture: a single-institution experience and literature review. Ulus Travma Acil Cerrahi Derg. 2017;23:421–6. https://doi.org/10.5505/tjtes.2017.78027.
92. Hammer MM, Raptis DA, Mellnick VM, Bhalla S, Raptis CA. Traumatic injuries of the diaphragm: overview of imaging findings and diagnosis. Abdom Radiol (NY). 2017;42:1020–7. https://doi.org/10.1007/s00261-016-0908-3.

93. Gooseman MR, et al. Unifying classification for transdiaphragmatic intercostal hernia and other costal margin injuriesdagger. Eur J Cardiothorac Surg. 2019;56:150. https://doi.org/10.1093/ejcts/ezz020.
94. Goh BK, Wong AS, Tay KH, Hoe MN. Delayed presentation of a patient with a ruptured diaphragm complicated by gastric incarceration and perforation after apparently minor blunt trauma. CJEM. 2004;6:277–80.
95. Testini M, et al. Emergency surgery due to diaphragmatic hernia: case series and review. World J Emerg Surg. 2017;12:23. https://doi.org/10.1186/s13017-017-0134-5.
96. Karmy-Jones R, Jurkovich GJ. Blunt chest trauma. Curr Probl Surg. 2004;41:211–380. https://doi.org/10.1016/j.cpsurg.2003.12.004.
97. McGillicuddy D, Rosen P. Diagnostic dilemmas and current controversies in blunt chest trauma. Emerg Med Clin North Am. 2007;25:695–711, viii–ix. https://doi.org/10.1016/j.emc.2007.06.004.
98. Scharff JR, Naunheim KS. Traumatic diaphragmatic injuries. Thorac Surg Clin. 2007;17:81–5. https://doi.org/10.1016/j.thorsurg.2007.03.006.
99. Chao PH, Chuang JH, Lee SY, Huang HC. Late-presenting congenital diaphragmatic hernia in childhood. Acta Paediatr. 2011;100:425–8. https://doi.org/10.1111/j.1651-2227.2010.02025.x.
100. Desir A, Ghaye B. CT of blunt diaphragmatic rupture. Radiographics. 2012;32:477–98. https://doi.org/10.1148/rg.322115082.
101. Mansour KA. Trauma to the diaphragm. Chest Surg Clin N Am. 1997;7:373–83.
102. Memon MA, Fitztgibbons RJ Jr. The role of minimal access surgery in the acute abdomen. Surg Clin North Am. 1997;77:1333–53.
103. Badillo A, Gingalewski C. Congenital diaphragmatic hernia: treatment and outcomes. Semin Perinatol. 2014;38:92–6. https://doi.org/10.1053/j.semperi.2013.11.005.
104. Antoniou SA, Pointner R, Granderath FA, Kockerling F. The use of biological meshes in diaphragmatic defects – an evidence-based review of the literature. Front Surg. 2015;2:56. https://doi.org/10.3389/fsurg.2015.00056.

Basics of Trauma Management Abdominal Trauma

18

George Tsoulfas

18.1 Introduction

The goal of this chapter is to present basic features of abdominal trauma, with a special emphasis on situations such as disasters and mass casualties, and the special challenges that these may present regarding the management of abdominal trauma. The first section of the chapter will present the basic features of abdominal trauma, including evaluation, diagnosis, and management for both penetrating and blunt injuries. Following that, the second section of the chapter will briefly present and discuss certain aspects of disasters and mass casualties, such as triage, blast injuries, crush and compartment injuries, wound management, damage control surgery, and the overall use of trauma laparotomy. Additionally, special consideration will be given to situations involving potentially more vulnerable patients, such as children and pregnant women. Although a lot of the points discussed in the second part of the chapter will be presented in more detail in other chapters, the goal here is to identify how they specifically affect the management of abdominal trauma. The most important point that should come out of this chapter is the critical need for a multidisciplinary and well-coordinated approach to abdominal trauma in patients in disasters or in mass casualty situations.

18.2 Basics of Abdominal Trauma Management

Any discussion of abdominal trauma management would be incomplete without emphasizing right from the beginning that this is **part** of the overall management of the trauma patient, which means that the first priority always remains the "ABCDE" approach. The key point here is that, for example, the abdominal bleeding that a

G. Tsoulfas (✉)
Surgery, Aristotle University of Thessaloniki, Thessaloniki, Greece

© Springer Nature Switzerland AG 2021
E. Pikoulis, J. Doucet (eds.), *Emergency Medicine, Trauma and Disaster Management*, Hot Topics in Acute Care Surgery and Trauma,
https://doi.org/10.1007/978-3-030-34116-9_18

patient may be experiencing from a blast injury, is of secondary importance if that same patient does not have a secure airway. Although the "ABCDE" remains the first priority, it should not take more than 10 min given the coordination and team-work that should take place. The primary survey will lead to the identification and treatment of those injuries that are considered life-threatening and do that in a timely manner, whereas the secondary survey will consist of a general and systemic examination to identify all occult injuries, as well as obtain an **A.M.P.L.E.** (Allergy, Medications, Past medical history, Last meal, Event) history. Regarding abdominal trauma, the two main types of injuries have their own intricacies and will be presented separately.

18.2.1 Blunt Abdominal Injuries

Blunt injury presents a more complex picture, as the areas or organs injured may not always be clear given the lack of entry or exit points. A variety of signs and symptoms or elements of the mechanism involved in the trauma or parts of the history of the event or of the clinical examination of the patient are criteria for a closer evaluation of the abdomen. Examples include unexplained hypotension, inability to obtain a reliable examination or history, inability to observe the patient (need to go to the operating room to address a non-abdominal injury), orthopedic injuries raising possibility of associated injuries, or high velocity injury (i.e., pelvic fracture, lower rib fractures, spine injury), among others. Apart from the clinical examination, and especially given the high potential for lack of reliability of that exam given coexisting distracting injuries or changes in cognitive status that can easily occur in large-scale disasters, it is imperative to have accurate tools to make the diagnosis of blunt abdominal injury. These include abdominal ultrasound (US), CT scan, and the use of deep peritoneal lavage (DPL). Each of them has advantages and disadvantages having to do with issues such as accuracy, sensitivity and specificity, ability to diagnose particular injuries or not (such as US missing bowel injuries), cost, ease of transfer/portability, speed, ability to repeat, invasiveness, dependency on an operator. Deep peritoneal lavage is a rapid, yet invasive, method of assessing the abdominal cavity through the placement of a percutaneous catheter and interpretation of the lavage results. In the appropriate setting, it can be performed expeditiously, and the only real contraindication is the need to go to the operating room for laparotomy, whereas relative contraindications include advanced (third trimester) pregnancy or multiple previous operations [1]. Ultrasound has been used in trauma in the form of Focused Assessment with Sonography in Trauma (FAST), which was first used in 1996 and is rapid and accurate with a sensitivity of 85–99% [2]. It can detect as little as 100 mL of fluid, and its cost-effectiveness and portability make it an invaluable companion for the trauma physician. The key aspect and what makes FAST so successful is the fact that the operator only has to look at four views (perihepatic, peripelvic, perisplenic, and pericardiac) in order to answer only one question: "Is there free fluid?" If that is the case in an unstable patient, then the patient has to go immediately to the operating room. The major deciding factors are the

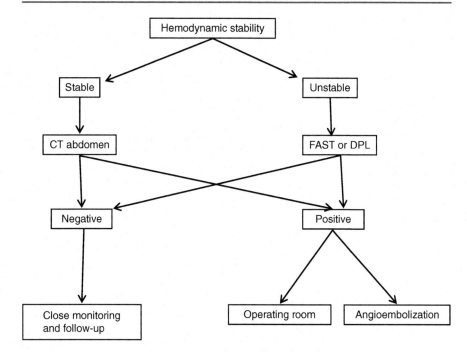

Fig. 18.1 Hemodynamic stability

hemodynamic stability of the patient and the availability of the diagnostic machine/ instrumentation. Specifically, as we can see in Fig. 18.1, a hemodynamically stable patient can undergo a CT scan which will provide significantly more detail regarding any abdominal injuries, including any extravasation of intravenous contrast that would be indicative of vascular injury. However, a patient who is hemodynamically unstable is not fit to be transferred anywhere (but the OR or wherever the definitive area of management of the cause of the instability is) and should undergo in the receiving area either a DPL or a FAST scan. The latter is preferred given its noninvasive nature and greater speed and ease.

Solid organ (spleen, liver, kidneys, pancreas) injuries are graded based on the presence and size of subcapsular hematoma, capsular tear, parenchymal lacerations, and avulsion of vascular pedicle. The major threat is bleeding which can be significant and in certain cases quite rapid. Certain cases involving a slower ooze may warrant careful observation and repeated assessment. Depending on the organ(s) injured and the type of the injury, the trauma team will have to decide on whether operative or conservative treatment is required.

18.2.1.1 Splenic Injury

The spleen is the most common abdominal organ injured (40–50%) with a strong association to left lower rib fractures. The grading of splenic injuries can be seen in Fig. 18.2. Conservative management of blunt splenic injuries was initiated in the

Fig. 18.2 Splenic injury
grading scale

Splenic injury grading scale	
Grade I	Laceration(s) <1 cm deep Subcapsular hematoma < 1cm diameter
Grade II	Laceration(s) 1-3 cm deep Subcapsular or central hematoma 1-3 cm diameter
Grade III	Laceration(s) 3-10 cm deep Subcapsular or central hematoma 3-10 cm diameter
Grade IV	Laceration(s) > 10 cm deep Subcapsular or central hematoma > 10 cm diameter
Grade V	Splenic tissue maceration or devascularization

pediatric population in order to avoid Overwhelming Post-Splenectomy Infection or Sepsis (OPSI or OPSS) [3]. This rapidly became the norm for adults as well, with the major criteria being a hemodynamically stable patient, absence of intravenous contrast extravasation in CT, and the lack of an associated hollow viscus injury [4, 5]. Conservative management is possible for Grades 1–3 of splenic injury with a success rate >80%. However, it is essential that these patients are monitored closely through clinical examination, hematocrit and overall hemodynamic evaluation, and if there are any changes then repeating an abdominal CT, or even proceeding to the OR in the case of instability is warranted. In the case of operative management for capsular tears, compression and application of hemostatic agents may be sufficient, whereas for deep lacerations horizontal mattress sutures or splenorrhaphy may be needed. For major lacerations not involving the hilum, a partial splenectomy may suffice, whereas for those involving the hilum total splenectomy is necessary. Grades 4–6 almost invariably require operative intervention, with a success rate of splenic salvage of 40–60%. An alternative to operative intervention in the case of bleeding is the use of angiographic embolization of the source of the bleeding. This obviously necessitates the immediate availability of an aggressive interventional radiology department.

18.2.1.2 Hepatic Injury

The liver is the largest organ in the abdomen and the second most commonly injured one (35–45%). A particular concern in the case of liver injury is that the bleeding is usually venous, and as a result the vast majority of patients with blunt hepatic injury are initially hemodynamically stable; the other side of the coin is that a significant number of hepatic injuries involving venous bleeding will have stopped bleeding by the time of the surgery [6, 7]. The grading of hepatic injuries can be seen in Fig. 18.3. Similar to splenic injuries, there is a similar tendency to make an effort for conservative management for hepatic injuries provided that the patient is hemodynamically

AAST grading of hepatic injury		
Grade	Type of injury	Description of injury
I	Hematoma	Subcapsular, <10% surface area
	Laceration	Capsular tear, < 1cm parenchymal depth
II	Hematoma	Subcapsular, 10-50% surface area, intraparenchymal < 10 cm in diameter
	Laceration	Capsular tear 1-3 parenchymal depth, <10 cm in length
III	Hematoma	Subcapsular, >50% surface area of ruptured subcapsular or parenchymal hematoma; intraparenchymal hematoma > 10 cm or expanding
	Laceration	Parenchymal laceration > 3 cm deep
IV	Hematoma	Parenchymal disruption involving 25-75% of the hepatic lobe or 1-3 Couinaud's segments
V	Laceration	Parenchymal disruption involving > 75% of hepatic lobe or > 3 Couinaud's segments within a single lobe
	Vascular	Juxtahepatic venous injuries; i.e. retrohepatic vena cava/central major hepatic veins
VI	Vascular	Hepatic avulsion

Fig. 18.3 AAST grading of hepatic injury

Fig. 18.4 Abdominal CT with blunt hepatic injury causing complete disruption of the parenchyma and active bleeding as evidenced by the free intravascular dye

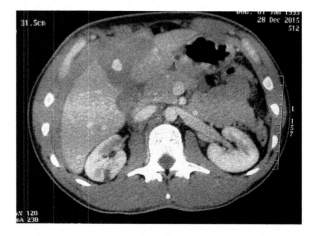

stable, there are no other intra-abdominal injuries that would warrant an operation, and the patient has required less than 2 units of red blood cells. This is usually possible for Grade I–III injuries, whereas with more advanced ones there is a need for operative management (Figs. 18.4 and 18.5). In general, injuries closer to the porta hepatis have a higher possibility of requiring operative intervention compared to more peripheral ones. The option of angiographic embolization also exists for cases with active bleeding, provided that an interventional radiology team is available. In cases requiring surgery, the first maneuver is packing of the abdomen and the hepatic area as well as using the Pringle maneuver, in order to allow the anesthesiologist to resuscitate the patient. Subsequently, a combination of pressure, application of

Fig. 18.5 Surgical
management of extreme
hepatic injury with active
bleeding

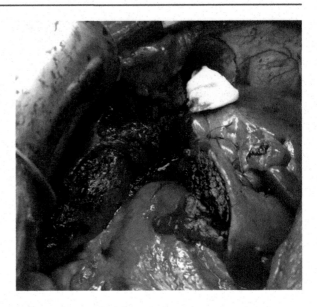

hemostatic agents, simple or deep mattress sutures, mesh hepatorrhaphy, and debridement can follow in order to control the bleeding. Techniques such as resection and/or
liver transplantation, although they may seem appealing, are not likely to succeed in
an already hemodynamically unstable patient who is in need of immediate control
and resuscitation. Leaving a drain is good practice, given the high likelihood of biliary leaks from the injured hepatic parenchyma. If the more conservative surgical
measures fail, then the trauma team should pack the area to temporarily control the
situation and move the patient to the intensive care unit with a plan to remove the
packs after 48 h should the situation improve and after the patient has been adequately resuscitated.

18.2.1.3 Pancreatic Injury

Pancreatic injury is relatively rare and is usually the result of crushing injuries or
injuries to the lumbar spine or seatbelt injury or direct blows to the abdomen. Due
to its anatomic location, pancreatic injury is usually associated with duodenal, vascular, and/or hepatic injury. Essentially, because of its retroperitoneal location, the
diagnosis requires a high index of suspicion and a careful examination of the
CT. There are often indirect signs, such as edema with pancreatic enlargement and
loss of lobulation, peripancreatic fluid or fat infiltration, concomitant duodenal
injury, or presence of fluid on the dorsal surface with densities indicative of blood.
The grading of pancreatic trauma can be seen in Fig. 18.6. Interestingly enough, the
management of pancreatic trauma, irrespective of whether it is the result of blunt or
penetrating injury, is managed in a similar manner, which is based on a "conservative operative" approach [8, 9]. Specifically, the location and the extent of the injury
determine the type of operative intervention needed, with the goal being to do the
least possible to ensure the safety of the patient, while avoiding further irritation or

AAST grading of pancreatic injury		
Grade	Type of injury	Description of injury
I	Hematoma	Minor contusion without duct injury
	Laceration	Superficial injury without duct injury
II	Hematoma	Major injury without duct injury or tissue loss
	Laceration	Major laceration without duct injury or tissue loss
III	Laceration	Distal transection or parenchymal injury with duct injury
IV	Laceration	Proximal transection or parenchymal injury with probable duct injury (not involving ampulla)
V	Laceration	Massive fragmentationof pancreatic head

Fig. 18.6 AAST grading of pancreatic injury

trauma to the area. If the pancreatic duct is not involved, then simple drainage of the area will suffice, whereas if the distal part of the duct is involved, then a distal pancreatectomy (with an effort to preserve the spleen) will be enough. The level of difficulty is increased when we move to proximal injuries of the pancreatic duct; there the issue becomes that of injury to adjacent organs, such as the duodenum. If the duodenum is unharmed, the ligation of the proximal duct and anastomosis with intestine of the distal one can provide a solution; alternatively, if the duodenum is damaged, then the possibility of requiring a pancreaticoduodenectomy is considered. However, the ideal setting for such a laborious and time-consuming procedure is not the first operation, and ideally every effort should be made to stabilize the patient and return to the OR after 24–48 h for the more definitive procedure. Obviously, in any surgery involving the pancreas, drain placement can be invaluable as possible postoperative and post-traumatic pancreatic fistulas can be diagnosed and managed.

18.2.1.4   Renal, Bladder, and Ureteral Injury

It is easy to overlook renal injury given the retroperitoneal position of the kidneys and the variety of reasons that can cause hematuria. It should be suspected in the case of lower rib fractures or fractures of the spinous process, abdominal crush and pelvic injuries, falls, motor vehicle accidents (MVA), and direct blows to the back

Classification of renal injury	
Grade I	Contusion or subcapsular hematoma
Grade II	Nonexpanding hematoma, <1 cm deep, no extravasation
Grade III	Laceration > 1 cm with urinary extravasation
Grade IV	Parenchymal laceration deep tothe corticomedullary junction
Grade V	Renovascular injury

Fig. 18.7 Classification of renal Injury

or the flanks. Diagnosis can be the result of symptoms/signs (pain and hematuria), X-ray, and US, as well as CT scan of the abdomen, which will also provide information about the vascular pedicle of the kidneys. There is a grading classification of renal injury as seen in Fig. 18.7. As renal preservation is a key goal, it is quite important that approximately 85% of blunt renal trauma can be managed conservatively [10]. Indications for operative exploration include deep cortico-medullary laceration with extravasation, large perinephric hematoma, renovascular injury, and uncontrolled bleeding; however, if salvage of the injured kidney is surgically not possible, it is important to assess the contralateral kidney before nephrectomy.

In the case of bladder injury, the majority are associated with pelvic fractures, given their anatomic proximity. Diagnosis can be made with retrograde vesicourethrogram (VCUG) or cystography, and the critical question is, in the case of a rupture, whether it is intra- or extra-peritoneal. In the former case, a transperitoneal closure and use of a suprapubic catheter is needed, whereas in the latter a simple Foley catheter placement for 2 weeks will suffice.

Ureteral injury is relatively uncommon with blunt injury and mostly associated with concomitant intra-abdominal or genitourinary injury. Diagnosis can be made with the use of intravenous pyelogram (IVP) or a retrograde VCUG. The treatment depends on the diameter, length, and location of the injury. Small and/or short injuries can usually be repaired over the use of a stent. Proximal and mid-ureter injuries require an end-to-end anastomosis over a stent, whereas distal ones are best managed with reimplantation of the ureter.

18.2.1.5 Diaphragmatic Injury

Diaphragmatic injury, as rare as it is, represents one of the bigger challenges of blunt (and sometimes penetrating) abdominal injury, given the fact that it is diagnosed early in only half of the cases. The reason for this delayed presentation is that it can usually be diagnosed only by indirect signs, such as a nasogastric tube or abdominal contents in the thorax, an elevated hemidiaphragm or distortion of the costodiaphragmatic angle among others, and as a result requires a high degree of suspicion. In addition to the already mentioned diagnostic measures, in this case there is a place for diagnostic laparoscopy [11]. Management is surgical repair with or without the use of a mesh, depending on the extent of the injury and the condition of the tissues.

18.2.1.6   Hollow Viscus Injury

In the case of hollow viscus injuries in blunt abdominal trauma, it usually involves the duodenum, small intestine, and colon and the stomach. The mechanism is usually one involving a significant force and a crushing injury against the spine or other fixed points. Despite the main diagnostic sign being free air in the abdomen or contrast extravasation in an abdominal CT, they frequently are characterized by delayed diagnosis [12]. Another feature is the coexistence with other intra-abdominal injuries, which is not surprising given the significant force required [13]. Primary repair and drainage is required in most cases, with resection and anastomosis in the case of small intestine. Duodenal injury represents one of the bigger challenges given the high risk of postoperative or post-trauma leaks and/or fistula creation. Primary repair if possible is a good option with the placement of drains in the surrounding area, while techniques such as pyloric exclusion or gastrointestinal bypass or a Thal patch are all options to safeguard the healing process [14].

18.2.2   Penetrating Abdominal Injuries

The most frequent scenarios for penetrating abdominal injuries are those involving gunshot wounds (GSW) or stab wounds, in addition to those occurring in mass disaster and mass casualty situations, which frequently have their own special features, as we will discuss later in the chapter. Overall, the most frequently involved organs are the small intestine, the liver, and the colon; they are frequently (20%) multiple and their management is "simplified" in the sense that deep penetrating injuries require operative management, whereas more superficial ones need to be investigated to identify whether the fascia has been penetrated. The basic points of the surgical management of abdominal injuries have been presented in the previous section; in this part the differences having to do with penetrating injuries will be discussed.

18.2.2.1   Stab Wounds

Stab wounds present the trauma team with a clear mechanism and a clear track for the injury. As helpful as this may be, the issue of the depth of the injury frequently poses a problem. Specifically, stab wounds to the anterior abdomen create no intra-abdominal injury in 20–40% of the cases, and as a result exploring all patients with these injuries would lead to an unacceptably high negative laparotomy rate. If this is limited to patients with hypotension or peritonitis or evisceration, there is still a negative laparotomy rate of 10–20%. All of this leads to the question of how to best decide which patients should undergo surgical exploration. Diagnostic methods such as FAST or DPL are not as accurate from the standpoint that fluid caused by a small hepatic or splenic parenchymal tear and which will respond to conservative management may lead to a positive diagnostic test. Additionally, they both present limitations when it comes to identifying small bowel injuries in this setting. Alternatives such as local exploration of the wound or diagnostic laparoscopy, as appealing as they may sound, have the disadvantages of either requiring anesthesia or not being sensitive enough [15]. The result is that in patients who are hemodynamically stable and without any abdominal signs a stab wound to the anterior abdomen may be managed conservatively with success, provided that close monitoring with serial abdominal exams is possible [16].

Stab wounds to the flank and the back represent more of a challenge in the sense that there is a bigger threat to retroperitoneal organs and the diaphragm. Based on this and in order to have a clear diagnosis these patients should undergo a triple contrast (intravenous, oral, and rectal) CT of the abdomen, and laparoscopy should be considered. Again, special emphasis and consideration should be given to the possibility of a diaphragmatic injury given the anatomic position and extent thereof of the diaphragm. This is a situation where laparoscopy can prove to be both diagnostic and therapeutic.

18.2.2.2 Gunshot Wounds
The concern with GSWs is that the mechanism involved is more complex given that there are differences based on whether it is a handgun, rifle, or shotgun, with the degree of injury depending on the amount of kinetic energy imparted by the bullet to the victim, the mass and type of the bullet, and the distance. The trajectory of the bullet (if it is a single one) is critical as far as being able to identify any associated injuries in the path, which however is less important in the case of hollow point bullets as there is no straight path in that case. One of the more interesting developments with increased understanding of trauma physiology, improvements in CT technology, as well as with increased experience from managing war-related wounds, has become clear that certain GSW could actually be managed conservatively in certain situations [17].

18.3 Abdominal Trauma and Mass Casualty Situations

In the first part of this chapter, we have seen the basic features of the diagnosis and management of abdominal trauma, both for blunt and penetrating. This second section of the chapter will present a series of special situations having to do with the specific challenges involved in the management of abdominal trauma in disaster situations with mass casualties. Although most of these will be presented in more detail in other chapters of the book, the goal here is to briefly present certain points relating to abdominal trauma.

18.3.1 Triage

Triage is the critical point where the most injured patients are identified on the scene and rapid treatment and rapid transfer to definitive care is provided. It should be stressed that the priorities based on which triage is conducted may differ between a civilian mass casualty scene and a combat zone; specifically, in a combat situation, priority is given to treating those that can get back to a fighting condition in the quickest possible time and with the least effort, something which is exactly the opposite from civilian life, where the more severely injured are given priority. Triage can be extremely complicated as most patients will have a variety of injuries with different mechanisms (heterogeneous bombs) producing unique injury patterns. Additionally, there is little room for errors, as under- or over-triage can either lead to unnecessary loss of life or overwhelm the medical system [18]. Moreover, triage is an active and evolving process, as patients are reevaluated when they arrive at the health care facility by a multidisciplinary, well-coordinated team. This last part is key as the arrival of the patients and triage needs to be a well-choreographed event where everybody has their role and where a senior member of the trauma team has the oversight of the whole situation [19]. The basics of the primary management remain the same with the ABCDE, but in the case of disasters and mass casualties there are some changes as the fact that although spine precautions should be considered by first-responders, full spine immobilization may not be always necessary given the time it takes. Another example is the effort to provide basic life support on the scene, rather than advanced, so that the patient can get to more definitive care in a timely fashion. These are examples of choices to be made and changes in strategy so that volume, together with the severity of the injuries, can also be accommodated.

18.3.2 Blast Injury

With the increasing appearance of bomb blast injuries in a noncombat setting as the result of terrorist acts, it is imperative for the health care team to be cognizant of the intricacies of these injuries. The specifics can vary depending on the type of explosives (high or low order), the material, the scene and other factors, all of which have a common mechanism. Specifically, the detonation leads to an instantaneous release of energy, which creates a shock wave blast in the form of expanding gases [20]. When these shock waves hit the tissues of the human body, they can have a variable effect depending on the density of the tissue of the different organs. As a result, hollow organs (stomach, duodenum, intestine) are more easily injured, compared to solid ones (liver, spleen), because of the different densities encountered [21]. Additionally, the location can also play a role, as in open spaces the velocity waves are dissipated in open air and the result is low, immediate mortalities, in contrast to closed spaces, where the blast waves can be reflected back, thus leading to repeated injuries [22].

Regarding abdominal injury, the most frequent pattern is that of the "blast abdomen" which is used to describe abdominal bleeding and perforation caused by the pressurized wave. The most frequently injured organ, as discussed in the previous paragraph and because of the difference in pressure densities, is the intestine. The signs and symptoms may be abdominal pain, emesis, and rectal bleeding, among others; however, given the fact that these injuries may not present in full force immediately, a high level of suspicion and close monitoring of these patients is needed. In addition to the small intestine, colonic injuries are also quite common, and again often with a delayed presentation, as mesenteric ischemia or an infarct can develop into full thickness necrosis and rupture [23]. In these cases and given the threat to the microcirculation, anastomosis is not the best choice and rather a colostomy should be performed [24]. Small, partial colonic tears can be repaired primarily, provided that the patient is hemodynamically stable, there has been no massive blood transfusion, no hypoxia or reperfusion injury, no other injuries and limited local tissue damage.

In the case of the solid abdominal organs (spleen, liver, kidney) in the case of significant blast forces, there can be rupture and tissue destruction, as well as hemorrhage. In the case of hemorrhagic shock, then the patient needs to go immediately to the operating room, or if there is doubt about the abdomen being the source, then a FAST can be performed expeditiously. In the case of bleeding from an abdominal wound, the initial management on the scene is based on the use of pressure as well as hemostatic dressings for nonextremity injuries (such as HemCon or Advanced Clotting Sponge, to name a few), which are applied directly to the wound and with direct 5 min pressure.

18.3.3 Crush Injury

Crush injuries can occur in situations where areas of the body are subjected to very high pressures, leading mainly to injuries involving muscles, bones, extremities, and the abdomen. The importance of crush injuries lies in the cascade of events that is set in motion by the initial insult, potentially culminating to rhabdomyolysis and ischemia/reperfusion injury [24]. The basic process of rhabdomyolysis involves the rapid breakdown of muscle tissue with the accompanying release of several products such as purines, lactic acid, phosphate, myoglobin, among others into the circulation and fluid entering the damaged cell, leading to intracellular swelling and eventually cell damage and death [25]. An electrolyte imbalance prevails with hyperkalemia and if the injury is managed in such a way so as to restore circulation, then the reperfusion that follows can lead to further cellular damage and swelling and ultimately cell necrosis. All of these changes, including the massive fluid shifts, the electrolyte abnormalities, the renal dysfunction, the lactic acidosis, and the possible disseminated intravascular coagulation form what is known as the "crush injury" [26]. Management includes excellent coordination between the first-responders and the receiving health trauma team, with emphasis on fluid resuscitation, as it is the best way to manage rhabdomyolysis.

The abdomen can be affected both from the crush injury itself, as well as from the cascade of events that follows and that can end in adverse situations such as a compartment syndrome [27]. The main problem with the compartment syndrome is that the pressures within a compartment (which is essentially a physiologically closed space) exceed the pressures of the circulatory system, thus cutting off circulation to tissues and organs. The abdominal compartment syndrome is an emergency when it occurs as it is associated with loss of renal function, labored respiration (due to the intra-abdominal pressure curtailing the movement of the diaphragm), and a lactic acidosis. The management includes immediate release of the compartment syndrome by a laparotomy to release the pressure. Additionally, disasters such as earthquakes involving crush injuries can lead to direct abdominal trauma with the most frequent types being injury to the abdominal wall, hepatic and splenic injury [28]. At the same time, the threat of the crush injury and the deadly sequence that it entails puts these patients at elevated risk, with a key priority being adequate fluid resuscitation.

A common aspect of both blast and crush injuries is the management of the abdominal wound. Given the setting and the mechanism involved, it is vital to perform wide wound debridement till healthy tissue is encountered, obtain fluid and tissue cultures to guide potential antibiotic use, and irrigate the wound sufficiently [29]. Abdominal wounds from blast or crush injuries should not be closed primarily, not even after the irrigation and debridement, but rather wound vacuum-assisted closure techniques should be used.

18.3.4 Special Considerations

Children and pregnant women represent groups that are particularly vulnerable when in the middle of a disaster or a mass casualty event. Experience from terrorist attacks has shown that intra-abdominal injuries in children require immediate surgical attention, given the fact that in a child a small loss of blood can lead to hemodynamic decompensation. Children have been shown to require more ICU and hospital resources given higher Injury Severity Scores, as well as prolonged hospitalizations [30]. In the case of pregnant women, the fetus is somewhat protected in its position, although abruption of the placenta can occur in the case of pressure waves from a blast injury. In the case of women in the second and third trimester, they should be admitted for fetal monitoring and an ultrasound performed to evaluate both the fetus as well as the mother's abdomen [31]. The overwhelming priority remains that in order to save the fetus the mother has to be saved first.

18.3.5 Damage Control Surgery

Damage control surgery is a key principle and a frequently employed strategy when dealing with mass casualties or disaster victims with abdominal injury. The basic concept is that "resuscitation takes precedence over surgery" and that "the operating room is not the best place to resuscitate a trauma victim." The decision to proceed with damage control means that the main goals of the surgical team are to stop any hemorrhage and control intestinal contamination; the latter means that any injured intestine is resected or stapled and no anastomosis are performed at this stage. The abdomen is closed in a rapid and temporary manner using either wound vacuum-assisted closure, an intravenous bag or a mesh, and the patient is transferred to the

ICU for resuscitation. Once that has occurred, then definitive surgery for any injuries can take place at a later time point with a more stable patient. The main threat and what we are trying to avoid is the trauma "triangle of death" which consists of hypothermia, lactic acidosis, and coagulopathy, since once that occurs, then there are limited options to overcome a critical situation [32]. Interestingly enough, there is evidence that damage control surgery may still be somewhat underused, even in combat situations [33].

It should be mentioned that a major trend in trauma is the increasing prevalence of conservative management of injuries (such as penetrating) that would have been immediately operated upon a decade ago. This is the result of improvements in the radiological diagnosis, as well as a better understanding of the physiology of trauma [34–36]. Although the ultimate goal is to reduce unnecessary laparotomies, patient selection should be very careful and strict so as to avoid missing an injury or not addressing it with the urgency required [37].

18.4   Conclusion

As difficult as the management of abdominal trauma can be, it becomes more of a challenge in disasters and in situations with mass casualties. Although the basic principles remain the same, as we have seen in this chapter, there are differences regarding the frequency and the types of injuries that can be encountered. Critical features in these situations are the ongoing triage and the ability to achieve multidisciplinary collaboration, which is no easy task if we consider the scale of these events [38].

References

1. Demetriades D, Velmahos G. Technology-driven triage of abdominal trauma: the emerging era of nonoperative management. Annu Rev Med. 2003;54:1–15.
2. Mohammad A, Hefny AF, Abu-Zidan FM. Focused assessment sonography for trauma (FAST) training: a systematic review. World J Surg. 2014;38:1009–18.
3. Okabayashi T, Hanazaki K. Overwhelming postsplenectomy infection syndrome in adults - a clinically preventable disease. World J Gastroenterol. 2008;14:176–9.
4. Feliciano DV. Abdominal trauma revisited. Am Surg. 2017;83:1193–202.
5. Coccolini F, Montori G, Catena F, Kluger Y, Biffl W, Moore EE, et al. Splenic trauma: WSES classification and guidelines for adult and pediatric patients. World J Emerg Surg. 2017;12:40–65.
6. Yu WY, Li QJ, Gong JP. Treatment strategy for hepatic trauma. Chin J Traumatol. 2016;19:168–71.
7. Ward J, Alarcon L, Peitzman AB. Management of blunt liver injury: what is new? Eur J Trauma Emerg Surg. 2015;41:229–37.
8. Johnsen NV, Betzold RD, Guillamondegui OD, Dennis BM, Stassen NA, Bhullar I, et al. Surgical management of solid organ injuries. Surg Clin North Am. 2017;97:1077–105.
9. Kilen P, Greenbaum A, Miskimins R, Rojo M, Preda R, Howdieshell T, et al. General surgeon management of complex hepatopancreatobiliary trauma at a level I trauma center. J Surg Res. 2017;217:226–31.

10. Van der Wilden GM, Velmahos GC, Joseph DK, Jacobs L, Debusk MG, Adams CA, et al. Successful nonoperative management of the most severe blunt renal injuries: a multi-center study of the research consortium of New England Centers for Trauma. JAMA Surg. 2013;148:924–31.
11. Justin V, Fingerhut A, Uranues S. Laparoscopy in blunt abdominal trauma: for whom? when? and why? Curr Trauma Rep. 2017;3:43–50.
12. Al-Hassani A, Tuma M, Mahmood I, Afifi I, Almadani A, El-Menyar A, et al. Dilemma of blunt bowel injury: what are the factors affecting early diagnosis and outcomes. Am Surg. 2013;79:922–7.
13. Swaid F, Peleg K, Alfici R, Matter I, Olsha O, Ashkenazi I, et al. Concomitant hollow viscus injuries in patients with blunt hepatic and splenic injuries: an analysis of a national trauma registry database. Injury. 2014;45:1409–12.
14. Bekker W, Kong VY, Laing GL, Bruce JL, Manchev V, Clarke DL. The spectrum and outcome of blunt trauma related enteric hollow visceral injury. Ann R Coll Surg Engl. 2018;100:290–4.
15. Lin HF, Wu JM, Tu CC, Chen HA, Shih HC. Value of diagnostic and therapeutic laparoscopy for abdominal stab wounds. World J Surg. 2010;34:1653–62.
16. Dayananda K, Kong VY, Bruce JL, Oosthuizen GV, Laing GL, Clarke DL. Selective non-operative management of abdominal stab wounds is a safe and cost effective strategy: a South African experience. Ann R Coll Surg Engl. 2017;99:490–6.
17. Salim A, Velmahos GC. When to operate on abdominal gunshot wounds. Scand J Surg. 2002;91:62–6.
18. Shea JM, Wei G, Donovan CM, Bryczkowski C, Chapleau W, Shah CN, et al. Medical management at the explosive incident scene. Ann Emerg Med. 2017;69:S20–8.
19. Gale SC, Shiroff AM, Donovan CM, Rhodes SC, Rhodes JS, Gracias VH. Medical management at the health care facility. Ann Emerg Med. 2017;69:S36–45.
20. Wightman JM, Gladish SL. Explosions and blast injuries. Ann Emerg Med. 2001;37:664–78.
21. Goh SH. Bomb blast mass casualty incidents: initial triage and management of injuries. Singap Med J. 2009;50:101–6.
22. Mayo A, Kluger Y. Terrorist bombing. World J Emerg Surg. 2006;1:33.
23. DePalma RG, Burris DG, Champion HR, Hodgson MJ. Blast injuries. N Engl J Med. 2005;352:1335–42.
24. Smith J, Greves I. Crush injury and crush syndrome: a review. J Trauma. 2003;54(5 suppl):S226–30.
25. Sever MS, Vanholder R, Lameire N. Management of crush-related injuries after disasters. N Engl J Med. 2006;354:1052–63.
26. Sever MS, Vanholder RL. RDRTF of ISN work group on recommendations for the management of crush victims in mass disasters. Recommendation for the management of crush victims in mass disasters. Nephrol Dial Transplant. 2012;27(Suppl 1):i1–i67.
27. Salomone JP, Pons PT. Musculoskeletal trauma. In: PHTLS: prehospital trauma life support. 6th ed. St. Louis, MO: Mosby JEMS Elsevier; 2007. p. 327.
28. Xu Y, Huang J, Zhou J, Zeng Y. Patterns of abdominal injury in 37387 disaster patients from the Wenchuan earthquake. Emerg Med J. 2013;30:538–42.
29. Hospenthal DR, Murray CK, Andersen RC, et al. Guidelines for the prevention of infection after combat-related injuries. J Trauma. 2008;64:S211–20.
30. Mikrogianakis A, Grant V. The kids are alright: pediatric trauma pearls. Emerg Med Clin North Am. 2018;36:237–57.
31. DePalma RG, Burris DG, Champion HR, et al. Blast injuries. N Engl J Med. 2005;352:1335–42.
32. Mitra B, Tullio F, Cameron PA, Fitzgerald M. Trauma patients with the 'triad of death'. Emerg Med J. 2012;29:622–5.
33. Fries CA, Penn-Barwell J, Tai NR, Hodgetts TJ, Midwinter MJ, Bowley DM. Management of intestinal injury in deployed UK hospitals. J R Army Med Corps. 2011;157:370–3.
34. Butt MU, Zacharias N, Velmahos GC. Penetrating abdominal injuries: management controversies. Scand J Trauma Resusc Emerg Med. 2009;17:19.

35. Demetriades D, Velmahos GC, Cornwell E III, Berne TV, Cober S, Bhasin PS. Selective nonoperative management of gunshot wounds to the anterior abdomen. Arch Surg. 1997;132:178–83.
36. Sharpe JP, Magnotti LJ, Weinberg JA, et al. Adherence to a simplified management algorithm reduces morbidity and mortality after penetrating colon injuries: a 15-year experience. J Am Coll Surg. 2012;214:591–7.
37. Morrison JJ, Poon H, Garner J, Midwinter MJ, Jansen JO. Nontherapeutic laparotomy in combat casualties. J Trauma Acute Care Surg. 2012;73(6 Suppl 5):S479–82.
38. Aschkenasy-Steuer G, Shamir M, Rivkind A, Mosheiff R, Shushan Y, Rosenthal G, et al. Clinical review: the Israeli experience: conventional terrorism and critical care. Crit Care. 2005;9:490–9.

Injuries to the Urinary Tract

19

Michael Chrisofos

Injury to the genitourinary tract occurs in 10% of abdominal trauma [1–3]. The kidney is the most commonly affected genitourinary organ during such traumas [1]. Ureteral trauma is relatively rare and mainly due to iatrogenic injuries or penetrating gunshot wounds (both in military and in civilian settings) [4]. Traumatic bladder injuries are usually due to blunt causes such as motor vehicle accidents (MVAs), and they are associated with pelvic fracture [5], although they may also be the result of iatrogenic trauma. The anterior urethra is most commonly injured by blunt or "fall-astride" trauma, whereas the posterior urethra is usually injured in pelvic fracture cases, the majority of which usually occur during MVAs [6]. Genital trauma is much more common in males due to the particular anatomical considerations and also their more frequent participation in physical sports, violent events, and war fighting [7].

19.1 Renal Trauma

Renal trauma occurs in approximately 1–5% of all trauma cases [8]. The kidney is the most commonly injured genitourinary organ at all ages, with a male-to-female ratio of 3:1 [9]. It is particularly vulnerable to deceleration injuries as the organ is fixed and supported spatially only by the renal pelvis and the vascular pedicle [10]. More than 80% of kidney injuries are due to blunt trauma [11]. Penetrating trauma is rare but is associated with more severe injury.

The evaluation of renal trauma is based on the patient's hemodynamic status (Grade A, EAU—European Association of Urology (EAU)), mechanism of injury, physical examination, and urine analysis [2]. Hematuria is present in 80–94% of

M. Chrisofos (✉)
3rd Urology Department, University Hospital "Attikon", Athens Medical School, National and Kapodistrian University of Athens, Athens, Greece

© Springer Nature Switzerland AG 2021
E. Pikoulis, J. Doucet (eds.), *Emergency Medicine, Trauma and Disaster Management*, Hot Topics in Acute Care Surgery and Trauma, https://doi.org/10.1007/978-3-030-34116-9_19

all cases [12]. Major injury (e.g., disruption of the ureteropelvic junction, pedicle injuries, segmental arterial thrombosis, and stab wounds) may also occur without hematuria being present.

Indications for radiographic evaluation are hemodynamically stable patients with gross hematuria (Grade B, AUA—American Urological Association (AUA), Grade A, EAU), nonvisible hematuria with hypotension, or major associated injuries [13]. Microscopic hematuria does not warrant imaging (Grade B, AUA) [1]. Patients with penetrating trauma to the torso have a high incidence of significant injuries, and imaging should be performed regardless of the degree of hematuria.

An ultrasound can identify who requires a more detailed investigation, and is useful for the follow-up of parenchymal lesions, hematomas, and urinomas, but cannot accurately assess renal lacerations [14].

Intravenous pyelography (IVP) is inferior to currently available CT imaging [15]. It may demonstrate nonfunction or extravasation. During an emergency laparotomy, a one-shot IVP (bolus intravenous injection of 2 ml/kg contrast followed by a single plain film after 10 min) may provide information on the presence and function of the contralateral kidney [16].

Abdominal/pelvic CT with IV contrast with immediate and delayed images is the imaging technique of choice for defining the location and the severity of injury (Grade C, AUA and SIU—Société Internationale d'Urologie (SIU); Grade A, EAU) [17, 18], as it provides a view of other abdominal and pelvic organs and also evaluates for pre-existing renal abnormalities. Also, CT provides visualization of the ureters and the contralateral kidney [19].

The American Association for the Surgery of Trauma (AAST) recommends the conservative management for Grade 1 or 2 injuries (Table 19.1, Fig. 19.1), with observation, bed rest, hydration, serial hematocrit monitoring, and the administration of antibiotics (Grade B, AUA, and EAU). Conservative management is also the recommended treatment for Grade 3 or 4 injuries (Grade B, AUA). The SIU guidelines make a specific recommendation of surgical repair for Grade 3 or 4 injuries if the patient is undergoing a laparotomy for other abdominal injuries (Grade C, SIU), while the EAU guidelines state that Grade 3 injuries should be managed expectantly (Grade B, EAU). With isolated Grade 4 injuries, the EAU states that treatment should be based solely on the extent of the renal injury. For Grade 5 injuries, the SIU recommends exploratory laparotomy (Grade C, SIU), while the EAU only

Table 19.1 American Association for the Surgery of Trauma (AAST), organ injury severity scale for renal trauma

Grade	Description of injury
1	Contusion of subcapsular hematoma
2	Cortical laceration <1 cm deep
3	Cortical laceration >1 cm without urinary extravasation
4	Laceration into collecting system, segmental vascular injury
5	Shattered kidney, renal pedicle injury, or avulsion

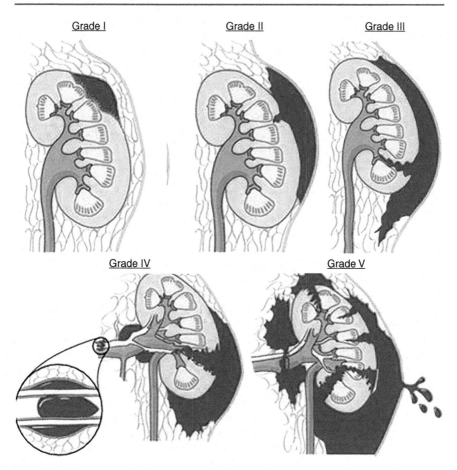

Fig. 19.1 Organ injury severity scale for renal trauma

recommends renal exploration in the case of the injury being vascular (Grade B, EAU). In contrast, the AUA recommends observation for hemodynamically stable patients regardless of AAST grade because of interobserver variability regarding the classification of Grade 4 and 5 injuries (Grade B, AUA). Patients diagnosed with urinary extravasation in solitary injuries can be managed without major intervention and with a resolution rate of >90% [20]. Unilateral main arterial injuries will normally be managed nonoperatively in patients who are stable, while surgical repair is reserved only for bilateral injuries or a solitary functional kidney in which the whole functioning renal mass is endangered. Conservative management is also advised in unilateral, complete, and blunt artery thrombosis, as well as in multiple trauma patients [21].

The goal of exploration is the control of hemorrhage and renal salvage. Immediate intervention is mandatory for hemodynamically unstable patients (Grade B, AUA, SIU and EAU). The SIU recommends only exploratory laparotomy (Grade B, SIU)

[17], while the more recent EAU and AUA guidelines also discuss angioemboliza-tion. The overall exploration rate for blunt trauma is <10% [22]. Absolute indications are life-threatening hemorrhage from renovascular injury, ureteropelvic junction avulsion, and urinoma unresponsive to ureteral stenting or perinephric drainage. Relative indications are laparotomy for other abdominal injuries or large, devascu-larized segments of the kidney. Unresponsive hemodynamic instability due to renal hemorrhage is an indication for exploration, regardless of the mode of injury, the existence of inconclusive imaging, or a pre-existing abnormality of the kidney [23]. Independent factors that increase the risk of surgical intervention are Injury Severity Score >16, increased transfusion needs, perirenal hematoma size >3.5 cm, intravas-cular contrast extravasation, and Grade 4–5 injuries [24] (Fig. 19.2).

Angiography with selective embolization is the first-line option in the absence of other indications for immediate open surgery. The main indications for angi-ography are embolization for active hemorrhage, pseudoaneurysm, and vascular fistulae [25].

The overall rate of nephrectomy is around 13%, usually in patients with penetrat-ing injury, higher rates of transfusion requirements, hemodynamic instability, and higher injury severity scores [26] (Fig. 19.3). Renorrhaphy is the most common reconstructive technique. Partial nephrectomy is required when nonviable tissue is

Fig. 19.2 Grade IV renal trauma

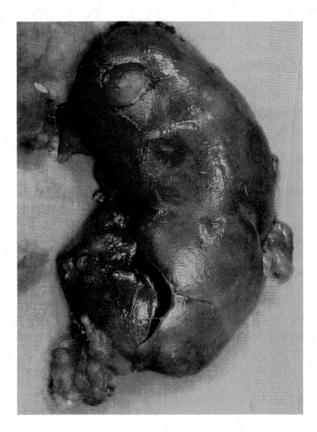

Fig. 19.3 Grade V
renal trauma

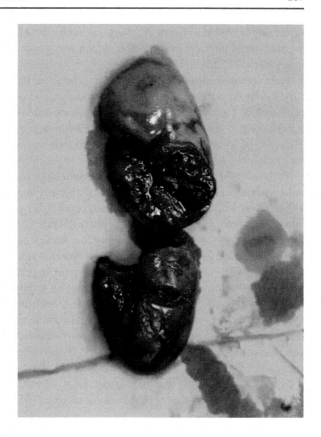

detected. Watertight closure of the collecting system is highly desirable. If the capsule is not preserved, an omental pedicle flap or perirenal fat bolster may be used instead.

Gunshot injuries should be explored only if they involve the hilum or if they are accompanied by signs of continued bleeding, ureteral injuries, or renal pelvis lacerations. Low-velocity gunshot and minor stab wounds may be managed conservatively and with a good outcome [27]. In contrast, tissue damage from high-velocity gunshot injuries can be more extensive, and a nephrectomy is often required. If the site of penetration by a stab wound is posterior to the anterior axillary line, 88% of such injuries can be managed nonoperatively. Stab wounds producing injuries of Grade 3 are associated with a higher rate of delayed complications if treated expectantly [28].

Iatrogenic renal injuries should be treated conservatively (Grade B, EAU). Significant injury is rare but requires immediate intervention with angioembolization which has excellent outcomes and lower complication rates when compared to surgery (Grade B, EAU) [18, 29].

For pediatric renal trauma, non-surgical conservative management has become the standard approach, even for high-grade injuries (Grade B, EAU) [30]. Absolute indications for surgery include hemodynamic instability, Grade 5 renal injuries, and expanding hematoma (Grade A). Surgical exploration is also indicated in a changing abdominal physical examination, which is suggestive of major intra-abdominal injury (Grade C, SIU) [17].

Early complications are bleeding, infection, perinephric abscess, sepsis, urinary fistula, hypertension, urinary extravasation, and urinoma. Delayed complications include bleeding, hydronephrosis, calculus formation, chronic pyelonephritis, hypertension, arteriovenous fistula (AVF), hydronephrosis, and pseudoaneurysms. The risk of complications following conservative management increases with the grade.

Follow-up CT is recommended if the patient has a fever, increasing flank pain, or falling hematocrit levels (Grade B, EAU). There is no need for imaging for Grade 1–3 injuries, while it is suggested that a repeat CT is made 36–72 h after a Grade 4 injury with damage to the collecting system (Grade C, SIU) [17]. The AUA guidelines also recommend follow-up imaging for Grade 4 or 5 injuries at 48 h (Grade C, AUA) [1]. Perinephric abscess formation is best managed by percutaneous drainage.

Patients with renal trauma at greatest risk of hypertension are those who have Grade 4 or 5 injuries. Patients with renal trauma should have periodic blood pressure monitoring after the injury (Grade C, AUA, SIU, and EAU). The post-traumatic hypertension rate is <5%. It may occur acutely due to compression from hematoma (Page kidney) or chronically because of scar formation; it is also renin dependent and is associated with parenchymal injury. Over the long term, etiologies include artery thrombosis or stenosis (Goldblatt kidney), devitalized fragments, and AVFs. If hypertension persists, medical management, excision of the ischemic segment, vascular reconstruction, or nephrectomy is required [31].

19.2   Ureteric Trauma

Trauma to the ureters is rare because they are protected from injury by their small size, mobility, and the adjacent vertebrae, bony pelvis, and muscles. Overall, it accounts for 1–2.5% of urinary tract trauma [32, 33].

Most ureteral injuries are iatrogenic and occur during open, laparoscopic, or ureteroscopic procedures, while less than 25% of ureteral injuries can be attributed to other causes [34–36].

Penetrating injuries account for most cases of ureteral injury. Among other causes of ureteric injuries are gunshot wounds, with the ureter being injured in between 2% and 5% of abdominal gunshot injuries [3]. The most common location for ureteral injuries is at the vesicoureteral junction and the upper part of the ureter [37]. Findings that increase the suspicion of ureteral injury on CT urography or IVP (Grade C, AUA) include delayed excretion of contrast, poor function on one side, hydronephrosis, failure to visualize the entire course of the ureter, and extravasation of the contrast material [37].

There are no specific signs and symptoms of ureteral injuries. Some of the patients may present a few days following the injury with lower abdominal pain, prolonged ileus, low-grade fever, nausea, vomiting, persistent hematuria, urinary

Table 19.2 American Association for the Surgery of Trauma (AAST), organ injury severity scale for ureteric trauma

Grade	Description of injury
1	Hematoma
2	Laceration <50% of circumference
3	Laceration >50% of circumference
4	Complete tear <2 cm of devascularization
5	Complete tear >2 cm of devascularization

tract infection (UTI), oliguria, and anuria, with laboratory investigations showing leukocytosis and raised inflammatory markers [38].

For children symptoms of a ureteric injury are often vague, so it is important to remain suspicious for potential ureteric injury after blunt abdominal trauma. The most sensitive diagnostic test to detect ureteric injury is retrograde urography (Grade A, EAU) [30].

The management of ureteral trauma depends on the nature, severity, and location of the injury. Partial injuries (Grade 2 or 3—Table 19.2) can be repaired immediately by primary closure over a stent [1, 39] (Grade C, AUA). For Grade 3–5 injuries, repair depends on the location of the injury (Grade C, AUA, and EAU). For injuries above the iliac vessels, ureteroureterostomy should be performed over a stent, if possible (Grade C, AUA). Injuries below the iliac vessels are typically repaired by re-implantation with psoas hitch and/or Boari flap (Grade C, AUA). Other less common surgical procedures include transureteroureterostomy, renal autotransplantation, and ureteral substitution with the ileum or appendix [40, 41].

In a case of delayed diagnosis or missed diagnosis of ureteral injuries, it is important to divert the urine. Surgical repair of the ureters in such cases is deferred for 6–8 weeks to allow any edema or inflammation to subside. However, there is no evidence to support that there is a worse outcome if the surgical repair is done immediately after identifying the injury [36].

Ureteral avulsion is a rare but serious complication; fortunately, its incidence is only 0.06–0.45% [42]. Risk factors for ureteral avulsion include symptomatic stones persisting >3 months, stones >5 mm, proximal ureteral distention, stones tightly encapsulated by granulation tissues, and a strong sense of tightness when the ureteroscope is moved. The muscle in the proximal ureteral tissue is weaker, and therefore, the use of a stone basket to remove the impacted stone in the upper third of the ureter increases the risk of avulsion [43]. For proximal ureteral avulsion, end-to-end anastomosis can be a good choice. Boari flap and psoas hitch are recommended for the middle third of ureteral avulsion. For distal ureteral injuries, ureteral re-implantation is recommended [44].

19.3 Bladder Trauma

Bladder injuries are frequently associated with pelvic fractures [45]. Bladder injuries can be divided into extraperitoneal (60%) and intraperitoneal (30%) (Table 19.3). Simultaneous extraperitoneal and intraperitoneal injuries occur in 10% of all traumatic bladder injuries [46]. Plain and computed tomography (CT) cystography

Table 19.3 American Association for the Surgery of Trauma (AAST), organ injury severity scale for bladder trauma

Grade	Description of injury
1	Hematoma, partial thickness laceration
2	Extraperitoneal bladder wall laceration <2 cm
3	Extraperitoneal bladder (>2 cm) or intraperitoneal (<2 cm) bladder laceration
4	Intraperitoneal bladder wall laceration >2 cm
5	Intraperitoneal or extraperitoneal bladder wall laceration extending into the bladder neck or ureteric orifice

(Grade B, AUA, and EAU), with bladder filling up to 350 mL, are the preferred diagnostic modalities for injury to the bladder [47–49]. Cystoscopy is the preferred method for detecting intraoperative bladder injuries (Grade B, EAU) [18, 39].

An uncomplicated extraperitoneal rupture can be managed safely via catheter drainage alone (Grade C, AUA; Grade B, EAU) [47, 48]. Follow-up cystography should be performed to confirm that the bladder injury has healed (Grade C, AUA) [50]. In case of bladder neck involvement, the presence of bone fragments in the bladder wall, concomitant rectal and/or vaginal injury, or entrapment of the bladder wall (e.g., by reduced pubic symphysis), early surgical repair is indicated to facilitate healing and prevent the formation of fistulae (Grade B, EAU) [1, 18]. Instances of blunt intraperitoneal rupture of the bladder should always be managed by surgical repair (Grade B, AUA, and EAU) [47, 51]. The rationale for this is that intraperitoneal extravasation of urine can lead to peritonitis, sepsis, and death.

Iatrogenic intraperitoneal bladder injuries can be managed with drainage if there is no ileus or peritonitis (Grade C, EAU) [18, 39]. Penetrating injuries to the bladder need emergency exploration with debridement of devitalized bladder detrusor and subsequent bladder repair [47, 52].

Pediatric bladder injuries can be evaluated by cystography (standard radiography or CT) with the bladder fully distended (Grade A, EAU). Management of intraperitoneal and extraperitoneal injuries in children (both uncomplicated and complicated) is the same as in adults with one difference: postoperatively, after the repair of an intraperitoneal injury, a suprapubic catheter is mandatory (Grade A, EAU) [18].

19.4   Urethral Trauma

Evaluation for urethral injuries is recommended for patients with blood at the meatus, with perineal or penile hematoma, who cannot void or who have had an injury that predisposes a straddle injury (Grade C, AUA) [1, 18].

Most urethral injuries occur in male patients. Blunt anterior urethral injuries are associated with spongiosal contusion which makes it more difficult to evaluate the limits of urethral debridement and define the accurate anatomy of adjacent structures. Acute or early urethroplasty is therefore not indicated [53]. Therapeutic options include suprapubic diversion or urethral catheter placement and delayed treatment, as the extent of injury is hard to discern (Grade B, AUA; Grade C, EAU) [46].

Penile fractures require early exploration and repair of the tear in the cavernosal tunica albuginea and, if involved, the urethra [54, 55]. A small laceration of the penis can be repaired by simple closure, while a complete rupture by anastomotic repair [55–57].

Immediate exploration of penetrating anterior urethral injuries is advised, except when this is precluded by other life-threatening injuries (Expert Opinion, AUA) [53, 54, 58]. For small lacerations and stab wounds, simple urethral closure might be sufficient [53]. Defects of up to 2–3 cm in the bulbar urethra and up to 1.5 cm in the penile urethra can be treated by anastomotic repair [58, 59]. In the case of larger defects or apparent infection (especially bite wounds), a staged repair with urethral marsupialization and a suprapubic catheter is needed [53, 58, 59], and a delayed repair with a graft or flap can occur at ≥3 months after the injury [18].

Pelvic fracture urethral injury (PFUI) is a disorder in urology often found in pelvic trauma, with an incidence ranging from 1.6% to 25% [60]. The pelvic fractures indicate a considerable strength in the lower abdominal area/pelvis. This energy can be transferred to the internal organs in the pelvic cavity including the lower urinary tract. Physical compression occurs, and the prostate is forced into the perineal membrane, causing stretching of the urethra, and it can be followed by rupture of the posterior urethra [61]. Prompt urinary drainage should be performed, whether via suprapubic or urethral catheter (Grade C, AUA).

For blunt posterior urethral injuries, it is important to distinguish between complete and partial rupture prior to proceeding with treatment.

The timing of an intervention is classified as [53, 59]: (1) immediate: <48 h after injury; (2) delayed primary: 2 days to 2 weeks after injury; or (3) deferred: >3 months after injury.

Although urinary diversion is not essential during the first few hours after the trauma, suprapubic catheterization is mandatory in urgent situations unless urethral catheterization can be achieved [54, 62, 63].

Therapeutic options for partial posterior urethral rupture are suprapubic or urethral catheterization [64–66]. Injuries may heal without significant scarring [65, 67]. Subsequent stricture should be managed with internal urethrotomy or urethroplasty, depending on the degree of narrowing and the stricture length [68].

Acute treatment options for complete posterior urethral rupture include: (1) realignment, with apposition of the urethral ends over a catheter; (2) exploration and primary repair; and (3) suprapubic catheterization alone.

The early realignment (ER) in the form of primary suturing/open urethra realignment is the best management for PFUI. Advancement in endoscopic techniques led to primary endoscopic realignment (PER) being established as an alternative management with good results (Grade C, AUA).

Patients with pelvic fractures present a high incidence of complications caused by the limited mobilization, and thus a delayed urethroplasty (DU) with cystostomy diversion may be preferred.

Treatment with early realignment can be done when the patient's condition is stable and life-threatening injuries have been treated [69]. In patients with vascular injury or other abnormalities that require exploration in the pelvic cavity, prostatourethral severe dislocation, or laceration of the neck of the bladder, early realignment could minimize the problems that may occur next [70].

The purpose of the early realignment is to pull down the proximal urethra properly/parallel to the distal side so that the healing process may occur with minimal strictures [71]. Realignment has a lower stricture rate than suprapubic catheter placement alone, for which stricture formation is almost certain. Realignment might thus avoid a prolonged period of suprapubic catheter drainage and a second operation for urethral reconstruction in some patients [48, 65, 68]. After a successful realignment, the catheter should remain in place for 4–8 weeks (EAU) [18].

Early realignment using endoscopic techniques may reduce the frequency of advanced urethrotomy procedures, something that provides a great advantage in the management of the complications and the costs [72]. Cystoscopy, either rigid or flexible, can be performed simultaneously through cystostomy and through the urethra in order to facilitate the process of realignment [73]. The success rate of realignment using endoscopy is very good, around 72–100% [65, 74].

In the absence of indications for immediate exploration, delayed primary realignment requires placement of a suprapubic catheter at the time of the initial injury, with endoscopic realignment performed within 14 days, when patients are stable and most of the pelvic bleeding has resolved (Clinical Principle, AUA) [67, 75].

Hemodynamically unstable patients should have suprapubic catheter placement and delayed management (Grade C, AUA).

Delayed urethral repair is indicated when the rupture is not complete, the separation of the urethra is minimal, there is critical condition of unstable patients, or when there is no facility to support it, and/or there is an absence of an experienced surgeon [66].

For a complete rupture treated with an initial period of ≥3 months of suprapubic diversion (Grade B, EAU), obliteration of the posterior urethra is almost inevitable [63, 67]. The stricture cannot be avoided and will be treated electively several months later [76]. The benefit of a delayed repair is that urinary diversion is easily done, optimizing the patient's general condition and management of other injuries that are more life-threatening. Exploration of the urethra in the acute phase of injury is difficult because of large hematomas, and with a significant loss of blood, resulting in a high risk of failure. For these patients, a delayed repair is an option [70, 76].

Treatment options for these posterior urethral stenoses are deferred urethroplasty and deferred endoscopic optical incision.

Most posterior urethral-distraction defects are short and can be treated with a perineal anastomotic repair. The key objective is to achieve a tension-free anastomosis between two healthy urethral ends. Restricture rates that have been reported amount approximately to 10% [53, 77–79].

For large distraction defects and/or complicated cases (bladder neck injuries, fistula, redo-urethroplasty), a sequential step repair with inferior pubectomy or corporal rerouting, or even a combined abdominoperineal approach, might be necessary, with similar results [80].

Deferred endoscopic treatment has been proposed for complete obliteration but with disappointing results [81, 82]. For short, non-obliterative strictures following realignment or urethroplasty, direct-visualization urethrotomy can be performed [80]. Repeated urethrotomies and/or dilations must be discouraged because these do not represent curative treatment [83]. Stents are not recommended for patients with strictures following pelvic trauma, as fibrotic tissue tends to grow through into the lumen of the stent [53].

The incidence of ED in PFUI patients secondary to pelvic fracture and/or perineal trauma ranges from 27.5% to 72% based on diagnostic abnormalities observed in nocturnal penile tumescence studies [84, 85]. Penile duplex Doppler ultrasound has documented that 48.7% of these patients had arterial ED, 14.6% had venous leak, and 36.5% had non-vascular ED, most likely secondary to neurogenic causes [86].

Erectile dysfunction of PFUI can be caused by vasculogenic factors and neurogenic factors. Stief et al. explain that impotence occurring after pelvic trauma is due to the damage of the autonomic plexus and the erigentes nerve as a result of the displacement of the prostate [87]. Armenakas et al. [88] evaluated the impotent patient with disruption of the prostate pars membranous before doing the reconstruction using MRI pelvis and ultrasound duplex; and it shows that 80% cases of erectile dysfunction are caused by vasculogenic factors. Husmann et al. reported that there was no significant difference in the degree of incontinence in patients treated with early realignment and delayed urethroplasty [89].

Surveillance strategies with uroflowmetry, RUG, cystoscopy, or a combination of these methods are recommended for at least 1 year (Grade C, AUA) [90].

Female urethral injuries are rare. They occur almost exclusively as a result of pelvic fractures and often occur together with bladder rupture. Proximal and midurethral disruptions need early exploration and primary repair via the retropubic and transvaginal route, respectively, with primary suturing of the urethral ends. Concomitant vaginal laceration is repaired transvaginally and at the same time [48, 59]. Distal urethral injuries can be managed vaginally by primary suturing or can be left untreated and hypospadiac.

Catheter placement is the most common cause of iatrogenic urethral trauma [91]. Iatrogenic urethral injuries also occur after radical prostatectomy, pelvic radiotherapy, and other abdominopelvic surgery [92]. The main consequence of iatrogenic trauma is urethral stricture. False passages should be treated with urethral catheter placement if possible, while strictures should be managed endoscopically with incision or resection initially, followed by urethral reconstruction, if endoscopic management fails [18, 39].

The recommended radiographic method for diagnostic evaluation of pediatric urethral trauma is RUG (Grade A, EAU). The first step in management according to the Pediatric EAU guidelines is to provide urinary drainage. Transurethral catheterization can be performed only if the patient can still void and the diagnostic evaluation is not suspicious for urethral rupture; a suprapubic catheter should be placed, otherwise. There is no singular accepted method for managing posterior urethral injuries; either immediate suprapubic drainage with late urethral reconstruction or immediate primary re-alignment can be performed (Grade C, EAU) [18].

19.5 External Genitalia Trauma

The most common injuries involving the external genitalia are penile fracture, testicular rupture, and penetrating penile injury.

19.5.1 Penile Trauma

About 20–30% of penile fractures may involve the corpus spongiosum, while only 10–20% of penile fractures involve the urethra [93]. It usually consists of the disruption of the tunica albuginea of one or both corpus cavernosum due to blunt trauma to the erect penis during sexual intercourse. It can be accompanied by partial or complete urethral rupture, or injury of the dorsal nerve and vessels [94, 95]. Tunica albuginea is one of the strongest fascias in the human body. One reason for the increased risk of penile fracture is that the tunica albuginea stretches and thins significantly during erection: in the flaccid state, it is up to 2.4 mm thick; during erection, it becomes as thin as 0.25–0.5 mm.

Common clinical findings of penile fracture are penile swelling, hematoma, ecchymosis, and deformity; suspicion of urethral injury increases with the presence of blood at the external meatus (Grade B, AUA) [1].

Corporal or urethral rupture contained by Buck's fascia leads to dissection of urine and blood along the penile shaft. Rupture through Buck's fascia results in extravasation of blood and urine through superficial layers (scrotum, suprapubic area, and perineum).

If the extravasation is contained by Colles' fascia, it may be shown by a characteristic "butterfly sign" in the perineum [96].

Regarding the role of imaging studies in the diagnosis of penile fracture, there is still some controversy. Some studies showed the usefulness of ultrasound, cavernosography, and MRI, with a superiority of MRI in identifying corporal injury [97]. When penile fracture with suspected concomitant urethral injury is present, an evaluation is performed with retrograde urethrography or urethroscopy (Grade B, AUA).

Conservative management with nonsteroidal analgesics and cold compresses is recommended for subcutaneous haematoma [18]. Closure of the tunica albuginea is recommended (Grade B, AUA, and EAU) to prevent erectile dysfunction and penile curvature [98]. Urethral injury should be repaired at the same time as the repair of the penile fracture [18].

Immediate intervention has been associated with shorter duration of hospital stay, higher levels of patient satisfaction, and improved outcomes including reduced incidence of erectile dysfunction, stricture and curvature, and with better functional outcome such as voiding capability and sexual activity [99, 100]. A palpable penile fibrosis is a common long-term complication with an incidence ranging from 41% up to 93% [101, 102].

For penetrating penile trauma, physical examination is sufficient for evaluation. Penetrating penile injury is accompanied by concomitant urethral injury in 11–29%

of cases [103]. Surgical exploration with conservative debridement and primary closure of the tunica albuginea is recommended. If there is extensive skin loss, reconstruction with a full-thickness skin graft is superior to a split-thickness skin graft [18, 104].

Animal and human bites are associated with high risk of wound infection. Besides debridement and closure, targeted antibiotics according to the most common associated pathogen should be given. Additionally, the rabies vaccine, hepatitis B vaccine, and/or HIV post-exposure prophylaxis should be considered [2, 18].

In case of traumatic penile amputation, the amputated appendage should be wrapped in saline-soaked gauze, placed in a plastic bag, and placed in a second bag filled with ice during transport. The appendage should then be re-implanted as soon as possible (Clinical Principle, AUA), within 24 h of amputation (EAU) [1].

19.5.2 Scrotal Trauma

Testicular rupture is found in approximately 50% of direct blunt trauma to the scrotum [105]. Testicular rupture is characterized by scrotal ecchymosis and swelling and also difficulty in identifying the contours of the testicle on examination. Scrotal ultrasound is recommended by the EAU for the evaluation of scrotal trauma. Surgical exploration is recommended for suspected testis rupture to prevent complications such as ischemic atrophy of the testis and infection (Grade B, AUA, and EAU). After conservative surgical debridement of non-viable tissue, the tunica albuginea should be closed. The tunica vaginalis can be used for closure if primary closure of tunica albuginea is not possible (Expert Opinion, AUA) [18].

Conservative management is recommended for minor intratesticular hematomas with observation, nonsteroidal analgesics, and ice packs [106]. If a major intratesticular hematoma is discovered, surgical drainage is indicated to prevent secondary infection or pressure atrophy [107]. If scrotal trauma results in skin defects, primary closure is typically possible due to the elasticity of scrotal skin [104]. Debridement should be limited to non-viable tissue as the patient may need multiple reconstructive procedures (Grade B, AUA).

19.5.3 Female External Genitalia Trauma

The first step in the evaluation of female external genitalia injury is the consideration of sexual abuse. The most common sign of external genitalia trauma is blood at the vaginal introitus. With an injury to the female external genitalia, imaging with ultrasound, CT, or MRI should be performed to evaluate for additional injuries. Primary closure of vaginal injuries is recommended to prevent fistula formation. Conservative management with nonsteroidal analgesics and ice packs is recommended if there is no vaginal tear [18].

References

1. Morey AF, Brandes S, Dugi DD III, et al. Urotrauma: AUA guideline. J Urol. 2014;192:327–35.
2. Santucci RA, Bartley JM. Urologic trauma guidelines: a 21st century update. Nat Rev Urol. 2010;7:510–9.
3. Bent C, Iyngkaran T, Power N, et al. Urological injuries following trauma. Clin Radiol. 2008;63(12):1361–71.
4. Pereira BM, et al. A review of ureteral injuries after external trauma. Scand J Trauma Resusc Emerg Med. 2010;18:6.
5. Bjurlin MA, et al. Genitourinary injuries in pelvic fracture morbidity and mortality using the National Trauma Data Bank. J Trauma. 2009;67:1033.
6. Dixon CM. Diagnosis and acute management of posterior urethral disruptions. In: McAninch JW, editor. Traumatic and reconstructive urology. Philadelphia, PA: WB Saunders; 1996.
7. Brandes SB, et al. External genitalia gunshot wounds: a ten-year experience with fifty-six cases. J Trauma. 1995;39:266.
8. Meng MV, et al. Renal trauma: indications and techniques for surgical exploration. World J Urol. 1999;17:71.
9. Paparel P, N'Diaye A, Laumon B, et al. The epidemiology of trauma of the genitourinary system after traffic accidents: analysis of a register of over 43,000 victims. BJU Int. 2006;97: 338–41.
10. Schmidlin F, Farshad M, Bidaut L, et al. Biomechanical analysis and clinical treatment of blunt renal trauma. Swiss Surg. 1998;5:237–43.
11. Santucci RA, McAninch JW, Safir M, Mario LA, Service S, Segal MR. Validation of the American Association for the Surgery of Trauma organ injury severity scale for the kidney. J Trauma. 2001;50:195–200.
12. Mendez R. Renal trauma. J Urol. 1977;118:698–703.
13. Miller KS, McAninch JW. Radiographic assessment of renal trauma: our 15-year experience. J Urol. 1995;154:352–5.
14. Gaitini D, Razi NB, Ghersin E, et al. Sonographic evaluation of vascular injuries. J Ultrasound Med. 2008;27:95–107.
15. Kawashima A, Sandler CM, Corl FM, et al. Imaging of renal trauma: a comprehensive review. Radiographics. 2001;21:557–74.
16. Morey AF, McAninch JW, Tiller BK, et al. Single shot intraoperative excretory urography for the immediate evaluation of renal trauma. J Urol. 1999;161:1088–92.
17. Santucci RA, Wessells H, Bartsch G, et al. Evaluation and management of renal injuries: consensus statement of the renal trauma subcommittee. BJU Int. 2004;93:937–54.
18. Summerton DJ, Djakovic N, Kitrey ND et al. Guidelines on urological trauma; 2015.
19. Ramchandani P, Buckler PM. Imaging of genitourinary trauma. AJR Am J Roentgenol. 2009;192:1514–23.
20. Elliott SP, Olweny EO, McAninch JW. Renal arterial injuries: a single center analysis of management strategies and outcomes. J Urol. 2007;178:2451–5.
21. Jawas A, Abu-Zidan FM. Management algorithm for complete blunt renal artery occlusion in multiple trauma patients: case series. Int J Surg. 2008;6:317–22.
22. Hammer CC, Santucci RA. Effect of an institutional policy of nonoperative treatment of grades I to IV renal injuries. J Urol. 2003;169:1751–3.
23. Armenakas NA, Duckett CP, McAninch JW. Indications for nonoperative management of renal stab wounds. J Urol. 1999;161:768–71.
24. Hardee MJ, Lowrance W, Brant WO, et al. High grade renal injuries: application of Parkland Hospital predictors of intervention for renal hemorrhage. J Urol. 2013;189:1771–6.
25. Nuss GR, Morey AF, Jenkins AC, et al. Radiographic predictors of need for angiographic embolization after traumatic renal injury. J Trauma. 2009;67:578–82, discussion 582.
26. Wright JL, Nathens AB, Rivara FP, et al. Renal and extrarenal predictors of nephrectomy from the national trauma data bank. J Urol. 2006;175:970–5, discussion 975.

27. Baniel J, Schein M. The management of penetrating trauma to the urinary tract. J Am Coll Surg. 1994;178:417–25.
28. Wessells H, McAninch JW, Meyer A, et al. Criteria for nonoperative treatment of significant penetrating renal lacerations. J Urol. 1997;157:24–7.
29. Breyer BN, McAninch JW, Elliott SP, Master VA. Minimally invasive endovascular techniques to treat acute renal hemorrhage. J Urol. 2008;179:2248–53.
30. Tekgül S, Dogan HS, Hoebeke P et al. Guidelines on paediatric urology; 2015.
31. Montgomery RC, Richardson JD, Harty JI. Posttraumatic renovascular hypertension after occult renal injury. J Trauma. 1998;45:106–10.
32. Elliott SP, McAninch JW. Ureteral injuries: external and iatrogenic. Urol Clin North Am. 2006;33:55–66.
33. Siram SM, Gerald SZ, Greene WR, et al. Ureteral trauma: patterns and mechanisms of injury of an uncommon condition. Am J Surg. 2010;199:566–70.
34. Pereira BM, Ogilvie MP, Gomez-Rodriguez JC, et al. A review of ureteral injuries after external trauma. Scand J Trauma Resusc Emerg Med. 2010;18:6.
35. Pirani Y, Talner LB, Culp S. Delayed diagnosis of ureteral injury after gunshot wound to abdomen. Curr Probl Diagn Radiol. 2012;41(4):138–9.
36. Abboudi H, Kamran A, Royle J, et al. Ureteric injury: a challenging condition to diagnose and manage. Nat Rev Urol. 2013;10(2):108–15.
37. Brandes S, Coburn M, Armenakas N, et al. Diagnosis and management of ureteric injury: an evidence based analysis. BJU Int. 2004;94:277–89.
38. Taqi KM, et al. Ureteral injury in penetrating abdominal trauma. Am J Case Rep. 2017;18:1377–81.
39. Summerton DJ, Kitrey ND, Lumen N, Serafetinidis E, Djakovic N, European Association of Urology. EAU guidelines on iatrogenic trauma. Eur Urol. 2012;62:628–39.
40. Holevar M, Ebert J, Luchette F, et al. Practice management guidelines for the evaluation of genitourinary trauma. Chicago, IL: The EAST Practice Management Guidelines Work Group; 2004.
41. Burks FN, Santucci RA. Management of iatrogenic ureteral injury. Ther Adv Urol. 2014;6(3):115–24.
42. Sevinc C, Balaban M, Ozkaptan O, et al. The management of total avulsion of the ureter from both ends: our experience and literature review. Archiv Ital Urol Androl. 2016;88(2):97–100.
43. de la Rosette JJ, Skrekas T, Segura JW. Handling and prevention of complications in stone basketing. Eur Urol. 2006;50:991–8.
44. Gupta V, Sadasukhi TC, Sharma KK, et al. Complete ureteral avulsion. Sci World J. 2005;28:125–7.
45. Sandler CM, Goldman SM, Kawashima A. Lower urinary tract trauma. World J Urol. 1998;16:69–75.
46. Brandes S, Borrelli J Jr. Pelvic fracture and associated urologic injuries. World J Surg. 2001;25:1578–87.
47. Gomez RG, Ceballos L, Coburn M, et al. Consensus statement on bladder injuries. BJU Int. 2004;94:27–32.
48. Figler BD, Hoffler CE, Reisman W, et al. Multi-disciplinary update on pelvic fracture associated bladder and urethral injuries. Injury. 2012;43:1242–9.
49. Shenfeld OZ, Gnessin E. Management of urogenital trauma: state of the art. Curr Opin Urol. 2011;21:449–54.
50. Inaba K, McKenney M, Munera F, et al. Cystogram follow-up in the management of traumatic bladder disruption. J Trauma. 2006;60:23–8.
51. Wirth GJ, Peter R, Poletti PA, Iselin CE. Advances in the management of blunt traumatic bladder rupture: experience with 36 cases. BJU Int. 2010;106:1344–9.
52. Cinman NM, McAninch JW, Porten SP, et al. Gunshot wounds to the lower urinary tract: a single-institution experience. J Trauma Acute Care Surg. 2013;74:725–30.
53. Chapple C, Barbagli G, Jordan G, et al. Consensus statement on urethral trauma. BJU Int. 2004;93:1195–202.

54. Mundy AR, Andrich DE. Urethral trauma. Part II: types of injury and their management. BJU Int. 2011;108:630–50.
55. Jack GS, Garraway I, Reznichek R, Rajfer J. Current treatment options for penile fractures. Rev Urol. 2004;6:114–20.
56. Kamdar C, Mooppan UM, Kim H, Gulmi FA. Penile fracture: preoperative evaluation and surgical technique for optimal patient outcome. BJU Int. 2008;102:1640–4.
57. Cavalcanti AG, Krambeck R, Araujo A, Rabelo PH, Carvalho JP, Favorito LA. Management of urethral lesions in penile blunt trauma. Int J Urol. 2006;13:1218–20.
58. Bjurlin MA, Kim DY, Zhao LC, et al. Clinical characteristics and surgical outcomes of penetrating external genital injuries. J Trauma Acute Care Surg. 2013;74:839–44.
59. Brandes S. Initial management of anterior and posterior urethral injuries. Urol Clin North Am. 2006;33:87–95.
60. Barret K. Primary realignment vs suprapubic cystostomy for the management of pelvic fracture associated urethral injuries: a systematic review and meta-analysis. Urology. 2014;83:924–9.
61. Hampson LA, McAninch JW, Breyer BN. Male urethral strictures and their management. Nat Rev Urol. 2014;11(1):43–50.
62. Rosenstein DI, Alsikafi NF. Diagnosis and classification of urethral injuries. Urol Clin North Am. 2006;33:73–85.
63. Mundy AR, Andrich DE. Urethral trauma. Part I: introduction, history, anatomy, pathology, assessment and emergency management. BJU Int. 2011;108:310–27.
64. Kielb SJ, Voeltz ZL, Wolf JS. Evaluation and management of traumatic posterior urethral disruption with flexible cystourethroscopy. J Trauma. 2001;50:36–40.
65. Leddy LS, Vanni AJ, Wessells H, Voelzke BB. Outcomes of endoscopic realignment of pelvic fracture associated urethral injuries at a level 1 trauma center. J Urol. 2012;188:174–8.
66. Koraitim MM. Effect of early realignment on length and delayed repair of postpelvic fracture urethral injury. Urology. 2012;79:912–5.
67. Koraitim MM. Pelvic fracture urethral injuries: evaluation of various methods of management. J Urol. 1996;156:1288–91.
68. Mouraviev VB, Coburn M, Santucci RA. The treatment of posterior urethral disruption associated with pelvic fractures: comparative experience of early realignment versus delayed urethroplasty. J Urol. 2005;173:873–6.
69. Asci R, Sarikaya S, Buyukalpelli R, et al. Voiding and sexual dysfunction after pelvic fracture urethral injuries treated with either initial cystostomy and delayed urethroplasty or immediate primary urethral realignment. Scand J Urol Nephrol. 1999;33:228–33.
70. Ku JH, Jeon YS, Kim ME, et al. Comparison of long term results according to the primary mode of management and type of injury for posterior urethral injuries. Urol Int. 2002;69:227–32.
71. Hadjizacharia P. Evaluation of immediate endoscopic realignment as a treatment modality for traumatic urethral injuries. J Trauma. 2008;64(6):1443–9; 1449–50.
72. Chang PC, Hsu YC, Shee JJ, et al. Early endoscopic primary realignment decreases stricture formation and reduces medical costs in traumatic complete posterior urethral disruptions in a 2 year follow up. Chang Gung Med J. 2011;34:179–85.
73. Santucci RA, Joyce GF, Wise M. Male urethral stricture disease. J Urol. 2007;177(5):1667–74.
74. Kim FJ, Pompeo A, Sehrt D, et al. Early effectiveness of endoscopic posterior urethra primary alignment. J Trauma Acute Care Surg. 2013;75:189–94.
75. Moudouni SM, Patard JJ, Manunta A, Guiraud P, Lobel B, Guille F. Early endoscopic realignment of post-traumatic posterior urethral disruption. Urology. 2001;57:628–32.
76. Qu Y, Zhang W, Sun N, et al. Immediate or delayed repair of pelvic fracture urethral disruption defects in young boys: twenty years of comparative experience. Chin Med J. 2014;127(19):3418–22.
77. Lumen N, Hoebeke P, Troyer BD, Ysebaert B, Oosterlinck W. Perineal anastomotic urethroplasty for posttraumatic urethral stricture with or without previous urethral manipulations: a review of 61 cases with long-term follow-up. J Urol. 2009;181:1196–200.
78. Koraitim MM. On the art of anastomotic posterior urethroplasty: a 27-year experience. J Urol. 2005;173:135–9.

79. Fu Q, Zhang J, Sa YL, Jin SB, Xu YM. Recurrence and complications after transperineal bulboprostatic anastomosis for posterior urethral strictures resulting from pelvic fracture: a retrospective study from a urethral referral centre. BJU Int. 2013;112:E358–63.

80. Cooperberg MR, McAninch JW, Alsikafi NF, Elliott SP. Urethral reconstruction for traumatic posterior urethral disruption: outcomes of a 25-year experience. J Urol. 2007;178:2006–10.

81. Levine J, Wessells H. Comparison of open and endoscopic treatment of posttraumatic posterior urethral strictures. World J Surg. 2001;25:1597–601.

82. Dogra PN, Ansari MS, Gupta NP, Tandon S. Holmium laser core through urethrotomy for traumatic obliterative strictures of urethra: initial experience. Urology. 2004;64:232–5.

83. Santucci R, Eisenberg L. Urethrotomy has a much lower success rate than previously reported. J Urol. 2010;183:1859–62.

84. Shenfeld OZ, Kiselgorf D, Gofrit ON, Verstandig AG, Landau EH, Pode D, Jordan GH, McAninch JW. The incidence and causes of erectile dysfunction after pelvic fractures associated with posterior urethral disruption. J Urol. 2003;169:2173–6.

85. Feng C, Xu YM, Yu JJ, Fei XF, Chen L. Risk factors for erectile dysfunction in patients with urethral strictures secondary to blunt trauma. J Sex Med. 2008;5:2656–61.

86. Fu Q, Sun X, Tang C, Cui R, Chen L. An assessment of the efficacy and safety of sildenafil administered to patients with erectile dysfunction referred for posterior urethroplasty: a single-center experience. J Sex Med. 2012;9:282–7.

87. Stief CG, Pohlemann T, Hagemann J, Schlote N, Truss M, Tscherne H, et al. Etiology of erectile dysfunction after pelvic trauma. Eur Urol. 1998;31(Suppl 1):12. (A48).

88. Armenakas NA, McAninch JW, Lue TF, Dixon CM, Hricak H. Post-traumatic impotence: magnetic resonance imaging and duplex ultrasound in diagnosis and management. J Urol. 1993;149(Part 2):1272–6.

89. Husmann DA, Wilson WT, Boone TB, Allen TD. Prostatomembranous urethral disruptions: management by suprapubic cystostomy and delayed urethroplasty. J Urol. 1990;144(1):76–8.

90. Follis HW, Koch MO, McDougal WS. Immediate management of prostatomembranous urethral disruptions. J Urol. 1992;147:1259–62.

91. Elliott SP, Meng MV, Elkin EP, McAninch JW, Duchane J, Carroll PR, et al. Incidence of urethral stricture after primary treatment for prostate cancer: data From CaPSURE. J Urol. 2007;178:529–34.

92. Polat O, Gül O, Aksoy Y, Ozbey I, Demirel A, Bayraktar Y. Iatrogenic injuries to ureter, bladder and urethra during abdominal and pelvic operations. Int Urol Nephrol. 1997;29:13–8.

93. Tsang T, Demby AM. Penile fracture with urethral injury. J Urol. 1992;147:466–8.

94. Haas CA, Brown SL, Spirnak JP. Penile fracture and testicular rupture. World J Urol. 1999;17:101–6.

95. Jagodic K, Erklavec M, Bizjak I, et al. A case of penile fracture with complete urethral disruption during sexual intercourse: a case report. J Med Case Rep. 2007;1:14.

96. Garofalo M, Bianchi L, Gentile G, et al. Sex-related penile fracture with complete urethral rupture: a case report and review of the literature. Arch Ital Urol Androl. 2015;87:3.

97. Raheem AA, El-Tatawy H, Eissa A, et al. Urinary and sexual functions after surgical treatment of penile fracture concomitant with complete urethral disruption. Arch Ital Urol Androl. 2014;86:15–9.

98. Phonsombat S, Master VA, McAninch JW. Penetrating external genital trauma: a 30-year single institution experience. J Urol. 2008;180:192–6.

99. Yapanoglu T, Aksoy Y, Adanur S, et al. Seventeen years' experience of penile fracture: conservative vs. surgical treatment. J Sex Med. 2009;6:2058–63.

100. Rivas JG, Dorrego JM, Hernández MM, et al. Traumatic rupture of the corpus cavernosum: surgical management and clinical outcomes. A 30 years review. Cent Eur J Urol. 2014;67:88–92.

101. Ateyah A, Mostafa T, Nasser TA, et al. Penile fracture: surgical repair and late effects on erectile function. J Sex Med. 2008;5:1496–502.

102. Zargooshi J. Sexual function and tunica albuginea wound healing following penile fracture: an 18-year follow-up study of 353 patients from Kermanshah, Iran. J Sex Med. 2009;6:1141–50.

103. Koifman L, Barros R, Junior RA, Cavalcanti AG, Favorito LA. Penile fracture: diagnosis, treatment and outcomes of 150 patients. Urology. 2010;76:1488–92.
104. Simhan J, Rothman J, Canter D, et al. Gunshot wounds to the scrotum: a large single-institutional 20-year experience. BJU Int. 2012;109:1704–7.
105. Fournier GR Jr, Laing FC, McAninch JW. Scrotal ultrasonography and the management of testicular trauma. Urol Clin North Am. 1989;16:377–85.
106. Cass AS, Luxenberg M. Value of early operation in blunt testicular contusion with hematocele. J Urol. 1988;139:746–7.
107. Cass AS, Luxenberg M. Testicular injuries. Urology. 1991;37:528–30.

Blunt Abdominal Trauma

20

Konstantinos Nastos

20.1 Introduction: Blunt Force Trauma

Trauma is a major cause of morbidity and mortality, especially in the age group under 35 years old. Although trauma patients vary in respect to the presenting severity, as well as the etiology of injury, blunt trauma seems to be the leading cause of the majority of serious traumatic injuries. The most frequent cause of blunt trauma is associated with motor vehicle accidents, involving passengers as well as pedestrians. Another major cause of injury associated with blunt trauma are falls, direct assaults either in terms of domestic violence or aggressive social behavior, and work accidents.

The general classification of blunt trauma involves contusion, abrasion, laceration, and fracture. The severity of these types of injury vary and is directly related to the causing mechanism and the associated impact force.

20.2 Liver Trauma

20.2.1 Introduction

Liver trauma is the second in frequency site of solid organ injury from blunt trauma in the abdominal cavity. Due to the mechanism of injury, liver trauma is most commonly associated with other injuries as well, most frequently with thoracic or pleural injuries. Three basic mechanisms of injury have been described in blunt non-penetrating liver trauma: acceleration injury, deceleration injury, and compression injury [1].

K. Nastos (✉)
Third Department of Surgery, Attikon University Hospital, National and Kapodistrian Univeristy of Athens, Athens, Greece

© Springer Nature Switzerland AG 2021
E. Pikoulis, J. Doucet (eds.), *Emergency Medicine, Trauma and Disaster Management*, Hot Topics in Acute Care Surgery and Trauma, https://doi.org/10.1007/978-3-030-34116-9_20

Acceleration injury is the type of injury that occurs after the force is applied in the anterior or lateral chest or abdominal wall. This moves the abdominal wall and forces the underlying liver to accelerate. Depending on the exact site and direction of the force, there are different resulting injuries associated with this type of trauma. The part of the liver most frequently involved in acceleration injury is the right lobe in over 60% of cases. This can be explained by the increased mass of the right lobe of the liver compared to the left lobe, and usually this type of injury is also associated with injury to the coastal margin and the rib cage, as in normal circumstances the right and the left lobes of the liver are protected by the ribs. When the direction of the injury involves the right lateral chest wall, the posterior lobe of the liver which is relatively immobilized by the right triangular ligament stays immobile while the right anterior lobe of the liver accelerates, thus creating lacerations in the margin between the right posterior and right anterior segments of the liver. When the direction of the force is from the anterior to the posterior part of the abdomen, the right lobe of the liver is accelerated and pushed backwards while the left lobe and the right posterior lobe are immobilized by the falciform ligament and the inferior vena cava (IVC), respectively. This creates a laceration along the plane of Cantlie's line. Injuries to the left lobe of the liver are more infrequent as the mass of the left lobe is relatively smaller and is in greater part protected by the sternum and the ribs. However, when acceleration injury occurs from the anterior of the abdominal and chest wall, the liver is lacerated in either side of the falciform ligament according to the direction of the force.

Deceleration injury occurs during an accident or a fall, when the liver which has the same velocity as the whole body continues to move after a sudden stop from impact due to inertia. When this happens, there are two distinct phases of the injury: the first one is associated with the crushing injury of the liver on the anterior abdominal/thoracic wall during the collision due to its inertia, and the second type of injury is associated with the collision of the liver after the impact to the posterior abdominal wall. In addition, during this sequence, the liver is torn from its ligaments usually at the right triangular ligaments involving the right posterior lobe of the liver [2].

The third mechanism of injury is crushing injury of the liver, which is associated with very high-speed accidents and with accidents of increased violence. Due to the increased mass of the right lobe of the liver and its incompressibility, when the rib cage is forced into the abdominal cavity, the liver parenchyma is compressed between the ribs and the vertebrae, crushing the parenchyma between these two structures. All the above mechanisms have been investigated and validated in biomechanical models of blunt abdominal trauma [3].

20.2.2 Classification of Blunt Liver Injury

Classification of liver injuries has been a major concern over the last decades, and there are multiple scoring systems that have been adopted through the years, including Moore's score which is based on the organ injury scale of the American Association for the Surgery of Trauma, which has been used as the classification system of choice for the description of liver injuries. For a long time, an attempt has been made to associate liver injuries with CT findings, in order to be able to classify the patients according to their need for immediate operative management or to an attempt for conservative nonoperative treatment. To date, the most important parameter for deciding if a patient is suitable for nonoperative management is hemodynamic stability and other concomitant injuries to organs that necessitate immediate operative intervention. This has not been incorporated to liver injury classification systems until recently [4]. In 2016, the World Society for Emergency Surgery has adopted a new classification system that allocates patients based on CT findings, in addition to hemodynamic stability and other related injuries.

The old American Association for the Surgery of Trauma (AAST) classification of liver injury [5] is depicted in Table 20.1:

The World Society for Emergency Surgery (WSES) has divided hepatic injury into three major categories: minor (Grade I), moderate (Grade II), and severe (Grade III and IV) hepatic trauma [6]. Table 20.2 summarizes the criteria for staging liver injuries according to the new classification system:

Table 20.1 The American Association for the Surgery of Trauma classification of liver injury

Grade	Type of injury	Description of injury
I	Hematoma	Subcapsular, <10% surface area
	Laceration	Capsular tear, <1 cm parenchymal depth
II	Hematoma	Subcapsular, 10–50% surface area, intraparenchymal <10 cm in diameter
	Laceration	Capsular tear 1–3 parenchymal depth, <10 cm in length
III	Hematoma	Subcapsular, >50% surface area of ruptured subcapsular or parenchymal hematoma; intraparenchymal hematoma >10 cm or expanding
	Laceration	>3 cm parenchymal depth
IV	Laceration	Parenchymal disruption involving 25–75% hepatic lobe or 1–3 Couinaud's segments
V	Laceration	Parenchymal disruption involving >75% of hepatic lobe or >3 Couinaud's segments within a single lobe
	Vascular	Juxtahepatic venous injuries; i.e., retrohepatic vena cava/central major hepatic veins
VI	Vascular	Hepatic avulsion

From Moore et al. [5]

Table 20.2 The World Society for Emergency Surgery classification for liver injury

	WSES grade	AAST	Hemodynamic	CT scan	First-line treatment
Minor	WSES Grade I	I–II	Stable		
Moderate	WSES Grade II	III	Stable	Yes + local exploration in SW#	Nonoperative management—serial clinical/laboratory/radiological evaluation
Severe	WSES Grade III	IV–V	Stable		
	WSES grade IV	I–VI	Unstable	No	Operative management

From Coccolini et al. [6]

Minor and moderate hepatic injuries include patients who are hemodynamically stable and include injuries classified as Grade I, II, III, according to the AAST classification system, while severe hepatic injuries include patients who were previously classified as Grade IV, V, and VI hemodynamically stable injuries according to the AAST grading system, as well as any injury that is associated with hemodynamic instability of the patient [6].

20.2.3 Management of Blunt Liver Injury

Management has shifted during the last decades from an aggressive operative approach in the majority of patients to a more conservative approach in most cases [7]. Aggressive strategy includes an attempt to stop hemorrhage as soon as possible in order to avoid the complications of shock and transfusion and reperfusion injury associated with shock liver syndrome. In addition, any possible bile leaks are addressed at the time of initial operation. However, evidence has shown that most patients with hemorrhage due to lacerations in the liver parenchyma stop bleeding spontaneously. In addition, bile leaks are not frequently seen in superficial lacerations, and as a result, patients can undergo conservative treatment, avoiding laparotomy in suboptimal conditions (hypothermia, acidosis, and coagulopathy). WSES classification has made the stratification of patients to either strategy more effective [6]. In addition, interventional radiology and the widespread use of endoscopic retrograde cholangiopancreatography (ERCP) with interventions in the biliary tract has made nonoperative management even more appealing and successful. Current evidence suggests that minor and moderate injuries according to the WSES classification can be treated conservatively with very good outcomes (success rates of over 92% for minor and 80% for moderate injuries have been reported) [8]. In addition, the bile leak rates for minor and moderate liver injuries have been reported to be from 0% to 12%, respectively [6]. The nomenclature of the recent WSES classification system takes into account the hemodynamic stability of patients, as patients with minor or moderate injuries can be hemodynamically unstable in some cases, and thus should be managed with an emergency laparotomy, whereas some of the more severe hepatic injuries can present with hemodynamic stability, and thus, a conservative management with the assistance of embolization techniques and ERCP interventions can lead to favorable outcomes, avoiding unnecessary hospital stay and intraoperative complications.

In a patient who is hemodynamically stable but requires continuous transfusions, angiographic embolization could also prevent an unnecessary emergency laparotomy. Naturally, conservative management should be employed in centers that can support such an approach, where an immediate access to the operating room and surgical intervention is possible in a 24-h basis, and when invasive radiology techniques are readily available. When a nonoperative approach is selected, the patient should be carefully followed up either clinically or radiographically with the use of CT scans for early identification of complications, which can occur in a significant portion of patients with major liver injuries, such as biloma formation, hepatic abscess, biliary peritonitis, and liver insufficiency [9]. In a conservatively treated patient, all of these complications should also be attempted to be treated conservatively.

Operative management of blunt liver trauma should be avoided and only be chosen in cases of severe grade injuries or in injuries accompanied with hemodynamic instability and other organ injuries, since the major cause of mortality and death in these patients is continuous hemorrhage that cannot be treated efficiently [10]. Intraoperatively, the surgeon should try to identify the source of bleeding; many times, this can be associated with injuries in multiple foci in the liver, especially in deceleration injuries. Minor lacerations and parenchymal tearing can be managed with simple techniques, such as manual compression of the liver until hemostasis has been achieved, by suturing liver parenchyma and by using energy sources such as electrocoagulation, argon beam coagulation, etc. When the liver parenchyma is massively injured leading to tearing of major hepatic veins, more advanced techniques are necessary [11]. However, in the setting of an emergency laparotomy, the nomenclature of damage control surgery should be applied [12]. The most commonly performed maneuver should be immediate packing of the liver if this can prevent further exsanguination. In any case, a simultaneous attempt to reverse the lethal triad should be pursued by the anesthetic team. In case of successful hepatic packing, the patient should be returned to the ICU (intense care unit) and resuscitated improving hemodynamical parameters and after 24 to 48 hours a more definitive form of repair should be attempted. If this is not possible during the initial operation, then other maneuvers such as emergency ligation of vessels in the level of the hepatic veins or the porta hepatis, balloon tamponade, shunting procedures, and vascular isolation of the liver either in the form of Pringle maneuver or complete vascular isolation should be performed [11]. Anatomic hepatectomies should be avoided in the emergency setting as atypical hepatic resections seem to be safer and more easily performed in the acute situation. When arterial hemorrhage cannot be managed inside the liver parenchyma, hepatic artery ligation can be performed in the porta hepatis. However, this is associated with late complication involving hepatic necrosis, abscess and biloma formation, in addition to intrahepatic stenosis of the bile tree. In these situations, mortality is high [13].

20.3 Splenic Injury

20.3.1 Introduction

The spleen is, by most studies, reported as the most commonly injured solid organ in trauma patients. The spleen has functions that render it indispensable for patients, especially during childhood. It is located in the left upper quadrant of the abdomen and protected by the left coastal margin. The splenic capsule is a thin layer and actually a continuity of the visceral peritoneum. The spleen is immobilized through its ligaments, which connect the splenic capsule to the parietal peritoneum. Intrasplenic vascular anatomy plays a significant role in the mechanics of splenic injury. In detail, arterial branches start from the hilum and enter the splenic parenchyma with a transverse course leading to separate segments within the spleen [14]. If any laceration occurs in parallel with these vessels, then usually there is no vascular injury or severe blood exsanguination (vascular blush) seen in the CT scan. If, however, the laceration of the spleen is perpendicular to the course of these vessels, then usually vascular involvement occurs. The spleen has a discrete physiology as it is part of the reticuloendothelial system; its role is to store and metabolize erythrocytes and platelets and has a major role in the function of the immune system by destroying encapsulated bacteria. Consequently, patients that undergo splenectomy are prone to infectious diseases, may need long-term antibiotic prophylaxis and are also prone to severe sepsis, mainly due to Streptococcus pneumoniae, Neisseria meningitidis, and Hemophilus influenza for which patients undergoing splenectomy are advised to be vaccinated [15].

20.3.2 Mechanism of Injury to the Spleen

The most common type of blunt injury to the spleen are automobile-related accidents, followed by falls and force applied directly on the abdominal cavity with physical contact. As in the case of the liver, the exact mechanisms involved vary according to the force and direction of the impacting force. Spleen is prone to acceleration, deceleration, and compression injury. Most usually, however, it is the result of deceleration injury. Injury occurs either in the form of parenchymal laceration with an intact capsule, or in the form of concomitant parenchymal and capsular rupture. The first type is associated with intraparenchymal hematomas, the second one is manifested with the presence of hemoperitoneum. The third type of injury is direct injury to the hilar vessels.

20.3.3 Imaging and Classification

Clinical diagnosis is based on radiographic findings and on the suspicion of a splenic injury based on the mechanism of the accident. The first imaging modality used, which is the gold standard for the initial evaluation of a splenic capsule rupture, is the ultrasound scan (FAST) which has a high sensitivity to detect splenic trauma that causes hemoperitoneum. However, this is not a definite diagnostic modality, as it does not describe the degree of the splenic injury and can sometimes not be reliable in detecting intraparenchymal injury that does not incorporate capsular tear and hemoperitoneum. Further evaluation with a CT scan is warranted, but only in the situation where the patient is hemodynamically stable, in order to further evaluate the degree of injury and guide further treatment. After the CT scan is performed, the patient is classified according to the AAST splenic injury scale as shown in the following Table 20.3:

As in the case of liver injuries, this is a classification which describes anatomically the injury to the spleen and the extent of this injury, in addition to the participation of vascular injury, either intraparenchymal or in the hilum of the spleen. More

Table 20.3 The American Association for the Surgery of Trauma classification for splenic injury

Grade	Injury type	Description of injury
I	Hematoma	Subcapsular, <10% surface area
	Laceration	Capsular tear, <1 cm parenchymal depth
II	Hematoma	Subcapsular, 10–50% surface area; intraparenchymal, <5 cm in diameter
	Laceration	Capsular tear, 1–3 cm parenchymal depth that does not involve a trabecular vessel
III	Hematoma	Subcapsular, >50% surface area or expanding; ruptured subcapsular or parenchymal hematoma; intraparenchymal hematoma ≥5 cm or expanding
	Laceration	>3 cm parenchymal depth or involving trabecular vessels
IV	Laceration	Laceration involving segmental or hilar vessels producing major devascularisation (>25% of spleen)
V	Laceration	Completely shattered spleen
	Vascular	Hilar vascular injury that devascularizes spleen

From Moore et al. [5]

Table 20.4 The World Society for Emergency Surgery classification for splenic injury

	WSES class	AAST	Hemodynamic status	CT scan	First-line treatment in adults
Minor	WSES I	I–II	Stable	Yes	Nonoperative management + serial clinical/laboratory/radiological evaluation
Moderate	WSES II	III	Stable		Consider angiography-angioembolization
	WSES III	IV–V	Stable		Nonoperative management All angiography/angioembolization + serial clinical/laboratory/radiological evaluation
Severe	WSES IV	I–V	Unstable	No	Operative management

From Coccolini et al. [16]

recently, the World Society of Emergency Surgery (WSES) has incorporated their own classification in order to further facilitate the management of patients with blunt splenic trauma and assign them to either a nonoperative management strategy or to immediate operative management [16]. In this more recent classification, the hemodynamic stability of the patient has been taken into account, and as a result, splenic trauma has been categorized into three categories of injury: minor, moderate, and severe (Table 20.4).

Minor splenic injuries consist of AAST Grade I and II injuries in hemodynamically stable patients; moderate splenic injuries correspond to AAST Grade III injuries, in addition to more severe injuries (Grade IV and V) in patients who are also hemodynamically stable; severe splenic injury consists of any type of injury (Grade I–V) which causes hemodynamic instability and in which the patient cannot be rendered stable after the initial resuscitation. Criteria of hemodynamic instability include systolic blood pressure (SBP) <90 mmHg with evidence of shock, altered level of consciousness and shortness of breath, and requirement of more than 4–6 units of packed red blood cells (PRBC) in the first 24 h [16].

20.3.4 Management of Patients with Splenic Trauma

As in other cases of intra-abdominal blunt trauma, a nonoperative approach has been employed gradually during the last decades, in order to avoid the complications associated with laparotomy. Although the nonoperative management of Grade I, II, and III splenic injuries has been established, recently, evidence has shown that a nonoperative management should be attempted even in high-grade splenic injury (Grades IV and V) as long as the patient is not hemodynamically unstable. This, of course, as in any other situation, should be performed only in a specialized hospital setting with the facility of interventional radiology providing angiography and angioembolization, as well as access to immediate surgical intervention [17].

During the last decades, studies have attempted to address issues that include the criteria for conservative treatment, the possibility of secondary bleeding after conservative treatment as well as the role of interventional radiology.

Recent guidelines from the WSES have attempted to elucidate the above issues. Nonoperative management of the majority of splenic injuries has led to a rate of success of nearly 90%. Although patient age, grade of injury, the volume of hemoperitoneum (260–500 mL), and the presence of vascular abnormalities of the spleen during imaging have been associated as risk factors for failure of nonoperative management, it seems that the findings of the studies addressing this issue are not uniform, and consensus cannot be found within the literature [18]. This is reflected in the guidelines, where a nonoperative approach is recommended undependably from the presence of any of these risk factors [16].

The use of angiography and angioembolization should be adopted when readily available in the hospital; however, this has not been shown to be effective for all cases of blunt splenic trauma [19]. Routinely performing an angiography after CT scan in all patients, including patients with Grade I and II injuries, has failed to show significant positive yield and further attempt to angioembolization, which seems to be lower than 10%. In contrary, in patients with Grade III, IV, and V injuries, angiography and possibly angioembolization, if a vascular injury is diagnosed, seems to be of benefit in increasing the success rate of nonoperative management [20]. In addition, it is not yet fully clear if an angioembolization should be performed routinely, even if a contrast blush is not seen during angiography, in patients that had a positive finding of contrast blush in the CT scan. Finally, angiography should be performed in patients that have been managed nonoperatively and although hemodynamically stable have a steady decrease in hemoglobulin or continue to require transfusions.

Operative management should be decided in patients that are hemodynamically unstable or that have other associated injuries that require surgical intervention [21]. Of course, an operative management should be decided early if the patient has high-grade injuries and intensive monitoring is not safe in the center that they are hospitalized. During the operation, although splenectomy is the traditional operation performed, there are reports of attempts to salvage damaged parenchyma in order to preserve the immunological function of the spleen. There is no evidence to date that supports this strategy. Finally, the use of minimally invasive techniques seems to be contraindicated in this setting.

In terms of follow-up, patients with moderate and severe lesions should be clinically and biochemically observed with immobilization in bed for at least 3 days. In Grade I and II injuries, a repeat CT scan is not always needed if the patient is hemodynamically stable and with no clinical signs of intraperitoneal hemorrhage or laboratory evidence of decreasing hematocrit levels. If these occur, a repeat CT scan should be performed in order to evaluate the healing process of the spleen. In addition, in moderate and severe lesions (AAST Grade III, IV, and V), a repeat CT scan seems to be appropriate. The recommended duration of hospital stay is at least 5 days, and this is recommended due to the fact that most emergency operations in patients that are initially treated conservatively occur within this time frame and in the majority of cases within the first 3 days. Return to normal physical activity can be recommended 3 weeks after operative management of splenic injury or after 8–12 weeks following nonoperative treatment [22].

20.4 Pancreatic Trauma

20.4.1 Introduction

Pancreatic injury is rarely seen in multitrauma patients, and its incidence is relatively low. Most commonly, pancreatic injury takes place in penetrating trauma, and only a few cases are caused by blunt trauma. The most common related mechanism is crushing injury of the pancreas due to compression of the upper abdomen from the steering wheel in car accidents upon the bodies of the patient's vertebrae. Late diagnosis is the most common problem associated with pancreatic injury, and this is caused by a lack of clinical signs and symptoms due to its location in the retroperitoneum. Most common site of injury is the body of the pancreas, followed by the head and the tail. Due to its position in the retroperitoneum and its surrounding retroperitoneal fat and other organs, blunt pancreatic injury is very commonly associated with other organ injuries. Likewise, any patient with multiple organ injuries should be considered a candidate for pancreatic injury [23].

20.4.2 Diagnosis and Classification of Pancreatic Injury

Apart from the typical pathophysiologic mechanism of injury, there are no other clear clinical signs of blunt pancreatic trauma. Diagnosis is made after clinical suspicion by the mechanism of injury and elevated serum amylase levels. However, this lacks specificity as increased amylase may be absent at the time of patient evaluation.

The clinical manifestation of blunt pancreatic trauma may vary and involves a wide spectrum from acute pancreatitis caused by soft tissue injury, to laceration and tearing of pancreatic parenchyma and major pancreatic duct disruption. The most common site of pancreatic duct disruption is at the junction of the body and tail, where the mechanical force of the impact shears the pancreas upon the bodies of the vertebrae.

Morbidity and mortality from blunt pancreatic trauma are increased due to misdiagnosis of injury to this organ. Laboratory investigations are not very helpful in diagnosing blunt pancreatic trauma, as raised amylase concentration in blood may be associated with injury of the salivary glands, the duodenum, and also be present in intoxicated patients that have undergone an accident. On the other hand, diagnostic peritoneal lavage may reveal increased amylase levels due to bowel or duodenal injury. Both conventional radiography and abdominal ultrasound scanning are not diagnostic of blunt pancreatic trauma. However, computed tomography (CT) scan may provide helpful information in order to diagnose this type of injury. CT is the examination of choice for any hemodynamically stable patient and can provide indirect signs of blunt pancreatic injury. These may include direct evidence of laceration or transection of the pancreatic body, or focal pancreatic edema, and nonhomogeneous enhancement in arterial phase. In addition, hematoma formation and fluid in the retroperitoneum should lead to the suspicion of this kind of injury. Although computed tomography may provide direct or indirect information suggesting pancreatic injury, usually it does not provide useful information about the continuity of the pancreatic duct [24]. For the diagnosis of major duct disruption, Magnetic Resonance Cholangiopancreatography (MRCP) should be used. MRCP has a high specificity for the diagnosis of this kind of injury, and if disruption is found, early Endoscopic Retrograde Cholangiopancreatography (ERCP) should be performed in order to attempt an intraductal stent placement to restore the continuity of a partially disrupted or even a fully disrupted major pancreatic duct [25]. This of course has to be performed in a hemodynamically stable patient, and in any other case, surgical exploration should be performed and pancreatic injury addressed intraoperatively.

The American Association for the Surgery of Trauma has classified pancreatic trauma, as shown in Table 20.5:

Although this classification describes the severity of pancreatic injury, management of blunt pancreatic trauma is also dictated from coexisting injuries to other organs [27].

Table 20.5 The American Association for the Surgery of Trauma classification of pancreatic injury

Grade	Type of injury	Description of injury
I	Hematoma	Minor contusion without duct injury
	Laceration	Superficial laceration without duct injury
II	Hematoma	Major contusion without duct injury or tissue loss
	Laceration	Major laceration without duct injury or tissue loss
III	Laceration	Distal transection or parenchymal injury with duct injury
IV	Laceration	Proximal transection or parenchymal injury involving ampulla
V	Laceration	Massive disruption of pancreatic head

From Moore et al. [26]

20.4.3 Management of Patients with Pancreatic Injury

Patients who present with intra-abdominal hemorrhage or intraluminal spillage in the abdominal cavity should be managed surgically for the coexisting injuries, and drainage should also be performed in the retroperitoneal region in the area of pancreatic injury. In case of a hemodynamically stable patient and no other major abdominal injuries, then pancreatic trauma should be managed according to its severity. In simple contusions or superficial lacerations (Grade I), conservative management should be performed according to the basic principles of pancreatitis management (bowel rest, nasogastric suction, and nutritional support). In cases where injury is more than a simple contusion and the main pancreatic duct has been injured (Grade III), then ERCP-guided stent placement is the procedure of choice [28]. However, if ERCP-guided stenting is not available, any transection of the pancreatic parenchyma involving ductal injury should be treated with surgery, and usually this consists of resecting the pancreas or draining the site [29]. Other more complex operations, including Whipple's procedure, could be used in injury of the pancreatic head, provided that the patient is hemodynamically stable. Other options in Grade III transections include conservation of pancreatic parenchyma, especially if the abdominal cavity is clean from any other contamination and there is no peritonitis present. In these cases, the patient can be subjected to full transection of the pancreas followed by a jejunal Roux-en-Y anastomosis to the distal pancreas. The central pancreas is sutured and drained. In Grade IV and V injuries, more complex operations involving the pancreatic head may be required. In case of a Grade IV injury with no compromise of the duodenum, simple drainage and washup can be attempted; however, in pancreatic head disruption, a pancreatoduodenectomy may be necessary. Finally, in Grade V injuries, a major parameter that dictates the surgeon's possible steps are the concomitant injuries to other organs, which also predict morbidity and mortality.

Recent reports have systematically reviewed the existing literature for an evidence-based approach to pancreatic injury. All of the above are summarized in recent guidelines [30]. It is recommneded that patients with Grade I or II injuries should be treated conservatively after diagnosis with a CT scan; patients with Grade III and IV injuries should be led to the operating theater, although this is not confirmed by all of the studies. If a patient is found to have a Grade I or II pancreatic injury during a laparotomy performed for damage control, then the suggestion is to perform simple drainage; whereas in patients with Grade III and IV injuries, resection of the injured pancreatic site should be performed in order to prevent fistula formation and septic complications [29]. Finally, in Grade V injuries, it is not clear if a formal pancreatoduodenectomy or simple drainage is the preferred treatment of choice, as evidence is quite limited for this patient group.

References

1. Jin W, Deng L, Lv H, Zhang Q, Zhu J. Mechanisms of blunt liver trauma patterns: an analysis of 53 cases. Exp Ther Med. 2013;5(2):395–8.
2. Rogers CB, Devera R. The forensic pathology of liver trauma. Acad Forensic Pathol. 2018;8(2):184–91.
3. Shao Y, Zou D, Li Z, Wan L, Qin Z, Liu N, et al. Blunt liver injury with intact ribs under impacts on the abdomen: a biomechanical investigation. PLoS One. 2013;8(1):e52366.
4. Slotta JE, Justinger C, Kollmar O, Kollmar C, Schafer T, Schilling MK. Liver injury following blunt abdominal trauma: a new mechanism-driven classification. Surg Today. 2014;44(2):241–6.
5. Moore E, Shackford S, Pachter H, McAninch J, Browner B, Champion H, et al. Organ injury scaling: spleen, liver, and kidney. J Trauma. 1989;29(12):1664–6.
6. Coccolini F, Catena F, Moore EE, Ivatury R, Biffl W, Peitzman A, et al. WSES classification and guidelines for liver trauma. World J Emerg Surg. 2016;11:50.
7. Noyola-Villalobos HF, Loera-Torres MA, Jimenez-Chavarria E, Nunez-Cantu O, Garcia-Nunez LM, Arcaute-Velazquez FF. [Non-surgical management after blunt traumatic liver injuries: a review article]. Cir Cir. 2016;84(3):263–6.
8. Hosseini M, Mousavie SH, Negahi AR, Majdsepas H, Nafissi N, Lundgren J, Hosseini SK, et al. Blunt trauma liver-conservative or surgical management? Int J Dev Res. 2018;8:10596.
9. Monnin V, Sengel C, Thony F, Bricault I, Voirin D, Letoublon C, et al. Place of arterial embolization in severe blunt hepatic trauma: a multidisciplinary approach. Cardiovasc Intervent Radiol. 2008;31(5):875–82.
10. Croce MA, Fabian TC, Menke PG, Waddle-Smith L, Minard G, Kudsk KA, et al. Nonoperative management of blunt hepatic trauma is the treatment of choice for hemodynamically stable patients. Results of a prospective trial. Ann Surg. 1995;221(6):744.
11. Peitzman AB, Marsh JW. Advanced operative techniques in the management of complex liver injury. J Trauma Acute Care Surg. 2012;73(3):765–70.
12. Leppäniemi AK, Mentula PJ, Streng MH, Koivikko MP, Handolin LE. Severe hepatic trauma: nonoperative management, definitive repair, or damage control surgery? World J Surg. 2011;35(12):2643–9.
13. Badger S, Barclay R, Campbell P, Mole D, Diamond T. Management of liver trauma. World J Surg. 2009;33(12):2522–37.
14. Stevens W, Bortier H, Van Meir F. 1 Anatomy, embryology, histology and physiology of the spleen. In: Medical imaging of the spleen. New York, NY: Springer; 2012.
15. Cadili A, de Gara C. Complications of splenectomy. Am J Med. 2008;121(5):371–5.
16. Coccolini F, Montori G, Catena F, Kluger Y, Biffl W, Moore EE, et al. Splenic trauma: WSES classification and guidelines for adult and pediatric patients. World J Emerg Surg. 2017;12:40.
17. Yiannoullou P, Hall C, Newton K, Pearce L, Bouamra O, Jenks T, et al. A review of the management of blunt splenic trauma in England and Wales: have regional trauma networks influenced management strategies and outcomes? Ann R Coll Surg Engl. 2017;99(1):63–9.
18. Zarzaur BL, Rozycki GS. An update on nonoperative management of the spleen in adults. Trauma Surg Acute Care Open. 2017;2(1):e000075.
19. Crichton JCI, Naidoo K, Yet B, Brundage SI, Perkins Z. The role of splenic angioembolization as an adjunct to nonoperative management of blunt splenic injuries: a systematic review and meta-analysis. J Trauma Acute Care Surg. 2017;83(5):934–43.
20. Hildebrand DR, Ben-Sassi A, Ross NP, Macvicar R, Frizelle FA, Watson AJ. Modern management of splenic trauma. BMJ. 2014;348:g1864.
21. El-Matbouly M, Jabbour G, El-Menyar A, Peralta R, Abdelrahman H, Zarour A, et al. Blunt splenic trauma: assessment, management and outcomes. Surgeon. 2016;14(1):52–8.
22. Yorkgitis BK. Primary care of the blunt splenic injured adult. Am J Med. 2017;130(3):365.e1–5.
23. Debi U, Kaur R, Prasad KK, Sinha SK, Sinha A, Singh K. Pancreatic trauma: a concise review. World J Gastroenterol. 2013;19(47):9003–11.

24. Gupta A, Stuhlfaut JW, Fleming KW, Lucey BC, Soto JA. Blunt trauma of the pancreas and biliary tract: a multimodality imaging approach to diagnosis. Radiographics. 2004;24(5):1381–95.
25. Bhasin DK, Rana SS, Rawal P. Endoscopic retrograde pancreatography in pancreatic trauma: need to break the mental barrier. J Gastroenterol Hepatol. 2009;24(5):720–8.
26. Moore E, Cogbill T, Malangoni M, Jurkovich G, Champion H, Gennarelli T, et al. Organ injury scaling, II: pancreas, duodenum, small bowel, colon, and rectum. J Trauma. 1990;30(11):1427–9.
27. Menahem B, Lim C, Lahat E, Salloum C, Osseis M, Lacaze L, et al. Conservative and surgical management of pancreatic trauma in adult patients. Hepatobil Surg Nutr. 2016;5(6):470–7.
28. Subramanian A, Dente CJ, Feliciano DV. The management of pancreatic trauma in the modern era. Surg Clin North Am. 2007;87(6):1515–32, x.
29. Degiannis E, Glapa M, Loukogeorgakis S, Smith M. Management of pancreatic trauma. Injury. 2008;39(1):21–9.
30. Ho VP, Patel NJ, Bokhari F, Madbak FG, Hambley JE, Yon JR, et al. Management of adult pancreatic injuries: a practice management guideline from the Eastern Association for the Surgery of Trauma. J Trauma Acute Care Surg. 2017;82(1):185–99.

Blast Injuries: Tips, Evaluation, and Management

21

Yoram Kluger, Hany Bahouth, and Assaf Harbi

21.1 Introduction

The term "blast" is used to define the anatomical lesions and the clinical syndrome caused by the exposure of the organism to the effects of a shock wave resulting from an explosion. An explosion is an exothermic chemical reaction that transforms, in a very short time, a liquid or solid body into gas, schematically with three components: the shock wave, the airflow, and the heat. This sudden release of gases causes a large increase in pressure, known as a blast wave, which radiates in all directions away from the source.

According to the environment in which the shock wave propagates, blast is distinguished in air, liquid, or solid environments: The medium in which the wave is traveling affects its propagation; liquids transmit a stronger pressure wave over a longer distance, thereby giving underwater explosions a different injury pattern [1, 2].

The explosions may be the result of domestic or industrial accidents, but recently, most of these events are due to terror acts or war, with blast injuries causing serious physical and psychological injuries. Most of the terror acts and war blast injuries are events with mass casualties. In such scenarios it is crucial to understand the pathophysiology of blast injuries to provide a better diagnosis and prompt treatment to the victims.

Y. Kluger (✉) · A. Harbi
Division of General Surgery, The Ruth & Bruce Rappaport Faculty of Medicine, Technion – Israel Institute of Technology, Haifa, Israel
e-mail: y_kluger@rambam.health.gov.il; A_harbi@rambam.health.gov.il

H. Bahouth
Trauma & Emergency Surgery, Division of General Surgery, The Ruth & Bruce Rappaport Faculty of Medicine, Technion – Israel Institute of Technology, Haifa, Israel
e-mail: H_bahouth@rambam.health.gov.il

© Springer Nature Switzerland AG 2021   289
E. Pikoulis, J. Doucet (eds.), *Emergency Medicine, Trauma and Disaster Management*, Hot Topics in Acute Care Surgery and Trauma,
https://doi.org/10.1007/978-3-030-34116-9_21

The knowledge and the early identification of the explosive type and nature can also help to provide a better clinical, diagnostic, and management approach.

21.2   Classification of Explosive

Explosives are classified as high-order explosives (HE) or low-order explosives (LE) due to their speed of detonation:

- High-order explosives produce an overpressure shockwave. This type of explosives does not burn, but instead detonates when a shock wave passes through the material with a high velocity, generating a substantial blast overpressure, even if unconfined. Among the high-order explosives: TNT, C-4, Semtex, nitroglycerin, dynamite, and ammonium nitrate fuel oil (ANFO) [1, 2].
- Low-order explosives cause a subsonic explosion and lack of shock wave overpressure of high explosives. Low-order explosives burn rapidly through a process of deflagration and produce large volumes of gas that only explode if confined. Among the low-order explosive: bombs, firearms, and most pure oil-based bombs, like Molotov cocktails [1, 2].

21.3   Mechanisms of Blast Injury

The effects of the shock wave are related to different factors like the initial size of the explosion, the surrounding medium (water is a dense medium with low elastic properties), and the distance from the explosion (the effect is inversely proportional to distance) [3].

Furthermore, pressure variations produced by the shock wave are accompanied by high-velocity winds that can accelerate light surrounding objects transforming them into potentially penetrating objects.

The nature of the blast injuries depends upon the tissue characteristics that are exposed to the blast wave phenomenon [4]. When the blast front (which is the leading edge of the blast wave) reaches an object or the human body itself, it causes an almost instantaneous rise in the atmospheric "static pressure" which creates an immediate positive pressure shift which is responsible for the tissue damage [4].

The human body tissue damage is directly proportional to the duration of the blast wave. As the blast wave moves in the air in the speed of sound, the damage is higher in a medium with reduced acoustic impendence such as water and close environments [4].

The following negative phase of the blast wave, called "blast wind," can also be responsible for blast injuries produced by stress and shear waves. Furthermore, in this phase, a partial vacuum is created, and air is sucked in. Turbulent movement of air following the blast wave can cause debris to be thrown to long distances from the explosive source [4].

Table 21.1 Classification and mechanism of blast injury

Category	Characteristics	Body part affected	Types of injuries
Primary	Unique to high-order explosives, results from the impact of the overpressurization wave with body surfaces	Gas-filled structures are most susceptible—lungs, GI tract, and middle ear	Blast lung (pulmonary barotrauma), TM rupture and middle ear damage, abdominal hemorrhage and perforation, globe (eye) rupture, concussion (TBI without physical signs of head injury)
Secondary	Results from flying debris and bomb fragments	Any body part may be affected	Affected, penetrating ballistic (fragmentation) or blunt injuries, eye penetration (can be occult)
Tertiary	Results from individuals being thrown by the blast wind	Any body part may be affected	Fracture and traumatic amputation, closed and open brain injury
Quaternary	All explosion-related injuries, illnesses, or diseases not due to primary, secondary, or tertiary mechanisms. Includes exacerbation or complications of existing conditions	Any body part may be affected	Burns (flash, partial, and full thickness), crush injuries, closed and open brain injury, asthma, COPD, or other breathing problems from dust, smoke, or toxic fumes, angina, hyperglycemia, hypertension
Quinary	Morbidity and injuries resulting from nonprojectile additives to explosives, as well as any environmental contamination	Any body part may be affected	Bacteremia from bacteria-laded bombs, radiation from dirty bombs

The lesions caused by the explosion are categorized into five categories of injuries associated with the shock wave, primary, secondary, tertiary, quaternary, and quinary, according to the American Department of Defense Directive [5] (Table 21.1).

The victims of a blast trauma usually will present with multiple injuries which will haze this classification and will create what has been defined as a multidimensional injury [1, 6].

21.3.1 Primary Blast Injury (PBI)

The primary blast injuries are due to overpressure blast wave that affects mainly the hollow organs or other body parts that are composed of structures with an interface of liquid air or air-filled structures like lungs, blood vessels, gastrointestinal tract, and tympanic membrane.

21.3.2 Secondary Blast Injuries

Secondary blast injuries are the injuries that are caused by flying objects, debris, or bomb fragments physically displaced by the overpressure wave or the wind wave and present as a combination between a penetrating organ injury and a blunt trauma [1]. These are common to any type of explosions and account for the largest class of injuries [4].

The secondary blast injuries are more common than the primary blast injuries due the fact that the distance over which the fragments travel is much longer than the distance that the blast wave propagates [2]. Therefore, secondary blast injuries can be seen in patients located hundreds and thousands of meters away from the explosion's site, while primary blast injury is usually seen in injured patients who were at the explosion's site [7].

21.3.3 Tertiary Blast Injuries

Tertiary blast injuries are caused when the person is physically displaced through the air and impacts on another standing object by the overpressure wave or the blast wind. The resulting injury can be either penetrating or blunt injury, such as skull fractures; orthopedic injuries; head injuries; chest, abdominal, and pelvic injuries; traumatic amputations; and spinal cord injuries.

Structural collapse and entrapment can cause crush injuries and compartment syndrome.

It is clear that the strength of the explosion will determine the severity of the injury.

21.3.4 Quaternary Blast Injuries

Quaternary blast injuries include all injuries that are not part of the primary, secondary, or tertiary blast injury categories. Those injuries can be caused by exposure to resulting fire (burn injuries), toxic substance exposures (e.g., radiation, carbon monoxide poisoning, cyanide poisoning), environmental exposure injury (thermic injuries) asphyxia, and psychological trauma.

21.3.5 Quinary Blast Injuries

Quinary blast injuries include illnesses, injuries, and diseases resulting from post-explosion environmental contaminants (e.g., bacteria, radiation). This category of blast injuries was suggested and inserts to the classification ultimately on the basis of a case series in which a hyperinflammatory state was seen in patients after a bombing in Israel [6, 8]. These patients manifested hyperpyrexia, diaphoresis, low central venous pressure, and a positive fluid balance [1].

21.3.6 Blast Injury of Specific Organs

21.3.6.1   Pulmonary Injury

"The explosion lung injury" is a direct consequence of the overpressure wave of high explosives because of its substantial air-tissue surface area. In consequence, the explosion can cause a pulmonary hemorrhage and contusions, vascular air embolism, and a direct barotrauma. The manifestation of a lung blast injury is caused by disruption of the pulmonary structure (capillary walls, alveolar, lung parenchyma) causing hemorrhage and pulmonary edema. Later in time after 12–24 h, an inflammatory response develops.

Thoraco-pulmonary lesions include hemorrhages and/or pulmonary contusions, alveolar rupture, pneumothorax, hemothorax, pneumomediastinum and subcutaneous emphysema, air embolism with possible departure of gaseous emboli, and cerebral infraction.

The pulmonary blast injury is the most common fatal injury among those who initially survive. About 17–47% of victims of explosions forces who died had pulmonary primary blast injuries. It is has been reported that 71% of critically injured patients involved in explosions have a pulmonary injury.

The mortality rates range from 3% to 25%. However, for those who survive, a prompt diagnosis and resuscitation efforts are imperative, and long-term prognosis seems to be good.

The signs of the pulmonary explosion lesion are generally present admission, but in some cases, they were reported even after 48 h from the explosion, possibly caused by the late inflammatory response.

The clinical signs of pulmonary explosion lesion are characterized by the clinical triad composed dyspnea, cough, and hypoxia, and they are secondary to altered gas exchange and vascular shunting.

The other consequence of the blast pulmonary injury is air embolism caused by possible disruption of the bronco-vascular tree creating bronco-vascular fistulas. Those air embolisms can be fatal if they are massive and can cause a myocardial infraction, stroke, bowel ischemia, hemorrhagic, shock and death.

The presence of an explosion lung lesion should be suspected in all cases where there is dyspnea, cough, hemoptysis, and chest pain following or evidence of any other primary blast injuries. The explosion lung injury is recognizable in chest X-ray and characterized by a typical "butterfly" pattern, caused by bilateral pulmonary infiltrates [1]. It is highly recommended to undergo an X-ray to all those who have been exposed to an explosion.

A chest CT scan should be considered if manifestations persist to avoid missed lesions on X-ray of the chest.

21.3.6.2   Auditory System Injury

The main explosion lesions of the ear system cause significant morbidity, but are often neglected. Auditory system lesions are the most frequently diagnosed in blast trauma.

The lesion strongly depends on the orientation of the ear relative to the point of detonation. Perforation of the tympanic membrane is the most severe injury of the middle ear. The signs of the auricular lesion are generally present at the time of the initial evaluation and should be suspected in those with reduced hearing, tinnitus, otalgia, vertigo, bleeding from the external canal, perforation of the tympanic membrane, or mucopurulent otitis.

A tympanic membrane perforation considered an indication for more prompt investigation for other primary blast injuries by either imaging or observation. On the other hand, asymptomatic patients without perforation of the tympanic membrane have a very low probability to have other major primary blast injuries.

All patients exposed to an explosion should undergo an otolaryngology visit and an audiometric check.

The prognosis of patient with a tympanic membrane perforation is good, and usually it does not necessitate any further intervention. However, up to 30% of patients with a tympanic membrane rupture will have a permanent hearing loss [9].

21.3.6.3 Gastrointestinal Injury

The gastrointestinal tract injuries are less common than auditory and pulmonary blast lesions although they have a similar rate of occurrence in open-air blast explosions.

Gastrointestinal injuries occur more often in a setting of a closed space explosions or underwater setting as blast waves travel more easily in water than air. Lesions of the gastrointestinal tract are commonly associated with thoraco-pulmonary lesions and tympanic lesions [4]. Generally gastrointestinal injuries involve the fixed parts of the colon with perforation but can include any part of the gastrointestinal tract, which contains a certain quantity of air [9].

The sections of the gastrointestinal tract that contain gas are the most vulnerable to the effects of the explosion, which can cause immediate perforation of the intestine, hemorrhage (from small petechiae and large hematomas) lesions to the mesenteric artery, lacerations of solid organs, and rupture of the testicles. The abdominal explosion lesions should be suspected in any patient exposed to an explosion and present abdominal pain, nausea, vomiting, hematemesis, rectal pain, tenesmus, testicular pain, hypovolemia without explanation, or any other signs that suggest an acute abdomen. Clinical signs may be absent until complications develop.

- Lesions of parenchymatous organs such as the spleen, the liver, or kidneys are associated with very high explosive pressures in patients placed at close distances from the source.

21.3.6.4 Occular Injuries

The incidence of eye blast injury is relatively high considering the small surface area of the eye.

Eye blast injury can be result of primary blast injury and can manifest as ocular hemorrhage, a globe rupture, or retinal detachment. However, eye injury is more often a consequence of a secondary blast injury mechanism induced by projectile fragments that cause corneal abrasions, lacerations, orbital fracture, etc.

21.3.6.5 Brain Injuries

Brain blast injuries are more common than they were thought or diagnosed and documented in the past. The mechanism of injury can be the result of diffuse axonal injury, shearing, and hemorrhage formation due to a rupture of cerebral vessels.

Primary shock waves can cause concussions or mild traumatic brain injuries (MTBI) even without a direct blow to the head.

Injuries that are more significant include subarachnoid hemorrhage, subdural hemorrhage, and hyperemia of the brain and meninges.

It is necessary to consider the proximity of the victim to the site of the explosion in particular when the injured patient complains of headaches, fatigue, poor concentration, lethargy, depression, anxiety, or insomnia.

21.3.6.6 Muscoloskeletal Injuries

Extremity and musculoskeletal injuries are extremely common and can be caused by any of the mechanisms of blast injury, but secondary blunt injury seems to be the most common cause.

Crash injuries and compartment syndrome are common and can be the consequences of bone fracture, burns, and direct soft tissue damage that can increase the compartment pressure. Compartment syndrome if not early diagnosed and treated can lead to rhabdomyolysis, acidosis, renal failure, and also death.

Although compartment syndrome classified as tertiary blast injury can be also diagnosed in patient without evident injury, this raises the suspicion of primary blast injury mechanism as responsible to the syndrome.

Traumatic amputations occur in 1–7% of the explosions victims. The prognosis of those is poor especially if the amputation is proximal to the wrist or to the ankle, lesions which suggests a concomitant other internal damage.

21.3.7 Management

The general approach to all blast injured patients is based on the Advanced Trauma Life Support (ATLS) [10]. Also all blast injury patients need evaluation for PBI of the lung, abdomen, and ears even in the absence of apparent lesions.

21.3.7.1 Pulmonary

Pulmonary blast injuries or "blast lung" can be difficult to manage as it can present with a variety of clinical characteristics.

Patients will present with symptoms of cough, dyspnea, chest pain and hemoptysis, tachypnea, reduced breath sounds, cyanosis, and subcutaneous emphysema.

The variety of clinical scenarios can be lung contusion that can be treated with only supportive care to a dramatic scenario of massive air embolism or acute respiratory distress syndrome (ARDS). The different injuries require a different strategy of management.

Oxygen should be given to all patients.

A chest X-ray is mandatory in all blast-exposed patients.

Unstable patients or patient who should undergo an emergent surgery should be intubated. In patient who present with pneumohemothorax, immediate thoracostomy is indicated.

A preventive decompressive thoracostomy should be taken in consideration in severe injuries that require a positive pressure ventilation or before air transportation [1].

Severe lung injury may require an elevated positive end-expiratory pressure (PEEP) and a positive pressure ventilation that may aggravate the injury of the lung parenchyma and may result in pneumothorax [11]. Therefore, it is important to consider preventive strategy before utilizing a mechanical ventilation in patient with lung injury.

It is highly important to emphasize that aggressive intravenous liquid resuscitation can aggravate the lung edema in patient with already severe lung injury [1, 12].

Acute gas embolism can be manifest with cardiac arrhythmias, cardiac ischemia, and central nervous system symptoms and can be detected by fundoscopy findings. The management is symptomatic, and a high flow oxygen should be initiated. Hyperbaric oxygen therapy has demonstrated to be effective in stable patient even after 24 h [13].

21.3.7.2 Auditory System

Most tympanic membrane perforation can be treated conservatively. Routine otoscopy is mandatory for all blast victims [14].

Removal of debris and sterile irrigation can be done in case of TM perforation, while surgical treatment is indicated in case of TM rupture of more than one third of the membrane [9].

21.3.7.3 Ocular Injuries

Eye-penetrating foreign bodies, shrapnels, and particles are common after blasts; therefore a routine ophthalmologic evaluation is mandatory in all casualties [14].

21.3.7.4 Gastrointestinal Injuries

All patients should be evaluated as in general abdominal trauma according to the ATLS [15].

Air and fluid containing organs are at higher risk for perforation and bleeding, especially the fixed colon and the mesentery, but also a parenchymatous organ injury should be highly suspected.

Patient may present symptoms like abdominal pain, abdominal wall contusion, tenesmus, and peritonitis [4].

Bowel contusion may be difficult to detect immediately and can manifest with secondary perforation which occurs after 3–5 days [10, 16]. If perforation is diagnosed, the management is surgical with laparotomy, and the decisions are based on the general physiology and the extent of the infectious process into the abdomen of the specific patient.

In patient who present with chest pain, dyspnea, and subcutaneous emphysema, esophageal perforation should be suspected [17].

21.3.7.5 Muscoloskeletal Injuries

Tetanus prophylaxis, antibiotics, and X-ray series are advocated in patient with blast skeletal injuries for evaluating fracture and debris penetration.

Small foreign bodies (less than 2 cm) that are not involving major structures like pleura, peritoneum, and vascular can be treated nonoperatively with irrigation and antibiotics. But this approach remains controversial [18].

Compartment syndrome must always be taken in consideration for every extremity injury for any cause [9]. If diagnosed, fasciotomy needs to be done.

References

1. Wolf SJ, Bebarta VS, Bonnett CJ, Pons PT, Cantrill SV. Blast injuries. Lancet. 2009;374:405–15.
2. Westrol MS, Donovan CM, Kapitanyan R. Blast physics and pathophysiology of explosive injuries. Ann Emerg Med. 2017;69(1S):S4–9. https://doi.org/10.1016/j.annemergmed.2016.09.005.
3. Adler OB, Rosenberger A. Blast injuries. Acta Radiol. 1988;29(1):1–5.
4. Kumar M. Blast injuries. Med J Armed Forces India. 2010;66(4):309–11. https://doi.org/10.1016/S0377-1237(10)80005-X.
5. United States of America Department of Defense. Department of Defence Directive. 2006. http://www.dtic.mil/whs/directives/corres/pdf/602521p.pdf. Accessed 29 Sep 2016.
6. Kluger Y, Nimrod A, Biderman P, Mayo A, Sorkin P. The quinary pattern of blast injury. Am J Disaster Med. 2007;2:21–5.
7. Wildegger-Gaissmaier A. Aspects of thermobaric weaponry. ADF Health. 2003;4:3–6.
8. DePalma RG, Burris DG, Champion HR, Hodgson MJ. Blast injuries. N Engl J Med. 2005;352:1335–42.
9. Mathews ZR, Koyfman A. Blast injuries. J Emerg Med. 2015;49(4):573–87.
10. Guzzi LM, Argyros G. The management of blast injury. Eur J Emerg Med. 1996;3:252–5.
11. Alfici R, Ashkenazi I, Kessel B. Management of victims in a mass casualty incident caused by a terrorist bombing: treatment algorithms for stable, unstable, and in extremis victims. Mil Med. 2006;171:1155–62.
12. Housden S. Blast injury: a case study. Int Emerg Nurs. 2012;20:173–8.
13. Dunbar EM, Fox R, Watson B, Akrill P. Successful late treatment of venous air embolism with hyperbaric oxygen. Postgrad Med J. 1990;66(776):469–7.
14. Stein M. Urban bombing: a trauma surgeon's perspective. Scand J Surg. 2005;94:286–92.
15. Ratto J, Johnson BK, Condra CS, Knapp JF. Pediatric blast lung injury from a fireworks-related explosion. Pediatr Emerg Care. 2012;28:573–6.
16. Yeh DD, Schecter WP. Primary blast injuries—an updated concise review. World J Surg. 2012;36:966–72.
17. Roan JN, Wu MH. Esophageal perforation caused by external airblast injury. J Cardiothorac Surg. 2010;5:130–2.
18. Bridges EJ. Blast injuries: from triage to critical care. Crit Care Nurs Clin North Am. 2006;18:333–48.

Basics of Trauma Management: Crush Injuries

22

Nikoletta Dimitriou

22.1 Introduction

Each year, millions of people must contend with earthquakes, cyclones, hurricanes, and other natural disasters (tornados, landslides, and flooding) or man-made disasters (wars, terrorist attacks, air and railway crashes, and collapsed poorly constructed buildings) [1]. In many of those disasters, people are entrapped and crushed in buildings. As a result, a lot of the victims suffered from crush injuries and their sequences.

Crush injury is defined as compression of extremities or other parts of the body that causes muscle swelling and/or neurological disturbances in the affected areas of the body [2]. Typically affected areas of the body include lower extremities (74%), upper extremities (10%), and trunk (9%) [3]. This definition avoids mention of the duration of crush, degree of pressure, size of muscle involved, or the presence of associated symptomatology, which all determines the seriousness of the injury [4].

Crush injuries occur most commonly after natural or man-made disasters such as earthquakes, mining, and industrial accidents and in war zones, where falling debris can crush hundreds of patients at once [4]. Earthquakes are estimated to have a 3–20% incidence of crushing injuries [5]. The collapse of a multistory building may cause crush injury in up to 40% of the extricated survivors [6]. This number becomes more relevant today in the advent of terrorist bombings [7]. Crush injures may also be caused by more common events, including vehicular crashes, industrial or mining mishaps, and farming incidents, where extremities become pinned in moving machine parts [8]. They can also occur after periods of unconsciousness from drug intoxication, anesthesia, trauma, or cerebral events [9].

N. Dimitriou (✉)
Department of Surgery, National and Kapodistrian University of Athens, Athens, Greece

© Springer Nature Switzerland AG 2021
E. Pikoulis, J. Doucet (eds.), *Emergency Medicine, Trauma and Disaster Management*, Hot Topics in Acute Care Surgery and Trauma,
https://doi.org/10.1007/978-3-030-34116-9_22

It is recorded that up to 80% of crush injury patients die due to severe head injuries or asphyxiation. Of the 20% that reach hospital, 10% make an uneventful recovery. The other 10% go into crush syndrome [10].

Crush syndrome was first reported in 1910 by German authors who described symptoms including muscle pain, weakness, and brown-colored urine in soldiers rescued after being buried in structural debris [7]. Crush syndrome was not well-defined until the 1940s when nephrologists Bywaters and Beall provided descriptions of victims trapped by their extremities during the London Blitz who presented with shock, swollen extremities, tea-colored urine, and subsequent renal failure [7, 8, 11, 12].

Crush syndrome is the systemic manifestation of muscular tissue injury (traumatic rhabdomyolysis) caused by compression, provoking the releasing of potentially toxic muscle cell components into the extracellular fluid [3]. It is a reperfusion injury phenomenon secondary to traumatic rhabdomyolysis.

Previous experience with earthquakes that caused major structural damage has demonstrated that the incidence of crush syndrome is 2–15% with approximately 50% of those with crush syndrome developing acute renal failure and over 50% needing fasciotomy. Of those with renal failure, 50% need dialysis [3].

22.2 Pathophysiology-Clinical Features

The likelihood of developing acute crush syndrome is directly related to the compression time; therefore victims should be released as quickly as possible, irrespective of how long they have been trapped [13, 14].

As already noted, most commonly in traumatic crush, the legs are affected and less frequently the arms, torso, and head. Many authors believe that crush injury of the head and torso significant enough to cause the syndrome is incompatible with life due to the inherent internal organ damage. However studies show that up to 10% chest trauma is associated with crush injuries [15].

The typical clinical features of crush syndrome are predominantly a result of traumatic rhabdomyolysis and subsequent release of muscle cell contents [13]. Muscle cells, as a response to the physical stimulus of being crushed, become stretched, and the sarcolemmal membranes start to leak contents out of the cells into the circulation [16]. These contents include myoglobin which gets converted to metmyoglobin and finally acid hematin, which is released into the circulation [15]. Muscles also contain potassium, magnesium, phosphate, acids, enzymes like creatine phosphokinase (CKMM), and lactate dehydrogenase (LDH), which are toxic when released into the circulation in large amounts. The leakiness of the sarcolemma membranes also allows passage of water, calcium, and sodium into the cells from the extracellular space, causing muscle swelling and intravascular volume depletion. The results from sarcolemma membranes are hypovolemic shock [4], hyperkalemia (which may precipitate cardiac arrest), hypocalcemia, metabolic acidosis, compartment syndrome (due to compartment swelling), and acute renal failure [13].

Acute renal failure is caused by hypoperfusion of the kidneys, which normally receive 25% of cardiac output [17]. This hypoperfusion compounds the toxicity caused by cast formation and mechanical blockage of the nephrons by myoglobin and underscores the importance of early, vigorous volume resuscitation to improve urine flow, which dilutes and clears toxins [8].

Crush injury also causes hypovolemia by hemorrhagic volume loss and the rapid shift of extracellular volume into the damaged tissues [8]. This may cause hypovolemia, as the intravascular volume is depleted. Electrolyte imbalances such as hyperkalemia, hypocalcemia, and a metabolic acidosis will have a negatively inotropic effect, and there is also evidence that there is direct myocardial depression from other factors released when muscle cells are damaged [13].

Cardiovascular instability is commonly seen as a result of crush syndrome and may be multifactorial, firstly as a result of hypovolemic shock either from the massive fluid shift from the extracellular space into the damaged muscle cells or by other associated injuries causing blood loss [4] and secondly from direct myocardial toxicity from electrolyte disturbance (hyperkalemia, hypocalcemia, acidemia (lactate), and hyperphosphatemia) [7].

Cardiovascular complications seen are arrhythmias secondary to the hyperkalemia and the associated acidosis. Simultaneous electrolyte abnormalities may also include hypocalcemia and hyperphosphatemia [7]. Hyperkalemia and its associated cardiotoxicity represent the second most common cause of early deaths after crush injury from the potassium released and from damaged cells, into the circulation. The effects of potassium are the result of cell membrane dysfunction allowing the leakage of intracellular potassium. Hyperkalemia at levels >6 mg/dL causes cardiotoxicity. The high potassium levels lead to dysrhythmias and eventually cardiac arrest. The leakage of phosphate from lysed cells results in hyperphosphatemia (<6 mg/dL). Levels of phosphate in this range can aggravate hypocalcemia. The stretch-activated channels in cell walls allow for influx of sodium and calcium into the cell. This results in a drop in the intravascular calcium concentration. Postreperfusion there is a calcium influx into cells. This can result in hypocalcemia (<8 mg/dL). This is usually asymptomatic and self-correcting but can be cardiotoxic and requires replacement. The resulting hypocalcemia may also lead to cardiac dysrhythmias. Hyperphosphatemia also follows rhabdomyolysis and exacerbates the effects of the hypocalcemia [7].

Another complication of crush injuries is the development of compartment syndrome, which occurs when pressures increase within a fascia-encased region, classically a muscle group or the abdomen. The fascia provides a nonexpendable space, and, as fluid is sequestered, the pressure within the compartment rises. With the rise in pressure, the microvascular circulation is compromised leading to tissue ischemia [8]. Increased pressure within this confined space leads to microvascular compromise and subsequent cellular death. Systemic hypotension, limb trauma, and interstitial tissue pressure of 30 mmHg have been suggested as threshold at which there is the diagnosis of compartment syndrome [8].

The signs and symptoms of compartment syndrome in an extremity include pain out of proportion to the injury or with passive motion, pallor, paresthesia,

pulselessness, and paralysis of the affected extremity. Attempts should be made to intervene before there is a loss of pulses, an ominous finding that will almost always reflect irreversible tissue necrosis. Compartment syndrome may also occur in the abdomen [8].

Physicians must have high suspect of crush syndrome in any victim of crush injury. Usually victims appear to be normal at rescue, without complaints of pain until after extraction, and then suddenly go into shock, secondary to reperfusion. Victims of crush injury may present with petechiae, blisters, and muscle bruising, and superficial injuries are seen. Myalgia, muscle paralysis, and sensory deficit are common. Fever, cardiac arrhythmia, pneumonia, "tea- or cola-" colored urine, oliguria, and renal failure are the sequence of events. Nausea, vomiting, agitation, and delirium are seen in the delayed rescue patients [15].

When compression involves the thorax, by direct chest pressure from debris, traumatic asphyxia can occur. Traumatic asphyxia can occur by any compression in the thorax and upper abdomen. The patient has limited chest extraction, which limits both oxygen intake and CO_2 exhalation. The direct pressure increases intrathoracic pressure and decreases the cardiac pump function [7, 9].

22.3 Diagnosis

Crush syndrome can be developed in any patient how had suffered a crush injury. High level of suspicion of crush syndrome is essential. Laboratory evaluation requires the clinician to monitor the urine myoglobin, serum creatine phosphokinase, and serum electrolytes [7].

A simple but rapid test for rhabdomyolysis can be done with a standard urine dipstick. The heme portion of myoglobin causes a positive reading for blood on the test strip and, in the absence of any red blood cells on microscopic examination, suggests myoglobinuria. However, dipstick findings are positive in only about half of patients with rhabdomyolysis. Accordingly, a normal urine dipstick does not rule out the condition, and a laboratory evaluation for myoglobin should be performed in patients suspected of having crush syndrome [8].

22.4 Management

As already mentioned crush injuries tend to present as mass casualty, after an earthquake, terrorist attack, collapse of poorly constructed buildings, etc. It is essential for the medical and paramedical staff to be familiarized with the diagnosis and management of crush injuries and crush syndrome. Because crush syndrome is a common cause of death in a mass casualty, hemodialysis facilities and their capacity should be identified in advance [18].

Patients crushed under rubble usually suffer multiple injuries, and their management must follow the principles of ABCDE paradigm. In a mass casualty setting, triage protocols must apply as well. Below, we present the differences or the extra precautionary measures that must be obtained for crush injury patients.

The management of crush injury patients involves rescue, resuscitation, recognition of the syndrome, treatment, and rehabilitation [15]. The first priority is volume resuscitation and repletion, which is critical to reverse hypovolemic shock, prevent acute renal failure, and thereby minimize lactic acidosis and hyperkalemia. The second priority is systemic alkalinization as a means to reduce acidosis and hyperkalemia. Reducing intracompartmental pressures to avoid compartment syndrome is also important [19].

Treatment of the crushed patient can be divided into two phases. The initial prehospital phase may (on the field), depending on the mechanism of injury, involves a prolonged extrication period. The second phase commences on reaching a definitive medical care facility [13].

22.4.1 Prehospital Management

22.4.1.1 Intervention Before Extrication

Safety is the first priority when approaching an accident-disaster scene. Extra caution is needed in scene with entrapped patients in falling buildings, as the risk of further collapse is present, especially in aftershocks [13, 20]. Medical and paramedical personnel, who is inexperienced in rescue procedures, should not participate in the direct extrication of victims from partially or totally collapsed buildings [20]. All personnel including rescue should be trained to recognize and treat problems associated with prolonged limb compression and have appropriate fluid and medications to treat potential complications [20].

Once the scene has been declared safe and contact is established with the entrapped victim, *medical assessment should start, even before extrication* [20]. Twenty percent of deaths after earthquakes happen shortly after extrication, probably due to consequence of reperfusion of the traumatized limbs and diffusion of tissue breakdown products into the systemic circulation [20].

Assessment needs to determine the physical status of the victim either by oral inquiry or by direct examination [21].

Fluid resuscitation must start as soon as possible, even before extrication [13, 20]. The principles of hypotensive resuscitation do not apply in the setting of extremity crush injury requiring extrication [22]. If possible, a large bore venous access in any limb should be placed, even while the victim is still under the rubble and fluid resuscitation should begin. Isotonic saline at a rate of 1000 mL/h for adults and 15–20 mL/kg/h for children; that is reducing to 500 mL/h in adults and 10 mL/kg/h in children, or even lower, is appropriate in most victims [20]. When peripheral venous access is impossible, intraosseous infusion using the same rate is possible. Other routes are oral intake of electrolyte solution and rectal infusion of electrolyte solution, in combination with oral intake [22]. Electrolyte solutions that can be used are [22]:

- World Health Organization (WHO) oral rehydration salts (ORS): preferred
- Pedialyte® (Abbott Laboratories, https://pedialyte.com)
- Per 1 L water: 8 tsp sugar, 0.5 tsp salt, 0.5 tsp baking soda
- Per quart Gatorade® (Stokely-Van Camp Inc, https://www.gatorade.com): 0.25 tsp salt, 0.25 tsp baking soda

Isotonic saline is the first option as it is readily available and highly effective for volume replacement [20]. Ringer's lactate solution contains potassium and has a theoretical disadvantage of exacerbating hyperkalemia [13].

Even if though fluid resuscitation is essential in the prevention of acute renal failure, fluid administration is and should be individualized based on time spent under the rubble, length of extrication procedure, volume status and urine flow, dimensions of the disaster, demographic characteristics of the victims, and environmental conditions [2]. Figure 22.1 shows algorithm for fluid resuscitation in crush victims of mass disasters before, during, and after extrication.

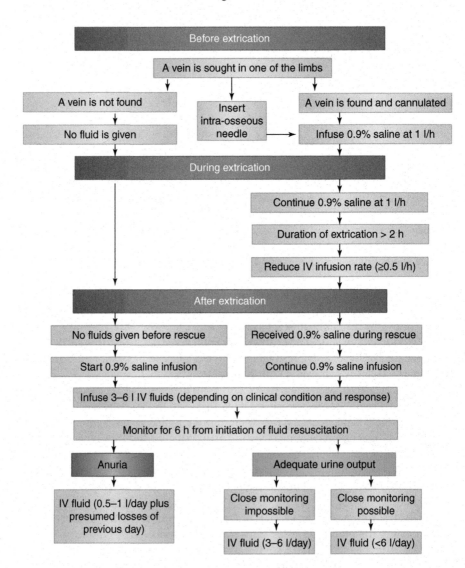

Fig. 22.1 Algorithm for fluid resuscitation in crush victims of mass disasters before, during, and after extrication. *IV* intravenous. (Modified from Sever et al. [20])

Pain management is also essential. Appropriate analgesia should be given as soon as possible; this may include the use of Entonox® initially, but most patients will require intravenous analgesia such as an opiate, titrated against response. The use of ketamine, with or without the concomitant use of a benzodiazepine, is also an effective means of relieving pain and may aid extrication [23].

22.4.1.2 Intervention During Extrication

During extrication (usually 45–90 min), *intravenous isotonic saline should be administered at a rate of 1000 mL/h*. If extrication takes longer than 2 h, the rate of fluid must be reduced so as not to exceed 500 mL/h and adjust its rate depending on age, body weight, trauma pattern, ambient temperature, urine production, and amount of overall estimated fluid losses [20].

On-site amputation is indicated only for life-saving interventions, i.e. to liberate the victim [13, 20]. Amputation should not be used as a prophylactic measure to prevent crush syndrome, firstly because amputation is associated with mortality by itself [20] and secondly because of reports from the literature which suggest that even severely crushed limbs can recover to full function [13].

22.4.1.3 General Approach Early After Extrication

After rescue, an initial-primary systematic assessment of the injured patient must be done, in order to identify and treat life-threatening injuries and to prioritize urgent therapeutic needs [20]. For each individual casualty, an assessment based on ABCDEs must be obtained. Patients with crush injuries may suffer from many additional problems, some of which may be life-threatening. Attention must be given to the possibility of spinal injury, and full spinal precautions should be maintained. Administration of high flow oxygen by mask should be a priority in treatment. The patient should be exposed as necessary to assess and manage injuries. In a hostile environment, or where there is a risk of hypothermia, exposure should be as limited as possible [13].

For uncontrollable otherwise life-threatening hemorrhage, tourniquet should be used. The use of *tourniquets* for the prevention of reperfusion injury following extrication, or in the prevention of washing of the products of rhabdomyolysis into the circulation, is still controversial. The latest guidelines suggest the placement of tourniquet if the length of entrapment exceeds 2 h and crush injury protocol cannot be initiated immediately [22].

Previous guidelines from the Faculty of Pre-Hospital Care of the Royal College of Surgeons of Edinburgh supported that there was no evidence to support the use of tourniquet for crush injury [13].

As soon as possible, secondary assessment must perform to diagnose and manage any injuries missed during the primary survey, including an inventory of injuries as well as prospective follow-up for late signs of crush syndrome.

After extrication, isotonic saline must either continue, or be started in the same regime. Urine output must be closely monitored [20]. The aim is to maintain a high urine output of 100–200 mL/h [22]. In established crush syndrome, urinary output should be at least 300 mL/h [24]. However, evidence suggests that mannitol is not superior to IV fluids alone, though it is indicated in a setting of compartment syndrome [25].

Experts advocate the use of urine dipsticks to check myoglobin and subclinical rhabdomyolysis [26].

If available, *5% dextrose + isotonic saline solution* should be administered, which may provide the advantage of supplying some calories and attenuating hyperkalemia.

Alkalization of urine above 6.5, with the addition of 50 mL of sodium bicarbonate in isotonic solutions, *is used to prevent renal tubular deposition of myoglobin and uric acid, to* improve metabolic acidosis and reduce hyperkalemia [27]. Alkaline solutions should be administered to all victims in small-scale disasters, unless symptomatic alkalosis, suggested by the presence of neuromuscular irritability, somnolence, or paresis, is present [19].

In case of *anuria*, after hypovolemia is excluded, fluids must restrict to 500–1000 mL/day in addition to a volume equivalent to all measured or estimated fluid losses of the previous day. In the case of *urinary response* to intravenous fluid administration (urine volume above 50 mL/h), fluids must restrict to 3–6 L/day if victims cannot be monitored closely. In case of close follow-up, more than 6 L/day of fluids can be administered [20].

Hyperkalemia as already mentioned is the second cause of early death after crush injury, so it must be diagnosed early in the field. Measurement of potassium in the blood is the best option for monitor hyperkalemia, but on the field is difficult, so portable electrocardiography (ECG) devices have been used for this purpose, although specificity and sensitivity of ECG findings in the case of hyperkalemia have been questioned [20]. If portable ECG is not available, close monitoring of vital signs and circulatory examination, every 15 min in the first 1–2 h, is essential [22]. Specific sings on the ECG that indicate hyperkalemia are sinus bradycardia (primary sign), peaked T waves, lengthening of PR interval (early signs), prolonged QRS interval, PVCs or runs of ventricular tachycardia, and conduction block (bundle branch, fascicular) are: On clinical examination premature ventricular contractions (PVCs; skipped beats), bradycardia, decreased peripheral pulse strength, and hypotension are all signs of hyperkalemia [22]. Urgent measures for the treatment of hyperkalemia are calcium gluconate, insulin + D50, sodium bicarbonate, and β-2 agonists, while second-line measures are dialysis and kayexalate [20, 22].

Patients with crush injuries should be transferred to a hospital with an intensive care facility and the equipment and expertise necessary to provide renal support therapy such as hemofiltration or dialysis [13].

22.4.2 Hospital Management

In the case of mass disaster, the rules of triage must apply. Patients should be assessed following normal Advanced Trauma Life Support (ATLS) guidelines. Baseline blood tests should be taken, these will include: full blood count, urea and electrolytes, creatinine kinase, amylase, liver function tests, clotting screen and group and save (cross match if deemed appropriate). The patient should be catheterized and hourly urine measurements commenced. Central venous pressure and invasive arterial monitoring should be considered [13].

In hospital, treatment of patients continues, with the involvement of nephrologists. As already mentioned many of the patients who develop crush syndrome needs dialysis. Predictive factors for dialysis are anuria, fluid overload, serum creatinine levels, BUN, and bicarbonate levels. Potassium >7 mEq/L is also an independent and important predictive factor of dialysis. At least twice or even thrice daily dialysis may be needed for up to 15 days. Prophylactic dialysis may be called for in patients at high risk for hyperkalemia [15].

Compartment syndrome is a secondary complication of crush syndrome. The traditional treatment of compartment syndrome is fasciotomy, but there is now evidence that initial treatment with mannitol may decompress compartment syndrome and avoid the need for surgery [13] (Fig. 22.2).

Mannitol administration reduces muscle edema, intracompartmental pressure, and pain. The results of mannitol can be detected within 40 min by the relief of

What Happens in Compartment Syndrome?

These illustrations show a cross-section of a normal calf and a cross-section of a calf with compartment syndrome. Compartment pressures over 30 mmHg often require surgical decompression with a fasciotomy.

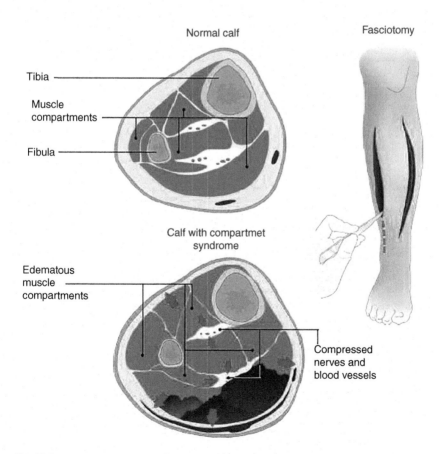

Fig. 22.2 Compartment syndrome and fasciotomies. (From Sahjian and Frakes [8])

symptoms, reduction of limb swelling, and recovery of motor function. Therefore, unless contraindicated mannitol can be used as a preventive measure in treating increasing intracompartmental pressures which have not yet reached critical levels [20]. Fasciotomy should be performed if mannitol causes no marked improvement within 1 h [20].

Recommendations suggest that fasciotomies should not be performed routinely to prevent compartment syndrome, but only when there are physical findings of compartment syndrome or when intracompartmental pressure is above 30 mmHg [20]. When pressure exceeds 30 mmHg and shows no tendency to decrease within 6 h, surgical fasciotomy should urgently be performed. In addition, fasciotomy should also be performed if compartmental pressure and diastolic blood pressure differ by less than 30 mmHg, since this condition will likely cause serious perfusion problems. When fasciotomy is indicated, it should be performed early, within the first 12 h of muscle swelling [20]. The risks of soft tissue and bone infection, delayed wound healing, subsequent amputation, and permanent functional sequelae are lower [20].

Wound infections increase the mortality in patients with crush injury, so broad-spectrum antibiotics are indicated as well as surgical debridement if needed. Immunization against tetanus is also indicated. Late complications of muscle contracture require rehabilitation. Rehabilitation should be not only physical but also psychiatric and is a long-term process [15].

References

1. Gibney RT, Sever MS, Vanholder RC. Disaster nephrology: crush injury and beyond. Kidney Int. 2014;85:1049–57.
2. Sever MS, Vanholder R. Management of crush victims in mass disasters: highlights from recently published recommendations. Clin J Am Soc Nephrol. 2013;8:328–35.
3. Centers for Disease Control and Prevention. Blast injuries: crush injury and crush syndrome. Atlanta, GA: Centers for Disease Control and Prevention; 2009.
4. Smith J, Greaves I. Crush injury and crush syndrome: a review. J Trauma. 2003;54:S226–30.
5. Pepe PE, Mosesso VN Jr, Falk JL. Prehospital fluid resuscitation of the patient with major trauma. Prehosp Emerg Care. 2002;6:81–91.
6. Better OS, Rubinstein I. Management of shock and acute renal failure in casualties suffering from the crush syndrome. Ren Fail. 1997;19:647–53.
7. Gonzalez D. Crush syndrome. Crit Care Med. 2005;33:S34–41.
8. Sahjian M, Frakes M. Crush injuries: pathophysiology and current treatment. Nurs Pract. 2007;32:13–8.
9. Mistovich JJ, Limmer D, Werman HA. Transition series: topics for the EMT. Part 5: soft tissue injuries: crush injury and compartment syndrome. EMS World. 2011;40:54–7.
10. Bywaters EG. 50 years on: the crush syndrome. BMJ. 1990;301:1412–5.
11. Better OS, Stein JH. Early management of shock and prophylaxis of acute renal failure in traumatic rhabdomyolysis. N Engl J Med. 1990;322:825–9.
12. Malinoski DJ, Slater MS, Mullins RJ. Crush injury and rhabdomyolysis. Crit Care Clin. 2004;20:171–92.
13. Greaves I, Porter K, Smith JE. Consensus statement on the early management of crush injury and prevention of crush syndrome. J R Army Med Corps. 2003;149:255–9.

14. Aoki N, Demsar J, Zupan B, Mozina M, Pretto EA, Oda J, Tanaka H, Sugimoto K, Yoshioka T, Fukui T. Predictive model for estimating risk of crush syndrome: a data mining approach. J Trauma. 2007;62:940–5.
15. Rajagopalan S. Crush injuries and the crush syndrome. Med J Armed Forces India. 2010;66:317–20.
16. Abassi ZA, Hoffman A, Better OS. Acute renal failure complicating muscle crush injury. Semin Nephrol. 1998;18:558–65.
17. Lameire N. The pathophysiology of acute renal failure. Crit Care Clin. 2005;21:197–210.
18. Johnson DW, Hayes B, Gray NA, Hawley C, Hole J, Mantha M. Renal services disaster planning: lessons learnt from the 2011 Queensland floods and North Queensland cyclone experiences. Nephrology (Carlton). 2013;18:41–6.
19. Sever MS, Vanholder R. Management of crush syndrome casualties after disasters. Rambam Maimonides Med J. 2011;2:e0039.
20. Sever MS, Vanholder R. Recommendation for the management of crush victims in mass disasters. Nephrol Dial Transplant. 2012;27(Suppl 1):i1–67.
21. Ashkenazi I, Isakovich B, Kluger Y, Alfici R, Kessel B, Better OS. Prehospital management of earthquake casualties buried under rubble. Prehosp Disast Med. 2005;20:122–33.
22. Walters TJ, Powell D, Penny A, Stewart I, Chung K, Keenan S, Shackelford S. Management of crush syndrome under prolonged field care. J Spec Oper Med. 2016;16:78–85.
23. Greaves I, Porter KM. Consensus statement on crush injury and crush syndrome. Accid Emerg Nurs. 2004;12:47–52.
24. Sever MS, Vanholder R, Lameire N. Management of crush-related injuries after disasters. N Engl J Med. 2006;354:1052–63.
25. Holt SG, Moore KP. Pathogenesis and treatment of renal dysfunction in rhabdomyolysis. Intensive Care Med. 2001;27:803–11.
26. Knapik JJ, O'Connor FG. Exertional rhabdomyolysis: epidemiology, diagnosis, treatment, and prevention. J Spec Oper Med. 2016;16:65–71.
27. Better OS, Rubinstein I, Reis DN. Muscle crush compartment syndrome: fulminant local edema with threatening systemic effects. Kidney Int. 2003;63:1155–7.

Missile and Fragment Injuries

23

Petros M. Kouridakis, Andreas Pikoulis, Fotios Stavratis, and Charalampos Theodoridis

23.1   Introduction

War trauma is not just a physical wound. Its scars are usually exceedingly greater than the injury itself. But in order to cure both evident and hidden traumas, an understanding of the nature of weapon-related injuries is necessary as well as the types of wounds caused in warfare. As war traumas are categorized basically according to the cause of injury, an overview of the nature of combat wounds draws special attention to their complexity and long-term prevalence.

23.2   Weapon Effects and War Wounds

Conventional or traditional warfare refers to an interstate conflict between rival armed forces, using:

> all types of weapons with the exception of weapons of mass destruction [1].

such as biochemical or nuclear weapons. However, a new type of combat has recently been introduced, that of *hybrid warfare* which is related to the usage of:

> coordinated military, political, economic, civilian and informational (MPECI) instruments of power that extend far beyond the military realm [2].

P. M. Kouridakis (✉)
2nd Surgical Department, 424 General Military Hospital of Thessaloniki, Thessaloniki, Greece

A. Pikoulis · F. Stavratis · C. Theodoridis
General Surgery, University General Hospital "Attikon", National and Kapodistrian University of Athens, Athens, Greece

© Springer Nature Switzerland AG 2021
E. Pikoulis, J. Doucet (eds.), *Emergency Medicine, Trauma and Disaster Management*, Hot Topics in Acute Care Surgery and Trauma,
https://doi.org/10.1007/978-3-030-34116-9_23

Although a war may be described as traditional, either sides may eventually implement unconventional warfare and battlefield tactics.

The typology of weapons in the course of a conventional war includes:

- Explosive ordnance consisting of all munitions containing explosives, including bombs, guided and ballistic missiles, artillery, mortar, rockets, mines, torpedoes, pyrotechnics, electro-explosive devices, as well as all similar explosive items or components [3]
- Portable firearms encompassing kinetic projectiles including pistols, rifles, and machine guns

Armed conflict may provoke blunt injuries and burns as well as traumas related to weapons and the circumstances of warfare [4]. The managing of combat wounds is challenging taken into account the severity of the trauma, the massiveness of the injured, the resources available, and overall working conditions. The International Committee of the Red Cross states that:

War wounds are different. The extent of tissue destruction and contamination seen in war injuries is nothing like what is seen in everyday trauma practice. [5]

The nature of warfare creates a particular epidemiology of the wounded, but basically, injuries are characterized as penetrating, blast, and thermal.

23.2.1 Penetrating Wounds

Penetrating (fragment) wounds are mainly caused by munitions both of modern warfare and those of a conventional battlefield [6]. Projectiles from such armaments may include material that was originally implemented in the device as well as the debris propelled as part of the blast effect. The latter may include objects such as nails, bolts, shrapnel, flying glass, or other foreign bodies [7], scattered to an unpredictably extended range depending on the type of the explosion or blast. Munitions, either highly sophisticated or improvised, release fragments that may vary in size and shape and depending on the construction of the weapon may consist of either preformed or asymmetrical particles.

Penetrating wounds caused by weapons of war not only are limited to bullets or pellets released from handguns, rifles, or other firearms, but also include exploding bombs, shells, rockets and grenades, landmines, as well as more sophisticated munitions, which are often referred to as *smart* or *state-of-the-art* or *next-technology* armament [8]. Exploding material produces metal fragments that derive from the weapon casing once is fired or discharged, usually regular in shape and size and weighting less than 1 g [4]. When other, usually improvised, weapons are used, nails, bolts, steel pellets, and other metallic debris are released along with the explosive material.

The amount of tissue damage and, consequently, the severity of injuries mainly depend on the transmitted energy and velocity of fragments and projectiles which is in turn influenced by the proximity of the wounded to the exposure [9]. Red Cross Wound Classification provides a scoring system of the wounds after initial assessment or surgery, which is based on characteristics such as the diameter of the entry wound (E), the diameter of the exit wound (X), the cavity (C), the type of fracture (F), the injury of the brain, viscera or major arteries (V), and bullet or fragments visible on X-rays (M) [10].

Further to war-related wounds, in the US firearm, injuries have a severe public healthcare impact as they cost more than 70$ billion annually to the US healthcare system [11]. They also make up for more than 32,000 deaths and over 67,000 injuries per annum in the country alone [12]. Morbidity and mortality is high with ballistic injuries, depending on the velocity, the efficiency of energy transfer, the physical characteristics of the projectile, the kinetic energy, stability, entrance profile and path traveled through the body, as well as the biologic characteristics of the tissues injured [13].

23.2.1.1 Mechanism of Injury

Bullet placement and the path followed by the projectile are the most important factors in causing acute injury or even death, depending on the regions of the body being hurt. The head and the torso are the most vulnerable parts of the human body because of the abundance of vital structures such as the CNS, spinal cord, lungs, and other vital organs which can be incapacitated, be destructed, or, once hit, produce extensive hemorrhage [14].

Laceration originating by penetration from explosively propelled fragments and bullets is common in combat injury [15]. When a moving projectile enters the human body, soft tissue damage is provoked through crushing, which, along with the release of kinetic energy, causes temporary cavity to the body [16]. The latter may either be a penetrating or perforating wound, depending on whether the bullet is retained in tissue or exits the body [17].

Once entering the body and shredding the tissue in its path, the bullet produces a temporary cavity considerably larger than its diameter [18]. According to existing bibliography, "this temporary cavity, which has a lifetime of 5–10 ms from initial rapid growth until collapse, undergoes a series of gradually smaller pulsations and contractions before it finally disappears, leaving the permanent wound track" [19].

The shape and construction of the bullet shape determine the extent of damage when interacting with human tissue. As the bullet moves through the body, the tissue is disrupted, crushed, and stretched; it then follows its path [20]. Certain organs, such as the brain and spleen, are prone to permanent damage due to their inelasticity [21].

Ballistic injury has a double effect on the human body as it creates both a permanent and temporary cavity:

- *Permanent cavity* is defined as:
  "localized area of cell necrosis, proportional to the size of the projectile as it passes through" [22]

- *Temporary cavity* refers to:
  "Transient lateral displacement of tissue, which is also known as a stretch cavity and occurs after the passage of a projectile. Elastic tissue, such as skeletal muscle, blood vessels and skin, may be pushed aside after passage of the projectile, but then rebound. Inelastic tissue, such as bone or liver, may fracture in this area" [23].

Bullet wounds seen in the injured are usually single with a small entry, and there may not always be an exit wound, which size is variable. Multiple bullet injuries are more likely to kill. According to international humanitarian law as documented by the Third Hague Convention of 1899:

all bullets used during armed conflict are supposed to remain intact. [24]

Military bullets with a full metal jacketing tend to pass through the body intact, thus producing less extensive injuries since they usually do not fragment in the body or shed fragments of lead while penetrating the body [19]. However, bullets used by civilian weapons, such as large-caliber shotguns or hunting rifles, do not require full metal jacket, and they therefore produce extensive and more severe wounds than those in combat [20].

23.2.2 Explosive Blast Injuries

Explosions, either accidental or intentional, may be the cause of severe injuries or even death on a mass scale, since they are simultaneously inflicting on many people [25]. Their effects are categorized in primary, secondary, tertiary, and quaternary injuries [26], depending on the type of the explosion (chemical, mechanical, nuclear), the material used, its proximity to the victim, the interfering objects, and the type of available protection [25].

According to the Federal Emergency Management Agency (FEMA) [27], an explosion:

is the rapid release of energy in form of light, heat, sound and shock wave.

When a high-order explosion is initiated, only one-third of the chemical energy is released during the detonation process, while the remaining two-thirds are slowly released as the detonation outputs mix with air and burn. The shock wave is followed by a blast wind which is the flow of superheated air interacting with people and objects and is the cause of injury or damage [28]. Research has shown that explosions in confined spaces are associated with a higher prevalence of primary blast injuries and a higher mortality rate in comparison with explosions in the open air [29].

A victim of a blast may not bear any external injury. When exposed to explosions, the human body may be subjected to injuries as described below. **Primary** injuries are related to the direct injuries caused by the blast, mainly damaging air-filled organs (lungs, auditory organs, the eye, brain, and gastrointestinal tract) whereas **secondary** by flying casing fragments or, according to existing literature:

> by debris carried by the blast wind and most often result in penetrating injury from small shrapnel. The shrapnel can also cause blunt trauma similar to that encountered in motor vehicle accidents, gunshot wounds, stabbings, and assaults [30].

Such injuries affect mainly the musculoskeletal system and, on occasion, may be the cause of limp amputations.

Tertiary injuries occur when victims are thrown against solid objects due to air displacement caused by the explosion, and **quaternary** are usually induced when exposed to fire, fumes, radiation, biological agents, smoke, dust, toxins, etc. and also involve the psychological impact of the event [28]. Bone fragments can also function as secondary projectiles causing further tissue disruption [31].

By either of the aforementioned type of injuries of a blast, multiple wounds may be caused to a single individual; the polytrauma patient is the defined as a casualty:

> whose injuries involve multiple body regions and in whom the combination of injuries would cause a life-threatening condition. [32]

Fragment injuries predominate in mixed injuries. However, epidemiological data referring to the primary injuries and effects of the blast include ear and ruptured tympanum, blast lung, arterial air embolism, visceral injury, eye and maxillofacial injuries, as well as musculoskeletal injuries mainly involving limps [5].

In addition, the experience of the war in Afghanistan and Iraq has shown that although a UN Weapons Convention in 1980 adopted specific rules on the use of land mines, antipersonnel landmines are still causing casualties long after the cease-fire [33]. Civilians, women and children among them, have either been killed or amputated since landmines are still to be found in agricultural fields, near water supplies, along roadways, and around villages [34].

23.2.3 Thermal Wounds

War burns have been recorded for more than 5000 years of written history [35]; the liquid fire which dates back in the seventh century BC, the napalm bomb, the white phosphate and mustard gas, and modern nuclear weapons consist of documented practices of burn threatening artillery used during armed conflicts.

Thermal wound is defined as traumatic injury to the skin or other tissues primarily caused by other acute exposures to thermal sources. Burns occur when some or all of the cells in the skin or other tissues are destroyed by heat, electrical discharge, friction, chemicals, or radiation [36].

Such wounds are in turn classified into six separate groups depending on the mechanism of injury: scalds, contact burns, fire, chemical, electrical, and radiation. These can be provoked by contact with liquid, gas, or grease and can be produced by either flash or flame burns [37]. Burn injuries can be extremely complex and severe, depending on the duration of exposure to the source of the associated trauma. Inhalation injuries are closely associated with the exposure to smoke or chemicals.

Thermal trauma causes injuries to the skin or other tissues, due to the exposure to heat, chemicals, radiation, high or other acute thermal sources, resulting to destruction of skin cells or other tissues. Burns are mostly classified into three degrees [38]:

- First degree: Erythema
- Second degree: Blistering of the skin leading to superficial ulceration
- Third degree: Tissue disorganization leading to a dry yellow crust

Historically, burns account for a 5–20% of combat casualties [39]. Treatment on-site consists of bandaging, alleviation of pain, and treatment of the consequent shock, along with the respiratory difficulties caused by smoke inhalation. Burn injuries also require fluid resuscitation [40] and occasionally a multidiscipline approach, including general, orthopedic, plastic-reconstructive, maxillofacial, ophthalmic, and neurological surgeons and general and intensive treatment unit anesthetists [35]. Similar corporal reactions are produced by exposure to extreme cold conditions which often results to nonfreezing and freezing injuries, depending on the conditions which the person is exposed to. These affect mostly the limbs as well as other exposed body parts, nose, ears, etc. [4] and need to be specifically addressed to in order to avoid hypothermia and amputation.

In case of combined thermodynamic injuries, the internal body compartments may suffer extensive trauma due to the sudden transitions caused by internal or external pressure and the direct and indirect effects related to the event itself [41]. Treatment is applied according to the severity of burns. The first 24 h are crucial in order to stabilize the patient and preserve their organ functions. From Day 3 surgical intervention is possible, if their general status allows such procedures and homeostasis has sufficiently normalized [41].

Skin graft may be required in order to avoid infection, when skin cells have been damaged and wounds extend deeper into the skin dermal layers where cells that would normally heal the wound have been destroyed [42].

When it comes to burn wounds, psychological support is often required, especially in cases of mass burn injuries where severe long-term impairment may be the cause of PTSD or other psychological disorders [43].

23.2.3.1 Mental Injury

Mental injury is common among combatants, due to exposure to stressful and unusual conditions and may additionally be consequence to the exposure to the aforementioned war traumas. Not only does it affect the daily routine after being at war, but may also be associated with various psychosomatic reactions. CSR (combat stress reaction) is an acute behavioral disorientation and is evident in cognitive, affective, and behavioral reactions [44]. PTSD prevalence is considerable for military personnel exposed in combat conditions—analyses have shown that PTSD in postwar periods increases suicide rates [45], cases of self-injury, and suicidal idealization, which may worsen the health status of combatants already exposed in combat traumas. The connection between physical impairment and mental injury remains close and extensively researched.

23.3   Conclusion

War wounds are far more complex than other types of injury encountered in civilian practice. They are also treated under stressful conditions and with limited resources. A review of the existing literature shows that the types of wounds encountered in warfare are generally classified in ballistic, blast, and thermal wounds, depending on the typology of weapons used in the course of the combat. Furthermore, somatic wounds are also associated with mental injuries and disorders, which may unfold, in a postwar period.

References

1. Dictionary of basic military terms, a soviet view. 1965. Published under the auspices of the United States Air Force, Translated by the DGIS Mulfilinguml Section Translation Bureau Secretary of State; Department Ottawa Canada.
2. Cullen P, Reichborn-Kjennerud E. Understanding hybrid warfare a multinational capability development campaign project. MCDC countering hybrid warfare project; 2016.
3. Handbook of defence land ranges safety JSP 403, vol. 4, 2 edn., Change 3 vol. IV by Command of The Defence Council GLOSSARY OF TERMS AND DEFINITIONS.
4. International Committee of the Red Cross; Giannou G, Baldan M. War surgery – working with limited resources in armed conflict and other situations of violence, vol. 1. 2010. https://www.icrc.org/en/doc/assets/files/other/icrc-002-0973.pdf.
5. International Committee of the Red Cross; Giannou G, Baldan M, Molde A. War surgery – working with limited resources in armed conflict and other situations of violence, vol. 2. 2010.
6. Bowyer GW, Cooper GJ, Rice P. Small fragment wounds: biophysics and pathophysiology. J Trauma. 1996;40:S159–64.
7. Lemonick D. Bombings and blast injuries: a primer for physicians. Am J Clin Med. 2011;8:3.
8. Mahajan CP, Motghare V. Smart munitions. Def Sci J. 2010;60(2):159–63.
9. Lerner A, Soudry M. Armed conflict injuries to the extremities, vol. 21. Berlin: Springer; 2011. https://doi.org/10.1007/978-3-642-16155-1_2.
10. Coupland R. FRCS. The Red Cross wound classification. http://icrcndresourcecentre.org/wp-content/uploads/2016/04/The_Red_Cross_Wound_Classification.pdf.
11. Tasigiorgos S, Economopoulos KP, Winfield RD, Sakran JV. Firearm injury in the United States: an overview of an evolving public health problem. J Am Coll Surg. 2015;221(6):1005–14.
12. Fowler KA, Dahlberg LL, Haileyesus T, Annest JL. Firearm injuries in the United States. Prev Med. 2015;79:5–14.
13. Bartlett CS, Helfet DL, Hausman MR, Strauss E. Ballistics and gunshot wounds: effects on musculoskeletal tissues. J Am Acad Orthop Surg. 2000;8(1):21–36.
14. Maiden N. Ballistics reviews: mechanisms of bullet wound trauma. Forensic Sci Med Pathol. 2009;5:204. https://doi.org/10.1007/s12024-009-9096-6.
15. Liu S, Xu C, Wen Y, et al. Assessment of bullet effectiveness based on a human vulnerability model. J R Army Med Corps. 2018;164:172–8.
16. Swift B, Rutty GN. The exploding bullet. J Clin Pathol. 2004;57(1):108.

17. Stefanopoulos PK, Pinialidis DE, Hadjigeorgiou GF, et al. Wound ballistics 101: the mechanisms of soft tissue wounding by bullets. Eur J Trauma Emerg Surg. 2017;43:579. https://doi.org/10.1007/s00068-015-0581-1.
18. Netto FS, Pannell D, Tien H. Hollow-point ammunition and handguns: the potential for large temporary cavities. Injury Extra. 2008;39:50–2.
19. Di Mayo VJM. Gunshot wounds – practical aspects of firearms, ballistics and forensic techniques. 2nd ed. Boca Raton, FL; New York, NY: CRC Press; 1999.
20. Hollerman J, Fackler M, Coldwell D, Ben-Menachem Y. Gunshot wounds 1. Bullets, ballistics and mechanisms of injury. AJR. 1990;155:685–90.
21. Dahistorm D, Powley K. Technical report – TR-01-95. Comparative performance of 9 mm Parabellum. 38 Special, 40 Smith & Wesson Ammunition in ballistic gelatin. Toronto, ON: Canadian Police Research Center; 1994.
22. Rockwood C, Bucholz R, Court-Brown C, Heckman J, Tornetta P. Rockwood and green's fractures in adults, vol. I. Philadelphia, PA: Wolters Kluwer Health; 2010.
23. Lichte P, Oberbeck R, Binnebösel M, Wildenauer R, Pape H, Kobbe P. A civilian perspective on ballistic trauma and gunshot injuries. Scand J Trauma Resusc Emerg Med. 2010;18:35. http://www.sjtrem.com/content/18/1/35.
24. Division of International Law of the Carnegie Endowment for International Peace. The Proceedings of the Hague Peace Conferences Translation of the Official Text. New York, NY: Oxford University Press; 1920. http://www.loc.gov/rr/frd/Military_Law/pdf/Hague-Peace-Conference_1899.pdf.
25. Jorolemon MR, Krywko DM. Blast injuries. 2017. In: StatPearls. Treasure Island, FL: StatPearls Publishing; 2018. https://www.ncbi.nlm.nih.gov/books/NBK430914/.
26. Pennardt A. Blast injuries. 2018. https://emedicine.medscape.com/article/822587-overview.
27. https://www.fema.gov/pdf/plan/prevent/rms/428/fema428_ch4.pdf, https://www.fema.gov/media-library-data/20130726-1455-20490-7465/fema426_ch4.pdf.
28. Jorolemon MR, Krywko DM. Blast injuries. 2018. In: StatPearls. Treasure Island, FL: StatPearls Publishing; 2018. https://www.ncbi.nlm.nih.gov/books/NBK430914/.
29. Leibovici D, Gofrit ON, Stein M, Shapira SC, Noga Y, Heruti RJ, Shemer J. Blast injuries in a bus versus open-air bombings: a comparative study of injuries in survivors of open-air versus confined-space explosions. J Trauma. 1996;41:1030–5.
30. Singh A, Ditkofsky N, York J, Abujudeh H, Avery L, Brunner J, Sodickson A, Lev M. Blast injuries: from improvised explosive device blasts to the Boston marathon bombing. 2016;36:295. https://doi.org/10.1148/rg.2016150114.
31. Maiden NR. The assessment of bullet wound trauma dynamics and the potential role of anatomical models. 2010. https://digital.library.adelaide.edu.au/dspace/bitstream/2440/99527/2/02whole.pdf.
32. Rau CS, Wu SC, Kuo PJ, Chen YC, Chien PC, Hsieh HY, Hsieh CH. Polytrauma defined by the New Berlin definition: a validation test based on propensity-score matching approach. Int J Environ Res Public Health. 2017;14(9):1045. https://doi.org/10.3390/ijerph14091045.
33. Jeffrey SJ. Antipersonnel mines: who are the victims? J Accid Emerg Med. 1996;13(5):343–6.
34. McIvor JD. Anti-personnel landmine injuries: a global epidemic. Work. 1997;8(3):299–304. https://doi.org/10.3233/WOR-1997-8310.
35. Atiyeh BS, Gunn SW, Hayek SN. Military and civilian burn injuries during armed conflicts. Ann Burns Fire Disast. 2007;20(4):203–15.
36. Rice PL, Orgill DP. Classification of burn injury. https://www.uptodate.com/contents/classification-of-burn-injury#H20.
37. Vorstenbosch J. Thermal burns. 2017. https://emedicine.medscape.com/article/1278244-overview.
38. Lee KC, Joory K, Moiemen NS. History of burns: the past, present and the future. Burns Trauma. 2014;2:20040169. https://doi.org/10.4103/2321-3868.143620.
39. Kauvar DS, Wolf SE, Wade CE, Cancio LC, Renz EM, Holcomb JB. Burns sustained in combat explosions in Operations Iraqi and Enduring Freedom (OIF/OEF explosion burns). Burns. 2006;32(7):853–7, ISSN 0305-4179.

40. Michaeli D. Medicine on the battlefield: a review. J R Soc Med. 1979;72:1979.
41. Franke A, Kollig E. Recommendations for the treatment of severe burn injuries in the field. https://military-medicine.com/article/3062-recommendations-for-the-treatment-of-severe-burn-injuries-in-the-field.html.
42. North Bristol NHS Trust. Skin grafts and donor sites following a burn injury-information for adults. 2016.
43. Willebrand M, Andersson G, Ekselius L. Prediction of psychological health after an accidental burn. J Trauma. 2004;57:367–74.
44. Benyamini Y, Solomon Z. Combat stress reactions, posttraumatic stress disorder, cumulative life stress, and physical health among Israeli veterans twenty years after exposure to combat. Soc Sci Med. 2005;61(6):1267–77. https://doi.org/10.1016/j.socscimed.2005.01.023, ISSN 0277-9536.
45. Rozanov V, Carli V. Suicide among war veterans. Int J Environ Res Public Health. 2012;9(7):2504–19.

Pelvic Injuries and Spinal Injuries

24

Olga Savvidou, Angelos Kaspiris,
and Panayiotis J. Papagelopoulos

24.1 Introduction

The sudden presentation of a large number of injured patients to hospitals to such an extent that leads to impaired ability of providing the appropriate treatment is characterized as a mass casualty situation [1]. Similarly, Emergency Management and Disaster Medicine (EMDM) Academy Consensus Group defines that disaster is the incident in which the medical need exceeds the response capabilities in the affected area, mainly due to a large number and/or severity of injured or ill victims. Alternatively to the word "disaster," the terms "emergency" and "mass casualty incident/event" are usually used [2]. A mega mass casualty situation has two characteristics: first, the large number of casualties which is accompanied by a tremendous medical need overwhelming the available local resources, e.g., rescue equipment and medical or nursing personnel and, secondly, the emergency event which is associated with dangerous environmental conditions that often prevent medical assistance [3]. The management of a patient during a mass casualty incident includes the following stages:

1. "The golden hour" that is defined as the time in the operating room where a patient does not exceed its physiologic limits and does not show the characteristic triad of hypothermia, acidosis, and coagulopathy [4]

O. Savvidou (✉) · P. J. Papagelopoulos
First Department of Orthopaedic Surgery, School of Medicine, "ATTIKON" University General Hospital, National and Kapodistrian University of Athens, Athens, Greece

A. Kaspiris
Department of Orthopaedic Research, Laboratory of Molecular Pharmacology, School of Health Sciences, University of Patras, Patras, Greece

© Springer Nature Switzerland AG 2021
E. Pikoulis, J. Doucet (eds.), *Emergency Medicine, Trauma and Disaster Management*, Hot Topics in Acute Care Surgery and Trauma,
https://doi.org/10.1007/978-3-030-34116-9_24

2. Damage control philosophy which is defined as the application of the limited surgical assistance that is able to save the patient's life [5]
3. The series of survival processes that are depend on a well-structured care approaches from the initial in-hospital management to rehabilitation [6]

24.2 Blast Injuries

The wide use of explosives in the combat fields and in terrorist's attacks on civilian targets has become very common recently leading to an increased requirement of expertized military personnel and civilians too. Interestingly, 70% of disasters that cause more than 20 dead at the scene are associated with explosions. The recent conflicts of the USA and their allies in Iraq and Afghanistan have shown that improvised explosive devices (IED) cause an array of very severe injuries to military personnel and civilians. Additionally, terrorist actions like Madrid commuter train bombing, London underground bombing, Oklahoma City bombing, and Boston marathon bombing are well-known examples of noncombat blast injuries. Explosives' mechanism of action is based on the instantaneous release of expanding gases unleashing large amount of energy. Consequently the surrounding air is heated and compressed by the released gases giving generation to a shock-blast wave [7]. These shock-blast waves apply different types of mechanical forces to the human body, causing stretching and tearing damages to the human organs [7]. The severity of the injury is also associated with the surroundings in which the blast occurs. Specifically, blasts in a close room are correlated with more severe injuries and increased mortality rate when compared to shock waves in an open environment [7]. Mechanism of blast injury is classified into five stages based on trauma physiological properties. The "primary blast injury" is the result of the energy from the crashing overpressure wave of the explosion, while the "secondary blast injury" is the result of a penetrating trauma caused by projectile fragments. "Tertiary blast injury" is the result of falling debris or spread of the casualty against surrounding structures, and "quaternary blast injury" is the consequences of the thermal injury or toxic inhalation. Finally, radiation exposure or bacterial contamination results in a "quinary blast injury."

24.3 Spinal and Pelvic Injuries

Musculoskeletal injuries are very common among the victims of blast events and are responsible for more than 80% of all the surgical procedures. Prehospital management priorities remain airway and spinal prophylaxis, breathing, circulation, stabilization of fractures, and transport.

In general the in-hospital management of blast-induced bony injuries includes plain films and CT imaging to evaluate for fractures and foreign bodies, tetanus prophylaxis, and broad-spectrum antibiotics in the cases of open fractures [7]. Initial evaluation with magnetic resonance imaging (MRI) should be avoided due to the possibility of metallic shrapnel presence that could be overheated or moved by the magnetic fields. For the great majority of the blast victims suffering from fractures, early external fixation is highly recommended. We have to underline the fact that any injury of the extremities must be examined for signs of compartment syndrome.

Concerning the evaluation and management of combat-related injuries, which also apply in bombing terrorists actions, the USA Ministry of Defense has published more than 25 clinical guidelines focusing on the management of a spinal trauma [8]. According to these guidelines, injured military personnel suffering of neck pain and demonstrating neurological complications should be immobilized in the field with a cervical collar. Moreover, a collar should apply in individuals with penetrating traumas from an explosion with the exception of conscious patients with isolated injuries without neurological symptoms or neck pain [8]. It must be highlighted that moving the injured personnel outside the battle field in a secure area takes priority over the cervical immobilization [8]. In the hospital, CT scan or three views (anteroposterior, lateral, and odontoid) must be performed. If radiological examination does not reveal any cervical pathology, the collar can be removed. In the cases of neck pain, limited range of neck motion, or paresthesia, the collar should be retained despite the negative radiographic data [8]. If a prolonged cervical immobilization is necessary, the collar may be replaced by an orthosis averting the ulcer development and providing adequate padding. Furthermore, spinal injuries management includes CT examination or orthogonal views of the thoracic and lumbar spinal zones [8, 9]. As an MRI is not indicated, a CT myelogram may be necessary in patients with spinal cord compression due to a vertebral fracture, post-traumatic disc herniation, or epidural hematoma [8, 9]. Interestingly, administration of high doses of methylprednisolone is not indicated, because steroids are associated with immunosuppression and thus may prevent would heal [9]. Individuals with severe thoracic or lumbar traumas should be immobilized in a vacuum spine board (VSB) before transfer despite the referred minor side effects like skin disruption, increased anxiety, or claustrophobia [8]. Regardless of the concerns about the infections from the implant application in order to stabilize or decompress the spine, the decompression and instrumentation in a hemodynamically stable patient, without contaminated spinal injury but with progressive neurological symptoms, may be performed [8]. Furthermore, in penetrating spinal traumas, surgical debridement and decompression is allowed in the cases of progressive neurological deficits, cauda equina syndrome, fragment presence within the spinal canal, and leakage of cerebrospinal fluid [8].

The beneficial effects of spinal immobilization in the battlefield have been described by Comstock et al. [10]. In their study regarding military personnel injured in Afghanistan, 29 patients out of 372 have suffered from spinal fractures (8%). Among them, 12 have been diagnosed with unstable fractures (41%) accompanied by foreign bodies or bony fragments in the spinal canal or impinging on vertebral artery [10]. The improvised explosive devices are linked to high incidence of spinal injuries, and the authors support the notion that spinal immobilization must be performed in all patients in the Tactical Field Care phase [10]. On the contrary, Bellamy et al. reported that only 1.4% of Vietnam War casualties who suffered penetrating injuries had beneficial effects of spinal immobilization [11]. In the survey of Blair et al. [12], a comparison between the severity of penetrating and blunt injuries was studied [12]. They reported that, despite the fact that blunt injuries are associated with increased rate of spinal fractures like transverse process and compression, penetrating injuries resulted in transverse, lamina, and spinous process fractures and accompanied by higher rate of spinal cord injury [12]. Kahraman et al. reviewed a series of 106 military patients with military penetrating spinal injuries in Western Europe [13]. In the acute surgical group, a 64% with neurological improvement was reported, compared to 60% to nonoperative group [13]. These results are in agreement with Klimo et al. that an approximate neurological improvement rate was 50% after the surgical stabilization of military spinal cord injuries. Klimo's study group also recommended that a decompression should be considered in hemodynamically stable patients, with incomplete neurological deficits or with clear spinal cord compressive pathology [13]. Complications associated with the military spine injuries are not uncommon [12], and their frequency is similar to the civilian literature [14]. Higher rate of the complication was observed in patients treated operatively including neurological deficits, pneumonia, perioperative death, wound laceration, deep wound infection, iliac screw malposition, hardware removal, instrumental failure, and pulmonary embolism. Both blunt and penetrating traumas were associated with complications [14].

Pelvic injuries were also reported during bombing attacks either in battle fields or in terrorist's attacks. Schoenfeld et al. reported that pelvic trauma comprised the 7% of the musculoskeletal wounds, compared to spinal trauma that was responsible for the 14% [15]. Pelvic injuries include acetabular fractures, pelvic fractures (Fig. 24.1a, b), and pelvic amputation [15]. Generally, an open blast pelvis is considered to be the most severe injury within the spectrum of battlefield trauma [16]. For these patients immediate transfer to the operation room is deemed necessary. In

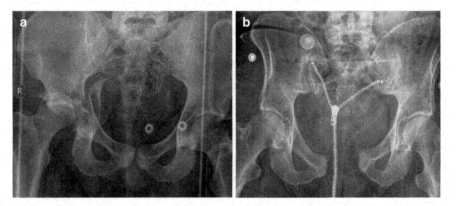

Fig. 24.1 (a) Anterior and posterior column fracture of the right acetabulum 2. (b) Type C (unstable) (vertical shear) according to tile classification of pelvic ring disruption

the operation theatre damage control resuscitation must be performed. Ramasamy et al. reported that the mean number of units of packed red cells transfused in the first 24 h after injury was 28.6. On the contrary, in civilians with open pelvic injuries following blunt trauma, the mean number of units of packed red cells transfused was 16.0. In these cases, the use of a massive transfusion protocol during the immediate management of severely injured trauma patients has been widely accepted and shown to have beneficial effects in the mortality rates [16]. IV antibiotics must be administered immediately after the arrival during pelvic packing and pelvic stabilization. External fixation is the preferred management of these fractures [16]. Notably, pelvic injuries are accompanied by soft tissue injuries. The most widely used classification of soft tissue injuries is the Faringer system that describes the anatomical location of the soft tissue injury dividing the body in three zones: Zone I includes perineum, anterior pubis, medial buttock, and posterior sacrum; Zone II includes the medial thigh and groin crease; and, finally, Zone III includes the posterolateral buttock and the iliac crest. Vascular structures, hollow viscera, and genitalia injuries are not uncommon [16]. Therefore, it became apparent that management of this injury pattern demands huge resources and remarkable multidisciplinary cooperation. The estimated survival is in about the range of 10–33%.

Severe injuries of the pelvic ring may lead to trauma-related hemipelvectomies, which are rare but massively destructive open ring disruptions caused by high-energy mechanism of injury. Hemipelvectomy is indicated in the cases of insufficient soft tissue coverage, complicated by life-threatening local infection like aggressive necrotizing infections of the pelvic girdle and a dysvascular hemipelvis. In the study of D'Alleyrand [17], 13 patients after a blast injury underwent hemipelvectomy due to vascular injury and associated lower extremity necrosis or ipsilateral vertically and rotationally unstable pelvic ring disruption with an associated acetabular fracture [17]. Care of these patients requires an interdisciplinary approach involving the orthopedic, general, urological, and plastic surgeon as well as with the infectious diseases, psychiatry, and prosthetic and rehabilitation services.

Analysis of data concerning children's blasts injuries reveals that predominant traumas in children younger than 15 years occur in the head and neck [18], while children younger than 7 years appears low incident of injury to the extremity or pelvic girdle. Additionally, pediatric patients show higher Injury Severity Score and prolonged intensive care unit stay. Children 9–14 years of age underwent significantly more procedures compared with adults, while children younger than 3 years underwent significant fewer procedures [18].

24.4   Earthquakes–Tsunamis

Earthquake is a natural disaster which can be characterized as a mega mass casualty situation. Compared to other natural disasters, earthquakes are much more harmful and unpredictable causing significant loss of lives and assets due to immense amount of energy released. It is mostly mechanical energy, and almost all the casualties are the result of a single episode concentrated in a very short period of time. Moreover, dramatic rise in the rate of complex injuries and related diseases has been reported within the first 72 h. In addition to direct injuries to vital organs, such as the head and heart and rupture of large vessels, crush injuries caused by prolonged pressing of the body by collapsed buildings are also major causes of death. The acute increase of muscle pressure can also lead to compartment syndrome.

The first step in spine, pelvis, and extremity injuries is the proper immobilization of the injured region along with an established and secure airway. Wide intravenous access is required for immediate hemodynamic stabilization. Spinal injuries of the cervical spine are clinically significant. Maintenance of cervical alignment at the scene with a cervical collar and a spine board is very important for a positive outcome. Pelvic fractures management under disaster situations constitutes a great challenge. The purpose of the emergency procedures at the scene is to check hemorrhage through stabilization of the fracture site by reducing pelvic diameter. This can be achieved through the application of anti-shock trousers or external fixation by a pelvic clamp. If the necessary equipment, like trousers or external fixation material, is not available, an improvised taping technique can be assessed for rigid fixation of the torso and pelvis after primary stabilization.

In the catastrophic earthquake at Yashu Prefecture in China on 2010, 3255 patients were admitted in the hospital [19]. The most frequent injuries were bone fractures that were diagnosed in the 55% of the patients. Seventeen percent of the patients had spinal fractures, and 15% had pelvic fractures [19]. Among the spinal fractures, the most common injuries were observed in the lumbar spine, and the majority of the patients (88.46%) had no neurological deficit according to the Frankel's classification. Similar numbers were noted in the Nicaragua, in Guatemala, and in Haiti earthquakes. However, many surveys have suggested that increased rates of fractures are observed during night earthquakes [19]. General treatment guidelines for the management of orthopedic injuries were proposed by the Israeli Defense Forces that were involved in the Haiti earthquake on 2010. They suggested that first priority has to be the treatment of the life-threatening infections with extensive debridement or by an amputation of unsalvageable limbs. Second all the closed fractures, with the exception of femoral fractures, have to be treated nonoperatively. Closed femoral fractures must be treated with external fixation, while open fractures must be treated by debridement and external fixation. IV antibiotics have to be administered immediately, and a second debridement must be performed after 2–3 days. Closed compartment syndromes may be encountered as chronic. Radiographic guidelines are as follows: only one anteroposterior (AP) view may be taken, and postoperative radiographs must be applied only in selected cases like doubts about a successful fixation.

In the same group study, the majority of the pelvic fractures were categorized as lateral compression, just as in Iran's earthquake in 2003, corresponding to 69.1% of the pelvic fractures. Treatment of choice to immobilize an unstable pelvis was the application of external fixation, while in a remarkable percentage of patients, stabilization with the application of iliosacral screw was performed [20].

Similarly, in the cases of spinal fractures, a proper immobilization is deemed necessary. Studies have shown that immobilization of patients with a board and collar and head immobilization between foam wedges provides the most stable biomechanical immobilization. It has been, also, reported that patients transported within 24 h to a proper health facility have better outcome than those who are transported after 24 h. Furthermore, early catheterization, analgesia, fluid resuscitation, and steroid administration are correlated with reduced mortality rate and neurological complications.

Tsunami is a natural phenomenon in which a series of large waves are generated after a displacement of submarine landslides caused by earthquakes. In 2004 during the Indian Ocean tsunami, thousands of people were severely injured [21, 22]. The main injuries of the surviving population were salt water aspiration and traumas. Orthopedic emergencies like fractures, dislocations, and tendon rupture were very common. Mechanism of orthopedic injuries was blunt trauma from floating debris or crashes injuries from large masses, e.g., vehicles, trees, or houses etch. Pelvic fractures were not common. Contrariwise, spinal fractures represented the 9.5% of all fracture types. Skeletal tractions for the extremities and external fixation were the treatments of choice. Spinal stabilization with posterior spinal fusion was also performed. Poor facilities, operating theatre sharing with other specialties, and uncertain hygiene conditions made the application of any implant or intramedullary nailing inappropriate. A fact that must be highlighted is that almost all tsunamis traumas are severely contaminated due to the body coverage of mud, dirt, and sand. Thus, it is proposed that, after a tsunami injury, all the minor wounds should be left open while penetrating traumas need detail exploration and lacerated wounds and open fractures, emergency dressing, debridement and exhausting cleaning is appropriate [21, 22].

24.5   Conclusions

Nowadays blast injuries are very common due to the increasing frequency of terrorists bombing attacks that led to high-volume pelvic and spinal traumas previously seen only in military conflicts. Similarly, natural disasters like earthquakes are associated with severe pelvic and spinal injuries. All the above traumas are multidimensional and can affect every organ system. Therefore, it is very important for either prehospital providers or emergency doctors to be familiar with the recognition and management of the injuries caused during mega mass casualty situations.

References

1. Aylwin CJ, König TC, Brennan NW, Shirley PJ, Davies G, Walsh MS, Brohi K. Reduction in critical mortality in urban mass casualty incidents: analysis of triage, surge, and resource use after the London bombings on July 7, 2005. Lancet. 2006;368(9554):2219–25.
2. Debacker M, Hubloue I, Dhondt E, Rockenschaub G, Rüter A, Codreanu T, Koenig KL, Schultz C, Peleg K, Halpern P, Stratton S, Della Corte F, Delooz H, Ingrassia PL, Colombo D, Castrèn M. Utstein-style template for uniform data reporting of acute medical response in disasters. PLoS Curr. 2012;4:e4f6cf3e8df15a.

3. Rega P, Burkholder-Allen K, Bork C. An algorithm for the evaluation and management of red, yellow, and green zone patients during a botulism mass casualty incident. Am J Disaster Med. 2009;4(4):192–8.

4. Newgard CD, Schmicker RH, Hedges JR, Trickett JP, Davis DP, Bulger EM, Aufderheide TP, Minei JP, Hata JS, Gubler KD, Brown TB, Yelle JD, Bardarson B, Nichol G. Resuscitation Outcomes Consortium Investigators. Emergency medical services intervals and survival in trauma: assessment of the "golden hour" in a North American prospective cohort. Ann Emerg Med. 2010;55(3):235–246.e4.

5. Cirocchi R, Abraha I, Montedori A, Farinella E, Bonacini I, Tagliabue L, Sciannameo F. Damage control surgery for abdominal trauma. Cochrane Database Syst Rev. 2010;1:CD007438.

6. Marchant J, Cheng NG, Lam LT, Fahy FE, Soundappan SV, Cass DT, Browne GJ. Bystander basic life support: an important link in the chain of survival for children suffering a drowning or near-drowning episode. Med J Aust. 2008;188(8):484–855.

7. Goh SH. Bomb blast mass casualty incidents: initial triage and management of injuries. Singap Med J. 2009;50(1):101–6.

8. Schoenfeld AJ, Lehman RA Jr, Hsu JR. Evaluation and management of combat-related spinal injuries: a review based on recent experiences. Spine J. 2012;12(9):817–23.

9. Hadley MN, Walters BC, Grabb PA, Oyesiku NM, Przybylski GJ, Resnick DK, Ryken TC, Mielke DH. Guidelines for the management of acute cervical spine and spinal cord injuries. Clin Neurosurg. 2002;49:407–98.

10. Comstock S, Pannell D, Talbot M, Compton L, Withers N, Tien HC. Spinal injuries after improvised explosive device incidents: implications for Tactical Combat Casualty Care. J Trauma. 2011;71(5 Suppl 1):S413–7.

11. Arishita GI, Vayer JS, Bellamy RF. Cervical spine immobilization of penetrating neck wounds in a hostile environment. J Trauma. 1989;29(3):332–7.

12. Possley DR, Blair JA, Schoenfeld AJ, Lehman RA, Hsu JR. Skeletal Trauma Research Consortium (STReC). Complications associated with military spine injuries. Spine J. 2012;12(9):756–61.

13. Kahraman S, Gonul E, Kayali H, Sirin S, Duz B, Beduk A, Timurkaynak E. Retrospective analysis of spinal missile injuries. Neurosurg Rev. 2004;27(1):42–5.

14. Bono CM, Heary RF. Gunshot wounds to the spine. Spine J. 2004;4(2):230–40.

15. Schoenfeld AJ, Dunn JC, Belmont PJ. Pelvic, spinal and extremity wounds among combat-specific personnel serving in Iraq and Afghanistan (2003-2011): a new paradigm in military musculoskeletal medicine. Injury. 2013;44(12):1866–70.

16. Ramasamy A, Evans S, Kendrew JM, Cooper J. The open blast pelvis: the significant burden of management. J Bone Joint Surg (Br). 2012;94(6):829–35.

17. D'Alleyrand JC, Lewandowski LR, Forsberg JA, Gordon WT, Fleming ME, Mullis BH, Andersen RC, Potter BK. Combat-related hemipelvectomy: 14 cases, a review of the literature and lessons learned. J Orthop Trauma. 2015;29(12):e493–8.

18. Edwards MJ, Lustik M, Carlson T, Tabak B, Farmer D, Edwards K, Eichelberger M. Surgical interventions for pediatric blast injury: an analysis from Afghanistan and Iraq 2002 to 2010. J Trauma Acute Care Surg. 2014;76(3):854–8.

19. Kang P, Zhang L, Liang W, Zhu Z, Liu Y, Liu X, Yang H. Medical evacuation management and clinical characteristics of 3,255 inpatients after the 2010 Yushu earthquake in China. J Trauma Acute Care Surg. 2012;72(6):1626–33.

20. Bar-On E, Lebel E, Kreiss Y, Merin O, Benedict S, Gill A, Lee E, Pirotsky A, Shirov T, Blumberg N. Orthopaedic management in a mega mass casualty situation. The Israel Defence Forces Field Hospital in Haiti following the January 2010 earthquake. Injury. 2011;42(10):1053–9.

21. Calder J, Mannion S. Orthopaedics in Sri Lanka post-tsunami. J Bone Joint Surg (Br). 2005;87(6):759–61.

22. Prasartritha T, Tungsiripat R, Warachit P. The revisit of 2004 tsunami in Thailand: characteristics of wounds. Int Wound J. 2008;5(1):8–19.

Burn Management

25

Gerasimos Tsourouflis, Andreas Pikoulis, and Nikos Pararas

25.1 Introduction

The skin, well known as the largest organ in the human body, presents an efficient, self-recovery barrier with its main goal being to protect the body from the external environment. Burn accidents disrupt the complicated tissue structure by abolishing some essential skin functions (Table 25.1) [1].

Burns are a major cause of mortality and morbidity due to the evident physiologic and catabolic changes that lead the human body in shock. Twenty-nine thousand patients were admitted to UK burn services between 2003 and 2007 [2]. A crucial portion of these patients were admitted to intensive care units upon presentation where successful management required multidisciplinary approach.

Table 25.1 Function of the skin

• Protection from infection and bacterial invasion
• Control of fluid and electrolyte loss
• Protection from harmful effects of ultra-violet radiation
• Production and synthesis of vitamin D
• Temperature regulation
• Sensory interface to touch, perception of pain and temperature
• Body image and non-verbal communication

G. Tsourouflis (✉)
Propaedeutic Surgery, Medical School, National and Kapodistrian University of Athens, Athens, Greece

2nd Department of Propaedeutic Surgery, Laiko General Hospital, Athens, Greece

A. Pikoulis
General Surgery, University General Hospital "Attikon", National and Kapodistrian University of Athens, Athens, Greece

N. Pararas
National and Kapodistrian University of Athens, Athens, Greece

© Springer Nature Switzerland AG 2021
E. Pikoulis, J. Doucet (eds.), *Emergency Medicine, Trauma and Disaster Management*, Hot Topics in Acute Care Surgery and Trauma,
https://doi.org/10.1007/978-3-030-34116-9_25

Burn injury, subsequent ischemia-reperfusion trauma, and sepsis, lead the body to a state of cardiogenic, hypovolemic, and distributive shock. Widespread increases to microvascular permeability, caused by the release of inflammatory mediators, lead to depletion of intravascular volume, interstitial edema and fluid shifts. Due to low intravascular colloid osmotic pressure, fluid escaping the vascular system results in oxygen utilization becoming impaired causing organ hypoperfusion. Adequate fluid resuscitation is marked as the critical therapeutic intervention in conjunction with supportive treatment.

25.2   Fluid Resuscitation

The most important intervention in the treatment of acute burn injury is appropriate fluid management. Burns involving greater than 15–20% of total body surface area (*TBSA*) can cause hypovolemic shock, while delaying resuscitation for longer than 2 h post-burn injury, increases mortality dramatically (Table 25.2) [3]. The main goal is to minimize the disruptive cascade of physiologic events and prevent a state of normovolemic hypoperfusion, also known as burn shock.

The use of formulas has been utilized to guide burn resuscitation while avoiding over-resuscitation, also known as a "*fluid creep*," described as pulmonary edema, acute respiratory distress syndrome (*ARDS*) and compartment syndrome in unburned limbs or abdomen. The resuscitation formulas include but are not limited to the Parkland and modified Brooke formula (Table 25.3) [4].

Recommendations for use of lactated Ringer's solution range from 2 to 4 mL/kg/% burn over a 24-h period. All the formulas guide resuscitation with the goal of titrating fluids to obtain a urine output of 0.3–0.5 mL/kg/h in adults and 1.0 mL/kg/h in children. Formula instructions further recommend that pediatric patients require more fluid for burns comparable to those of adults due to the increase in body surface area-to-weight ratio. Maintenance fluids, including a source of glucose, should also be added to pediatric patient resuscitation fluid as hepatic glycogen stores will be depleted after 12–14 h of fasting [4].

Though there is limited evidence on burn resuscitation, the Parkland formula is widely used when initiating treatment. These principles, although useful, are used

Table 25.2 Estimating Total Body Surface Area (*TBSA*) burned

Area	Percentage (%)	Total %
Head and neck	9	9
Each forelimb	9	18
Each rear limb	18	36
Dorsal trunk	18	18
Ventral trunk	18	18
Perineum	1	1
TOTAL		100

Table 25.3 Resuscitation formulas for estimating adult burn patient fluid needs

Colloid formulas	Electrolyte	Colloid	D5W
Evans	Normal saline 1.0 cm³/kg/% burn	1.0 cm³/kg/% burn	2000 cm³
Brooke	Lactated Ringer's 1.5 cm³/kg/% burn	0.5 cm³/kg	2000 cm³
Slater	Lactated Ringer's 2 L/24 h	Fresh frozen plasma 75 cm³/kg/24 h	
Crystalloid formulas			
Parkland	Lactated Ringer's	4 cm³/kg/% burn	
Modified Brooke	Lactated Ringer's	2 cm³/kg/% burn	
Hypertonic saline formulas			
Hypertonic saline solution (Monafo)	Volume to maintain urine output at 30 cm³/h Fluid contains 250 mEq Na/L		
Modified hypertonic (Warden)	Lactated Ringer's + 50 mEq NaHCO₃ (180 mEq Na/L) for 8 h to maintain urine output at 30–50 cm³/h Lactated Ringer's to maintain urine output at 30–50 cm³/h beginning 8 h post-burn		
Dextran formula (Demling)	Dextran 40 in saline—2 cm³/kg/h for 8 h Lactated Ringer's—volume to maintain urine output at 30 cm³/h Fresh frozen plasma—0.5 cm³/kg/h for 18 h beginning 8 h post-burn		

as a guide and should be adjusted depending on the physiologic needs of the individual patient. In particular, patients received 150% of recommended fluid based on the emergency department TBSA estimation increasing to 200% after TBSA estimation by the burn unit. Therefore, initial fluid resuscitation is often inappropriate. Other parameters such as burn type, inhalation injury as well as onset of resuscitation response may influence fluid requirements.

While correcting acidosis attention should be given to base deficit and lactate since there is strong correlation associated with mortality and fluid resuscitation volumes. Clinicians should highly regard urine output as it is an essential parameter in resuscitation attempts. American Burn Association recommends a urine output of 0.5–1 mL/kg/h with intensive monitoring of vital signs [5].

To date, there is no single tool to guide resuscitation attempts, making complications such as over-resuscitation and under-resuscitation a matter of focus by experienced burn teams. Inaccuracies in calculating fluid requirement often results in over-resuscitation, causing excess fluid loading. Another matter of consideration is the types of fluids administered, colloids vs. crystalloids. No increase in multiple organ failure rates or mortality was found following the administration of 5% human albumin solution (*HAS*) for burn shock resuscitation, while patients who received albumin resuscitation did not significantly reduce mortality compared with those who did not receive albumin [6].

Although there is no gold standard regarding the timing of colloid initiation, early administration appears to have a pulmonary volume-sparing benefit, making it essential in burn shock management. Further studies could be key in determining the necessary type and volume needed to reduce edema related complications and over-resuscitation.

An alternative to colloid is hypertonic saline. Although it is rarely used in routine practice due to the unknown risk-benefit ratio, it potentially reduces fluid shift to the interstitium.

25.3 Inhalation Injury

The nature of respiratory failure is complex in burn patients, therefore airway management, ventilatory support, and oxygen therapy is a primary concern. Thermal inhalation injury can cause primary injury to the lungs and upper airway directly. Secondary injury can be immediate due to an inflammatory response or delayed following sepsis.

Mechanical ventilation can aggravate any pulmonary injury, so it should be adjusted to provide adequate oxygenation at low tidal volumes. Though the exact pathophysiological response to inhalation injury remains unclear, the classic complement cascade is thought to be activated, followed by intrapulmonary leukocyte aggregation and oxygen free radical release resulting in pulmonary edema [7].

Carbon monoxide poisoning should be considered in all serious burn cases. It binds to hemoglobin causing impaired availability for oxygen molecules at the local tissue level. When suspected, it should be treated with endotracheal intubation and ventilation with high inspired oxygen concentration. There is little consensus regarding parameters or indications for hyperbaric oxygen, and availability is limited [8].

Heparin can reduce airway obstruction by potentiating antithrombin-III-mediated inactivation of thrombin. The effect of nebulized heparin in reducing airway obstruction is quite confirmed. Further knowledge on the use of pharmaceuticals to treat inhalation injury is unavailable due to the lack of commercial access to some agents, the lack of human trials and contradicting experimental outcomes.

25.4 Blood Transfusion

Over the years a restrictive transfusion strategy has gained popularity, after a multiple-center cohort analysis reported an increased mortality in burn patients with multiple blood transfusions [9]. It's worth mentioning that patients receiving more transfusions had also more extensive burn injuries. Therefore increased transfusion requirements may simply be a substitute for the severity of burn injury.

When planning a large excision where major transfusion is required, the patient needs to be prepped for surgery, meaning a low hematocrit level may be ill-advised since it can lead to additional blood loss. If patients are entering the rehabilitation phase of treatment, anemia compromising pertinent activities should be avoided since the consequences of delayed or impaired recovery are immense.

Attempts to minimize perioperative bleeds and transfusion requirements have brought focus on tranexamic acid, however there is not enough data to prove conclusive benefits when used in this patient group.

25.5   Burn Related Sepsis

Patients exhibiting progressive tachycardia, tachypnoea, and rise in baseline core temperature following a severe burn injury, essentially meet the criteria for systemic inflammatory response syndrome (*SIRS*). The American Burn Association has produced consensus guidelines suggesting modified definitions for utilizing the SIRS criteria in burn patients [5]. In addition to the physiologic and metabolic responses, additional markers for diagnosing sepsis include, but are not limited to white cell count, C-reactive protein and erythrocyte sedimentation rate.

Sepsis prevention is crucial in the management of a burn patient. Early excision and skin grafting is now common practice. An analysis of studies comparing early debridement vs. conservative treatment showed that the early debridement group required a shorter duration of antibiotic therapy and had fewer positive wound cultures.

When grafting is limited due to extensive burn damage, wound treatment should be optimized using a dermal substitute, synthetic or biological, or a silver dressing. Meshing of grafts allows for greater wound coverage, especially when dealing with a limited donor area.

In adults, there is no indication for treatment with antibiotics without signs of infection, due to the possibility of adverse events and the development of antimicrobial resistance. Early detection and utilization of appropriate antibiotics is key in the treatment of burn sepsis. With fungal infections and multidrug resistant organisms being a major complication of large burns, antifungal or combination therapy with topical antibiotics may be required. Physiologic changes following burns may affect the efficacy of administered drugs. Adjusted dosage, especially regarding infusions, timing, and appropriate monitoring should be considered to ensure therapeutic levels.

There is inconclusive data to support routine use of corticosteroids in burn patients with sepsis although it is not recommended due to the possibility it could lead to secondary infection. Moreover, the use of enteral glutamine supplementation has been recommended for burn patients [10].

25.6   Wound Treatment

The first step toward infection prevention, safe healing, and eventually curing a burn injury is proper wound cleansing (Fig. 25.1) [11]. All systematic reviews conducted to date did not find any significant correlation between the solution used, water included, and the rate of infection or healing. The importance therefore lies in the method of applying the agent rather than its nature. Mechanical cleansing by irrigation is the factor that was significantly correlated to decreasing the bacterial count in the wound as well as promoting sound healing. Even in cases where the swabbing and irrigation did not show a significant difference in terms of wound contamination and healing, patient satisfaction, and cost-effectiveness were significantly better with irrigation [12].

Fig. 25.1 An adult male patient with a second to third degree extended burn injury covering about 85% of TBSA after initial supportive and resuscitation interventions: intratracheal intubation and ventilation, nasogastric catheter, urinary catheter, venous catheter of left femoral vein and arterial line. (*Under the auspices of Plastic Surgeon Marios Frangoulis, MD*)

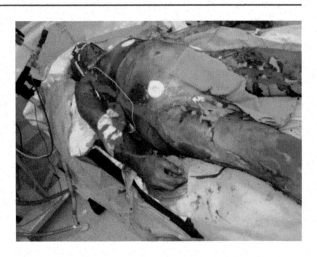

25.7 Nutrition and Hypermetabolism

Metabolism is significantly affected following a severe burn injury. The body enters a hypermetabolic state characterized by hyperglycemia, loss of protein and lean body mass. This hypermetabolic state ultimately leads to immune dysfunction, sepsis and organ failure. Hyperglycemia in the first 2 days after burn injury has been demonstrated as a poor prognostic factor [13].

These results, in addition to the additional immunomodulatory effects of insulin led hyperglycemia control to become standard care in burn patients. Insulin has nourishing effects on mucosal and dermal barriers, improves wound matrix formation, reduces bacterial invasion, and inhibits proinflammatory mediator production.

When the body's nutritional demands go unmet, the healing process is abruptly interrupted. Since it is essential for calorific needs to be fulfilled, enteral, and parenteral nutrition are greatly favored in relation to outcome measures and cost.

Nasogastric and nasojejunal feeding each have their proponents, with the advocates of duodenal feeding citing the ability to continue nourishment during surgical procedures without risk of aspiration, although reduced aspiration with intestinal feeding has not been proven. After early enteral feeding, aggressive fluid resuscitation and proton pump inhibitors, the incidence of Curling's ulcer decreased from 15% to 3%, with a following decrease in mortality of 70% [14].

25.8 Acute Kidney Injury

Burn injury is often followed by acute kidney injury (*AKI*) with an incidence as high as 30% associated with a high mortality rate. One-half of patients, particularly those with a severe burn injury, developed AKI during the first week post injury and the remaining patients during the second week. In many of these patients, AKI was preceded by other organ dysfunction due to over-resuscitation complications such as intra-abdominal hypertension and abdominal compartment syndrome. In the past, late-onset AKI has been strongly associated with sepsis, though exposure to nephrotoxic antibiotics and intravenous contrast may also be contributing factors [15].

25.9 Conclusion

Advances in critical care have led to significant improvements in outcome following burn injuries. The introduction of fluid resuscitation protocols, early burn excision and closure, infection control, nutritional support, and regulation of the metabolic response have led to increased survival rates.

Burn management is a rapidly evolving field with treatment options still to be explored. Hopefully the numerous studies underway will provide further guidance for the management of these critically ill patients.

References

1. Stiles K. Emergency management of burns: part 1. Emerg Nurse. 2018;26(1):36–42.
2. UK burn injury data 1986–2007. First report of the iBID. http://www.ibidb.org/downloads.
3. Snell JA, Loh NH, Mahambrey T, Shokrollahi K. Clinical review: the critical care management of the burn patient. Crit Care. 2013;17(5):241.
4. Warden GD. Chapter 9: Fluid resuscitation and early management. In: Total burn care. Amsterdam: Elsevier; 2012.
5. Pham TN, Cancio LC, Gibran NS. American Burn Association practice guidelines. Burn shock resuscitation. J Burn Care Res. 2008;29:257–66.
6. Cochran A, Morris SE, Edelman LS, Saffle JR. Burn patient characteristics and outcomes following resuscitation with albumin. Burns. 2007;33:25–30.
7. Enkhbaatar P, Traber DL. Pathophysiology of acute lung injury in combined burn and smoke inhalation injury. Clin Sci. 2004;107:137–43.
8. Kealey GP. Carbon monoxide toxicity. J Burn Care Res. 2009;301:146–7.
9. Palmieri TL, Caruso DM, Foster KN, Cairns BA, Peck MD, Gamelli RL, Mozingo DW, Kagan RJ, Wahl W, Kemalyan NA, Fish JA, Gomez M, Sheridan RL, Faucher LD, Latenser BA, Gibran NS, Klein RL, Solem LD, Saffle JR, Morris SE, Jeng JC, Voigt D, Howard PA, Molitor F, Grennhalgh DG. Effect of blood transfusion on outcome after major burn injury: a multi-centre study. Crit Care Med. 2006;34:1602–7.
10. Kurmis R, Parker A, Greenwood J. The use of immunonutrition in burn injury care: where are we? J Burn Care Res. 2010;31:677–91.
11. Lundy JB, Chung KK, Pamplin JC, Ainsworth CR, Jeng JC, Friedman BC. Update on severe burn management for the intensivist. J Intensive Care Med. 2016;31(8):499–510.
12. Tricco AC, Antony J, Vafaei A, Khan PA, Harrington A, Cogo E, et al. Seeking effective interventions to treat complex wounds: an overview of systematic reviews. BMC Med. 2015;13:89–102.
13. Holm C, Horbrand F, Mayr M, von Donnersmarck GH, Muhlbauer W. Acute hyperglycaemia following thermal injury: friend or foe? Resuscitation. 2004;60:71–7.
14. Mentec H, Dupont H, Bocchetti M, Cani P, Ponche F, Bleichner G. Upper digestive intolerance during enteral nutrition in critically ill patients: frequency, risk factors, and complications. Crit Care Med. 2001;29:1955–61.
15. Mustonen KM, Vuola J. Acute renal failure in intensive care burn patients. J Burn Care Res. 2008;29:227–37.

Endovascular Damage Control and Management of Vascular Injuries

26

Efthymios D. Avgerinos

Trauma remains the leading cause of death in the 15- to 44-year-old age group in the Western World, as a consequence of a motor vehicle accident, unintentional injury, terrorism, homicide, and suicide. In many ways, all life-threatening trauma other than that to the brain or heart is vascular trauma. One-third of the patients are dying from exsanguination driven by major vascular trauma (typically penetrating) and a lot more suffer a limb loss [1, 2]. Military experience, damage control (DC) strategies and new technologies, have altered the overall management of both peripheral and truncal vascular trauma.

26.1 Pathophysiology of Vascular Injury

As noted by the preponderance of penetrating injury in the published medical literature, the vascular tree, both arterial and venous, appears to have some limited natural protection from stretching and bending, which results in fewer blunt injuries to the extremity vasculature following trauma. The smooth muscle of the arterial media protects the patient from both stretch-type injuries and minor puncture wounds, which heal spontaneously in most cases. The smooth-muscle layer also offers mild protection from death due to ongoing hemorrhage.

When the arterial vessel is transected, vascular spasm coupled with low systemic blood pressure appears to promote clotting at the site of injury and to preserve vital organ perfusion better than is the case with ongoing uncontrolled hemorrhage. For example, not infrequently bleeding from a popliteal or even an iliac artery

E. D. Avgerinos (✉)
Department of Surgery, University of Pittsburgh Medical Center, Pittsburgh, PA, USA

Department of Vascular Surgery, University of Athens, Athens, Greece

Clinic of Vascular and Endovascular Surgery, Athens Medical Center, Athens, Greece
e-mail: avgerinose@upmc.edu

© Springer Nature Switzerland AG 2021
E. Pikoulis, J. Doucet (eds.), *Emergency Medicine, Trauma and Disaster Management*, Hot Topics in Acute Care Surgery and Trauma,
https://doi.org/10.1007/978-3-030-34116-9_26

transection can sometimes self-limit by strong vessel contracture and clotting. This partially explains the improved outcomes by limited prehospital fluid resuscitation (permissive hypotension).

26.2   Trauma Prehospital/Preoperative Damage Control

Trauma DC is an established strategy to optimally manage injured patients targeting to minimize morbidity and mortality (Fig. 26.1). It includes DC resuscitation and DC surgery. Damage control resuscitation includes rapid hemorrhage control, permissive hypotension, and appropriate fluid administration [3]. Damage control surgery in vascular trauma is used to control exsanguinating hemorrhage or temporarily reperfuse a threatened ischemic limb till definite repair is feasible.

Existing literature estimates that up to 20% of deaths after trauma are preventable, the majority of these being due to uncontrolled hemorrhage. Hemorrhage can be ongoing in up to 25% of trauma admissions due to associated coagulopathy, increasing mortality by threefold [4]. The concept of DC resuscitation based on infusion of blood products was developed by military physicians in the early 2000s. Subsequently, drastic improvement in postoperative coagulopathy and reduction of edema made it popular among civilian trauma centers [5, 6].

26.2.1 Fluid Resuscitation

Hemorrhage is an etiologic factor of mortality in 30–40% of trauma patients, and many of these deaths happen before the patient reaches the hospital. Advanced trauma life support recommends the prehospital assessment of a patient's circulation status and resuscitation with intravenous fluids. Fluid resuscitation is aimed at replacing lost volume to maintain perfusion of vital organs until definitive care [7].

Traditionally, the concept of "early and aggressive" fluid administration has been applied to patients with severe trauma, in order to restore circulating blood volume

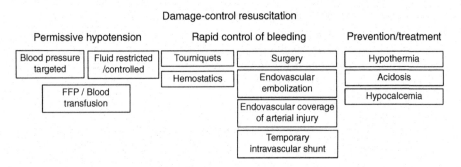

Fig. 26.1 Damage control strategy algorithm

and maintain tissue perfusion. However, this treatment approach may increase hydrostatic pressure in injured vessels, dislodge hemostatic blood clots, induce dilutional coagulopathy, and result in hypothermia. The concept of "permissive hypotension" refers to managing trauma patients by restricting the amount of fluid resuscitation administered while maintaining blood pressure in the lower than normal range if there is still active bleeding during the acute period of injury. Although this treatment approach may avoid the adverse effects of early and high-dose fluid resuscitation, it carries the potential risk of tissue hypoperfusion.

For patients with major trauma, defined as having an Injury Severity Score of more than or equal to 16, the American College of Surgeons' Advanced Trauma Life Support guidelines currently advocate "balanced" resuscitation with an initial 1–2 L of crystalloids before definitive/surgical control of bleeding. The mechanism of injury, whether penetrating or blunt, and injury site is not specifically described. Permissive hypotension and restricted fluid resuscitation strategies are stated in the fourth edition of the European guideline on management of major bleeding and coagulopathy following trauma [8].

Fluid therapy can be achieved by administering crystalloid solutions, colloidal solutions, or blood products [9]. Aqueous fluids used for resuscitation are termed based on additional elements found within the solutions. Fluids which contain electrolytes (crystal-forming elements) are termed crystalloids, while those which contain electrolytes and large organic molecules are termed colloids.

26.2.1.1 Crystalloids

Crystalloid resuscitation occurs when electrolytes pass through the endothelial membrane followed by water. The flow of water from the intravascular space into the extracellular space eventually reaches an equilibrium when concentrations are similar in both spaces. Solutions may contain an assortment of organic anions and inorganic cations. Organic anions include acetate, bicarbonate, gluconate, lactate, or Cl^-, while K^+, Ca^{2+}, and Mg^{2+} constitute the commonly used inorganic cations.

Commonly used crystalloids include normal saline (NS), Ringer's lactate (LR), Hartmann's solution, and Plasma-Lyte. Despite its nomenclature, normal saline is not physiologic as an electrolyte solution. The solution contains an equal amount of Na^+ and Cl^- making it hypernatremic, hyperchloremic, and slightly hypertonic. A hypernatremic, hyperchloremic, metabolic acidosis can occur with substantial NS infusions. Patients at risk of morbidity from these metabolic derangements (e.g., compromised renal function) may benefit from an alternative crystalloid solution [10].

Solutions such as Hartmann's solution, Plasma-Lyte, and LR more closely resemble the electrolyte composition of plasma. A key characteristic of these solutions is that they are isotonic relative to blood. Although these solutions are more balanced or physiologic, several randomized trials have failed to prove superiority in outcomes of acute kidney injury (AKI), major adverse kidney events, or mortality [11, 12].

26.2.1.2 Colloids

Large organic macromolecules and electrolytes contained within colloid solutions are better maintained within the intravascular space. It is postulated that the large size of the macromolecules limits their ability to cross the endothelial membrane. Water is thus retained within the intravascular space due to the increased intravascular oncotic pressure.

The oldest and most commonly used solution is albumin. Concentrations ranging from 4% to 25% are used clinically. Presently synthetic colloids such as dextran, gelatins, and starches (HES) are increasingly being used due to the varying cost of albumin solutions. Gelatins and albumin exist in hypo-oncotic concentrations, while dextran, HES, and albumin exist in hyper-oncotic solutions [9].

The Saline versus Albumin Fluid Evaluation (SAFE) trial randomized 6997 patients to receive either 4% albumin or NS resuscitation for 28 days in the intensive care unit (ICU). No significant differences in ICU days, hospital days, mechanical ventilation days, or renal replacement therapy days were found throughout the study period [11]. Similar results have been shown by other studies comparing the two resuscitation modalities [13, 14].

26.2.1.3 Blood Products

Recent literature has also led to changes in the tenets of hemostatic resuscitation. A "1:1" transfusion ratio of fresh frozen plasma (FFP) and red blood cells (RBCs) has been shown to reduce mortality in military literature [4]. Several studies have aimed at evaluating whether a specific FFP:RBC ratio best reduces morbidity and mortality in patients with polytrauma, though a consensus has yet to be reached [15]. There is a growing body of literature which suggests that in patients requiring massive transfusion (MT), increased use of FFP and platelets (PLT) improves survival and decreases ventilator and ICU days [16, 17]. While increased FFP and PLT administration ratios may provide benefit in patients who require massive transfusion, euvolemic patients requiring less than 10 units of RBCs do not seem to gain any benefit in survival rates [18, 19].

European guidelines recommend patients with traumatic injuries be maintained at target hemoglobin (Hb) levels between 7 and 9 g/dL [8]. Several randomized controlled trials (RCTs) have shown that liberal transfusion strategies (Hb $\geq$9 g/dL) are not as safe as restrictive transfusion strategies (Hb 7–9 g/dL) in critically ill patients [20, 21]. As of now, no prospective RCTs exist which compare liberal and restrictive transfusion strategies in trauma patients specifically.

Adequate tissue oxygenation remains the mainstay of goal-directed resuscitation. Historically, aggressive fluid resuscitation with a normotensive target (systolic blood pressure (SBP) above 100 mmHg) was used. This commonly resulted in dilution of coagulation factors, hypothermia, and reversal of vasoconstriction, thus leading to the use of a permissive hypotension strategy (goal SBP 50–100 mmHg).

26.2.2 Tourniquets

Increasingly available, accessible, and early tourniquet application has limited isolated limb exsanguination from the leading cause of preventable wartime death.

Subsequently, one of the earliest assessments of penetrating extremity injuries in civilians postulated that adequate hemorrhage control, i.e., with a tourniquet, may prevent limb loss and deaths. The use of tourniquets in civilian trauma scenarios has been increasing since 2008 [22].

For the patient with significant extremity hemorrhage, the failure to place a tourniquet and stop bleeding may potentially result in exsanguination within minutes. The best evidence for tourniquet use in the prehospital environment comes from the experience of military hospitals. A prospective study analyzing 428 tourniquets placed on 309 injured limbs showed that early tourniquet use before the onset of shock was associated with a 90% survival rate versus 10% survival if the application was delayed until the casualty was in shock [23].

Retrospective studies have examined the use of prehospital tourniquets in civilian trauma. In a 2007 review of tourniquet use in the prehospital setting, it was found that immediate application of a tourniquet may be justifiable in (a) life-threatening limb hemorrhage, amputation, or a mangled extremity, (b) life-threatening limb hemorrhage not controlled by simple methods, (c) entrapment of a limb preventing access to a point of hemorrhage, (d) multiple casualties with extremity hemorrhage and inability to perform simple methods of hemorrhage control, or (e) benefits of prevention of death which outweigh limb loss from ischemia caused by use of a tourniquet [24].

When studied in the urban emergency medical service (EMS) setting, prehospital tourniquet use appeared to be safe. The Boston EMS experience with prehospital tourniquets reported that 91% (95/98) of cases resulted in successful control of hemorrhage, and they were in place for an average of 14.9 min prior to hospital arrival. Tourniquets were removed in the emergency department in 54.7% (52/95) of cases and in the operating room in 31.6% (30/95) of cases. Of the 30 tourniquets removed in the operating room, 14 did indeed have a documented vascular injury which required repair. A complication rate of 2.1% was reported in that study, showing that effective tourniquet application may be used in the prehospital setting safely [25]. Despite this, complications of tourniquet use are well documented including arterial injury and thrombosis, deep venous thrombosis, and neuronal injury. It has been documented in literature that up to 65% of tourniquet gauges are inaccurate and inappropriate pressures up to 500 mmHg have been applied to limbs improperly [26]. Regardless of these potential complications, the use of tourniquets in the prehospital setting has been shown to be effective and potentially life-saving. Education on proper tourniquet use is a key to the success of this strategy.

Currently, both the American College of Surgeons Committee on Trauma (ACS-COT) and the American College of Emergency Physicians (ACEP) now recommend that tourniquets be used when extremity hemorrhage presents a threat to life emphasizing that tourniquet use should be avoided if the bleeding from an extremity injury is minor [27].

Recent initiatives in the United States have aimed at educating citizens to provide bleeding control for those in need. The "Stop the Bleed" campaign encourages citizens to learn how to prevent or slow potentially life-threatening hemorrhage as well as have access to and learn to use bleeding control kits.

26.2.3 Hemostatic Agents

Ideal characteristics for hemostatic dressings were previously described as able to stop severe arterial and/or venous bleeding in under 2 min, be without systemic or local toxicity/side effects, cause no pain or thermal injuries, pose no risk to provider applying the dressing, be ready to use, be easily packed into wounds, be inexpensive and cost-effective, and have a long shelf life [28]. The use of topical hemostatic dressings in the prehospital setting for the control of massive hemorrhage has the potential to alter the current standard of care for exsanguinating patients and improve the clinical outcome in heavy injured patients.

Prior to Operation Enduring Freedom and Operation Iraqi Freedom, the Army Field Bandage (AFB) was the foundation of hemorrhage control. A thick layer of cotton wrapped in layers of gauze was the simple premise to the AFB. This could be wrapped around an injured extremity to absorb blood as well as compress the wound. Since that time many hemostatic agents have been developed including the dry fibrin sealant dressing (American Red Cross Holland Laboratory, Rockville, MD), Fibrin Patch (Ethicon, Inc., Somerville, NJ), Rapid Deployment Hemostat (Marine Polymer Technologies, Inc., Danvers, MA), HemCon Bandage (Oregon Medical Laser Center, Portland, OR), and QuikClot (Z-Medica Corp., Wallingford, CT). The HemCon bandage consists of freeze-dried chitosan, which appears to strongly adhere to wet tissues and seal injured vessels. QuickClot functions as a mineral-based hemostatic agent. The zeolite minerals cause rapid water absorption which may concentrate clotting proteins and cells into the wound. The newer-generation mineral-based hemostatic agents QuikClot Combat Gauze (Z-Medica Corp, Wallingford, CT) and Celox (MedTrade Products Ltd., Crewe, UK) have shown improved hemostatic efficacy over prior topical hemostatic dressings [28]. Previously, efficacy and safety concerns arose with the HemCon and QuikClot dressings [29]. Improvements in the current formulations of these dressings have since made them safer and more effective for clinical use [30–32].

Currently approved topical hemostatic agents can be categorized under four functional categories: biologically active agents, fibrin sealants, mechanical barrier agents, and flowable sealants (thrombin plus a mechanical barrier). Mechanical barriers block blood flow and create thrombogenic surfaces. QuikClot remains the most commonly used of this category [32, 33]. Biologically active agents are indicated for minor bleeding and oozing. Thrombin and fibrinogen-thrombin-containing agents do not depend on patients' intrinsic clotting mechanism. Flowable sealants are delivered in a paste-like mixture and combine thrombin with a mechanical hemostatic agent. Fibrin sealants combine human fibrinogen with thrombin immediately before use and cause more rapid clot formation than a patient's own coagulation cascade. Fibrinogen concentrations up to 25 times greater than physiologic concentrations may be produced at sites of hemorrhage [34].

The use of topical hemostatic agents in combination as an adjunct to surgical bleeding control has been identified as a Grade 1B recommendation in European guidelines [8]. Like many tenants of the care of patients with traumatic injuries, military experiences in the use of topical hemostatic agents have advanced the care of civilians.

26.3   Damage Control Surgery

Surgical intervention for damage control in trauma involves an abbreviated exploratory laparotomy in an unstable patient. The triad of hypothermia, acidosis, and coagulopathy as well as shock physiology would lead to acute decompensation in these patients if not immediately intervened upon.

The damage control laparotomy may be divided into three phases. Phase I is based on acute hemorrhage control, repair of visceral injuries using stapling methods, abdominal packing, and transport to an intensive care unit. Phase II is based on aggressive resuscitation as described in previous sections. The basis of Phase III involves a return to the operating room within 72 h for removal of packing and reestablishment of intestinal continuity. While indications for damage control laparotomy may differ among level 1 trauma centers, institutional algorithms are a mainstay of treatment in the trauma population [35, 36].

26.3.1   Resuscitative Endovascular Balloon Occlusion of the Aorta (REBOA)

Patients with life-threatening hypotension and hypovolemia secondary to hemorrhage may require aortic occlusion to facilitate resuscitation. Aortic occlusion is thought to preserve coronary filling and cerebral perfusion in the setting of physiologic collapse due to hemorrhage although most of the data collected on clinical use has been limited and retrospective in nature [37–39]. Traditionally, aortic occlusion was achieved by cross-clamping the descending thoracic aorta via thoracotomy; however, newer strategies such as the use of resuscitative endovascular balloon occlusion of the aorta (REBOA) have become more common in level 1 trauma centers. Interestingly, REBOA has been even suggested as a measure to control torso hemorrhage in the prehospital setting by specialized emergency medical services teams.

REBOA is not a definitive hemorrhagic control maneuver but instead works as a bridge while transfusions are initiated and the source of bleeding can be identified and stopped. In this context, REBOA is used for a brief period of time, either pre- or intraoperatively, until open or endovascular hemorrhage control can be accomplished. Depending on the source of bleeding, a REBOA catheter can be positioned either in the descending thoracic aorta (Zone 1) or the infrarenal aorta (Zone 3). Zone 1 deployment is necessary for intraperitoneal sources of bleeding such as high-grade solid organ injury (i.e., liver, kidney, spleen) or bleeding from a named visceral vessel. Zone 3 deployment is reserved for bleeding and shock associated with a high-grade pelvic fracture or from the junctional femoral area. Although the exact source of bleeding is often unknown, using the physical exam and a few basic imaging modalities can provide enough information to inform the provider whether to position the balloon in Zone 1 or 3 (Fig. 26.2).

Use of REBOA has been shown to improve hemodynamics, increase survival as compared to historical controls who underwent thoracotomy (21.1% vs. 7.4%), and preserve neurological outcome in survivors [40]. Access-site complications and

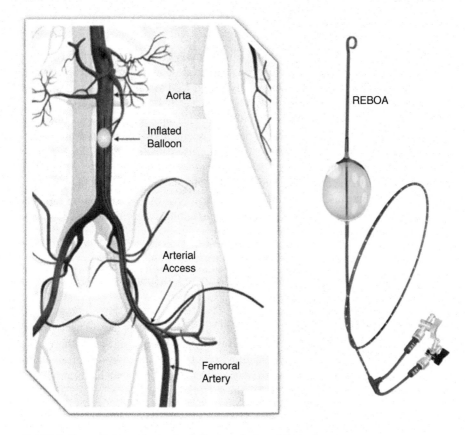

Fig. 26.2 Resuscitative endovascular balloon occlusion of the aorta

limb-related adverse events remain low, and the use of smaller systems (7 Fr) may aid in increasing safety [40–42]. Increasing use of this strategy may require a shift in the training paradigm of acute care and trauma providers to include endovascular skills.

26.4 Shunts

The use of temporary intravascular shunts (TIVS) has been well documented in the military literature. The civilian sector later caught up with the military experience albeit under different circumstances. Due to the widespread availability of Level 1 trauma centers where definitive management is possible, some controversy exists over the use of TIVS in civilian trauma; however, there may be specific patient populations or injury patterns in which TIVS may provide benefit. The mechanisms of injury, indications, and incidence of use are quite different, and as such it is difficult to extrapolate data from the military. The incidence of shunt use in civilian vascular trauma is otherwise lower and ranges between 3% and 9% [43, 44].

Temporary intravascular shunting is indicated in (1) open extremity fractures with extensive soft tissue injury and concurrent arterial injury (Gustilo IIIC), (2) need for perfusion during complex vascular reconstruction, (3) damage control for patients in extremis, (4) perfusion prior to limb replantation, (5) truncal vascular control, and (6) complex repair of Zone 3 neck injuries. The two most common indications are damage control and as a temporizing measure for orthopedic fixation.

The high limb salvage and relatively low complication rates associated with shunts make them quite appealing. Compared to ligation, TIVS reduced amputation, fasciotomy, and mortality rates from 47% to 0%, 93–43%, and 73–43%, respectively, in patients with iliac artery injuries [45]. An earlier 10-year analysis from a Level I trauma center looking at 99 shunted vascular injuries showed a 9% shunt incidence rate. Damage control (44%) and orthopedic-vascular injuries (42%) were the most frequent shunt indications. Shunts were more commonly used in extremity (65–94%) and arterial (70–100%) injuries compared to truncal and venous injuries, respectively. The most commonly shunted extremity vessels were the superficial femoral artery (25%) followed by the popliteal artery (19%) [43, 44].

Although no differences among shunt types have been reported, the Argyle shunt (C.R. Bard, Billerica, MA) followed by the Pruitt-Inahara shunts (LeMaitre Vascular, Burlington, MA) have been the most commonly utilized conduits [43, 44]. Chest tubes have been used for larger vessels with the majority being for truncal aortic injuries [44]. Nasogastric tubes were used to fashion shunts in one study from South Africa [46]. There was no association between shunt thrombosis and the use of noncommercial shunts (chest tube/feeding tube). However, noncommercial shunts and "damage control" shunt indication were associated with higher odds of subsequent graft failure (OR = 6.2, OR = 3.3, $p < 0.05$, respectively) [44].

Venous injury adds more treatment heterogeneity to vascular trauma. One study reported ligating all venous injuries [46]. There is evidence, however, that vein shunting and repair is associated with lower incidences of compartment syndromes, fasciotomies, and amputations [47, 48]. Shunt diameter is another critical consideration; oversizing causes intimal injury, while undersizing might cause shunt dislodgement. Shunt dwell time has not been associated with thrombosis; 86.5% of shunts were removed at 24 h in one study, while the mean "dwell" time was 24 h in another [43, 44]. Current shunt configuration is in a straight position (vs. looped) inserted to a depth of 2 cm into the injured vessel [47, 49] (Fig. 26.3).

There is no consensus surrounding the factors associated with shunt thrombosis although shunt sizing and vessel caliber have been implicated. One series demonstrated a shunt thrombosis rate of 5% all occurring in small-caliber vessels (superior mesenteric and brachial arteries) [43]. This is relevant since the majority of shunts (78%) are placed in larger-caliber vessels [44].

While the aforementioned shunting series portray favorable outcomes, the absence of a control group (primary or definitive vascular repair without prior vascular shunting) is a major limitation in most studies describing vascular shunt use. While it is true that compared to ligation shunting has superior outcomes, the same cannot be extrapolated when we compare shunts to definitive surgical repair [50–52]. One would assume that shunts would be most needed in small, rural centers

Fig. 26.3 Poplliteal artery and vein transection following tibial fracture and knee dislocation after a motor vehicle accident. Patient was transferred to thee emergency room with a 4 hour delay and an ischemic foot. Figure indicates arterial and venous shunt in place to allow time to the orthopedic surgeons to realign the knee and fixate the fracture

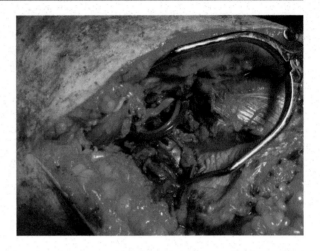

with limited access to vascular surgeons and appropriate resources, yet most of the literature supporting shunts comes from Level I trauma centers which are well-equipped and capable of definitive vascular surgical repair.

Trauma societal guidelines recommend minimizing the ischemic time to less than 6 h to allow for maximum limb salvage [53, 54]. Restoration of blood flow through temporary shunting is suggested in the presence of a concomitant bone injury, while immediate vascular repair is advised for "stable skeletal injuries" [55].

26.5   Overview of Vascular Injuries

26.5.1 Neck Vascular Injuries

Neck trauma is a leading cause of death among younger trauma persons, posing to surgeons the dilemma whether to proceed with reconstruction of the vascular injuries in the presence of coma or severe neurological deficit. Most patients presenting with vascular neck injuries will pass away during injury or immediately after transportation to the emergency department. For better evaluation and approach of the injury, the neck is separated into three anatomical zones: Zone 1 (sternal notch to cricoid cartilage), Zone 2 (cricoid cartilage to angle of the mandible), and Zone 3 angle (mandible to the base of skull). Most injuries are found in Zone 2 (47%), whereas a smaller amount of injuries will be found in Zone 3 (19%) and Zone 1 (18%) [56].

The main vascular structures in this zone are the common carotid artery, the internal carotid artery, the external carotid artery, the vertebral artery, and the internal jugular vein. The patient presents often in the emergency room with "hard signs" that require immediate exploration or "soft signs" that need further diagnostic evaluation and observation of the patient's hemodynamic status. Hard signs are defined as shock, pulsatile bleeding mass, souffle, expanding hematoma, and loss of pulse with stable or developing neurological deficit. Soft signs include stable hematoma and history of bleeding at the scene of injury. Carotid injury is associated with a high mortality rate (~50%) and high incidence of neurological deficit development (~80%) [56–58].

The management of Zone II injuries has been an object of debate over the previous decades. Conventionally, injuries in this zone would mandate immediate surgical exploration due to the accessible anatomy and high mortality of missed injuries. More recently mandatory exploration has been questioned compared to selective or nonoperative management with serial examination and further diagnostic testing in asymptomatic, hemodynamically stable patients. Several studies from experienced trauma centers confirmed that Zone II injuries can be reliably evaluated with physical examination. An injury to the vertebral artery from blunt trauma or active hemorrhage from penetrating wound can be evaluated with CTA in the hemodynamically stable patient. The stroke risk is 20% irrespective of lesion grade. Medical management has no role for penetrating injuries, but it does have a role for blunt injuries identified during the diagnostic evaluation. Injuries to the jugular veins occur in 20% of penetrating neck trauma. Isolated injuries are manifested with hard or soft signs of a vascular injury, but patients are rarely unstable [57, 58].

26.5.2 Thoracic Aortic Injuries

Blunt traumatic thoracic aortic injury of the aortic isthmus is the second most frequent cause of trauma-related mortality.

Isthmus is the segment of the aorta affected in the vast majority of blunt thoracic injury cases, reaching 80% of these patients. Other aortic segments, such as the aortic arch and the ascending and the descending aorta, are affected significantly less frequently [59].

Patients who make it to the emergency room have typically a "contained" rupture as the ones with free rupture will expire at the trauma scene. Diagnosis is typically done with a CT angiogram. In the past, these lesions were routinely treated on an emergency basis right after the diagnosis was established, but in recent years, treatment has been shifted toward a more expectant strategy in combination with thorough radiological surveillance and proper pharmaceutical regime, aiming at a strict blood pressure control [59–61].

Despite the lack of high-level evidence, endovascular repair with a thoracic aortic stent is considered "standard of care," as the advantages of this procedure in terms of operative complexity, complications, and associated mortality when compared to open surgical repair are clear [60, 61] (Fig. 26.4).

26.5.3 Abdominal/Pelvic Vascular Injuries

The mortality rate of abdominopelvic trauma varies widely and may reach 90%. More than 70% of deaths can be expected to occur within the first day, whereas late-stage mortality may be attributed to secondary complications such as sepsis and/or

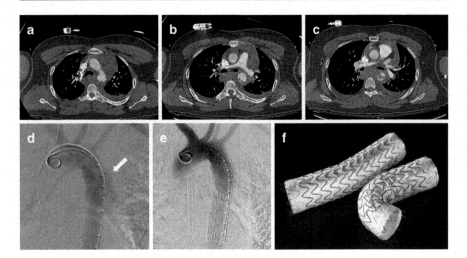

Fig. 26.4 (**a–c**) Advanced traumatic injury of the thoracic aorta at the isthmus,. Large traumatic intimal flap, intramural hematoma and periaortic hematoma extending along the thoracic aorta. Associated moderate size mediastinal hematoma. Small left hemothorax; (**d**) aortogram indicating the aortic transection / contain aortic rupture; (**e**) coverage of the injured aorta with a thoracic endograft; (**f**) thoracic aortic endograft TAG Gore Medical (Flagstaff, Arizona, USA)

multiple organ failure due to trauma [62, 63]. Blunt injuries predominate in rural areas, while penetrating ones are more frequent in urban settings.

Although, the management of acute traumatic vascular injuries was, until recently, restricted to traditional open surgical techniques, the use of endovascular techniques provides a reliable alternative.

The major sites of hemorrhage in patients are the viscera, following the mesentery, and the major abdominal vessels. For a better estimation and management of the injuries, the abdomen is conventionally divided into three zones:

- **Zone 1**: Midline retroperitoneum (extending from the aortic hiatus to the sacral promotore). This zone is subdivided into the supramesocolic (suprarenal aorta (SA), celiac axis (CA), superior mesenteric artery (SMA), renal arteries (RAs), the supramesocolic area of inferior vena cava (IVC), superior mesenteric vein (SMV)) area and the inframesocolic area that contains the infrarenal aorta and the IVC.
- **Zone 2**: Upper lateral retroperitoneum (left and right, which contains the kidneys and their vessels)
- **Zone 3**: Pelvic retroperitoneum (including the iliac vessels)

Abdominal vascular trauma presents as free intraperitoneal hemorrhage, intraperitoneal/retroperitoneal hematoma, or thrombosis of the vessel. Under these circumstances, the hemodynamic status of the patients should be rapidly evaluated in order to divide them in two groups, those with ongoing hemorrhage and those without (hematoma/thrombosis). In cases of active hemorrhage, the patients arrive at the emergency department hypotensive and "nonresponding" to fluid resuscitation. Immediate transfer to the operating room for definitive repair of their vascular injuries is essential.

Vascular injury is also frequent in pelvic fractures, and it is usually of venous origin, but in unstable pelvic fractures and particularly in hemodynamically unstable patients, arterial bleeding should be suspected. Arterial bleed is typically combined with venous. Percutaneous angioembolization (typically of internal iliac arterial branches) is preferred for treatment of hemodynamically unstable pelvic fractures. Venous bleeding and hemorrhage from fracture sites are effectively controlled by preperitoneal pelvic packing in conjunction with pelvic stabilization. Angioembolization for active arterial bleeding in PI has a high success rate (85–100%) and can be repeated in case of ongoing bleeding [64].

26.5.4 Extremity Vascular Injuries

Upper or lower extremity arterial injury in trauma patients has the potential to progress to ischemia and limb loss if not promptly recognized and treated. Lower extremity injuries are more frequent than those of the upper extremity, and penetrating trauma is more prevalent than blunt.

When damage is severe or ischemia has been prolonged, primary amputation is often performed at the discretion of the trauma team. Patients who do not require an immediate primary amputation, however, may continue on to require a delayed amputation as a result of irreversible or progressive ischemia, extensive unreconstructable soft tissue, or skeletal damage, or electively for intractable pain or a nonfunctional limb.

Outcomes of lower extremity injuries in the global civilian population are difficult to quantify due to the low rate of injuries in the general population: despite the large number of patients in some studies, results have been non-homogenous because the injury characteristics of many study populations differ substantially in mechanism and injury location, with amputation rates ranging from 2% to 33% [64].

Vascular injuries can be classified clinically into hard signs and soft signs of injury on the basis of examination. Classic so-called hard signs of vascular injury include the following:

- Observed pulsatile bleeding
- Arterial thrill (i.e., vibration) by manual palpation
- Bruit over or near the artery by auscultation
- Signs of distal ischemia
- Visible expanding hematoma

Soft signs of vascular injury include the following:

- Significant hemorrhage found on history
- Decreased pulse compared to the contralateral extremity

- Bony injury or proximity penetrating wound
- Neurologic abnormality

In general, hard signs of injury (e.g., a change in pulse quality compared to the opposite extremity or a loss of pulse in the extremity) are absolute indications for further diagnostic studies (e.g., arteriography or exploration and direct visualization in the operating room). Softer signs (e.g., temperature change, color change, delayed capillary refill, or neurologic deficit) should alert the clinician to the need for close observation and monitoring.

The physical examination may be augmented by measurement of the ankle-brachial index (ABI).

Imaging studies (e.g., CT angiogram) can be performed when patient is stable and/or the limb is not severely ischemic; otherwise the surgeon can perform on-table angiography in the operating room with minimal risk to the patient.

Treatment is often complex due to the involvement of trauma to multiorgan systems and concomitant local musculoskeletal injuries. Management of lower extremity injuries is best accomplished using a multidisciplinary approach among trauma, orthopedic, and vascular surgeons. Various scoring systems have been proposed for assessing the severity of the mangled extremity, with the MESS score the most commonly used in vascular trauma. This score has classically been used with a cutoff score of 7 to predict future viability of any limb salvage procedures. Irrespectively, the decision regarding whether or not to amputate should be made individually on the basis of clinical signs and intraoperative findings of irreversible limb ischemia.

Medical therapy alone is rarely an option in penetrating or blunt trauma to the extremity vasculature when hard signs of injury are present. Patients who are asymptomatic or who have only soft signs can often be observed, but such observation is best performed by a surgeon who is prepared to operate if changing circumstances require it. The observation must be performed with the understanding that if the examination findings change or if hard signs develop, surgical intervention is necessary. The timing of surgical intervention can be critical to outcome in extremity vascular injury. Vascular reconstruction that occurs within 3 h of injury is generally accepted to have the best outcome [65].

Surgical intervention when suspecting peripheral vascular injuries can be as minor as operative visualization of normal vascular anatomy for diagnostic purposes or as extensive as reconstruction and replacement of entire segments of injured vessels. As a general rule while arteries need to be reconstructed, veins can be generally ligated with minimal morbidity. If patient is too unstable, damage control by placement of a temporary intravascular shunt can allow time for optimization before definite repair (see previous section on shunts).

26.6 The Role of Endovascular Techniques in the Management of Vascular Injuries

While open surgical management has always been the gold standard, the use of endovascular techniques is becoming more prominent for selected indications. This trend is in part due to advancements in numerous technologies such as embolization materials and covered stents from the aorta to the periphery.

A full account of endovascular techniques used to manage vascular injuries, hemorrhage, and shock is beyond the scope of this article. However, like REBOA, catheter-based management of intraperitoneal hemorrhage is best performed by a team (e.g., technicians, nurses, physicians) and guided by protocols that standardize the rapid evaluation, movement, and treatment of these injury patterns, whether treatment takes place in an interventional radiology suite, an operating room, or a hybrid endovascular operating room.

The decision for endovascular or open intervention can be difficult and should be guided by the patient's clinical condition and anatomy of the injury. When patients are unstable, there is little debate that open surgery takes precedence; however, in the reasonably stable patient, the traditional thinking of mandatory surgical exploration is now challenged. Blunt traumatic vascular injuries are largely amenable to endovascular therapy, and some previously high-mortality, penetrating injuries like those to the visceral vessels can now sometimes be successfully treated with covered stenting. Thoracic aortic and axillosubclavian injuries are associated with favorable endovascular outcomes and have the most robust data supporting their use. If solid organ bleeding is amenable to endovascular treatment, it most commonly requires selective or semiselective embolization using one or more modalities, such as coils, plugs, or thrombotic material (Fig. 26.5). As such, having the inventory and practiced operating or interventional room staff who understand these devices is critical to their rapid and effective use. Lastly, because these patients are unstable and prone to cardiovascular collapse, use of endovascular devices to control intraperitoneal bleeding should include preestablished bailout options such as REBOA and/or laparotomy if the catheter-based approach is unsuccessful [5, 58, 62, 63, 66].

Hybrid operating rooms offer several advantages to using portable C-arms, particularly for complex endovascular aortic or cerebrovascular procedures, and can be integrated into the trauma pathway as an alternative to a traditional operating room. The hybrid room can be useful with concomitant orthopedic injuries as well as visceral bleeding amenable to embolization.

Ideally a multidisciplinary team is required to make appropriate treatment decisions and weigh the risks and benefits of available treatment modalities.

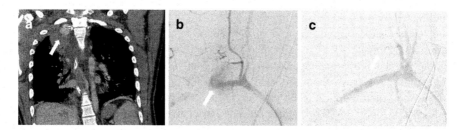

Fig. 26.5 26 year old male who suffered multiple gunshot wounds to neck transported from trauma scene. The patient has a 1 cm wound over his right anterior neck at the apex of the sternocleidomastoid triangle. (**a**) CT scan shows pseudoaneurysm of a right subclavian branch versus blast injury to the top of his lung with minimal hemothorax; (**b**) selective angiogram of the thyrocervical trunk showed extravasation from the suprascapular artery and the transverse cervical artery; (**c**) injured arterial branches were coiled embolized and bleeding has been controlled

26.7   Management of Bleeding in Austere Environments

Remote, isolated, and austere locations without the benefit of relying on local medical infrastructure necessitate development of dedicated medical units and capabilities to provide this care. Current knowledge comes from military practice.

"Remote" or "forward" has been proposed to define the prehospital phase of resuscitation, and "austere" or "far-forward" as "the environment where professional healthcare providers normally do not operate, and basic equipment and capabilities necessary for resuscitation are often not available" [10]. The translation of hospital-based damage control resuscitation techniques to remote and austere settings forms the crux of remote damage control resuscitation (RDCR). RDCR is applicable in a wide range of settings: rural, frontier/wilderness, ships at sea, and mass casualty incidents. Given the inherent logistical and resource limitations in these settings, however, translation of damage control to RDCR is challenging [67, 68].

As discussed earlier permissive hypotension improves outcomes. This holds true in urban environments where prehospital transport times are relatively short. In remote and austere environments, permissive hypotension will undoubtedly lead to some accumulation of oxygen debt.

Plasma is used as the primary volume expander in urban damage control resuscitation. Storage conditions and therefore immediate availability of plasma products differ with implications for RDCR. Fresh frozen plasma and thawed plasma are ill suited for RDCR; liquid plasma has fewer constraints, enabling wider use. Freeze-dried (lyophilized) plasma (FDP) has been "rediscovered" as a more suitable plasma product for RDCR. FDP was used extensively during World War II, but production was stopped in the United States due to heightened risk of disease transmission. Currently, FDP is manufactured by updated processes in France, Germany, and South Africa. The French product has been in continuous production since World War II, albeit in small quantities. Advantages of FDP include its long shelf life (up to 2 years), room temperature storage, rapid reconstitution within minutes, and relative stability at temperature extremes. The French and South African products are produced from pooled plasma. The advantages of pooling include uniform factor concentrations and universal ABO compatibility, while transmissible disease risk is minimized by pathogen inactivation [67].

Platelets are an important part of hemostatic resuscitation, but logistical constraints make platelets essentially unavailable in remote and austere settings. Cold storage of platelets, which appears to preserve hemostatic function better than room temperature storage without the need for agitation, appears viable. Another hemostatic resuscitation option when platelets are unavailable is whole blood, including fresh whole blood (FWB) obtained as needed from the "walking blood bank." Being fresh, the well-described "storage lesion" of aged RBCs and platelets is avoided. Transfusion of bag of FWB in lieu of three to four bags of components is logistically simpler (reducing risk of administrative error) and reduces donor exposure (lowering the risk of disease transmission) [67, 69].

In the civilian sector, pilot trials have reported successful use of cross-matched modified whole blood (leukoreduced, platelets removed) and uncross-matched cold-stored whole blood (leukoreduced, containing platelets) in the initial resuscitation of civilian trauma patients. Norwegian Naval Special Operations have published their simplified protocol for whole blood "buddy" transfusions in the field, and a similar protocol for US forces has been proposed.

Tranexamic acid (TXA) inhibits tissue plasminogen activator and fibrinolysis, potentially making it an important damage control resuscitation adjunct. It is recommended for hospitalized trauma patients within 3 h of injury if possible, and it reduces blood loss without increased risk of venous thromboembolism. Prehospital TXA is given by several military and civilian aeromedical transport services, at the point of injury, so far with no apparent increase in adverse events [70]. A recent matched cohort study found that prehospital TXA was associated with reduced 24-h mortality (5.8% vs. 12.4%) in 516 patients transported by the German Air Rescue Service without increased VTE incidence [71].

As far as mechanical control of hemorrhage is concerned, hemorrhage can be classified as compressible (controllable with external pressure) or noncompressible (torso hemorrhage). Tourniquets, hemostatic dressings, and sponges and the REBOA balloon have substantially reduced exsanguination from torso or extremity hemorrhage. These have been thoroughly described in the previous sections of this chapter. Finally, specifically for vascular injuries, should damage control surgery is performed in the austere setting, use of a temporary intravascular shunt can allow reperfusion of an ischemic limb till patient is transferred to an urban facility with the appropriate resources.

As the future unfolds, the benefits and detriments of these contemporary strategies are constantly reevaluated targeting optimal care, minimal limb, and life losses. Currently, we still do not have enough evidence to make robust recommendations in austere situations.

Acknowledgments This chapter is partially based on the following open access articles: "Damage Control for Vascular Trauma from the Prehospital to the Operating Room Setting," © 2017 Pikoulis, Salem, Avgerinos, Pikouli, Angelou, Pikoulis, Georgopoulos and Karavokyros; "Vascular Shunts in Civilian Trauma," © 2017 Abou Ali, Salem, Alarcon, Bauza, Pikoulis, Chaer and Avgerinos. Both articles are distributed under the terms of the Creative Commons Attribution License (CC BY)

References

1. Evans JA, van Wessem KJ, McDougall D, Lee KA, Lyons T, Balogh ZJ. Epidemiology of traumatic deaths: comprehensive population-based assessment. World J Surg. 2010;34(1):58–163.
2. Roberts DJ, Ball CG, Feliciano DV, Moore EE, Ivatury RR, Lucas CE, et al. History of the innovation of damage control for management of trauma patients. Ann Surg. 2017;265(5):1034–44.
3. Curry N, Davis PW. What's new in resuscitation strategies for the patient with multiple trauma? Injury. 2012;43(7):1021–8.
4. Cotton BA, Reddy N, Hatch QM, Lefebvre E, Wade CE, Kozar RA, et al. Improvement in survival in 390 damage. Control. 2013;254(4):1–15.

5. Pikoulis E, Salem KM, Avgerinos ED, Pikouli A, Angelou A, Pikoulis A, et al. Damage control for vascular trauma from the prehospital to the operating room setting. Front Surg. 2017;4:73.
6. de Crescenzo C, Gorouhi F, Salcedo ES, Galante JM. Prehospital hypertonic fluid resuscitation for trauma patients. J Trauma Acute Care Surg. 2017;82(5):956–62.
7. Rossaint R, Bouillon B, Cerny V, Coats TJ, Duranteau J, Fernández-Mondéjar E, et al. The European guideline on management of major bleeding and coagulopathy following trauma: fourth edition. Crit Care. 2016;20(1):100.
8. Bedreag OH, Papurica M, Rogobete AF, Sarandan M, Cradigati CA, Vernic C, et al. New perspectives of volemic resuscitation in polytrauma patients: a review. Burn Trauma. 2016;4(1):5.
9. Lira A, Pinsky MR. Choices in fluid type and volume during resuscitation: impact on patient outcomes. Ann Intensive Care. 2014;4(1):38.
10. Finfer S, Bellomo R, Boyce N, French J, Myburgh J, Norton R, et al. A comparison of albumin and saline for fluid resuscitation in the intensive care unit. N Engl J Med. 2004;350(22):2247–56.
11. Semler MW, Wanderer JP, Ehrenfeld JM, Stollings JL, Self WH, Siew ED, et al. Balanced crystalloids versus saline in the intensive care unit: the SALT randomized trial. Am J Respir Crit Care Med. 2016;195(10):rccm.201607-1345OC.
12. Perel P, Roberts I, Ker K, Perel P, Roberts I, Ker K. Colloids versus crystalloids for fluid resuscitation in critically ill patients (Review) Colloids versus crystalloids for fluid resuscitation in critically ill patients. Cochrane Collab. 2013;3:1–71.
13. Cronhjort M, Wall O, Nyberg E, Zeng R, Svensen C, Mårtensson J, et al. Impact of hemodynamic goal-directed resuscitation on mortality in adult critically ill patients: a systematic review and meta-analysis. J Clin Monit Comput. 2018;32(3):403.
14. Zehtabchi S, Nishijima DK. Impact of transfusion of fresh-frozen plasma and packed red blood cells in a 1:1 ratio on survival of emergency department patients with severe trauma. Acad Emerg Med. 2009;16(5):371–8.
15. Zink KA, Sambasivan CN, Holcomb JB, Chisholm G, Schreiber MA. A high ratio of plasma and platelets to packed red blood cells in the first 6 hours of massive transfusion improves outcomes in a large multicenter study. Am J Surg. 2009;197(5):565–70.
16. Holcomb JB, Wade CE, Michalek JE, Chisholm GB, Zarzabal LA, Schreiber MA, et al. Increased plasma and platelet to red blood cell ratios improves outcome in 466 massively transfused civilian trauma patients. Trans Meet Am Surg Assoc. 2008;126(3):97–108.
17. Johansson I, Stensballe J, Oliveri R, Wade CE, Ostrowski SR, Holcomb JB. How I treat patients with massive hemorrhage. Blood. 2014;124(20):3052–9.
18. Inaba K, Branco BC, Rhee P, Blackbourne LH, Holcomb JB, Teixeira PGR, et al. Impact of plasma transfusion in trauma patients who do not require massive transfusion. J Am Coll Surg. 2010;210(6):957–65.
19. Hébert PC, Wells G, Blajchman MA, Marshall J, Martin C, Pagliarello G, et al. A multicenter, randomized, controlled clinical trial of transfusion requirements in critical care. N Engl J Med. 1999;340(6):409–17.
20. Holst LB, Haase N, Wetterslev J, Wernerman J, Guttormsen AB, Karlsson S, et al. Lower versus higher hemoglobin threshold for transfusion in septic shock. N Engl J Med. 2014;371(15):1381–91.
21. Scerbo MH, Holcomb JB, Taub E, Gates K, Love JD, Wade CE, Cotton BA. The trauma center is too late: major limb trauma without a pre-hospital tourniquet has increased death from hemorrhagic shock. J Trauma Acute Care Surg. 2016;83(6):1165–72.
22. Kragh JF, Littrel ML, Jones JA, Walters TJ, Baer DG, Wade CE, et al. Battle casualty survival with emergency tourniquet use to stop limb bleeding. J Emerg Med. 2011;41(6):590–7.
23. Lee C, Porter KM, Hodgetts TJ. Tourniquet use in the civilian prehospital setting. Emerg Med J. 2007;24(8):584–7.
24. Kue RC, Temin ES, Weiner SG, Gates J, Coleman MH, Fisher J, et al. Tourniquet use in a civilian emergency medical services setting: a descriptive analysis of the Boston EMS experience. Prehosp Emerg Care. 2015;19(3):399–404.

25. Saied A, Ayatollahi Mousavi A, Arabnejad F, Ahmadzadeh Heshmati A. Tourniquet in surgery of the limbs: a review of history, types and complications. Iran Red Crescent Med J. 2015;17(2):e9588.
26. Bulger EM, Snyder D, Schoelles K, Gotschall C, Dawson D, Lang E, Sanddal ND, Butler FK, Fallat M, Taillac P, et al. An evidence-based prehospital guideline for external hemorrhage control: American College of Surgeons Committee on Trauma. Prehosp Emerg Care. 2014;18(2):163–73.
27. Kheirabadi B. Evaluation of topical hemostatic agents for combat wound treatment. US Army Med Dep J. 2011;(June):25–37.
28. McManus J, Hurtado T, Pusateri A, Knoop KJ. A case series describing thermal injury resulting from zeolite use for hemorrhage control in combat operations. Prehosp Emerg Care. 2007;11(1):67–71.
29. Harjai MM. A salmon thrombin-fibrinogen dressing controls hemorrhage in a Swine model compared to standard kaolin-coated gauze. Med J Armed Forces India. 2012;68:239.
30. Rothwell SW, Reid TJ, Dorsey J, Flournoy WS, Bodo M, Janmey PA, et al. A salmon thrombin-fibrin bandage controls arterial bleeding in a swine aortotomy model. J Trauma Inj Infect Crit Care. 2005;59(1):143–9.
31. Causey MW, McVay DP, Miller S, Beekley A, Martin M. The efficacy of Combat Gauze in extreme physiologic conditions. J Surg Res. 2012;177(2):301–5.
32. Littlejohn L, Bennett BL, Drew B. Application of current hemorrhage control techniques for backcountry care: Part Two, hemostatic dressings and other adjuncts. Wilderness Environ Med. 2015;26(2):246–54.
33. Shander A, Kaplan LJ, Harris MT, Gross I, Nagarsheth NP, Nemeth J, et al. Topical hemostatic therapy in surgery: bridging the knowledge and practice gap. J Am Coll Surg. 2014;219(3):570–579.e4.
34. Baghdanian AA, Baghdanian AH, Khalid M, Armetta A, LeBedis CA, Anderson SW, et al. Damage control surgery: use of diagnostic CT after life-saving laparotomy. Emerg Radiol. 2016;23(5):483–95.
35. Walker ML. The damage control laparotomy. J Natl Med Assoc. 1995;87(2):119–22.
36. Markov NP, Percival TJ, Morrison JJ, Ross JD, Scott DJ, Spencer JR, et al. Physiologic tolerance of descending thoracic aortic balloon occlusion in a swine model of hemorrhagic shock. Surgery. 2013;153(6):848–56.
37. Biffl WL, Fox CJ, Moore EE. The role of REBOA in the control of exsanguinating torso hemorrhage. J Trauma Acute Care Surg. 2015;78(5):1054–8.
38. Rhee PM, Acosta J, Bridgeman A, Wang D, Jordan M, Rich N. Survival after emergency department thoracotomy: review of published data from the past 25 years. J Am Coll Surg. 2000;190(3):288–98.
39. DuBose JJ, Scalea TM, Brenner M, Skiada D, Inaba K, Cannon J, et al. The AAST prospective Aortic Occlusion for Resuscitation in Trauma and Acute Care Surgery (AORTA) registry. J Trauma Acute Care Surg. 2016;81(3):409–19.
40. Teeter WA, Matsumoto J, Idoguchi K, Kon Y, Orita T, Funabiki T, et al. Smaller introducer sheaths for REBOA may be associated with fewer complications. J Trauma Acute Care Surg. 2016;81(6):1039–45.
41. Taylor JR, Harvin JA, Martin C, Holcomb JB, Moore LJ. Vascular complications from resuscitative endovascular balloon occlusion of the aorta. J Trauma Acute Care Surg. 2017;83:S120–3.
42. Subramanian A, Vercruysse G, Dente C, Wyrzykowski A, King E, Feliciano DV. A decade's experience with temporary intravascular shunts at a civilian level I trauma center. J Trauma. 2008;65(2):316–24, 326.
43. Inaba K, Aksoy H, Seamon MJ, Marks JA, Duchesne J, Schroll R, et al. Multicenter evaluation of temporary intravascular shunt use in vascular trauma. J Trauma Acute Care Surg. 2016;80(3):359–65. http://content.wkhealth.com/linkback/openurl?sid=WKPTLP:landingpage&an=01586154-201603000-00001.

44. Ball CG, Feliciano DV. Damage control techniques for common and external iliac artery injuries: have temporary intravascular shunts replaced the need for ligation? J Trauma. 2010;68(5):1117–20. https://pubmed.ncbi.nlm.nih.gov/20453767/.

45. Oliver JC, Gill H, Nicol AJ, Edu S, Navsaria PH. Temporary vascular shunting in vascular trauma: a 10-year review from a civilian trauma centre. S Afr J Surg. 2013;51(1):6–10.

46. Hornez E, Boddaert G, Ngabou UD, Aguir S, Baudoin Y, Mocellin N, et al. Temporary vascular shunt for damage control of extremity vascular injury: a toolbox for trauma surgeons. J Visc Surg. 2015;152(6):363–8.

47. Barros D'Sa AAB, Harkin DW, Blair PHB, Hood JM, McIlrath E. The belfast approach to managing complex lower limb vascular injuries. Eur J Vasc Endovasc Surg. 2006;32(3):246–56.

48. Ding W, Wu X, Li J. Temporary intravascular shunts used as a damage control surgery adjunct in complex vascular injury: collective review. Injury. 2008;39(9):970–7.

49. Gifford SM, Aidinian G, Clouse WD, Fox CJ, Porras CA, Jones WT, et al. Effect of temporary shunting on extremity vascular injury: an outcome analysis from the Global War on Terror vascular injury initiative. J Vasc Surg. 2009;50(3):549–56. https://doi.org/10.1016/j.jvs.2009.03.051.

50. Rasmussen TE, Dubose JJ, Asensio JA, Feliciano DV, Fox CJ, Nunez TC, et al. Tourniquets, vascular shunts, and endovascular technologies: esoteric or essential? A report from the 2011 AAST Military Liaison Panel. J Trauma Acute Care Surg. 2012;73(1):282–5.

51. Abou Ali AN, Salem K, Alarcon L, et al. Vascular shunts in civilian trauma. Front Surg. 2017;4:39.

52. Fox N, Rajani RR, Bokhari F, Chiu WC, Kerwin A, Seamon MJ, et al. Evaluation and management of penetrating lower extremity arterial trauma: an Eastern Association for the Surgery of Trauma practice management guideline. J Trauma Acute Care Surg. 2012;73(5 Suppl 4):S315–20.

53. Feliciano DV, Moore EE, West MA, Moore FA, Davis JW, Cocanour CS, et al. Western Trauma Association critical decisions in trauma: evaluation and management of peripheral vascular injury, part II. J Trauma Acute Care Surg. 2013;75(3):391–7.

54. Reber PU, Patel AG, Sapio NL, Ris HB, Beck M, Kniemeyer HW. Selective use of temporary intravascular shunts in coincident vascular and orthopedic upper and lower limb trauma. J Trauma. 1999;47(1):72–6.

55. Karaolanis G, Maltezos K, Bakoyiannis C, Georgopoulos S. Contemporary strategies in the management of civilian neck zone II vascular trauma. Front Surg. 2017;4:16.

56. Tisherman SA, Bokhari F, Collier B, Cumming J, Ebert J, Holevar M, et al. Clinical practice guideline: penetrating zone II neck trauma. J Trauma. 2008;64:1392–405. https://doi.org/10.1097/TA.0b013e3181692116.

57. Shiroff AM, Gale SC, Martin ND, Marchalik D, Petrov D, Ahmed HM, et al. Penetrating neck trauma: a review of management strategies and discussion of the 'No Zone' approach. Am Surg. 2013;79:23–9.

58. Patelis N, Katsargyris A, Klonaris C. Endovascular repair of traumatic isthmic ruptures: special concerns. Front Surg. 2017;4:32.

59. Lee WA, Matsumura JS, Mitchell RS, Farber MA, Greenberg RK, Azizzadeh A, et al. Endovascular repair of traumatic thoracic aortic injury: clinical practice guidelines of the Society for Vascular Surgery. J Vasc Surg. 2011;53(1):187–92. https://doi.org/10.1016/j.jvs.2010.08.027.

60. Riambau V, Böckler D, Brunkwall J, Cao P, Chiesa R, et al. Editor's choice – management of descending thoracic aorta diseases: clinical practice guidelines of the European Society for Vascular Surgery (ESVS). Eur J Vasc Endovasc Surg. 2017;53(1):4–52. https://doi.org/10.1016/j.ejvs.2016.06.005.

61. Feliciano DV, Moore EE, Biffl WL. Western Trauma Association critical decisions in trauma: management of abdominal vascular trauma. J Trauma Acute Care Surg. 2015;79:1079–88. https://doi.org/10.1097/TA.0000000000000869.

62. Bakoyiannis C, Karaolanis G, Moris D, Georgopoulos S. Contemporary strategies in the management of civilian abdominal vascular trauma. Front Surg. 2018;5:7.

63. Ptohis ND, Charalampopoulos G, Abou Ali AN, Avgerinos ED, Mousogianni I, Filippiadis D, et al. Contemporary role of embolization of solid organ and pelvic injuries in polytrauma patients. Front Surg. 2017;4:43.
64. Liang NL, Alarcon LH, Jeyabalan G, Avgerinos ED, Makaroun MS, Chaer RA. Contemporary outcomes of civilian lower extremity arterial trauma. J Vasc Surg. 2016;64:731.
65. Bjerke S, Suhlmiller DFE. Extremity vascular trauma. https://emedicine.medscape.com/article/462752-overview. Accessed 1 Jul 2018.
66. Avgerinos ED, Pikoulis E. Editorial: Contemporary strategies in the management of civilian vascular trauma. Front Surg. 2018;5:43.
67. Chang R, Eastridge BJ, Holcomb JB. Remote damage control resuscitation in austere environments. Wilderness Environ Med. 2017;28:S124–34.
68. Jenkins DH, Rappold JF, Badloe JF, et al. Trauma hemostasis and oxygenation research position paper on remote damage control resuscitation: definitions, current practice, and knowledge gaps. Shock. 2014;41(Suppl 1):3–12.
69. Nessen SC, Eastridge BJ, Cronk D, et al. Fresh whole blood use by forward surgical teams in Afghanistan is associated with improved survival compared to component therapy without platelets. Transfusion. 2013;53(Suppl 1):107S–13S.
70. Morrison JJ, Dubose JJ, Rasmussen TE, Midwinter MJ. Military application of tranexamic acid in trauma emergency resuscitation (MATTERs) study. Arch Surg. 2012;147:113–39.
71. O'Reilly DJ, Morrison JJ, Jansen JO, Apodaca AN, Rasmussen TE, Midwinter MJ. Prehospital blood transfusion in the en route management to severe combat trauma: a matched cohort study. J Trauma Acute Care Surg. 2014;77(3 Suppl 2):S114–20.

Prevention and Treatment of Traumatic Brain Injury Due to Rapid-Onset Natural Disasters

27

Paul Brady, Shishir Rao, and Panagiotis Varelas

27.1 Introduction

Traumatic brain injury (TBI) is the leading cause of death and disability in children and young adults in the United States. TBI is also a major concern for elderly individuals, with a high rate of death and hospitalization due to falls among people age 75 and older. Depending on the severity of injury, TBI can have a lasting impact on quality of life for survivors of all ages, impairing thinking, decision-making and reasoning, concentration, memory, movement, and sensation and causing emotional problems (personality changes, impulsivity, anxiety, and depression) [1]. TBI can also lead to epilepsy.

Annually, TBI-related injuries cost an estimated $76 billion in direct and indirect medical expenses. The US Centers for Disease Control and Prevention (CDC) statistics for 2010 showed TBIs were a factor in the deaths of more than 50,000 people in the United States; more than 280,000 people with TBI were hospitalized and 2.2 million people with TBI visited an emergency department [1].

A TBI occurs when physical, external forces impact the brain from either a penetrating object or a bump, blow, or jolt to the head. Generally, not all blows or jolts to the head will result in a TBI. For those that do, TBIs can range from mild (a brief change in mental status or consciousness) to severe (an extended period of unconsciousness or amnesia after the injury) [1]. There are two broad types of head injuries: penetrating and non-penetrating. Penetrating TBI, or open TBI, occurs when

P. Brady · S. Rao
Henry Ford Hospital, Detroit, MI, USA

P. Varelas (✉)
Neuro-Critical Care Services, Neurosciences Intensive Care Unit, Neurology & Neurosurgery, Department of Neurology, Henry Ford Hospital, Detroit, MI, USA

Neurology, Wayne State University, Detroit, MI, USA
e-mail: PVARELA1@hfhs.org

© Springer Nature Switzerland AG 2021
E. Pikoulis, J. Doucet (eds.), *Emergency Medicine, Trauma and Disaster Management*, Hot Topics in Acute Care Surgery and Trauma,
https://doi.org/10.1007/978-3-030-34116-9_27

the skull is pierced by an object such as a bullet, shrapnel, or a blunt object including a hammer or knife. With this injury, the object enters the brain parenchyma. Non-penetrating TBI (also known as closed head injury or blunt TBI) is caused by an external force that produces movement of the brain within the skull. Non-penetrating TBIs include falls, motor vehicle crashes, sports injuries, or being struck by an object. Blast injuries due to explosions are also a cause of non-penetrating TBIs and have been the focus of intense study as this is a common injury sustained by soldiers and the underlying injury to the brain is not fully known. Some accidents such as explosions, natural disasters, or other extreme events can cause both penetrating and non-penetrating TBIs in the same patient.

The most common cause of TBIs, according to data from the CDC, is falls, and they occur most frequently among the youngest and oldest age groups. The second and third most common causes of TBI are unintentional blunt trauma, followed closely by motor vehicle accidents [1]. Less commonly, TBIs can be seen during and after natural disasters. Although the frequency and severity of rapid-onset natural disasters varies spatially and temporally, a review of the historical record demonstrates that earthquakes, floods, hurricanes or typhoons, tornadoes, and tsunamis are not rare events globally [2].

In this chapter we will be discussing classifications of TBIs; the pathophysiology and effect TBI has on the brain; TBI due to natural disasters, specifically looking at earthquakes and hurricanes; and prevention and treatment of TBI due to natural disasters.

27.2 Classification of Traumatic Brain Injuries

TBI has traditionally been classified using injury severity scores; the most commonly used is the Glasgow Coma Scale (GCS) [3]. A GCS score of 13–15 is considered mild injury, 9–12 is considered moderate injury, and 8 or less is considered as severe TBI. The GCS is universally accepted as a tool for TBI classification because of its simplicity, reproducibility, and predictive value for overall prognosis. However, it is limited by confounding factors such as medical sedation and paralysis, endotracheal intubation, and intoxication. An alternative scoring system, the Full Outline of UnResponsiveness (FOUR) Score, was developed as an attempt to obviate these issues, primarily by including a brainstem examination (Table 27.1) [4]. However, the FOUR score lacks the long track record of the GCS in predicting prognosis and is more complicated to perform, which may be a barrier for care providers who are not neurologists [5].

Neuroimaging provides an additional modality for TBI grading. Two currently used CT-based grading scales are the Marshall Scale and Rotterdam Scale. The Marshall Scale uses CT findings to classify injuries in six different categories (Table 27.2) [6]. The Rotterdam Scale is a more recent CT-based classification developed to overcome the limitations of the Marshall Scale (Table 27.3) [7].

Table 27.1 Glasgow Coma Scale and Full Outline of UnResponsiveness Score

Glasgow Coma Scale (GCS)	
Eye opening	
– Does not open eyes.	1
– Opens eyes in response to noxious stimuli.	2
– Opens eyes in response to voice.	3
– Opens eyes spontaneously.	4
Verbal output	
– Makes no sounds.	1
– Makes incomprehensible sounds.	2
– Utter inappropriate words.	3
– Confused and disoriented.	4
– Speaks normally and oriented.	5
Motor response (best)	
– Makes no movements.	1
– Extension to painful stimuli.	2
– Abnormal flexion to painful stimuli.	3
– Flexion/withdrawal to painful stimuli.	4
– Localized to painful stimuli.	5
– Obeys commands.	6
Full Outline of UnResponsiveness (FOUR) Score	
Eye response	
– Eye lids open or opened, tacking, or blinking to command.	4
– Eyelids open but not tracking.	3
– Eyelids closed but open to loud voice.	2
– Eyelids closed but open to pain.	1
– Eyelids remain closed with pain.	0
Motor response	
– Thumbs up, fist, or peace sign.	4
– Localizing to pain.	3
– Flexion response to pain.	2
– Extension response to pain.	1
– No response to pain or generalized myoclonus status.	0
Brainstem reflexes	
– Pupil and corneal reflexes present.	4
– One pupil wide and fixed.	3
– Pupil or corneal reflexes absent.	2
– Pupil and corneal reflexes absent.	1
– Absent pupil, corneal and cough reflex.	0
Respiration	
– Not intubated, regular breathing pattern.	4
– Not intubated, Cheyne-Stokes breathing pattern.	3
– Not intubated, irregular breathing.	2
– Breathes above ventilatory rate.	1
– Breathes at ventilatory rate or apnea .	0

Table 27.2 Marshall CT classification of traumatic brain injury

Category	Definition
Diffuse injury I (no visible pathology)	No visible intracranial pathology seen on CT scan
Diffuse injury II	Cisterns are present with midline shift of 0–5 mm and/or lesions densities present; no high or mixed density lesion >25 cm³ and may include bone fragments and foreign bodies
Diffuse injury III (swelling)	Cisterns compressed or absent with midline shift 0–5 mm; no high or mixed density lesion >25 cm³
Diffuse injury IV (shift)	Midline shift >5 mm; no high or mixed density lesion >25 cm³
Evacuated mass lesion V	Any lesion surgically evacuated
Non-evacuated mass lesion VI	High or mixed density lesion >25 cm³; not surgically evacuated

Table 27.3 Rotterdam CT classification of traumatic brain injury

Predictor value	Score
Basal cisterns	
– Normal	0
– Compressed	1
– Absent	2
Midline shift	
– No shift or shift ≤5 mm	0
– Shift >5 mm	1
Epidural mass lesion	
– Present	0
– Absent	1
Intraventricular blood or subarachnoid hemorrhage	
– Absent	0
– Present	1
Sum score	Total + 1

27.3 The Pathophysiology of Traumatic Brain Injury and the Effect It Has on the Brain

TBI-related damage can be confined to one area of the brain, known as a focal injury, or it can occur over a more widespread area, known as a diffuse injury. The type of injury is another determinant of the effect on the brain. Some injuries are classified as primary, indicating that the damage is immediate. Other consequences of TBI can be secondary and will occur gradually over the course of hours, days, or weeks. These secondary brain injuries are the result of reactive processes that occur after the initial head trauma.

Primary injuries lead to diffuse axonal injury (DAI), concussion, hematomas, contusions, coup and contrecoup lesions, and skull fractures. DAI is one of the most common types of brain injuries. DAI refers to widespread damage to the brain's white matter. It is the result of shearing forces which stretch or tear the underlying axons found in white matter. This damage commonly occurs in auto accidents, falls, or sports injuries and is usually a result of rotational forces or sudden deceleration. It commonly results in a disruption of neural circuits and a breakdown of overall communication among neurons in the brain. Patients with severe DAI typically present with profound coma without elevated intracranial pressure (ICP) and often have a poor outcome. The injuries associated with DAI can cause temporary or permanent damage and recovery can be prolonged.

A concussion is a type of mild TBI that may be considered a temporary injury to the brain but could take minutes to several months to heal. Individuals who suffer a concussion either suddenly lose consciousness or have an altered state of consciousness or awareness and can be characterized as being "dazed." A second concussion closely following a first one causes further brain damage and can lead to permanent damage or even death in some instances. This is known as the "second-impact syndrome" or "second-hit" phenomenon and can occur minutes to weeks after the initial concussion.

Extra-axial hematomas are generally encountered when forces are distributed to the cranial vault and the most superficial cerebral layers. Different types of hematomas form depending on where the blood collects relative to the meninges which include (from outer to inner) dura mater, arachnoid mater, and pia mater.

- Epidural hematomas (EDHs): Involve bleeding into the area between the skull and the dura mater. They are typically associated with torn dural vessels such as the middle meningeal artery and are almost always associated with a skull fracture. EDHs are lenticular-shaped and tend not to be associated with underlying brain damage (Fig. 27.1).

Fig. 27.1 CT head showing left parietal epidural hematoma with mass effect on the brain

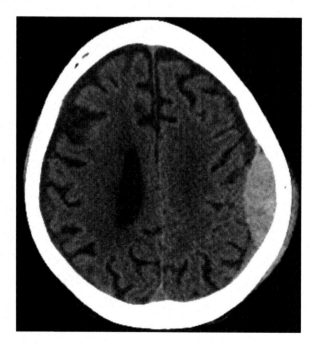

- Subdural hematomas: Involve bleeding between the dura and the arachnoid mater. They, like epidural hematomas, exert extra-axial pressure on the brain. They result from damage to bridging veins, which drain the cerebral cortical surfaces to dural venous sinuses, or from the blossoming of superficial cortical contusions. They tend to be crescent-shaped and are often associated with underlying cerebral injury (Fig. 27.2).
- Subarachnoid hemorrhage: Involves bleeding between the arachnoid mater and the pia mater. Effects vary on the amount of bleeding (Fig. 27.3).
- Intracerebral hematoma: Bleeding in the brain parenchyma itself with damage to surrounding tissue (Fig. 27.4).

Contusions are bruising or swelling of the brain that occurs when very small blood vessels bleed into the brain. Contusions can occur directly under the impact site, which is referred to as a coup injury, or, more often, on the complete opposite side of the brain from the impact, which is a contrecoup injury. These types of injuries are seen in high-velocity injuries, including motor vehicle accidents, and are also commonly seen in shaken baby syndrome. Skull fractures are also a common primary injury found in TBI patients and can cause damage to the underlying areas of the skull including the membranes, blood vessels, and brain.

Secondary injuries in TBI are usually considered a cascade of molecular injury mechanisms that are initiated at the time of the initial trauma and continue for hours or days. The hemorrhagic progression of a contusion contributes to secondary injuries. A hemorrhagic progression of a contusion occurs when the initial contusion from the primary injury continues to bleed and expands over time. This in turns

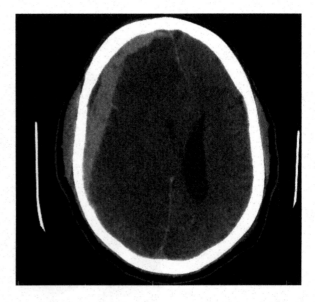

Fig. 27.2 CT head showing right frontoparietal subdural hematoma with midline shift

Fig. 27.3 CT head showing subarachnoid hemorrhage with right temporal hematoma

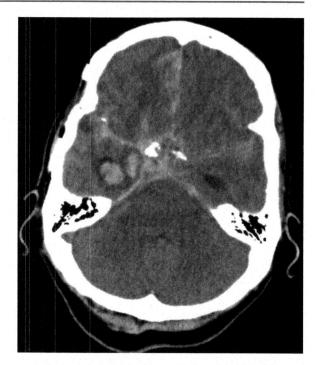

Fig. 27.4 CT head showing left parietotemporal hematoma with surrounding edema

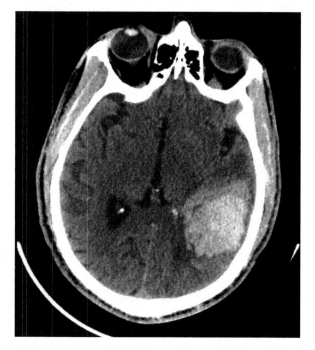

creates a new or larger lesion. Subsequently, this causes increased exposure to blood, which is toxic to brain cells through oxidative stress and leads to more swelling and further brain cell loss.

Breakdown in the blood-brain barrier (BBB) may also lead to secondary damage. Once disruption of the BBB occurs through a TBI, blood, plasma proteins, and other foreign substances leak into the space between neurons in the brain and trigger a chain reaction which causes the brain to swell. It also induces over activity of multiple biological system processes, including the systemic inflammatory response, which are harmful to the body and central nervous system if they continue for an extended period. Additionally, neurotransmitter mediation injury can occur caused by glutamate excitotoxicity and free radical injury to cell membranes. These molecular processes ultimately lead to apoptosis and cell death and eventually worsening of cerebral edema and ICP elevation, which will decrease cerebral perfusion pressure and further perpetuate the cycle.

27.4 Traumatic Brain Injury Due to Natural Disasters

As was previously discussed, the most common cause of TBIs is falls, particularly in the youngest and oldest age groups. However, natural disasters are a unique cause of TBIs which may occur more commonly than expected. The World Health Organization collaborating center for research on the epidemiology of disasters maintains an Emergency Events Database (EM-DAT) that contains information about the occurrence and effects of more than 18,000 mass disasters that have happened in the world since 1900 [2]. A search of the EM-DAT reveals that the total number of rapid-onset natural disasters and slow-onset crises (drought and armed conflict) reported each year, which either kill ≥ 10 people or leave ≥ 100 people injured, homeless, displaced, or evacuated as well as events that result in a country formally declaring a natural disaster and/or requesting international assistance reported each year, has been steadily increasing in recent decades. For example, tropical cyclones are estimated to have caused 1,330,000 deaths between 1900 and 2014. Within that overall period, approximately 1080 tropical cyclones occurred between 1980 and 2014, resulting in 412,644 deaths and 290,654 injuries. In part, the change in deaths and injuries reported reflects patterns of population migration to, as well as population density in, disaster-prone areas within developing countries in Africa, Asia, and Oceania. Rapid onset natural disasters have also caused significant damage in developed countries. This is illustrated by the fact that in the United States, there were approximately 58,169 tornadoes between 1950 and 2014 resulting in 6697 deaths and 104,597 injuries. Globally, there were 125 earthquakes that are known to have caused more than 1000 deaths per event between 1900 and 2014. The total number of deaths caused by these 125 earthquakes is estimated to be 2,309,716 [2].

Injury from rapid-onset natural disasters occurs due to high kinetic energy released, resulting in traumatic injuries that occur due to overpressure, penetrating wounds, and crushing including mild, moderate, and severe TBI. Chaotic environments as a result of the aftermath of major natural disaster, poses more challenges to diagnosis and treatment of TBI [2]. Providing immediate emergency care to disaster victims helps reduce development of secondary brain injuries. While it seems plausible in some of the developed countries, it seems to be fairly difficult in developing countries to provide such specialized care. Patients who survive rapid-onset natural disasters and sustain a mild or moderate TBI frequently require long-term care, thus increasing demand for more specialty medical care and also increasing demand for general medicine and nursing care while increasing utilization of mental health services as well [2]. It is also noted that the incidence of inflicted and non-inflicted childhood TBI can increase in regions affected by natural disasters such as earthquakes, tornadoes, hurricanes, and floods. The non-inflicted injuries were particularly attributed to increase in risk associated with driving, environmental hazard, and lodging displacement and a possible decrease in the quality of adult supervision. Child abuse was also seen to be higher in certain areas with natural disasters [8, 9].

Earthquakes are among the most devastating natural disasters, and this is exemplified by the earthquake which struck the Sichuan Province of China on May 12, 2008, registering a 7.8 on the Richter scale. More than 85,000 people were killed or reported missing, with >370,000 injured [7]. Thirty days after the earthquake, the medical records of 242 patients with seismic craniocerebral trauma were retrospectively analyzed, and their clinical features were summarized. In the entire cohort, there were 137 men and 105 women. More than 85% of patients were injured by falling objects. Most of the patients suffered mild head injuries (GCS score, 13–15), constituting 172 of the cases. For moderate head injury (GCS score, 8–12), there were 42 cases. Fifteen cases were severe head injury, and another 13 patients suffered from extremely severe head injuries with a GCS score < 5 [7]. The survival rate of the patients with a GCS < 5 was zero. The two leading causes of death were asphyxiation and intracranial injuries, which may cause immediate death on site and minimize the time window for rescue. Therefore, people seriously injured could hardly undergo proper treatment and survive [7]. One hundred sixty-six patients had scalp lacerations and contusions, which was reported to be associated with roofing materials and falling clay tiles. Another cause of injury was falling precast concrete planks, which caused fracture of skull bones and intracranial injuries [10].

A second earthquake struck Athens, Greece, on September 7, 1999. The earthquake was reported by the National Earthquake Planning and Protection Organization as 5.9 on the Richter scale, with its epicenter 17 km deep. The magnitude of the earthquake and its shallowness and close proximity of the epicenter to the city were the main factors implicated in the massive loss of human life and damage to property. One hundred and forty-three lives were lost, and more than 700 citizens were injured [11]. The vast majority of the deaths were consequent to the collapse of 32 buildings, including 3 factories leading to blunt injuries, asphyxia, and myocardial infarction. Long extrication times precluded treatment of most of the victims. These delayed extrication times were due to relatively limited rescue forces at the initial, but critical, time of the earthquake. A combination of blunt fatal injuries is a typical feature in individuals buried or trapped in collapse buildings. In Athens, 22.5% of the victims had head injuries not compatible with life. The most common fatal injuries were blunt injuries to the head, thorax, and abdomen. Those injuries affecting the face and neck commonly threaten the airway. Additionally, minor chest injuries, pneumothorax, rib fractures, and hemothorax are common and impair ventilation.

The temporal relation of TBIs and natural disasters, at times, can be unusual, as many of the injuries occur after the natural disaster has occurred. On September 16, 1999, Hurricane Floyd, a storm extending 300 miles with sustained winds of 96–110 miles per hour, made landfall in North Carolina. The hurricane dropped 20 in. of rain in eastern regions of the state, affecting an estimated 2.1 million people [8]. To monitor illness and injury related to the hurricane and subsequent flood, emergency department surveillance was established at 20 hospitals in 18 flood-affected counties in Eastern North Carolina. The medical examiner determined that 52 deaths were associated directly with the storm. The leading cause of death was drowning. However, comparing a week 1 month after Hurricane Floyd with same period in 1998 showed a significant increase in violence, particularly toward children.

The flooding and subsequent loss of, and disruption to, lives, property, and community ties may have contributed to an increase in parental stress and depression, thus contributing to an increase in child maltreatment [9]. Physical child maltreatment is the leading cause of death from injury among infants [12]. Inflicted TBI is a common form of child abuse in the first year of life, estimated at about 30 per 100,000 infants and approximately 17 per 100,000 child-years in the first 2 years of life [9]. Families at highest risk appear to be those with a first child, low maternal education, and minority status. During a 40-month study period following Hurricane Floyd, a total of 245 children were identified as having a TBI. Incidentally, the rate of both inflicted and non-inflicted injuries rose dramatically in the first 6 months after Hurricane Floyd in the counties which were severely affected. The rate of inflicted injuries returned close to baseline in the same counties 6 months post-hurricane. However, the rate of non-inflicted injuries appeared to remain elevated for the entire post hurricane period. This persistent elevation in non-inflicted injuries may reflect increased injury risk due to prolonged stress. These findings are consistent with a study of mental health effects performed following the Mt. Saint Helen's eruption. This study showed that patients in a high exposure group, meaning those who had experienced significant property loss or death of a family member, exhibited more psychiatric morbidity (generalized anxiety disorder, major depression, and post-traumatic stress disorder) when compared to low-exposure groups [13].

Ultimately, natural disasters can cause immediate and delayed TBIs to patients, similar to the ones seen during the Sichuan Province and Athens earthquakes and following Hurricane Floyd in North Carolina. Commonly, during earthquakes, TBIs are caused by blunt injuries. Many of the injuries sustained during earthquakes cause immediate death and minimize the time window for rescue. Whereas many injuries occur immediately in the wake of a natural disaster, there are also patients who sustain TBIs in a delayed manner, after the natural disaster has stopped or passed. This is an unfortunate consequence of natural disasters which causes increased stress and disrupts the social fabric of communities. Many of the victims, as in the aforementioned example of Hurricane Floyd, are children.

27.5 Prevention and Treatment of TBI Due to Natural Disasters

The immediate diagnosis and treatment of natural disaster victims with head injuries is essential to minimize the development of secondary brain injuries. This is the premiere challenge associated with delivery of emergency medical care when that category of natural disasters happens, especially in developing countries with limited communication means, roads, and medical infrastructure capacity that may be further degraded by the disaster [2]. This reality becomes clear in the event of a major rapid-onset natural disaster where neurosurgeons will be overwhelmed by the surge in injured patients requiring specialized care [2]. For example, there are approximately 140 neurosurgeons for 250 million people in Indonesia, whereas in the United States, there are 3500 neurosurgeons for a population of 299 million [2].

As a potential remedy to dampen the injuries caused by natural disasters, countries, such as Indonesia, have created interfaces to deliver telemetric, point-of-care treatment to help natural disaster victims with TBIs [14]. This interface allows neurosurgeons, surgeons, general practitioners, and nurses to evaluate patients and fill in the knowledge gaps of emergency first responders. The development and use of telemedicine allows for treatment of patients in remote areas, and it has its greatest impact when it is used to deliver highly specialized care that may otherwise be unavailable.

Long-term care also presents a challenge for those patients who have suffered TBIs during natural disasters. As described earlier in this chapter, many patients during natural disasters do not survive their injuries. However, those that do generally have suffered a mild to moderate TBI and, in some instances, a severe TBI. These injuries lead to an increase in local demand for neurological specialists who are capable of delivering long-term care for these types of nonlethal injuries [2]. This demand is likely to persist across the lifespan of the local TBI population, especially if the affected region experiences multiple disasters [2]. In addition to the need for neurological care, there will also be an increase in need of physical therapy, occupational therapy, nursing care, and mental health services for those patients who have suffered post-traumatic stress disorder.

A specific subset of patients who are particularly affected by the psychosocial stressors or natural disasters are children. The aftermath of Hurricane Floyd likely produced an increase in psychiatric symptoms as well as financial hardship and loss of social ties for families caught in the worst flooding [8]. Unfortunately, children become susceptible targets to physical abuse during times of social stress and this abuse, in turn, can lead to TBIs. To prevent excess financial burden and social stress, interventions should take place immediately after the disaster when families are gathered at shelters or are applying for assistance. When initiated prenatally, programs of intensive home visitation by nurses that address both the social and physical environments have been found to be efficacious in preventing child abuse and neglect, as well as childhood injury, in disadvantaged populations [8]. These interventions, if implemented appropriately and promptly, may be effective in preventing the number of TBIs suffered by children following a natural disaster.

27.6 Summary

This chapter has shown that natural disasters, although less common than falls, blunt trauma, and motor vehicle accidents, are a unique and common cause of TBIs. It has also shown the use of injury severity scores to classify TBIs. The most common is the Glasgow Coma Scale which can categorize the injuries as mild, moderate, and severe. Traumatic brain injuries can also be graded through neuroimaging, using both the Marshall and Rotterdam Scales. Patients who suffer TBIs can have both primary injuries, which include diffuse axonal injury, concussion, hematomas, contusions, coup and contrecoup lesions, as well as secondary injuries that are produced by a cascade of molecular injury mechanisms initiated at the time of the initial trauma and continued for hours or days.

Injury from rapid-onset natural disasters occurs due to high kinetic energy released, resulting in traumatic injuries that occur due to overpressure, penetrating wounds, and crushing. These injuries can be devastating and occur at the time of the natural disaster as seen during the earthquakes in China and Greece. However, patients can also suffer TBIs in the aftermath of a natural disaster. This was seen following Hurricane Floyd in North Carolina. The financial and social impact of the hurricane lead to increased parental stress and depression which subsequently lead to increased child maltreatment.

A few methods may be employed to minimize the injuries sustained and the debility caused by natural disasters. Telemedicine can provide point-of-care treatment for patients in remote areas, and it has its greatest impact when it is used to deliver highly specialized care that may otherwise be unavailable. Employing neurologists and providing adequate nursing care and mental health services for patients who live in areas where natural disasters are prevalent may be beneficial in reducing the morbidity associated with natural disaster injuries, including TBIs. Furthermore, programs which address both the social and physical environments following a natural disaster would be efficacious in preventing child abuse and neglect, as well as childhood injury. Future research on these models of disaster intervention may be worthwhile as the total number of rapid-onset natural disasters and slow-onset crises that result in countries formally declaring a natural disaster and/or requesting international assistance has been steadily increasing in recent decades.

References

1. Traumatic brain injury: hope through research. National Institute of Neurological Disorders and Stroke. 2015. (NIH Publication No. 15-2478).
2. Regens JL, Mould N. Prevention and treatment of traumatic brain injury due to rapid-onset natural disasters. Front Public Health. 2014;2:28. PubMed PMID: 24783188. Pubmed Central PMCID: 3995068.
3. Teasdale G, Jennett B. Assessment of coma and impaired consciousness. A practical scale. Lancet (London, England). 1974;2(7872):81–4. PubMed PMID: 4136544. Epub 1974/07/13. eng.
4. Stead LG, Wijdicks EF, Bhagra A, Kashyap R, Bellolio MF, Nash DL, et al. Validation of a new coma scale, the FOUR score, in the emergency department. Neurocrit Care. 2009;10(1):50–4. PubMed PMID: 18807215. Epub 2008/09/23. eng.
5. Saatman KE, Duhaime AC, Bullock R, Maas AI, Valadka A, Manley GT. Classification of traumatic brain injury for targeted therapies. J Neurotrauma. 2008;25(7):719–38. PubMed PMID: 18627252. Pubmed Central PMCID: PMC2721779. Epub 2008/07/17. eng.
6. Marshall LF, Marshall SB, Klauber MR, Van Berkum CM, Eisenberg H, Jane JA, et al. The diagnosis of head injury requires a classification based on computed axial tomography. J Neurotrauma. 1992;9(Suppl 1):S287–92. PubMed PMID: 1588618. Epub 1992/03/01. eng.
7. Maas AI, Hukkelhoven CW, Marshall LF, Steyerberg EW. Prediction of outcome in traumatic brain injury with computed tomographic characteristics: a comparison between computed tomographic classification and combinations of computed tomographic predictors. Neurosurgery. 2005;57(6):1173–81; discussion 82. PubMed PMID: 16331165.
8. Centers for Disease Control and Prevention (CDC). Morbidity and mortality associated with Hurricane Floyd--North Carolina, September-October 1999. MMWR Morb Mortal Wkly Rep. 2000;49(17):369–72. PubMed PMID: 10821481. Epub 2000/05/23. eng.
9. Keenan HT, Marshall SW, Nocera MA, Runyan DK. Increased incidence of inflicted traumatic brain injury in children after a natural disaster. Am J Prev Med. 2004;26(3):189–93. PubMed PMID: 15026097.
10. Wang L, Lei DL, He LS, Liu YP, Long Y, Cao J, et al. The association between roofing material and head injuries during the 2008 Wenchuan earthquake in China. Ann Emerg Med. 2009;54(3):e10–5. PubMed PMID: 19398243. Epub 2009/04/29. eng.
11. Papadopoulos IN, Kanakaris N, Triantafillidis A, Stefanakos J, Kainourgios A, Leukidis C. Autopsy findings from 111 deaths in the 1999 Athens earthquake as a basis for auditing the emergency response. Br J Surg. 2004;91(12):1633–40. PubMed PMID: 15505869. Epub 2004/10/27. eng.
12. Overpeck MD, Brenner RA, Trumble AC, Trifiletti LB, Berendes HW. Risk factors for infant homicide in the United States. N Engl J Med. 1998;339(17):1211–6. PubMed PMID: 9780342. Epub 1998/10/22. eng.
13. Shore JH, Tatum EL, Vollmer WM. Evaluation of mental effects of disaster, Mount St. Helens eruption. Am J Public Health. 1986;76(3 Suppl):76–83. PubMed PMID: 3946730. Pubmed Central PMCID: PMC1651694. Epub 1986/03/01. eng.
14. Sutiono AB, Suwa H, Ohta T, Arifin MZ, Kitamura Y, Yoshida K, et al. Development traumatic brain injury computer user interface for disaster area in Indonesia supported by emergency broadband access network. J Med Syst. 2012;36(6):3955–66. PubMed PMID: 22773106. Epub 2012/07/10. eng.

Hemorrhage Control

28

David L. Carter, Patrick D. Melmer,
and Christoph R. Kaufmann

Hemorrhage from traumatic injuries remains one of the most frequent reasons for loss of life in both military and civilian populations. The morbidity and mortality from hemorrhage come not only from blood loss itself but also from the physiologic derangements that occur as a consequence of that blood loss. Thus, hemorrhage control continues to be a mainstay in the preservation of life and remains challenging even with modern advances in surgery.

Hemorrhagic injuries are second only to brain injuries as the leading cause of death from trauma in the United States [1]. Proper management of the trauma patient from the time of injury through the hospital setting includes early identification of bleeding source (external, internal, or both), measures to stop or minimize continued bleeding, definitive control of bleeding, and restoration of blood flow to tissues to return hemodynamic stability to the patient.

"The fate of the wounded lies in the hands of the ones who apply the first dressing," as Dr. Nicholas Senn, founder of Association of Military Surgeons of the United States, so astutely pointed out in 1897 [2]. Many injured victims die from hemorrhage before they can reach a higher level of care. Thus, improving hemorrhage control at the scene of injury should improve the proportion of patients reaching the next level of care. Hemorrhage is the leading cause of death in the first hour of arrival at trauma centers. Furthermore, in trauma patients who survive to receive hospital care, hemorrhage is responsible for 80% of operative deaths and nearly 50% of all deaths during the first 24 h.

Bleeding noted from open wounds is either arterial, venous, or both, with regard to source. Precise identification of the exact source is not necessary in the field; rather, the focus should be on stopping the bleeding. To ensure optimal outcomes, familiarity with multiple techniques is required. Application of direct pressure at the

D. L. Carter · P. D. Melmer · C. R. Kaufmann (✉)
Grand Strand Medical Center, Myrtle Beach, SC, USA
e-mail: zerotrauma@icloud.com

© Springer Nature Switzerland AG 2021
E. Pikoulis, J. Doucet (eds.), *Emergency Medicine, Trauma and Disaster
Management*, Hot Topics in Acute Care Surgery and Trauma,
https://doi.org/10.1007/978-3-030-34116-9_28

bleeding site is always an appropriate first step. Tourniquets are a mainstay in the management of external bleeding from extremities. Compression at proximal pressure points (such as the femoral or brachial artery) is a technique that can be lifesaving, while large bleeds from the scalp or head may require temporary suture or staple closure until more definitive fixation is performed in the operating room. Neurosurgical Raney clips can also be useful for control of bleeding scalp wounds, even in the emergency department setting.

Physical exam remains the mainstay of the rapid assessment of the bleeding trauma patient. The pulse rate and character (slow, strong, and easily palpable versus rapid, thready, and difficult to palpate), color and temperature of the skin (warm versus mottled, cool, or cyanotic), and mental status (alert versus somnolent or lethargic) are all used to assess adequacy of perfusion. Blood pressure should be taken at the outset to define a baseline, with frequent rechecking every 5–10 min as clinically indicated. Hospital adjuncts such as central venous catheters can help assess central venous pressure, and monitoring of urine output over a time interval can further define adequacy of perfusion.

The first vital sign to classically change in the bleeding patient is the pulse rate. Tachycardia suggests hypovolemic shock until proven otherwise. Several factors may blunt the normal tachycardic response to bleeding, including rate-controlling cardiac medications and cardiac disease requiring a pacemaker. The pulse character is suggestive as well, with strong, regular pulses indicative of a relatively higher cardiac output as opposed to a thready pulse. Peripheral vasoconstriction, as mediated by catecholamines, can be present as a response to hypovolemia, so cyanotic, pale, and sweaty or clammy skin should also be presumed to represent bleeding until proven otherwise. Normal mentation implies adequate cerebral perfusion, whereas decreased mentation can be the result of several etiologies, ranging from shock to brain injury or other metabolic imbalances. Of note, blood pressure can be a misleading number in the assessment of a possible bleeding patient, as vasoconstrictive compensatory forces may be present. Up to 30% of the circulating blood volume may be lost before a noticeable drop in blood pressure occurs. A clue may be provided by the narrowing of the pulse pressure, the numeric difference between the systolic and diastolic pressures.

Advanced Trauma Life Support® (ATLS) defines four separate classes of hemorrhage based on blood loss both in terms of absolute volume and percent blood volume [3]. Many signs and symptoms are typically noted in the bleeding patient based on blood loss depending on class of hemorrhage. Class I hemorrhage represents the least blood loss, up to 15% or approximately 750 mL for a 70 kg man. Vital signs are essentially normal, with perhaps a mild anxiousness noted in the patient. Class II hemorrhage, 15–30% blood loss (750–1500 mL), is the first class of blood loss with noted changes in vital signs, tachycardia, and decreased pulse pressure. Class III hemorrhage continues with 30–40% loss and more significant derangement including increased tachycardia, tachypnea, and hypotension. Class IV hemorrhage, >40% blood volume loss (greater than 2 L), demonstrates effects including lethargy and profound hypotension. Table 28.1 highlights these distinctions [3].

Table 28.1 Signs and symptoms of hemorrhage by class. Adapted from American College of Surgeons Advanced Trauma Life Support Student Course Manual, Tenth Edition. Chicago: American College of Surgeons; 2018. p. 49

Parameter	Class I	Class II (mild)	Class III (moderate)	Class IV (severe)
Approximate blood loss	<15%	15–30%	31–40%	>40%
Heart rate	↔	↔/↑	↑	↑/↑↑
Blood pressure	↔	↔	↔/↓	↓
Pulse pressure	↔	↓	↓	↓
Respiratory rate	↔	↔	↔/↑	↑
Urine output	↔	↔	↓	↓↓
Glasgow Coma Scale score	↔	↔	↓	↓
Base deficit[a]	0 to −2 mEq/L	−2 to −6 mEq/L	−6 to −10 mEq/L	−10 mEq/L or less
Need for blood products	Monitor	Possible	Yes	Massive Transfusion Protocol

[a]Base excess is the quantity of base (HCO_3^-, in mEq/L) that is above or below the normal range in the body. A negative number is called a base deficit and indicates metabolic acidosis

Shock is currently defined at the level of cellular oxygen delivery and utilization. Aerobic metabolism, the physiologic set point, is replaced by anaerobic metabolism in the setting of poor oxygen delivery to tissues. $Q \times SaO_2 \times Hg$ defines oxygen delivery to tissues, based on cardiac output (Q), oxygenated hemoglobin percentage (SaO_2), and hemoglobin g/dL (Hg). Physiologic mechanisms exist to augment oxygen delivery during periods of homeostatic derangement secondary to blood loss. These include the ability for hemoglobin to increase unloading of O_2 to starving tissues. Central or mixed venous oxygen saturations are approximately 70% at rest, but can decrease as oxygen utilization is increased in accordance with the oxygen-hemoglobin dissociation curve. Cardiac mechanisms themselves can help affect this change as well. As heart rate and/or stroke volume increases, so does cardiac output and thus O_2 delivery. Reserve exists in that the average resting heart rate is approximately 50% that of the maximum [4]. Catecholamines and other biochemical mediators can augment the heart rate in response to hemorrhage. At the more distal portions of the cardiovascular system, peripheral vascular resistance is altered to preferentially shunt blood flow to more central, vital organs, most obviously noted in the cool and clammy extremity skin indicative of intravascular depletion. Oncotic forces also shift as bleeding ensues, such that interstitial and intracellular fluids are drawn into the intravascular space to help maintain volume. Renal mechanisms via antidiuretic hormone and the renin-angiotensin system decrease the amount of fluid removed in urine. These hallmarks of compensation also allow the physician to monitor response to resuscitation, the so-called endpoints. Normalization of cardiac function, warmth of extremities, increase in urine output, normal mentation, and other such evidence can signify restoration of the physiologic set point.

The first step in hemorrhage control should be identification of the location of the injury and the type of bleeding. Differentiating an arterial bleed from venous bleeding is a crucial step in control of hemorrhage. Bleeding from an artery is typically bright red in color and should spurt or pump blood from the wound. This type of bleeding can be immediately life-threatening, with complete exsanguination possible in as little as 3 min. A venous bleed can be differentiated as usually dark red in color, with a steady flow from the wound. Venous bleeding may also be life-threatening if a large vein is damaged. Capillary bleeding is the third type and can be seen as dark red in color with an ooze from the injury site. Serious bleeding from an extremity is the most frequent cause of preventable death from injury. As such, life-threatening bleeding always warrants immediate intervention.

After identification of external bleeding, the first responder should quickly control the hemorrhage. The most basic and sometimes most successful control of bleeding is manual pressure. The wound should be exposed, and a clean cloth or piece of clothing can be used to help cover the bleeding area as focused manual pressure is applied. A common mistake is to believe that larger bleeding requires a larger area of pressure for control. If the blood is seen to be coming from a single specific visible blood vessel, a fingertip judiciously applied to the correct spot can stop the bleeding. One common circumstance seen that responds well to single finger hemorrhage control is bleeding from a dialysis fistula source. This bleeding can be impressive because this is an arterial-equivalent bleed. But a fingertip placed very gently exactly on the bleeding site easily stops the bleeding and allows for vascular surgery consultation and repair. This is much more comfortable for the patient than a tourniquet for this specific source of bleeding.

An excellent method for controlling exsanguinating extremity hemorrhage is the tourniquet. Reports of tourniquets date to the fourth century BC with Alexander the Great's military conquest, where tourniquets were reportedly used to stop the bleeding of wounded soldiers. They were used frequently throughout history up until World War II, at which time their use began to become controversial. Many of the medical practitioners of the time condemned the use of tourniquets due to unnecessary applications and prolonged tourniquet times from delayed evacuations, which led to unnecessary amputations of limbs. After World War I, Major Dwight Tuttle of the Army Medical Corps described a set of rules for the use of the tourniquet which are still accurate today: "Never cover over or bandage a tourniquet; write plainly on the emergency medical tag the word 'tourniquet'; if the injured man is conscious, he should be instructed to tell every medical officer with whom he comes in contact that he has a tourniquet on; and if the tourniquet is left on for greater than 6 hours the limb shall surely die [5]."

The tourniquet is a simple and efficient method to adequately control active extremity hemorrhage and can be effectively placed by responding personnel [6]. The tourniquet should be applied immediately if life-threatening bleeding is seen on an arm or a leg. Clothing can be left in place, and the tourniquet should be applied well above the site of bleeding. The tourniquet should be tightened until all bleeding has stopped. Tourniquets should neither be applied directly over joints nor should they be applied over pockets that contain bulky items. The patient should be aware prior to placement if at all possible that the tourniquet will cause a considerable amount of pain. Pain does not indicate a mistake, rather that the tourniquet is being applied effectively. Limb ischemia can be caused by a tourniquet applied too long, though it is important to note that no amputations have been caused by tourniquets that have been left in place for less than 2 h and limb salvage has been successful for some applications up to 6 h [7]. With proper use under the right conditions, a tourniquet may save a life [8].

Some common mistakes seen with tourniquet use are not applying a tourniquet when life-threatening bleeding exists, waiting too long to apply a tourniquet, using a tourniquet for minor non-life-threatening bleeding, or placing the tourniquet distal to the injury. Some tourniquet failures have been because the tourniquets were not applied tightly enough to stop arterial outflow, but were only tight enough to obstruct the large superficial veins that return blood to the heart. This results in increased bleeding from the extremity rather than decreased. A tourniquet is a commitment and must be tight enough to stop flow through the arteries which may be deep within the extremity. Other causes of tourniquet failure include (1) when providers periodically loosen the tourniquet to allow blood flow to extremity, which only serves to waste red cell mass, and (2) not using a second tourniquet adjacent to the first if bleeding remains uncontrolled (typically only required when tourniquets are used on the thigh).

Junctional hemorrhages are those that occur in places where standard tourniquets do not work: the groin, perineum, axilla, base of neck, and buttocks. Techniques to control junctional wounds begin with pressure. Additional techniques include packing the wound with gauze or hemostatic dressings. Hemostatic dressings include substances that are designed to help blood rapidly clot to help stop bleeding. They are not definitive answers for bleeding but can provide additional time to allow for definitive control or as adjuncts for use with vascular control within the operating room. Multiple commercial hemostatic dressings, utilizing incorporated agents such as kaolin or chitosan, are available today.

To pack a junctional hemorrhage site, the clothing around the wound should be removed, and the wound should be rapidly cleaned without removing any formed clot. The site of the most active bleeding should be focused on first, with packing the dressing directly at the source of bleeding. Pressure should be held for a minimum of 3 min with hemostatic agents and 10 min with plain gauze. The wound should be reassessed, and if initial packing fails, a second layer should be applied and pressure repeated. The packing should remain in place and wound secured with compression bandage or roll of gauze.

Once brought to the trauma bay by emergency medical trained personnel, the resuscitation of the bleeding trauma patient continues. The trauma bay vitally allows for assessment by a traumatologist where the patient's extent of trauma and potential for ongoing hemorrhage is assessed. The physician will be able to assess the extent of traumatic injury taking into account the mechanism of injury, anatomical injury pattern, and the patient's response to initial resuscitation to help guide the best possible care for the patient. As part of the initial "ABCs of trauma," vascular access must be rapidly established. Two large bore peripheral lines should be established. As fluid flow is directly proportional to the fourth power of the radius and inversely to the length of the intravenous catheter, the largest bore and shortest IVs will result in the potential for the most rapid fluid resuscitation. Typically, upper extremity lines are placed, ideally one in each arm. A 16 gauge catheter will flow approximately twice the volume over time as will an 18 gauge catheter of the same length (30 mm), 220 vs. 105 mL/min, respectively. Sometimes, peripheral access is not possible for various reasons. In these cases, central venous catheters can be lifesaving. It is important to note that a single large bore central catheter is preferred to a multi-lumen central venous catheter because of the potential need for high flow rates in a trauma patient—multi-lumen catheters flow slowly.

In some circumstances, less common vascular access adjuncts are used. Intraosseous access is useful particularly in children 6 and under and is usually placed in the proximal tibia about one fingerbreadth below the tibial promontory and can also be placed in the proximal humerus for adults. Venous cutdown is often a method of last resort given the considerably longer period of time needed for access. Greater saphenous venous cutdown may be performed at the ankle anterior to the medial malleolus or at the groin.

The standard ATLS® approach to resuscitation of the adult trauma patient with hemorrhage has been to begin with two liters of intravenous crystalloid (LR or NS). The physiologic response to this initial bolus of fluid places the patient in one of three groups: responders, transient responders, and nonresponders. This response is primarily in terms of the patient's blood pressure and heart rate. Mental status, respiratory rate, and urine output are also indicators of response to fluid resuscitation. Nonresponders do not show a difference in their shock state following a crystalloid bolus of 2 L and remain in shock. These patients need blood which should be administered without delay. Continuing resuscitation with crystalloids has been associated with comparative poor outcomes in patients with severe hemorrhage [9, 10]. Responders are usually patients who have lost an aliquot of blood and then stopped bleeding; a typical example is the patient with a femur fracture that has been splinted. Intravascular repletion with crystalloid is all that is required. Transient responders are difficult to manage. The primary problem is the rapid and accurate diagnosis of the patient's injuries. If they respond to the first fluid boluses and later blood administration, they have either a larger than expected initial blood loss or, more likely, ongoing slow bleeding; this bleeding must be localized.

Resuscitation importantly includes replacing what is lost in the bleeding patient. Given that blood is the fluid lost in hemorrhagic shock, it is the most logical replacement fluid. The current concept for the trauma patient suspected to be suffering from hemorrhagic shock is to start resuscitation with blood rather than crystalloid, if blood is immediately available. This logic is mitigated by inconsistent availability of blood in the emergency department and also by potential problems with infectious agents, cost, compatibility, and shelf life. When possible, the mantra "the patient is bleeding whole blood, therefore the ideal replacement is whole blood" is ideal. Although whole blood has not been routinely available in US hospitals for the past 30 years, there are now US blood banks making whole blood available to their local trauma centers.

Depending on the mechanism, blunt vs. penetrating, bleeding can be obviously external, insidiously internal, or a combination of both. The chest, abdomen, pelvis, and even certain parts of the extremities can hold a large proportion of the body's total blood supply. In addition to paying close attention to the patient's physical exam as detailed above, imaging modalities can provide a clue as to the source of bleeding. Chest and pelvic radiographs and abdominal/chest ultrasound (FAST exam) can quickly be completed in the trauma bay [11]. The FAST exam in the trauma bay has been shown to be effective with larger prospective observational studies showing high specificity and low sensitivity in adults and children [12, 13]. A stable patient can be taken to the CT scanner for a more definitive look.

Beginning in the ED, the physician should also begin to determine if additional resources should be considered to control hemorrhage. For example, a trauma patient with pelvic fractures and extravasation in the pelvis on CT scan may benefit from embolization by an interventional specialist. Known vascular injuries may benefit from vascular surgery involvement. These decisions should be rapidly made, and not delay a patient that requires operative intervention. Of note, for the moribund patient in whom an intra-abdominal or intrathoracic hemorrhagic catastrophe is suspected, ED thoracotomy or the newer-modality resuscitative endovascular balloon occlusion of the aorta (REBOA) may be required in an effort to save a life [4, 14].

If initial attempts to identify the sources of hemorrhage and to control them are not rapidly successful in the emergency department and neither ED thoracotomy nor REBOA are considered appropriate in the current clinical scenario, the patient must be immediately transported to the operating room. Patients not responding to initial resuscitation efforts require operative control of hemorrhage and simultaneous resuscitation that is best achieved in the operative suite. It has been clearly demonstrated that there is a survival benefit from decreasing the elapsed time between traumatic injury and the time the patient is placed on the OR Table [15, 16].

In the operating room, the trauma patient should be prepped and draped from chin to knees. For known or suspected abdominal hemorrhage, a generous abdominal midline incision should be made, typically from xiphoid to pubis. It should be noted that when opening the abdominal cavity, the release of elevated intra-abdominal pressure that may have served to tamponade bleeding may result in immediate increased hemorrhage and more severe hypotension. Immediate bleeding control is necessary, and this can be facilitated by four-quadrant packing with multiple readied abdominal packs. Once all four quadrants are packed, the main source of bleeding should be identified and controlled. Control of bleeding may require organ removal, such as splenectomy, or packing of the pelvis or liver. Many specific hemostatic agents, both topical and intravenous, are available to surgeons to aid in intraoperative hemostasis, but are too numerous to be described here. Additionally, specific blood vessels frequently need to be ligated or repaired. In the most severely injured and unstable patients, a vascular shunt may be left in place to maintain flow and oxygen delivery to vital organs while the patient is rewarmed and his/her acidosis and coagulopathy are corrected.

Over recent decades, the surgical community has developed a new appreciation of factors that increase mortality, the trauma "lethal triad." Understanding the lethal triad of hypothermia, acidosis, and coagulopathy has led to a change in the initial operative goals of the trauma surgeon when providing operative care for the most critically injured patients. The operative goal today is to accomplish definitive management in a calculated stepwise fashion based on the patient's physiological tolerance. Stone was the first to describe a technique for abbreviated surgery; he described the techniques of abbreviated laparotomy, packing to control hemorrhage and deferred definitive repair until normal coagulation was re-established [17]. This has led to the concept of damage control surgery: a brief initial laparotomy, subsequent ICU resuscitation, and planned definitive reoperation. The simple concept of ending up with a live patient above all other priorities is the driving force behind damage control procedures. This philosophy includes rapidly achieving hemostasis and preventing ongoing contamination from within the gastrointestinal tract by the fastest means possible, including staple closure of bowel ends without restoration of continuity. The abdominal fascia should not be closed during the initial damage control procedure. Rather the peritoneal cavity contents should be protected using methods such as a silo bag or commercial vacuum-type dressing device until reoperation [18].

Definitive vascular repair and restoration of bowel continuity is typically performed at 24–36 h, after the patient has stabilized. Damage control surgery is supported by retrospective studies which have shown reduced morbidity and mortality rates in selective populations [19, 20].

Once the initial operation is completed, the patient is taken to the ICU for continued resuscitation with planned definitive reoperation, ideally within 36 h or less. The goal for the resuscitation in the ICU is restoring circulating volume and red cell mass, correcting coagulopathy, restoring normothermia, and reversing acidosis, again, correcting for the lethal triad. If the patient has additional bleeding while in the ICU, the patient may require prompt return to OR.

Trauma remains a major public healthcare issue faced by modern society, and better public awareness is needed. Uncontrolled bleeding is the leading cause of potentially preventable death among trauma patients [21, 22]. The management of the massively bleeding trauma patient includes the early identification of bleeding sources followed by prompt measures to minimize blood loss. Sometimes the initial response to the severely injury patient is by civilian bystanders who have minimal to no medical training. It has recently been recognized that training nonmedical personnel in simple techniques such as application of pressure to a bleeding wound or application of a tourniquet will save lives. To that end there is now a nationwide initiative in the United States to teach just such techniques. Among the first targeted "students" are policemen and teachers. The "STOP THE BLEED" campaign is a campaign with simple primary principles of trauma care response aimed at the general public. The campaign teaches the ABCs of bleeding control: (1) alert proper authorities; (2) bleeding, identify where the bleeding is coming from; (3) compress, apply pressure to the bleeding through direct pressure with hands, tourniquet, or packing with gauze or clean cloth. While basic, the "STOP THE BLEED" campaign hopes to teach early life-saving measures that can be provided by civilian bystanders to help decrease prehospital deaths from hemorrhage. In fact, according to the Stop the Bleeding Coalition, 35% of prehospital deaths are a result of bleeding [23].

Hemorrhage remains at the forefront of concern for the injured patient as it always has. As evidenced above, history is replete with examples of surgeons, scientists, and many other involved parties focusing on the study of bleeding, how to stop it, and how to prevent it. Furthermore, its interrelationship with shock continues to be an area of much research. Nearly 100 years later, Dr. Walter B. Cannon's dictum (passed along to him by those surgeons who trained him) that "shock is hemorrhage and hemorrhage is shock" continues to ring true [24]. From the prehospital provider to the attending surgeon, the nature of bleeding and its effect on the critically injured patient is a matter of great importance.

References

1. Sauaia A, Moore FA, Moore EE, Moser KS, Brennan R, Read RA, Pons PT. Epidemiology of trauma deaths: a reassessment. J Trauma. 1995;38(2):185–93.
2. Schwartz RB, McManus JG, Swienton RE. Tactical emergency medicine. Philadelphia: Lippincott Williams & Wilkins; 2008. p. 192. ISBN 978-0-7817-7332-4.
3. American College of Surgeons. Advanced trauma life support student course manual. 10th ed. Chicago: American College of Surgeons; 2018. p. 49.
4. Oliveira RK, Agarwal M, Tracy JA, et al. Age-related upper limits of normal for maximum upright exercise pulmonary haemodynamics. Eur Respir J. 2016;47(4):1179–88. https://doi.org/10.1183/13993003.01307-2015. Epub 2015 Dec 17.
5. Tuttle AD. Handbook for the medical soldier. New York: William Wood; 1927.
6. Kragh JF Jr, Walters TJ, Baer DG, Fox CJ, Wade CE, Salinas J, Holcomb JB. Survival with emergency tourniquet use to stop bleeding in major limb trauma. Ann Surg. 2009;249:1–7. https://doi.org/10.1097/SLA.0b013e31818842ba.
7. Dayan L, Zinmann C, Stahl S, Norman D. Complications associated with prolonged tourniquet application on the battlefield. Mil Med. 2008;173:63–6.
8. Beekley AC, Sebesta JA, Blackbourne LH, Herbert GS, Kauvar DS, Baer DG, Walters TJ, Mullenix PS, Holcomb JB. Prehospital tourniquet use in Operation Iraqi Freedom: effect on hemorrhage control and outcomes. J Trauma. 2008;64:S28–37. ; discussion S37. https://doi.org/10.1097/TA.0b013e318160937e.
9. Duchesne JC, Heaney GC, et al. Diluting the benefits of hemostatic resuscitation: a multi-institution analysis. J Trauma Acute Care Surg. 2013;75:76.
10. Neal MD, Hoffman MK, Cuschieri J, et al. Crystalloid to packed red blood cell transfusion ratio in the massively transfused patient: when a little goes a long way. J Trauma Acute Care Surg. 2012;72:892.
11. Gillman LM, Ball CG, Panebianco N, Al-Kadi A, Kirkpatrick AW. Clinician performed resuscitative ultrasonography for the initial evaluation and resuscitation of trauma. Scand J Trauma Resusc Emerg Med. 2009;17:34. https://doi.org/10.1186/1757-7241-17-34.
12. Richards JR, Schleper NH, Woo BD, Bohnen PA, McGahan JP. Sonographic assessment of blunt abdominal trauma: a 4-year prospective study. J Clin Ultrasound. 2002;30:59–67. https://doi.org/10.1002/jcu.10033.
13. Richards JR, Knopf NA, Wang L, McGahan JP. Blunt abdominal trauma in children: evaluation with emergency US. Radiology. 2002;222:749–54. https://doi.org/10.1148/radiol.2223010838.
14. Brenner M, Teeter W, Hoehn M, et al. Use of resuscitative endovascular balloon occlusion of the aorta for proximal aortic control in patients with severe hemorrhage and arrest. JAMA Surg. 2018;153(2):130–5. https://doi.org/10.1001/jamasurg.2017.3549.
15. Hill DA, West RH, Roncal S. Outcome of patients with haemorrhagic shock: an indicator of performance in a trauma centre. J R Coll Surg Edinb. 1995;40:221–4.

16. Hoyt DB, Bulger EM, Knudson MM, Morris J, Ierardi R, Sugerman HJ, Shackford SR, Landercasper J, Winchell RJ, Jurkovich G, Coffey SC, Chang M, O'Malley KF, Lowry J, Trevisani GT, Cogbill TH. Death in the operating room: an analysis of a multi-center experience. J Trauma. 1994;37:426–32. https://doi.org/10.1097/00005373-199409000-00016.
17. Stone HH, Strom PR, Mullins RJ. Management of the major coagulopathy with onset during laparotomy. Ann Surg. 1983;197:532–5. https://doi.org/10.1097/00000658-198305000-00005.
18. Kaufmann CR, Cooper GL, Barcia PJ. Polyvinyl chloride membrane as a temporary fascial substitute. Curr Surg. 1987;44(1):31–4.
19. Rotondo MF, Schwab CW, McGonigal MD, Phillips GR, Fruchterman TM, Kauder DR, Latenser BA, Angood PA. 'Damage control': an approach for improved survival in exsanguinating penetrating abdominal injury. J Trauma. 1993;35:375–82; discussion 373–382.
20. Johnson JW, Gracias VH, Schwab CW, Reilly PM, Kauder DR, Shapiro MB, Dabrowski GP, Rotondo MF. Evolution in damage control for exsanguinating penetrating abdominal injury. J Trauma. 2001;51:261–9. ; discussion 269–271. https://doi.org/10.1097/00005373-200108000-00007.
21. Cothren CC, Moore EE, Hedegaard HB, Meng K. Epidemiology of urban trauma deaths: a comprehensive reassessment 10 years later. World J Surg. 2007;17:1507–11. https://doi.org/10.1007/s00268-007-9087-2.
22. World Health Organisation. World health statistics 2009: cause-specific mortality and morbidity.
23. BleedingControl.org. Bleeding control. www.bleedingcontrol.org/.
24. Cannon W. Traumatic shock. New York: D. Appleton and Company; 1923.

Trauma Management in Children

29

Elias Degiannis and Aidona Tsepelaki

29.1　Introduction Epidemiology: Differences from Adults

Trauma is the leading cause of death in children aged 1–14 years in the developed world; it is estimated that it is responsible for approximately one million deaths of children under the age of 18 years [1, 2]. According to most reports, so-called accidental injuries account for the vast majority (90%) of these cases, while the remainder (10%) is estimated to be due to violence or maltreatment [3]. Traffic-related accidents account for the majority of trauma resulting in death childhood and account for 48% of mortality from accidental trauma. The child can be injured as pedestrian, as a bicyclist, or as poorly secured motor vehicle passenger. Falls are also very common cause for trauma but less frequently result in death. Burns, sports, gunshot wounds, and child abuse are less frequent events with the latter being a significant cause of morbidity and mortality and especially important in children less than 1 year old where it accounts for the majority in deaths [1–4].

Due to the child's body habitus, greater force is applied per unit of body area leading to more multisystem injuries; therefore, in a child with significant trauma, assume that all organs are injured [4]. There are also other differences of the child's anatomy and physiology that the attending physician needs to be aware. The ratio body surface area/mass is large placing the child at greater risk for hypothermia and dehydration. Head injury is the most common cause of morbidity and mortality in pediatric trauma due to the relatively large head size, less neck control, and plasticity of brain tissues [5]. The pediatric skeleton has not fully calcified yet therefore

E. Degiannis (✉)
Department of Surgery, University of the Witwatersrand, Johannesburg, South Africa

Academic Trauma Unit, Milpark Hospital, Johannesburg, South Africa
e-mail: degiannis@yebo.co.za

A. Tsepelaki
Psychiatric Hospital of Attica "Dafni", Athens, Greece

© Springer Nature Switzerland AG 2021
E. Pikoulis, J. Doucet (eds.), *Emergency Medicine, Trauma and Disaster Management*, Hot Topics in Acute Care Surgery and Trauma,
https://doi.org/10.1007/978-3-030-34116-9_29

remains elastic, and internal injuries are possible without external injuries or fractures. This is true particularly for pulmonary contusion which can be significant without rib fractures, and when rib fractures are seen in a child, that means a massive amount of force has been applied [4].

Tongue and tonsils in children are large and may obstruct airway and make intubation difficult. Epiglottis is less stiff (risk of esophageal intubation), and larynx is funnel shaped and lies more cephalad and anteriorly. The narrowest point of the child's airway is at the cricoid cartilage providing a natural seal of the endotracheal tube. Trachea is short, and extra care should be taken not to intubate the right main bronchus [1, 4]. When resuscitating the pediatric patient, remember that its blood volume is 80 mL/kg [4, 6].

29.2 Primary Survey

Initial assessment of the injured child follows the same pattern as for adults, and adherence to the ABCDE protocol is important. Knowledge of the "normal" vital signs according to the age group (Table 29.1) is essential in order to recognize any compromise [1–4].

First priority is the child's airway. Do not forget that the child's occiput is larger and when placed like an adult on a spinal board, passive flexion of the cervical spine occurs. In order to correct this, spinal malalignment backboards modified with occipital recess or reinforced with a mattress pad under the child's body only (not the head) should be used [4]. This way the midface is parallel to the spine board in the "sniffing position" which is the proper position to maintain a patent airway.

Due to the anatomic differences mentioned earlier, handling pediatric airway requires expertise. Initially the child should be placed in the "sniffing" position and use standard airway maneuvers (chin lift or jaw thrust) to keep airway open while maintaining cervical spine alignment and immobilization. Always assume cervical spine injury, especially if there is head injury, until proven otherwise. If the child is unconscious, the oropharyngeal airway can also be helpful and should be gently inserted using a tongue depressor. If a patent airway cannot be maintained with the above and the child's ventilation may compromise, endotracheal intubation is indicated. The size of the endotracheal tube can be calculated by using the formula, ETT internal diameter = age/4 + 4 (>1 year), or by approximating the child's little finger to the tube diameter [1, 4]. Until the age of 9 uncuffed endotracheal tubes are used,

Table 29.1 Vital signs according to age

Age	Weight (kg)	Heart rate (beats/min)	Blood pressure (mmHg)	Respiratory rate (breaths/min)
0–1	<10	120–160	>60	<60
1–3	10–14	<150	>70	<40
3–5	14–18	<140	>75	<35
6–12	18–36	<120	>80	<30
>12	>36	<100	>90	<30

and nasotracheal airway should not be performed [4, 6]. Before attempting endotracheal intubation, always oxygenate the child. Most trauma centers have a protocol for intubation in major trauma referred to as rapid sequence intubation.

Orotracheal intubation is the method of choice for establishing an airway in an injured child, but when it cannot be achieved and the obstruction is not complete, a laryngeal mask airway can be used until expert help is available. When airway obstruction is complete and ventilation of the child cannot be accomplished otherwise, needle cricothyroidotomy should be considered [1, 4]. Needle jet insufflation through a cannula connected to a three-way tap and oxygen at 15 L/min via the cricothyroid membrane is a temporary measure (max 2 h) until tracheostomy is established. Surgical cricothyroidotomy is contraindicated in children younger than 12 years old [4].

Evaluation of breathing is next. High-flow supplemental oxygen should be administered to all children with major trauma. When examining the chest, keep in mind that rib fractures are rare in children, but there could be significant pulmonary injury without rib fracture [1–4]. Respiratory rate according to age is listed in Table 29.1. Tachypnea, agitation, and nasal flaring are signs of hypoxia which should be addressed aggressively by identifying the chest injury that is causing it [2]. Pneumothorax of hemothorax should be identified during the primary survey. In small children tension pneumothorax is better tolerated due to increased tissue elasticity, but once the clinical signs develop, the cardiovascular collapse is imminent. Any pleural disruption should be managed with the insertion of chest tube [4]. Smaller pediatric chest tubes should be easily available in the emergency department. The point of insertion is the same as in adults, the fifth intercostal space in the anterior axillary line [1, 4]. The skin incision should be placed one intercostal space below the intended space of chest entry to ensure a tunneled subcutaneous tract.

Next priority is the evaluation of circulation. Children have increased cardiac reserve, and 30% of their blood volume could be lost until any signs of hypovolemia appear. Pay close attention to the first signs of hypovolemic shock which are tachycardia, lethargy, peripheral shut down, and narrowing of pulse pressure. By the time hypotension appears, more than 45% of blood volume has been lost, and the child has decompensated [1, 2, 4]. If tachycardia changes to bradycardia, the situation is grave, and rapid infusion of both crystalloid and blood should take place. Therefore fluid resuscitation starts early with the first signs of shock. A warmed fluid bolus of 20 mL/kg should be administered, and if the child fails to hemodynamically normalize, a second 20 mL/kg bolus should follow. If after the second bolus the situation does not improve, a third bolus should start and consider giving blood (packed red blood cells 10 mL/kg) [4]. The blood should be warmed, and it is best if it is type specific, but if there is not enough time, group O-negative blood can be given. In the latest edition (10th) of ATLS, the initial 20 mL/kg bolus of isotonic crystalloid should be followed by weight-based blood product resuscitation with 10–20 mL/kg of RBC and 10–20 mL/kg of FFP and platelets. Because children have small blood volumes, they can lose significant amount of blood usually from scalp or other lacerations which can be controlled easily by applying direct pressure on the wound.

Peripheral venous access in a hypovolemic child can be particularly challenging. If after two or three attempts peripheral venous access cannot be established, the intraosseous route is an excellent alternative. Fluids and drugs can be given, but when venous access becomes available, it should be discontinued. The preferred site for cannulation is the proximal tibia distally to the tibial tuberosity, but if the tibia is fractured, it can be placed into the distal femur [1, 2, 4]. Central venous access should be attempted by personnel with expertise in children.

After clearing the ABC, next is assessing disability (D). In children the AVPU scale is used which stands for *a*lert, responsive to *v*erbal stimuli, responsive to *p*ainful stimuli, or *u*nresponsive. Also note pupillary size and reaction to light.

To complete primary survey, exposure should take place. While undressing the child to inspect the whole body, care should be taken to maintain normal temperature. Children are very prone to hypothermia due to the increased ratio of body surface area to body mass, thin skin, and decreased subcutaneous tissue. Fluids should be warmed, and warm blankets and overhead heat lamps can be used. Do not expose a child longer than needed.

29.3 Secondary Survey

During the secondary survey, the child is examined from head to toe. Complete history should be obtained. The child should be thoroughly examined for any injuries, and any further investigations needed apart from the standard trauma X-rays (chest and pelvis) should be obtained. Specialist examination and advice should take place. At the same time resuscitation and monitoring should continue, and if any deterioration occurs, the secondary survey should be abandoned and return to the ABC.

29.4 Management of Specific Trauma and Other Situations

29.4.1 Abdominal Trauma

The majority of abdominal injuries are a result of blunt trauma. Penetrating trauma is less frequent and usually the result of accidental gunshot discharges in small children or homicide attempts during adolescence. In children with a gunshot wound in the abdomen, laparotomy is mandatory, whereas stab wounds can be initially managed nonoperatively provided:

(a) The child is hemodynamically stable and cooperative.
(b) No signs of peritonitis exist.
(c) No intestinal of omental evisceration [4, 6].

Laparoscopy can also be an option in a *stable* child to evaluate the presence of intra-abdominal extension of a penetrating wound or diagnose a hollow viscus injury when diagnostic uncertainty remains despite radiology studies [3].

Intravenous contrast-enhanced CT (computer tomography) is the preferred diagnostic modality following abdominal trauma. It does require the child to be hemodynamically stable, cooperative, or sedated [1, 2, 4, 7].

CT allows expeditious evaluation of abdominal injuries. In children with solid abdominal organ injury, the preferred management is nonoperative which is now the standard of care. Children do better than adults when managed conservatively for all grades of splenic injury and the majority of liver and renal injuries with excellent outcomes. Nonoperative management is particularly important for spleen preservation to avoid the risk of overwhelming post-splenectomy sepsis [7, 8]. When managing nonoperatively a child who stabilized after having suffered hypovolemia, a pediatric ICU bed should be available.

On the other hand, when hemodynamic stability cannot be achieved despite aggressive resuscitation and blood in the abdomen has been confirmed by CT or FAST (focused assessment with sonography for trauma), a prompt laparotomy is indicated. No published prospective studies have identified a maximum transfusion volume at which children fail nonoperative management and need laparotomy. Consensus studies suggest that 40 mL/kg is a reasonable breakpoint at which failure is more likely. Other indications for urgent laparotomy are hollow viscus rupture and diaphragmatic rupture.

Very few children fail nonoperative management. In a retrospective study by Holmes [8] and colleagues, the rate of failure for nonoperative management at pediatric trauma centers was overall 5%. For isolated injuries the rate of failure for nonoperative management was 3% for liver and kidney, each respectively, 4% for spleen and 18% for pancreas. Failure of nonoperative management typically occurred within the first 12 h after injury and associated with injury severity and multiplicity, as well as isolated pancreatic injuries.

Transcatheter embolization techniques, first popularized in the early 1970s, are now a key component in the treatment of traumatic vascular injuries to solid abdominal organs in adults and can increase the proportion of patients treated nonoperatively. There have been reports of children with solid abdominal injury treated with angiography and embolization to achieve nonoperative management, but evidence-based guidelines for its use in the pediatric population have yet to be established [6, 7].

Conservative management includes hospital admission for 2–5 days of bed rest, intravenous hydration, antibiotic therapy, and monitoring of hemoglobin and vital signs. Young children and infants swallow large amounts of air when distressed. Even in minor trauma, significant gastric distention can occur which can cause abdominal tenderness and complicate the abdominal examination. Therefore, decompression of the stomach with a gastric tube is important due to the increased likelihood of vomiting and aspiration as well [2, 4, 7].

29.4.2 Head Trauma

More than 50% of deaths from trauma in the pediatric population result from head injury [5]. The disproportional large head and weak neck of children puts them in greater risk of head injury even in low velocity. Nevertheless the functional outcome is better in children than in adults [4].

Primary brain injury is the injury that occurs at the time of impact and it cannot be altered. Secondary brain injury is caused by the complications of primary brain injury (hypoxia due to cerebral edema) and exacerbated from hypoxia/hypovolemia caused by other injuries in the body. Secondary brain injury is preventable, and its prevention is of paramount importance for the outcome of the injured child [3, 5]. Therefore, to minimize brain damage, resuscitation should start the earliest possible and should be aggressive to ensure adequate blood volume circulation and oxygenation of the injured brain. Early intubation and ventilation is indicated to avoid hypoxia and progressive brain damage [4, 5]. Four to five percent of head injuries have an associated cervical spine injury, most often at C1–C3, so cervical spine should be immobilized until a C-spine injury has been excluded [2, 4].

In the initial assessment of child with a head injury, the Glasgow Coma Scale (GCS) should be measured to determine the severity of brain injury and monitor any deterioration with an objective scale. In young children the V (verbal) component has been modified as in Table 29.2. Emergency CT scan and early neurosurgical consultation should be sought if brain injury is suspected.

Hypoglycemia may also cause further brain damage especially in infants and should be monitored and corrected. Children are more susceptible to post-traumatic seizures even after minor trauma, and antiepileptic medication should be easily available [2, 4].

In infants bleeding into the subdural or epidural space can be significant enough to cause hypotension. This happens due to the open cranial sutures and fontanelle. Initial treatment is to restore the circulating blood volume as if the infant was bleeding from other body parts [4]. Subdural hematomas in infants generally have a poor outcome and many times are due to nonaccidental injury.

Despite adequate resuscitation brain edema and raised intracranial pressure (ICP) can take place. If this is the case, measures to decrease ICP should be taken. Most recommendations for the treatment of raised ICP are supported by level of evidence (III) and some by level of evidence (II). These include ICP monitoring in infants and children with severe brain injury (GCS < 9) and moderate hypothermia (32–33 °C) beginning within 8 h after severe brain injury for up to 48 duration and hypertonic treatment with hypertonic saline 3%. (Dosing range is 6.5–10 mL/kg h), Prophylactic hyperventilation is not recommended, and normocarbia should be

Table 29.2 Pediatric verbal score of GCS [4]

Verbal response	Score
Appropriate words, smile, fixes and follows	5
Cries but consolable	4
Persistently irritable	3
Restless, agitated	2
None	1

maintained with $PaCO_2 > 30$ mmHg, particularly during the first 48 h after injury [5]. Hyperventilation should be reserved only for patients with refractory intracranial hypertension, and when used, advanced neuromonitoring for evaluation of cerebral ischemia may be considered [5].

Other medications used to reduce ICP include diuretics (Mannitol 0.5–1.0 g/kg). Mannitol may worsen hypovolemia and therefore should be used with extreme caution in the early phases of resuscitation [4]. Also, high-dose barbiturate therapy may be considered in hemodynamically stable patients with refractory intracranial hypertension despite maximal medical and surgical management [9]. The use of corticosteroids is not recommended to improve outcome or reduce ICP [5]. Prophylactic use of antiseizure therapy is not recommended for preventing late post-traumatic seizures in children with severe brain injury but may be considered as a treatment option to prevent early post-traumatic seizures in young pediatric patients and infants. CSF drainage through an external ventricular drain may be considered for management of elevated ICP. Decompressive craniectomy can also be considered in intracranial hypertension resistant to medical therapy, but evidence supporting it is still limited [5]. Intracranial hematomas which can be extradural, subdural, and rarely intracerebral if producing a mass effect will need surgical drainage. Note that children may suffer intracranial hematoma, and at the time of injury, they may not have had any alteration in consciousness which is common in adults.

29.5 The Abused Child

Nonaccidental trauma is increasingly being recognized as a major mechanism for childhood injury and accounts for more than 1000 deaths annually in the United States. In the first year, nonaccidental injury is the commonest cause of major head injuries, and although nonaccidental trauma occurs in children of all ages, children between the ages 0 year and 3 years are at the greatest risk for death. Intentional injury should be considered in all children who present with trauma and have no clear history of accidental injury. No care provider wants to miss nonaccidental trauma and potentially expose a child to additional harm, but unfortunately a significant proportion of child abuse cases remain undetected placing the child at risk. Half of the abused children who return to the hospital dead were examined before, but the abuse was not reported [4].

Red flags for nonaccidental trauma should be raised if one of the following applies:

- Delays in seeking treatment.
- Inconsistent stories between historians.
- Caregivers who have an inappropriate affect.
- A pattern of injury that does not match what caregivers say happened.
- History of repeated trauma treated in different emergency departments.

If the physical exam reveals any of these symptoms, care providers should be suspicious and conduct a very detailed exam [4, 9]:

- Retinal hemorrhage.
- Torn frenulum, perioral injuries.
- Bruises, bite marks, burns.
- Multiple fractures, especially in long bones in children younger than 3 years.
- Subdural hematoma especially without skull fracture.
- Trauma to the genital or perianal area.
- Fractures of the ribs, skull, scapulae, or sternum.
- Metaphyseal corner fractures.
- Visceral injury without previous major trauma.
- Telltale marks to the skin from instruments or burns [4].

When child abuse is suspected, the child should be thoroughly examined, and documentation should be detailed. To protect the child, admit him or her to the hospital, and report the case to the police and the child protection services.

Bibliography

1. Browne GJ, Cocks AJ, McCaskill ME. Current trends in the management of major paediatric trauma. Emerg Med (Fremantle). 2001;13(4):418–25.
2. Dykes EH. Paediatric trauma. Br J Anaesth. 1999;83(1):130–8.
3. Sebastian van As AB. Paediatric trauma care. Afr J Paediatr Surg. 2010;7(3):129–33.
4. American College of Surgeons. Committee on trauma (2004) ATLS: advance trauma life support for doctors. 7th ed. Chicago: American College of Surgeons; 2004. p. 243–61, 275–81.
5. Lam WH, MacKersie A. Paediatric head injury: incidence, aetiology and management. Paediatr Anaesth. 1999;9(5):377–85.
6. Kochanek PM, Carney N, Adelson PD, Ashwal S, Bell MJ, Bratton S, Carson S, Chesnut RM, Ghajar J, Goldstein B, Grant GA, Kissoon N, Peterson K, Selden NR, Tasker RC, Tong KA, Vavilala MS, Wainwright MS, Warden CR, American Academy of Pediatrics-Section on Neurological Surgery, American Association of Neurological Surgeons/Congress of Neurological Surgeons, Child Neurology Society, European Society of Pediatric and Neonatal Intensive Care, Neurocritical Care Society, Pediatric Neurocritical Care Research Group, Society of Critical Care Medicine, Paediatric Intensive Care Society UK, Society for Neuroscience in Anesthesiology and Critical Care, World Federation of Pediatric Intensive and Critical Care Societies. Guidelines for the acute medical management of severe traumatic brain injury in infants, children, and adolescents--second edition. Pediatr Crit Care Med. 2012;13(Suppl 1):S1–82.
7. Notrica DM, Linnaus ME. Nonoperative management of blunt solid organ injury in pediatric surgery. Surg Clin North Am. 2017;97(1):1–20.
8. Holmes JH, et al. The failure of nonoperative management in pediatric solid organ injury: a multi-institutional experience. J Trauma. 2005;59(6):1309–13.
9. Lee JK, Brady KM, Deutsch N. The anesthesiologist's role in treating abusive head trauma. Anesth Analg. 2016;122(6):1971–82.

Trauma Management in Pregnant Women

30

Elias Degiannis and Aidona Tsepelaki

30.1 Introduction

When dealing with a pregnant trauma patient, the challenge is great since the orchestration of trauma care has the addition of obstetric complications. Every female trauma patient of reproductive age should be considered pregnant until proven otherwise [1]. Once the patient is identified as pregnant, the doctor must remember there two patients that need proficient evaluation and management. Nevertheless, initial treatment priorities for an injured pregnant patient remain the same as for the nonpregnant patient. During pregnancy physiologic and anatomic changes occur in the body, and familiarity with these normal changes is essential since they can mimic or mask an injury making diagnosis difficult. Except the maternal complications of trauma, there are also unique pregnancy-related complications including abruptio placentae, fetomaternal hemorrhage, and the possibility of isoimmunization, preterm labor, fetal injury, and death.

30.2 Incidence and Etiology of Injury

Trauma in pregnancy is the leading nonobstetric cause of maternal death and the most common cause of fetal demise [2, 3]. Up to 6–7% of pregnancies are complicated by some degree of trauma, 0.4% will require hospital admission, and 0.1% of cases will be victims of major trauma. Fetal mortality is also a considerable issue,

E. Degiannis (✉)
Department of Surgery, University of the Witwatersrand, Johannesburg, South Africa

Academic Trauma Unit, Milpark Hospital, Johannesburg, South Africa
e-mail: degiannis@yebo.co.za

A. Tsepelaki
Psychiatric Hospital of Attica "Dafni", Athens, Greece

© Springer Nature Switzerland AG 2021
E. Pikoulis, J. Doucet (eds.), *Emergency Medicine, Trauma and Disaster Management*, Hot Topics in Acute Care Surgery and Trauma,
https://doi.org/10.1007/978-3-030-34116-9_30

with 3–7 fetal deaths per 100,000 live births as a result of trauma [3]. The most common causes of trauma during pregnancy are motor vehicle accidents (49%), falls (25%), assaults (18%), guns (4%), and burns (1%) [4]. Fetal deaths have a different etiology: motor vehicle accidents (82%), gunshot (6%), and falls (3%) with maternal death accounting for 11% of the fetal deaths [5].

In a retrospective analysis of 321 pregnant trauma patients, blunt trauma was noted to be ten times more common than penetrating trauma. However, maternal mortality was noted to be higher in the penetrating trauma group (7%) than the blunt trauma group (2%) [3, 6]. The fetal mortality difference in penetrating and blunt trauma was even more pronounced at 73% and 10%, respectively [3, 6]. Penetrating trauma should immediately raise concern for impending fetal demise. Fetal loss is much less common with minor injuries (1–5%), but these injuries are much more common than major trauma. As a result, the majority of fetal losses follow relatively minor trauma.

30.3 Anatomic and Physiologic Changes in Pregnancy
(Table 30.1)

30.3.1 Anatomic

The uterus is limited to the pelvis only for the first 12 weeks of gestation. By week 20 it is at the umbilicus, and at 34–36 weeks, it reaches the costal margin (Fig. 30.1). As the gravid uterus enlarges, the bowel is pushed cephalad encased by the lower rib cage and lying anterior to the retroperitoneal organs. This results to the bowel being protected, whereas the uterus and its contents are more vulnerable [1]. However, penetrating trauma to the upper abdomen during last weeks of gestation can result in more complex intestinal injury [1]. During the second trimester of pregnancy, the uterus rises above the pelvis, but the fetus is well protected by a generous amount of amniotic fluid. If the amniotic fluid gains access to the intravascular space because of trauma, it can be a source of amniotic fluid embolism and disseminated intravascular coagulation. During the third trimester, the uterus is large and thin walled, and the fetal head is usually within the pelvis which can be injured if pelvic fractures occur [1].

The dextrorotation of the enlarging uterus can cause right-sided ureteral dilation, and the bladder is also pushed superiorly, and this can cause bilateral ureteral dilation [1]. Other anatomic alterations include the slight widening of the pubic symphysis and an altered center of balance which predisposes to falls. The diaphragm is raised approximately 4 cm, and the thoracic anteroposterior diameter increases [7].

The enlarged uterus can cause aortocaval compression reducing venous return and consequently cardiac output. This diminished cardiac output may result in significant hypotension, which often results in vasovagal-type symptoms. To avoid this, it is important to remember placing the pregnant woman in the left lateral decubitus position during her evaluation and monitoring.

Table 30.1 Alterations during pregnancy

Parameter	Change during normal pregnancy	Normal range during pregnancy
Systolic blood pressure	Decreases by an average of 5–15 mmHg	110–110 mmHg
Diastolic blood pressure	Decreases by 5–15 mmHg	50–70 mmHg
Mean arterial pressure	Decreases by 10 mmHg	80 mmHg
Central venous pressure	Slightly decreases or no change	2–7 mmHg
Heart rate	Increases by 10–15 beats/min	75–95 beats/min
Cardiac output	Increases by 30–50%	6–7 L/min at rest
Blood volume	Increases by 30–50%	4500 mL
Red blood cell volume	Increases by 30%	
Hematocrit	Decreases	32–34%
White blood cell count	May increase	5000–15,000 mm^{-3}
Fibrinogen	Increases	300–600 mg/dL
Factors I, II, V, VII, X, XII	Increases	
Upper airway	Increased edema; capillary engorgement	
Diaphragm	Displaced 4 cm cephalad	
Respiratory rate	Slightly increases in the first trimester	
Oxygen consumption	Increases 15–20% at rest	
PaCO$_2$	Decreases	27–32 mmHg
PaO$_2$	Increase	100–108 mmHg
Tidal volume	Increases 40%	600 mL
Minute ventilation	Increases 40%	10.5 L/min
Functional residual capacity	Decreases 20–25%	
Intra-abdominal organs	Compartmentalization and cephalad displacement	
Gastrointestinal tract	Decreased gastric emptying; decreased motility	
Peritoneum	Small amounts of intraperitoneal fluid normally present	
Musculoskeletal system	Widened symphysis pubis and sacroiliac joints	
Kidneys	Mild hydronephrosis (right > left)	
Renal blood flow and GFR	Increases by 60%	
Serum creatinine	Decreases	0.6–0.7 mg/dL
Serum urea nitrogen	Decreases	3–3.5 mg/dL

30.3.2 Changes in Physiology

30.3.2.1 Cardiovascular

One of the most prominent changes during pregnancy takes place in the cardiovascular system. First there is decreased peripheral vascular resistance due to progesterone-related smooth muscle relaxation. During the second trimester, blood pressure gradually declines by 5–15 mmHg and returns to normal prepregnancy values at the end of third trimester [7]. There is an increase in heart rate by 10–15 beats per minute due to increase in alpha receptors of the myometrium stimulated

Fig. 30.1 Uterine size by week of gestation

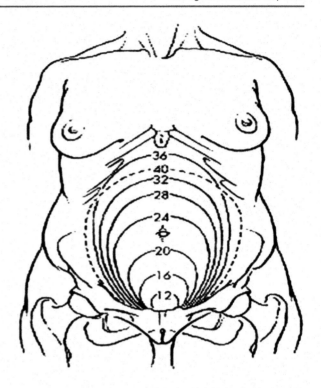

by estrogens [1]. The decrease in vascular resistance of the uterus and the placenta along with the increase in plasma volume results in an increased cardiac output up to 45% than normal. During labor there is an additional increase in cardiac output as each uterine contraction results in blood transfer from the uterus back into circulation. Electrocardiographic changes include flat or inverted T waves in leads III, aVF, V1, and V2 and Q waves in leads III and aVF [1, 8] . All the above changes mimic the first stages of shock, making the distinction from the normal physiologic changes of pregnancy challenging. However, do not be misled into attributing tachycardia or hypotension in the pregnant trauma patient to normal physiologic changes until a thorough workup for traumatic injury is complete.

30.3.2.2 Hematology

Blood volume increases during pregnancy by 30–50%. However, the increase in plasma volume is greater than the increase in red cell mass, and that results in the physiologic anemia of pregnancy (hematocrit of 31–35%). A pregnant woman can lose up to 1500 mL of blood and exhibit no signs of hypovolemia, but the fetus might be in distress since the uterine blood flow which comprises up to 20% of maternal cardiac output has no autoregulation and is totally dependent on maternal mean arterial pressure [1, 6, 8].

There is also an increase in white blood cells and in nearly all coagulation factors. This hypercoagulable state helps to protect from hemorrhage during delivery but on the other hand predisposes to thromboembolism or disseminated intravascular coagulation in case of massive hemorrhage or infection [6–8].

30.3.2.3 Respiratory

Oxygen consumption increases by 15–20% [1, 7, 8] during pregnancy, so it is crucial during the resuscitation process to keep the patient adequately oxygenated. The diaphragm is pushed cephalad, and the rib cage adjusts by increasing its anteroposterior and lateral diameters. Functional residual capacity decreases, but tidal volume and minute ventilation increase about 40% as the respiratory rate, which slightly increases in the first trimester, returns to baseline. Due to hyperventilation caused by progesterone, $PaCO_2$ decreases (at about 30 mmHg), but despite the slight respiratory alkalosis, pH remains normal due to metabolic compensation by the renal tubules excreting bicarbonate [1]. Keep in mind that a normal $PaCO_2$ of 40 mmHg in a pregnant patient may indicate respiratory failure, and since the pregnant patient has little oxygen reserve, rapid hypoxia can occur when respiratory stress is introduced. Fetal oxygenation remains constant provided the maternal PaO_2 remains above 60 mmHg. Below this PaO_2 level, fetal oxygenation drops precipitously [7].

The mucosa throughout the respiratory tract is swelled including that of nasal, oropharynx, larynx, and trachea putting the pregnant patient at a greater risk for airway management problems and difficult intubation than the nonpregnant patient [7].

30.3.2.4 Urinary

As mentioned before there is dilatation of the ureters and renal pelvises usually more pronounced on the right side due to the dextrorotation of the uterus [1]. Due to the increase of blood volume, renal perfusion increases and so does the glomerular filtration rate resulting in a significant decrease in serum creatinine and serum urea nitrogen [8]. Therefore if the values of creatinine and urea nitrogen are "normal," this should alert for a possible renal compromise.

30.3.2.5 Gastrointestinal

Smooth muscle relaxation induced by progesterone leads to delayed gastric emptying and lower esophageal sphincter tone [8]. This along with the cephalad displacement of the stomach places the pregnant patient at high risk for aspiration [1]. Therefore, placement of nasogastric tube early is important. Due to the gradual growth of the uterus and the chronic stretching of the parietal peritoneum, it is desensitized to irritation, and physical examination may not reveal tenderness and guarding despite intraperitoneal bleeding.

30.4   Assessment and Management

When managing the pregnant patient, it is recommended to early and aggressively resuscitate the mother to achieve the best outcome for her and the fetus. Assess the fetus after finishing primary survey of the mother.

30.4.1 Primary Survey

The ABCDEs of the initial assessment are the same as for the nonpregnant trauma patient [1].

Assuring a patent airway is essential, and keep in mind that pregnant women with an unsecured airway are at increased risk for aspiration of gastric contents. Intubation is more difficult in pregnant patients, with failed intubations being eight times more likely [2]. Adherence to the algorithm is essential, immediate administration of high-flow oxygen is very important, and ensuring adequate ventilation and circulating blood volume for oxygenation of the mother and fetus is of paramount importance. Log roll the pregnant patient to the left lateral position, and manually displace the uterus to the left side to relieve pressure from the inferior vena cava. If you need to insert a chest tube, this should be done one or two intercostal spaces higher due to the cephalad displacement of the diaphragm and the increase in the anteroposterior diameter of the rib cage [8]. Due to the increased maternal blood volume, signs of hypovolemia may not be present until one third of blood is lost; therefore fluid resuscitation must be aggressive, and if transfusion is indicated, it should be done with type-specific packed red blood cells. If there is not enough time, O Rh (−) blood can be used [8]. Remember that the fetus might be in distress even when the mother is hemodynamically normal. Because of their adverse effect on uteroplacental perfusion, vasopressors in pregnant women should be used only for intractable hypotension that is unresponsive to fluid resuscitation. The abdominal portion of military anti-shock trousers should not be inflated on a pregnant woman because this may reduce placental perfusion [5, 7].

Abdominal pain, tenderness, and guarding can suggest abruptio placentae or uterine rupture. The above situations can be accompanied by shock. Abnormal fetal position, palpation of fetal parts, and inability to palpate uterine fundus suggest uterine rupture which mandates operative exploration. Uterine tenderness and irritability, vaginal bleeding, and preterm labor are signs of abruptio placentae. Abruption may follow even minor trauma, and treatment should never be delayed for ultrasound confirmation because ultrasonography is not reliable in diagnosing the lesion [1, 4, 7].

30.4.2 Adjuncts to Primary Survey and Resuscitation

In pregnant women with a viable fetus (≥23 weeks) and suspected uterine contractions, placental abruption, or traumatic uterine rupture, urgent obstetrical consultation is recommended. All pregnant women at 20 weeks' gestation or longer should have cardiotocographic monitoring for 2–6 h after a traumatic injury which should be prolonged if uterine contractions are occurring [2]. Fetal heart rate ranges from 120 to 160 beats/min. Any abnormality in the fetal heart rate or frequent uterine activity may be a sign of fetal distress and maternal decompensation [1].

X-rays should be performed without delay as indicated with the uterus shielded. Focused assessment with sonography in trauma (FAST) examination is useful in pregnancy [1, 2]. Most studies have been able to report a sensitivity of approximately 80% and a specificity of 100% for detecting major abdominal injury [6]. Direct peritoneal lavage using an open technique is feasible during pregnancy and appears to be without any specific pregnancy-related complications; the catheter should be placed above the umbilicus.

30.4.3 Secondary Survey

The pregnant secondary survey should be thorough, and in addition to the routine history, obstetric history should be included. During physical examination all body parts of the pregnant trauma patient should be exposed and thoroughly examined, and an evaluation of the pregnancy should be included with a pelvic examination to identify vaginal bleeding, ruptured membranes, or a bulging perineum. In cases of vaginal bleeding at or after 23 weeks, speculum or digital vaginal examination should be deferred until placenta previa is excluded. Vaginal bleeding may indicate disruption of the placenta, preterm labor, or uterine rupture [1].

Further X-ray imaging and CT scan, if indicated, they should be performed. There have been no reported adverse fetal outcomes with regard to less than 5 rad of exposure, and all common trauma imaging falls well below this threshold (Table 30.2) [7]

Laboratory testing in the pregnant trauma patient should include hemoglobin, hematocrit, coagulation studies, typing and cross matching, and urine test [2, 4, 9]. Fibrinogen values are often more than 400 mg/dL during pregnancy; therefore the normal values of 250–300 mg/dL for a nonpregnant patient may actually signify mild hypofibrinogenemia, and levels below 200 mg/dL may indicate disseminated intravascular coagulation which develops rapidly after extensive placenta separation or amniotic fluid embolism. Treatment consists of rapid uterine evacuation and replacement of platelets, fibrinogen, and clotting factors [2, 4, 9]. Kleihauer-Betke test should also be obtained for patients in their second or third trimester to determine if there is any fetal blood in the maternal circulation. A negative Kleihauer-Betke test does not exclude minor degree of fetomaternal hemorrhage which is capable of sensitizing the Rh (−) mother, so Rh immunoglobulin therapy should be administered to all Rh (−) negative women following abdominal trauma. In Rh-negative pregnant trauma patients, quantification of maternal-fetal hemorrhage

Table 30.2 Radiation exposure to an unshielded uterus/fetus [8]

Examination	Fetal exposure (rad)
Chest X-ray	0.000045
Pelvis X-ray	0.04
Cervical spine X-ray	0.002
Abdomen CT	1–4
Head CT	<0.05
Chest CT	<0.01

by tests such as Kleihauer-Betke should be done to determine the need for additional doses of anti-D immunoglobulin [2, 6, 7].

Hospital admission and cardiotocographic monitoring is recommended for pregnant patients who exhibit the following: uterine tenderness, significant abdominal pain, vaginal bleeding, sustained contractions (>1/10 min), rupture of the membranes, atypical or abnormal fetal heart rate pattern, high-risk mechanism of injury, or serum fibrinogen <200 mg/dL [2].

30.5 Additional Considerations for Etiologies of Trauma and Other Conditions

30.5.1 Penetrating Trauma

Penetrating trauma in pregnancy is caused mainly by gunshot or stab wounds. Stab wounds tend to have better prognosis as in the nonpregnant population. As the gravid uterus enlarges, the bowel is pushed upward; therefore penetrating injury to the abdomen can result in more complex bowel injury if it is in the upper abdomen, but on the other hand, the uterus provides protection to the mother from anterior penetrating wounds [1, 2, 7, 8]. The uterine musculature can absorb great amount of the projectiles velocity, and it is rare to penetrate the posterior wall of the uterus; therefore the maternal viscera are often not involved [8]. Unfortunately, with penetrating trauma the fetus more often sustains significant injury (60–70%) and subsequently dies (40–65%) [1, 2, 8]

Management and resuscitation of pregnant women with penetrating trauma follow the same principles of ATLS and everything described previously in the chapter apply.

Nonoperative management should be considered if the following criteria are fulfilled:

1. Stable maternal vital signs
2. No evidence of fetal distress in the case of a viable fetus
3. Anterior entry wound below the level of the uterine fundus
4. Radiographic visualization of the foreign body, if any [8]

Close monitoring of both mother and fetus in an intensive care setting is required. A viable fetus demonstrating evidence of distress is an indication for immediate caesarean delivery regardless of the site of injury. Such an approach should be carried out only in high-level trauma centers.

The same indications for laparotomy apply as in the nonpregnant patient. If the decision made is to proceed with laparotomy, that does not mean that Caesarean section should be carried out at the same time. If it is known that the fetus is dead because of the penetrating trauma, it is better to proceed by inducing labor and deliver vaginally several hours later because Caesarian section spends time and blood at the time of laparotomy [8]. If, however, the fetus is in distress, the uterus has significant injuries that need repair, or the gravid uterus prevents surgical exposure for repair of maternal injuries, Caesarean section should be considered. The decision to proceed with Caesarean section should be weighed against the likelihood for fetal survival and long-term complications of prematurity and should be made in consultation with the trauma surgeon, neonatologist, and pediatric surgeon [8]. Tetanus vaccination is safe in pregnancy and should be given according to the usual protocol.

30.5.2 Domestic Violence

Domestic violence is common during pregnancy, and its incidence is clustered in the third trimester [2]. A pregnant woman is more likely to suffer domestic abuse than preeclampsia. The most commonly struck body area is the abdomen. These attacks can result in death and disability [6, 7]. When managing a pregnant woman with trauma, particularly penetrating abdominal trauma, there should be a high index of suspicion of domestic violence, and the woman should be asked specifically and in the absence of the partner. The most effective strategies for identifying domestic violence are screening questionnaires followed by in-person interviews by highly trained individuals [1, 6, 7]. Everything should be documented carefully and with detail. If domestic violence is suspected, consultation with social services should not be delayed [1].

30.5.3 Perimortem Caesarean Section

Perimortem C-section is defined as a Caesarean section performed in the face of maternal cardiac arrest. Unfortunately, there is little evidence regarding the perimortem C-section in pregnant trauma patients, and recommendations are mostly based on expert opinions and experience [1]. It should be emphasized that many studies and case reports relate to nontraumatic cardiac arrests in which the maternal resuscitation efforts were the major indication for delivery. Trauma patients with cardiac arrest are less likely to respond to resuscitation; in these cases, perimortem Caesarean is performed primarily for fetal salvage. Considering the fact that the fetus can be in distress due to hypovolemia even when the maternal vital signs are normal, by the time there is maternal cardiac arrest, the fetus has suffered prolonged hypoxia [1, 2, 5, 8].

A perimortem Caesarean section is recommended for viable pregnancies ($\geq$23 weeks, or fundal height 2 or more fingerbreadths above the umbilicus), and this should be performed within 4 min of maternal cardiac arrest and properly performed cardiopulmonary resuscitation for any acceptable outcome [1, 2, 8]. After 5 min of maternal cardiac arrest, perimortem C-section is unlikely to result in a viable normal infant, and since it is an extremely emotional practice, much consideration should be taken when acting outside this time frame [2]. No fetal survival has been reported in the absence of fetal heartbeats before the perimortem C-section.

Bibliography

1. American College of Surgeons. Committee on trauma (2004) ATLS: advance trauma life support for doctors. 7th ed. Chicago: American College of Surgeons; 2004. p. 243–61, 275–81.
2. Jain V, Chari R, Maslovitz S, Farine D. Guidelines for the management of a pregnant trauma patient. J Obstet Gynaecol Can. 2015;37(6):553–71.
3. Battaloglu E, McDonnell D, Chu J, Lecky F, Porter K. Epidemiology and outcomes of pregnancy and obstetric complications in trauma in the United Kingdom. Injury. 2016;47(1):184–7.
4. Mirza FG, Devine PC, Gaddipati S. Trauma in pregnancy: a systematic approach. Am J Perinatol. 2010;27:579–86.
5. Mattox KL, Goetzl L. Trauma in pregnancy. Crit Care Med. 2005;33(10 Suppl):S385–9.
6. Lucia A, Dantoni SE. Trauma management of the pregnant patient. Crit Care Clin. 2016;32(1):109–17.
7. Muench MV, Canterino JC. Trauma in pregnancy. Obstet Gynecol Clin North Am. 2007;34(3):555–83.
8. Velmahos GC, Degiannis E, Doll D. Penetrating trauma a practical guide on operative technique and peri-operative management. 2nd ed. Berlin: Springer; 2017. p. 565–70.
9. Mendez-Figueroa H, Dahlke JD, Vrees RA, Rouse DJ. Trauma in pregnancy: an updated systematic review. AJOG. 2013;209(1):1–10.

Blood Transfusion in Trauma

31

Panteleimon Vassiliu

31.1 The Problem

Trauma is the leading cause of death in ages until 44 years. Exsanguination is responsible for many of those deaths, accounting for >80% of deaths in the operating room and half of the deaths within 24 h from injury. When blood loss is >150 mL/min or 50% of blood volume in 20 min, mortality peaks. Fortunately 90% of trauma patients will not require any transfusion and their mortality is less than 1%. For this majority, blood transfusion is required only as an exception, and with the leisure that hemodynamic stability offers. We focus on the 3–5% of trauma patients that bleed massively (MB) (>10 units of PRBC within 24 h) and require massive transfusion (MT) (replace 100% of patient's blood in <24 h, or administration of 50% of the patient's blood volume in 1 h) [1].

31.2 How You Identify Patients Needing MT Early?

Definition of MB requires 24 h before establishing the criterion, and this is far too late for action. Early identification of these patients is feasible with clinical judgement coming with experience, which lacks from the readers of this book. Objective criteria to identify on admission the patient in need for MT have been proposed [2]. Assessment of Blood Consumption (ABC) [3] is a simple and effective score:

- Heart rate on arrival >120 bpm (no = 0, yes = 1)
- Blood pressure on arrival <90 mmHg (no = 0, yes = 1)

P. Vassiliu (✉)
University of Athens (NKUA), 4th Surgical Department, "Attikon" University Hospital, Athens, Greece

© Springer Nature Switzerland AG 2021
E. Pikoulis, J. Doucet (eds.), *Emergency Medicine, Trauma and Disaster Management*, Hot Topics in Acute Care Surgery and Trauma,
https://doi.org/10.1007/978-3-030-34116-9_31

- Penetrating mechanism (no = 0, yes = 1)
- Positive abdominal fluid (blood) on ultrasound (no = 0, yes = 1)

If two or more of those criteria are met, a MT protocol (MTP) should be initiated.

31.3   What Is Massive Transfusion Protocol (MTP)?

An algorithm of coordinated action from many hospital departments (surgery, blood bank, ICU, anesthesiology) activated upon arrival of a MB trauma patient. The protocol provides roles for the personnel, actions to be taken, medications and blood products to be transfused. Target is the increase of survival of the MB patient. Fountain of MTP is the recently acquired knowledge in modern battlefields, which has dramatically changed the way we manage these patients. Some of this knowledge is exposed at this chapter.

31.4   What Should We Transfuse?

It took half a century and a couple of wars to understand the self-evident: "Humans bleed FRESH WHOLE BLOOD (FWB), and not starch (also known as colloid, transfused for its oncotic effect on depleted intravascular space) or other fluid."

Logistics rather than choice compelled us to break blood into components [Packed Red Blood Cells (PRBC), Fresh Frozen Plasma (FFP), Platelets (PLT)] and store it, to have it available on demand.

31.5   Why WHOLE blood?

Human is O_2 depended organism and O_2 depletion creates within minutes major damage due to hypoxia. Thus, naturally, we prioritize hypoxia reversal in an exsanguinating patient, so we transfuse massively PRBC. Lethal mistake. Evidences from the Iraqi war and recently from studies in civil trauma, highlighted the advantage of FWB in the resuscitation and survival of the exsanguinating patient [1]. The rational behind it is that blood has more functions than O_2 carrier:

- Oncotic pressure (from plasma, stored FFP)
- Coagulation function (clotting factors in FFP, and PLT)
- Temperature homeostasis (warm circulating fluid)

Our practise to transfuse excessively crystalloids and PRBC dilute native clotting factors causing hypocoagulation [4]. This aggravates the coagulopathy initiated from the moment of injury due to:

1. The injury itself, and in proportion to its extent: (Hypoperfusion → ↑activated protein C → ↑*tissue* plasminogen activator → ↑fibrinolysis)

2. Loss of warm blood and replacement with cooler fluid → ↓ body temperature
3. Hypoperfusion → Anaerobic metabolism → Lactate production → ↓pH

Biochemical reactions within the body need specific, narrow temperature and pH range to proceed. Coagulation cascade doesn't proceed even in the presence of all the clotting factors, when tissue pH and temperature are out of that range.

This is defined as Acute Coagulopathy of Trauma-Shock (ACoTS) [5], and differs from Disseminated Intravascular Coagulopathy (DIC), which may develop after hours or days, when the septic component adds its consequences to trauma.

FWB offers warmth, and PRBC, FFP, PLT in natural proportions to cover the need of the exsanguinating patient for oxygen, oncotic pressure, and blunt most of the ACoTS. A 500 mL unit of FWB has a hematocrit of 38–50%, 150,000–400,000 fully functional PLT/mm^3, and 100% activity of clotting factors diluted only by the 70 mL of anticoagulant. In addition, the viability and flow characteristics of fresh RBC are better than their stored counterparts that have metabolic depletion and membrane dysfunction [6]. FWB unless in a military environment with a lot of healthy, screened, young blood carriers, it is not available. What is available is blood components. So next quest is what are the optimal proportions of those components to be transfused. No class I evidences on that. Military clinical research [2, 6] and newer studies on civil trauma [2] suggest transfusion of PRBC:FFP:PLT in a proportion of 1:1:1. Consider the mixture of one PRBC unit (335 mL) with a hematocrit of 55%, one unit of platelets (50 mL) with 5.5×10^{10} platelets, and one unit of FFP (275 mL) with 80% coagulation factor activity. This combination results in 660 mL of fluid with a hematocrit of 29%, 88,000 PLT per microliter, and 65% coagulation factor activity [6]. Comparison favors largely FWB but the blood components transfusion is the best feasible alternative.

31.6 Why FRESH Blood?

1. FWB if warm can be transfused within 24 h. It is considered still fresh if stored at 4 °C for 48 h [4]. If less than 8 h old can be refrigerated for 3 weeks [6], remaining transfusable but not fresh.
   (a) Levels of clotting factors V and VIII decline quickly for 24 h after collection. The rate of decline slows until clinically subnormal levels are reached within 7–14 days. It is because FWB contains these factors that it is recommended for massive transfusion and is so effective in correction of ACoTS. The other clotting factors remain stable in stored blood.
   (b) FWB has lost most of its platelets after 3 days of storage.
2. Stored PRBC (max 42 days with current FDA-approved storage solutions) [4] develops defects, proportionate to the duration of storage, that assume greater clinical significance when transfused rapidly, or in large quantities, that is in critically ill patients:
   (a) ↓ ATP

(b) Degradation of 2,3Diphosphoglycerate (2,3DPG), after 7–10 days in storage. 2,3DPG is an enzyme affecting Hgb affinity to O_2. After 7 days of storage Hgb oxygen transporting ability drops by 2/3. Adenine added to PRBC may restore levels of 2,3DPG in vivo after transfusion, although no level 1 evidences on that.

(c) Red cell membrane instability leading to cell rupture.

(d) ↑ potassium (K^+) release, hyperkalemia after 5–7 days of storage: Serum potassium levels rise in stored blood as the efficiency of the Na^+/K^+ pump decreases. Transfused blood may have a potassium concentration of 40–70 mmol/L. Transient hyperkalemia may occur as a result.

(e) ↑ ammonia release, due to release of intracellular protein.

(f) Age of PRBC >14–28 days independently relates with [4]:
  • Increase of microaggregates (platelet/leukocyte/fibrin thrombi) in buffy coat (a 1% fraction of the whole blood laying after centrifugation between red cells and plasma, containing white blood cells, usually contaminating PRBC) which cause:
    – Impaired pulmonary gas exchange, adult respiratory distress syndrome (ARDS), TRLI (transfusion related lung injury)
    – Reticulo-endothelial system (RES) depression
    – Activation of complement, coagulation cascades, DVT
    – Vaso-active substances, impaired vasoregulation, perfusion issues
    – Inflammatory mediators, immune dysfunction, infections
    – Antigenic stimulation
    – Acute phase response
    – MOF
    – DVT
    – DEATH

3. FFP. Contains all clotting factors of the coagulation cascade. Thawed plasma is FFP brought to 1–6 °C and stored for 5 days. This timeline is based on lifetime of factors V and VIII. Recent study shows that thawed plasma stored at 4 °C retains significant clotting function for up to 14 days [4].

4. PLTs have also minimal lifetime and usually are lost after 3–5 days of storage.

Despite above evidences, average age of PRBC in the USA is 21 days [2], while in combat theatres of Southeast Asia is >30 days [2].

31.7 Other RISKS of Blood Transfusion

1. PRBC
   Transfusion transmitted infections
   (a) Hepatitis A, B, C, and D
   (b) HIV "window period"
   (c) CMV
   (d) Atypical mononucleosis and swinging temp 7–10 days post transfusion

(e) Malaria

(f) Brucellosis

(g) Yersinia

(h) Syphilis

Hemolytic transfusion reactions

(a) Incompatibility: ABO, Rh (Type), and 26 others (Screen)

(b) Frozen blood, overheated blood, pressurized blood

(c) Immediate generalized reaction (plasma)

Immunological complications

(a) Major incompatibility reaction (usually caused by "wrong blood" due to administrative errors)

Post-transfusion purpura.

Graft-versus-host disease.

(a) Transfusion-related acute lung injury

Immunomodulation

(a) Reports on transplant and oncology patients have provided evidence that transfusion induces a regulatory immune response in the recipient that increases the ratio of suppressor to helper T cells.

(b) These changes may render the trauma patient more susceptible to infection.

Hemostatic Failure

(a) Hypothermia (1 unit 4 °C → 37 °C) = 1255 kJ

(b) Acidosis (Citrate, Lactate)

2. FFP [4]

(a) Allergic reactions

(b) Transfusion-associated acute lung injury (TRALI)

(c) Transfusion-associated cardiac overload (TACO)

(d) Acute respiratory distress syndrome (ARDS)

3. PLT [4]

(a) Bacterial contamination

(b) DVT

(c) Febrile reactions

(d) Transfusion of pooled platelets carries a greater risk of infection, as several donors have contributed to a single pack of platelets

Despite the aforementioned extensive list, there are *no* level 1 evidences regarding PRBC transfusion risks. There are level 2 evidences that PRBC transfusion is independent risk factor for [7]:

1. Increased nosocomial infection (wound infection, pneumonia, sepsis) rates.
2. MOF and SIRS.
3. Longer ICU and hospital length of stay, increased complications, and increased mortality.
4. There is no definitive evidence that prestorage leukocyte depletion of RBC transfusion reduces complication rates, but some studies have shown a reduction in infectious complications.
5. There is a relationship between transfusion and ALI and ARDS.

So blood is "bad" but there is no alternative so far. The less "bad" blood is the WFB, and is surrogate the components transfusion to reconstitute whole blood.

31.8   How You Monitor Your MT Effort?

It is evident so far that reversing hypoxia and acidosis is as important as to reverse coagulopathy. Blood gas analyzer at bedside is a valuable device that gives within 1 min the value of Hgb, pH, Lactic acid.

Regarding coagulation status things are not that simple. The classical coagulation panel that evaluates quantitatively intrinsic and extrinsic clotting paths and fibrinogen is of little practical value in the exsanguinating patient. The limitations are:

1. Time consuming. Blood specimen is centrifuged for 10 min, and then is introduced in the analyzer. Modern analyzers have the ability to process up to 120 specimens within 10–120 min. Result is a quantitative estimation on pT, aPTT, and INR. An equally time-consuming procedure evolving simultaneously gives a quantitative result on fibrinogen concentration and PLT number (not function). Utilizing an apparatus that can process 120 specimens for only 1 is not cost effective but it is ethical in a case of exsanguination. The complete coagulation panel including transportation of blood specimens requires 20–30 min to give result. This is equivalent to "light years" for the critically ill, and in addition the result is obsolete as the coagulation status changes every minute due to the evolving coagulopathy, and the resuscitation efforts.
2. Thermal effect. The coagulation panel is performed by warming the specimen at 36.6 °C. The effect of hypothermia on the coagulation enzymes is reversed, and as long as all clotting factors are present in the blood specimen, the blood clots in the lab, while fails in vivo due to the hypothermia.
3. Quantitative result: Number of platelets even if normal do not contain the information on their ability to clot. Qualitative, functional result is more important that the absolute numbers and classic metabolic panel don't give this result.

In practice your options for effective monitoring of coagulation status are two:

1. If MT criteria are fulfilled and have no way to measure coagulation status *real time*, you transfuse empirically:
   (a) Control during a damage control operation all surgical bleeding.
   (b) Start from the first moment, with 2 U of PRBC.
   (c) For every additional PRBC, give 1 unit of FFP (+/−2 mL/kg), and one simple unit of PLT. The adult dose of PLT transfusion is 6 simple units, or the equivalent, 1 apheresis Mega unit derived from concentration of 6 simple PLT units. If apheresis PLT is available, transfuse it after 6 units of PRBC, and 6 units of FFP (6:6:1).

(d) If bleeding continues, because clot is not formed clinically (surgical bleeding has been controlled), give 10 units of cryoprecipitate (concentrated clotting factors, carrying in a unit of 15 mL: 100 IU of factor VIII, 250 mg Fibrinogen, additionally factor XIII, and von Willebrand factor (vWF)).

(e) When the result of the classical coagulation panel arrives (after 30 min), you may:

   i. If PT or aPTT >1.5 * normal give 4 U of FFP.

   ii. If fibrinogen is <1 g/mL, give 10 U of cryoprecipitate (the only blood product containing fibrinogen). If cryo is not available, and you want to avoid loading the patient with FFP, **Beriplex®** is an alternative containing concentrated human prothrombin, the "father" of fibrinogen in the coagulation cascade.

   iii. Give in addition 1 A Cacl$_2$ 10%, if (i) and (ii) are required, or if calcium is low in serum. Calcium is previously known as IV factor, which stimulates as a coenzyme every single step of the coagulation cascade, and also activates platelets.

   iv. Platelet number is indicative, while function is crucial for the coagulation. In the presence of ongoing bleeding and if PLT count is <70,000/mm^3, give additional units of PLT. Options are:

- A simple PLT unit with a volume of 50–70 mL, which carries $5.5 * 10^{10}$ PLT and increases PLT count upon transfusion by 5–10,000 PLT/mm^3.
- An apheresis mega unit of PLT, which in a volume of 150 mL carries $3 * 10^{11}$ platelets and increases PLT count in blood by 35,000 PLT/mm^3.

Thrombocytopenia is defined as <50,000 PLT/mm^3. If you plan to operate on such a patient have PLT available. Spontaneous bleeding rarely occurs if the platelet count is greater than 30,000/mm^3. Petechiae (dry bleeding) appear when PLT is <10,000, and spontaneous (wet) bleeding when PLT is <5000. Thrombocytopenia appears after the replacement of 1–2 times the whole blood volume, and results from dilution. Despite this, the tissues seem to have large reserves of PLTs, which deployed to the blood stream in a bleeding patient. Platelet counts required after transfusion of every ten units of blood.

Adjuncts: The following medications have no routine use in trauma. Physician should be aware of their specific indications and give them accordingly when bleeding continues:

- Aprotinin has no indication in trauma, and it's out of market since 2008.
- Tranexamic acid is indicated for prolonged bleeding (empirically) or with evidences of hyperfibrinolysis (measured with TEG, see below). Dose 10 mg/kg, every 6 h.
- Desmopressin (DDAVP), indicated only for functional PLT disorder (aspirin), renal or hepatic failure, hemophilia-A and von Willebrand's disease.
- Recombinant factor VIIα [8]; Factor VII starts the extrinsic coagulation cascade and its active form (VIIα) actuates directly factor X, the last step before thrombin. The idea is that if you give the activated form you bypass steps of the coagulation cascade going directly to the final product, the

thrombin. Works with hemophilics and this is the official indication. There are evidences that reduce transfusion requirements in trauma (specifically blunt) [8], if you give it early (in presence of pH >7.1, hypothermia, thrombocytopenia does not work) that is after control of surgical bleeding, and the first 2–3 U of PRBC transfused. Recent strategies of transfusing FWB or components have diminished transfusion requirement either way, so the patients needed to prove the efficacy of factor VIIIα are much more than initially anticipated making the cost of such a study leaden.

2. Use of thromboelastography (TG or ROTEM) [9]. A portable bedside device that gives qualitative result on the coagulation function. Accept one specimen at a time and process it immediately in room temperature before the natural temperature of the specimen changes. The result is available within 3–10 min, at a form of a curve (see Fig. 31.1). Clinician is informed if the bleeding is surgical or pathological, which clotting factors are missing, the function of platelets, if fibrinolysis evolves normally. Transfusion of blood components, coagulation factors, and additional medications is elective based on these results (Table 31.1).

31.9   Additional Ways to Preserve Blood

1. **Reduce the need for transfusion**. Blood is a scarce (and expensive) resource and is also not universally safe. Reducing the need for transfusion is the best way to limit the complications.

   (a) Hypotensive resuscitation: SBP of 90 mmHg, effectively perfuse neural tissue, while protects from dislocation the fresh blood clot and rebreeding. Before the surgical control of bleeding it is advisable the resuscitation effort to target the limit of 90 mmHg, and not a normal SBP.

   (b) Treat the cause, i.e., urgent surgery to stop bleeding, avoid hypothermia and acidosis.

   (c) In the MB patient we do not rely on Hgb/Hct values. In a human with steady metabolic rate, a Hgb of 9 (Hct 27) gives rheological advantage in the circulating blood, while it covers all needs on O_2 demand. Hg 3 (Hct 10) is the limit where oxygen delivery (DO_2) marginally covers the needs of myocardium in a steady metabolic rate of a healthy individual. A patient in hemorrhagic shock is by definition metabolically unstable and need to be transfused with other criteria. Rapid and simple indicator of efficiency of oxygen delivery and uptake is cell's anaerobic metabolism by-products like the lactate. Decisions based solely on Hgb level for the rescusitation of trauma patients, apply only in stable patients [10].

   (d) Follow a restrictive transfusion policy in ICU. A recent multicenter trial documented a significantly lower mortality rate for critically ill patients managed with a restrictive transfusion strategy. However, this assumes normovolemia, absence of ongoing bleeding, and the absence of pre-existing cardiovascular disease. In such cases, transfusion indications are based on Hgb levels [7]. Intensivists favorable number to initiate transfusion in patients with the aforementioned status, is Hgb of 7 g/dL.

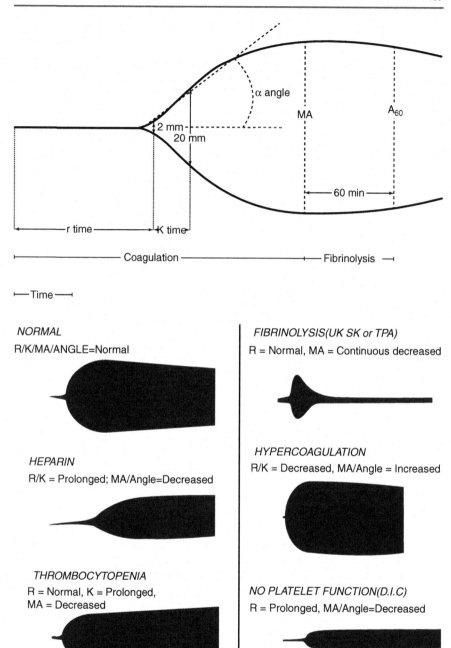

Fig. 31.1 The qualitative coagulation evaluation with the thromboelastogram (TG) [9]

Table 31.1 Primary and secondary treatment options for TEG-directed hemostatic resuscitation for children with traumatic injuries and significant bleeding [9]

Abnormal TEG value[a]	Primary treatment	Secondary treatment
R-time		
8–10 min	FFP (10 mL/kg)	
10–14 min	FFP (15 mL/kg)	rFVIIa (90 µg/kg)[b]
>14 min	FFP (20 mL/kg)	rFVIIa (120 µg/kg)[b]
K-time		
>4 min	Cryoprecipitate (0.1 units/kg)	FFP (10–15 mL/kg); rFVIIa (90 µg/kg)[b]
Alpha angle		
<45°	Cryoprecipitate (0.1 units/kg)	FFP (10–15 mL/kg); rFVIIa (90 µg/kg)[b]
Maximum amplitude		
49–54 mm	DDAVP (0.3 µg/kg) or apheresis platelets (10 mL/kg)	
40–48 mm	Apheresis platelets (10 mL/kg)	Cryoprecipitate (0.1 units/kg)
<40 mm	Apheresis platelets (15–20 mL/kg)	Cryoprecipitate (0.1 units/kg)
Lysis at 30 min		
>7.5% and $G < 6$	Consider Amicar (200 mg/kg IV)	

TEG thromboelastography, *FFP* fresh frozen plasma, *rFVIIa* recombinant activated factor VII, *DDAVP* desmopressin acetate
[a]Abnormal values reported for kaolin activated samples. Secondary treatment may be given with primary-treatment if immediate life threatening injury
[b]The use of rFVIIa should be reserved for life-threatening bleeding only. If bleeding not resolved clinically repeat TEG 30 min after treatment given

2. **Develop a capacity for cell salvage: Autotransfusion.**
   There are level 2 evidences that intraoperative and postoperative blood salvage and alternative methods for decreasing transfusion may lead to a significant reduction in allogenic blood usage [7], which rises up to 45% reduction in the use of banked blood [2]. The cell saver device has been introduced since 1990. Autotransfusion is generally contraindicated in the presence of bacterial or malignant cell contamination (e.g., open bowel, infected vascular prostheses, etc.) unless no other red blood cell source is available and the patient is in a life-threatening situation. Practically bleeding from the chest seems ideal for autotransfusion as contents of thoracic cavity are sterile. In the contrary, abdominal bleeding were hollow viscous injury and contamination may co-exist, autotransfusion is used with causion or contraindicated. Modern autotransfusion devices are basically of two types:
   (a) Collection of blood, mixing with an anticoagulant, typically citrate, and returned.
   (b) The blood is collected, anticoagulated with heparin, and then run through a system in which it is washed and centrifuged, before being re-transfused.
   To a degree, the simpler the system, the less likely it is that problems will occur. In elective situations, nurses, technicians, or anesthesia personnel can participate in the autotransfusion process. In emergency situations without additional personnel, such participation may not be possible.

Reinfusion after filtration is less labor intensive and provides blood for transfusion quickly. Whole blood is returned to the patient with platelets and proteins intact; but free hemoglobin and procoagulants are also reinfused. A high proportion of salvaged blood is returned to the patient and the most recent devices do not require mixing of the blood with an anticoagulant solution. In-line filters are essential when autotransfusion devices are used. These filters remove gross particles and macroaggregates during collection and reinfusion, thus minimizing microembolization [11].

The simplest effective method is to use the sterile chest drain container. Use saline to create the fluid valve at the end of a chest draining tube, and add 1000 U of heparin. Collect 1500 cc (if you delay to collect more, DIC is on the way) of drained blood, reverse the container, and using a microfilter to collect microaggregates, reintroduce immediately IV.

3. **Red blood cell substitutes**

Significant effort has been made to find a suitable substitute, which, essentially, should be treated as an artificial O_2 carrier. The ideal blood substitute is cheap, has a long shelf life, is universally compatible, has low viscosity, minimal infectious risks or concerns about immunogenicity and has an oxygen-delivery profile identical to blood. These products may also deliver more oxygen per unit mass than an equivalent amount of Hb from RBCs, providing the potential to sustain life in certain clinical situations. A number of problems remain, including short biological half-life, which may limit the application to times when the patient is most acutely anemic (i.e., in the intraoperative or immediate perioperative period) or for emergent use.

Artificial O_2 carriers can be grouped into perfluorocarbon emulsions (PFC), which showed discouraging results, and Hgb-based oxygen carriers (HBOCs).

Hemoglobin-based oxygen carriers (HBOCs) are undergoing investigation for use in critically ill and injured patients but are not yet approved for use in the United States. (Level 2) [7]. Two HBOCs are evaluated with clinical trials:

(a) PolyHeme (human HBOC derived from outdated human RBCs) has been studied in Phase II and Phase III in-hospital clinical trials [12]. Comparisons were performed between HBOC vs. PRBC. There was no significant difference between 30-day mortality, prevalence of MOF, adverse events, except MI (3% MI in HBOC vs. 1% PRBC group among 714 patients). Never the less the benefit/risk ratio of PolyHeme is favorable when blood is needed but not available [13].

(b) Hemopure (bovine HBOC) has completed Phase II and Phase III in-hospital clinical trials, which confirmed the reduction of allogeneic transfusion requirement [14].

The nanotechnology currently produces nanobubbles of O_2, which can dissolve in a liquid solvent. This innovation may be capable to transfer oxygen in a different way than the two currently patented by nature (the red blood cell and the oxygen dissolved in arterial blood). If research proves the efficiency of nanobubbles to oxygenate hypoxic tissue a new era in resuscitation rises, allowing oxygen to be injected directly in blood stream.

31.10 When Do You Stop Transfusion?

Endpoint of transfusion is when bleeding stops, so it's a clinical decision.

If you insist on numbers, and with the prerequisite of hemodynamic stability:

When Hgb is >8 g/dL, PT, aPTT <1.5 times normal, fibrinogen >1.5 g/L, pH>7.3, temperature >35 °C.

31.11 What You Need to Establish an Effective MTP in Your Hospital?

Quoting pioneers on this effort [2]: "To make this system work requires the cooperation and input of multiple specialties [2].The trauma patient will rapidly move through the system from emergency department (ED) to the operating room and if still alive, finally settle in to the intensive care unit. Physicians from each of these departments should be actively involved in the development of MT protocols. It is also essential that personnel from the BB are involved from the protocol's inception; this should include personnel from the hematology and pathology departments as well as BB technicians and managers." Although the MTP is established within the last 5 years in more than 80% of the USA hospital in most of them conditions are not mature to function properly [15] . This raises the issue of evaluation of compliance and "real-time" protocol adjustments from the MTP hospital team [2].

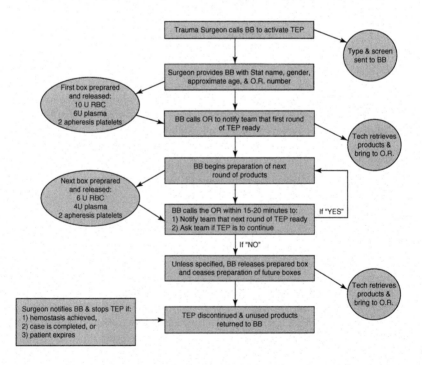

Algorithm 31.1 Flow diagram of massive transfusion protocol activation [2]

Bibliography

1. Holcomb J, Hess J. Early massive trauma transfusion: state of the art. J Trauma Acute Care Surg. 2006;60(6):S1–2.
2. Nunez TC, Young PP, Holcomb JB, Cotton BA. Creation, implementation, and maturation of a massive transfusion protocol for the exsanguinating trauma patient. J Trauma. 2010;68:1498–505.
3. Nunez TC, Voskresensky IV, Dossett LA, Shinall R, Dutton WD, Cotton BA. Early prediction of massive transfusion in trauma: simple as ABC (assessment of blood consumption)? J Trauma. 2009;66:346–52.
4. Spinella PC, Holcomb JB. Resuscitation and transfusion principles for traumatic hemorrhagic shock. Blood Rev. 2009;23:231–40.
5. Hess JR, Brohi K, Dutton RP, et al. The coagulopathy of trauma: a review of mechanisms. J Trauma. 2008;65:748–54.
6. Kauvar DS, Holcomb JB, Norris GC, Hess JR. Fresh whole blood transfusion: a controversial military practice. J Trauma. 2006;61:181–4.
7. Napolitano LM, Kurek S, Luchette FA, et al. Clinical practice guideline: red blood cell transfusion in adult trauma and critical care. Crit Care Med. 2009;37:3124–57.
8. Boffard KD, Riou B, Warren B, et al. Recombinant factor VIIa as adjunctive therapy for bleeding control in severely injured trauma patients: two parallel randomized, placebo-controlled, double-blind clinical trials. J Trauma. 2005;59:8–15; discussion 8.
9. Nylund CM, Borgman MA, Holcomb JB, Jenkins D, Spinella PC. Thromboelastography to direct the administration of recombinant activated factor VII in a child with traumatic injury requiring massive transfusion. Pediatr Crit Care Med. 2009;10:e22–6.
10. Holcomb JB, del Junco DJ, Fox EE, Wade CE, Cohen MJ, Schreiber MA, et al. The prospective, observational, multicenter, major trauma transfusion (PROMMTT) study: comparative effectiveness of a time-varying treatment with competing risks. JAMA Surg. 2013;148:127–36.
11. Hughes LG, Thomas DW, Wareham K, Jones JE, John A, Rees M. Intra-operative blood salvage in abdominal trauma: a review of 5 years' experience. Anaesthesia. 2001;56:217–20.
12. Gould SA, Moore EE, Hoyt DB, et al. The life-sustaining capacity of human polymerized hemoglobin when red cells might be unavailable. J Am Coll Surg. 2002;195:445–52; discussion 52–5.
13. Moore EE, Moore FA, Fabian TC, et al. Human polymerized hemoglobin for the treatment of hemorrhagic shock when blood is unavailable: the USA multicenter trial. J Am Coll Surg. 2009;208:1–13.
14. Napolitano LM. Hemoglobin-based oxygen carriers: first, second or third generation? Human or bovine? Where are we now? Crit Care Clin. 2009;25:279–301, Table of Contents.
15. Schuster KM, Davis KA, Lui FY, Maerz LL, Kaplan LJ. The status of massive transfusion protocols in United States trauma centers: massive transfusion or massive confusion? Transfusion. 2010;50:1545–51.

Part III

Management of Specific Incidents

The Acute Care Surgeon in Pandemics: Lessons from COVID-19

32

Amy E. Liepert and Jay Doucet

32.1 Introduction

A pre-pandemic survey of acute care surgeons performed by the American Association for the Surgery of Trauma (AAST) Disaster Committee in the summer of 2019 indicated that they felt significantly less prepared to deal with pandemics as compared to mass trauma events [1].

At the time of writing, the coronavirus disease 2019 (COVID-19), a contagious disease caused by severe acute respiratory syndrome coronavirus 2 (SARS-CoV-2), had infected over 65 million people causing 1.5 million deaths with continued exponential growth in case numbers in many parts of the world. The front line of hospitals' defense against COVID-19 is staffed by anesthesiologists, pulmonologists, infectious disease physicians, epidemiologists, and allied nursing and technologist disciplines. However many surgeons have been involved in the management of COVID-19 patients, using their experience either in looking after critically ill patients or in managing complications of COVID-19 disease.

Surgeons may anticipate responding to man-made disasters such as terrorist bombings or mass shootings, where the acute disruption to local trauma system processes may last several hours, or natural disasters such as earthquakes or cyclones, where regional disruptions may last for weeks or months. However, pandemics are global by nature and last for years. The COVID-19 pandemic has had economic, health, social, and cultural impacts on the entire world's population. The impact of surgical care delivery has been profound. Surgeons have been called on to perform leadership roles in reorganizing surgical care in the face of

A. E. Liepert (✉) · J. Doucet
Division of Trauma, Surgical Critical Care, Burns and Acute Care Surgery, Department of Surgery, University of California San Diego Health, San Diego, CA, USA
e-mail: aliepert@ucsd.edu; jdoucet@ucsd.edu

© Springer Nature Switzerland AG 2021
E. Pikoulis, J. Doucet (eds.), *Emergency Medicine, Trauma and Disaster Management*, Hot Topics in Acute Care Surgery and Trauma,
https://doi.org/10.1007/978-3-030-34116-9_32

shortages of personnel and equipment and increased risks of disease transmission to perioperative staff.

32.2 Surgical Considerations

32.2.1 Aerosol-Generating Procedures

In the first months of the pandemic, there were significant gaps in knowledge of COVID-19 disease effects, diagnostic testing, therapeutics, and outcomes. Even whether the disease was transmitted by droplet or airborne spread remained a public controversy for months. As in the 2003–2004 SARS outbreak, inadequate use of personal protective equipment (PPE) or inadequate PPE was blamed as the cause of many healthcare workers contracting COVID-19 [2, 3]. This has now again been a principal cause of transmission of COVID-19 to healthcare workers (HCWs) [4]. An area of great concern was aerosol-generating procedures (AGPs) such as intubation, tracheostomy, endoscopy, laparoscopy and use of electrocautery, which were known since the 2003–2004 SARS outbreak to have significant risk of transmission of coronavirus to HCWs. In general, those performing and assisting in AGPs require higher levels of PPE.

Initial advice on AGPs and surgery was sometimes contradictory or changed rapidly—for instance, the American College of Surgeons (ACS) in March 2020 had first recommended avoidance of laparoscopic surgery, or any surgery in COVID-19 patients. This included IV antibiotic management of appendicitis and percutaneous cholecystostomy for acute cholecystitis not responding to nonoperative management. This was surprising news to many surgeons as percutaneous cholecystostomy actually has worse outcomes with longer stays and simply shifts the risks and use of PPE from the operating room to interventional radiology suite [5]. Within 2 days, after feedback from acute care surgeons some responding via social media, the ACS policy was revised with the understanding that AGP risks were manageable and early surgery and discharge would avoid prolonged hospital stays and was a better use of resources. Paranoia about AGPs led to many initially perceived "good ideas" such as construction and distribution of intubation boxes, which actually made endotracheal intubation more difficult without any proven risk reduction and while possibly increasing risk to the HCW [6–8]. Similarly, much effort was expended on creating devices to allow two patients to use one ventilator, or to create expedient ventilators, neither of which saw significant use in the USA.

Tracheostomy is another example where several studies attempted to address fears over AGP by modifying usual techniques or creating physical barriers such as plastic tents to improve the safety of the procedure. Others advocated delay or complete avoidance of tracheostomy in intubated COVID-19 patients, despite known benefits of early tracheostomy over prolonged ventilation [9]. Over 230 articles on tracheostomy in COVID-19 were published in 2020. In actual fact, most of these mitigation attempts actually made the procedure more difficult. Subsequently a clinical study in 164 patients showed, independent of the severity of COVID-19 illness, that 30-day survival was higher and ICU stay shorter receiving standard early tracheostomy, without any HCW infections occurring [10].

In a similar fashion, there was concern regarding laparoscopic procedures on COVID-19 patients. Theoretically, laparoscopic port exhaust gases and smoke could contain infectious particles. Editorials appeared for and against laparoscopy in COVID-19 [11, 12]. The controversy erupted despite no prior reports of transmission of disease to HCWs from laparoscopic smoke or gases. Several reviews have subsequently suggested there is no apparent increased risk of laparoscopic versus open surgery for COVID-19 [13–15]. It is recommended to use filtered smoke and gas evacuation systems, especially for desufflation to avoid smoke exposure according to guidelines, but there is no prohibition of laparoscopic procedures in COVID-19 patients [16].

The AGP procedures most associated with risk of COVID-19 transmission are intubation and endoscopic procedures such as bronchoscopy, which are procedures performed in the operating room and intensive care unit by anesthesiologists and surgical intensivists. In the 2003–2004 SARS outbreak, transmission of coronavirus to HCWs was significantly associated with performance of intubation [17]. However, with appropriate PPE and technique, there have been a least one series of intubations of COVID-19 patients without any nosocomial infection of proceduralists [18]. Guidelines exist for the safe performance of endoscopy for COVID-19 patients with considerations what appropriate PPE should be worn and when immediate versus delayed procedures should be done [19, 20]. Unfortunately, in many regions there have been severe shortages of required PPE, which increases risks for HCW infection [21].

32.2.2 COVID-19 Surgical Presentations

The typical illness produced by SARS-CoV-2 is a viral upper respiratory infection, sometimes complicated with pneumonia, However, predominantly gastrointestinal presentations of COVID-19 have been described. About 61.5% of hospitalized COVID-19 patients had gastrointestinal symptoms at hospital admission, and 14.5% had abdominal pain [22]. There was also a significant association between anosmia and gastrointestinal symptoms at presentation. In some cases, the gastrointestinal symptoms of COVID-19 may mimic surgical conditions such as acute cholecystitis, requiring careful evaluation and preoperative SARS-CoV-2 testing to avoid a non-therapeutic procedure and increased risk of postoperative complications due to COVID-19 [23].

Increased postoperative morbidity and mortality in COVID-19 surgical patients was noted early in the pandemic when testing for SARS-CoV-2 was not available or timely. A review of 4 studies showed 14 postoperative deaths in 51 asymptomatic surgical patients (27.5%) and severe, mostly pulmonic complications [24]. In another series of 34 asymptomatic elective surgical cases, there was a 20% postoperative death rate, 44% ICU admission rate, and 100% rate of postoperative pneumonia [25]. These alarming results led to calls to delay elective surgery and obtain screening tests for SARS-CoV-2 for asymptomatic adult preoperative cases whenever possible [26]. However, safe performance of urgent EGS procedures, even with positive SARS-CoV-2 tests, is possible, especially when operating room workers are properly trained and have appropriate PPE. Most facilities designated at least operating room as a COVID-19 OR to avoid exposing patients to SARS-CoV-2-contaminated spaces and equipment.

32.2.3 COVID-19 and Emergency General Surgery

Given the high prevalence of COVID-19 cases, it should not be surprising that some COVID-19 positive patients will present with acute abdomens and other acute surgical issues, including burns and trauma. In these cases, delay of surgery is usually not feasible.

An early international cohort study of 235 hospitals in 24 countries included all patients undergoing surgery who had SARS-CoV-2 infection confirmed within 7 days before or 30 days after surgery. It included 1128 patients, 835 (74.0%) had emergency surgery, and 280 (24.8%) had elective surgery. SARS-CoV-2 infection was confirmed preoperatively in 294 (26.1%) patients. Thirty-day mortality was 23.8% overall. Pulmonary complications occurred in 577 (51.2%) patients; 30-day mortality in those patients was 38.0%, accounting for 81.7% of all deaths. The authors recommended that thresholds for surgery during the COVID-19 pandemic should be higher than during normal practice, particularly in men aged 70 years and older [27].

Such results could lead to fears of performing EGS during the pandemic; however later published results indicate that conventional approaches to EGS can lead to reasonable survival. A UK retrospective study of 103 EGS patients aged 17–88, 49% of whom had a preoperative COVID-19 test, all negative, had only 1 death (1%). Morbidity was 16%, with 11/16 having non-pulmonary complications. Postoperatively, 7% tested COVID-19 positive; these patients had longer lengths of stay.

A study of 141 patients with severe ARDS and COVID-19 showed that they were more likely to develop gastrointestinal complications compared with those without COVID-19 (74% vs. 37%; $P < 0.001$; OR 2.33 [95% CI, 1.52–3.63]) [28]. Four patients (3.8%) developed bowel ischemia, three went for laparotomy, and pathology findings demonstrated fibrin thrombi in the microvasculature underlying areas of necrosis of the intestine. Patients with severe COVID-19 disease develop a highly inflammatory and prothrombotic state that leads to increase death and complications, including thrombotic complications. A meta-analysis of thromboembolism (TE) in COVID-19 patients identified 42 studies enrolling 8271 patients. The overall venous TE rate was 21%, the deep vein thrombosis rate (DVT) was 20%, and the pulmonary embolism rate was 13%. Arterial TE rate was seen in 2%. The mortality rate among patients with TE was 23% versus 13% among patients without TE. Clinical trials are underway to determine the impact of thromboprophylaxis on TE and mortality risk of COVID-19 [29]. Careful assessment of coagulation status and stratification of VTE risk with appropriate prophylaxis is prudent in perioperative COVID-19 patients.

Trauma surgery has been successfully performed, before and after the availability of rapid preoperative SARS-CoV-2 testing. A trauma patient with persistent fever, thrombocytopenia, elevated transaminases, or diarrhea could be SARS-CoV-2 positive, as the usual leukopenia and hypoxia may arrive in a delayed fashion [30]. Universal testing should be done for all trauma patients and appropriate PPE worn until tests return negative. Rapid (<1 h) RNA amplification tests for SARS-CoV-2 unfortunately have limited availability in many areas and may suffer from somewhat decreased sensitivity (80–90%) compared to batched reference RT-PCR tests (97%) [31].

Cancer surgery cannot be delayed indefinitely during the pandemic but can be completed successfully. A series of 520 cancer procedures, 494 of which were elective, was accomplished in March and April 2020 in an area of moderate COVID-19 prevalence in India without any deaths [32].

32.3   Systems of Surgical Care

32.3.1   Impact on Trauma Center/EGS Access

An unfortunate phenomena in many US cities during the 2020 pandemic was an increase in trauma center admissions due to interpersonal violence, including gun violence [33]. While many types of elective surgery were on hold to allow hospitals to deal with COVID-19 admissions, the spike in gun violence cases was tragic and most unhelpful. Possible reasons for the escalation include increased unemployment, increased alcohol consumption, and increased gun sales. The initial shutdown of many surgical services and lockdown orders was accompanied by a significant decrease in overall trauma admissions during March–June, 2020, in many US cities, especially for elderly falls, road traffic accidents, and non-intentional mechanisms [34, 35]. However trauma admissions increased to pre-pandemic levels in most US centers by September, 2020. Any hope that later lockdowns would decrease utilization of hospital resources by trauma patients during the November–December 2020 surges has not been realized.

Another tragic effect on the pandemic seen in trauma centers was an increase in intimate partner violence (IPV). Nine US cities reported increases in IPV from 20 to 30% and as high as 60% [36]. There is serious concern about mental health issues during the pandemic, and the risk of further health crisis including depression, suicide and homicides. Child abuse and neglect is another concern. With the prolonged closure of schools, children are often confined at home with potential abusers, and may not have access to teacher witnesses, nurses, or school-based social workers. Increased vigilance by trauma surgeons and allies treating injured children is warranted [37].

Delays in presentation of EGS patients were seen early in the pandemic and led to increased morbidity with increased postoperative complications. A Spanish study noted a monthly decrease in EGS presentations of 58.9% and an increase in time between symptom onset and presentation, with morbidity increasing from 34.7% to 47.1% of cases [38]. Many surgical patients expressed fear of going to the hospital due to a perceived risk of exposure to COVID-19. However, hospitals were quick to implement masking, social distancing, and limited visitation resulting in a rather safe environment. As such, many centers performed outreach efforts in the media to encourage patients to feel safe seeking care.

Elective surgeries were canceled by public health agencies to preserve PPE and to allow for development of processes surrounding the operating rooms both in the inpatient and ambulatory settings. In many facilities, these areas have physical space overlap, and the operating rooms have common space where healthy and COVID-19-infected patients have potential to overlap. Active management was required to both cancel and track patients affected by OR shutdowns; to ensure postoperative care was delivered, new consultations were triaged, and canceled cases were rescheduled. Surveillance of cancelled cases was necessarily re-evaluated to ensure no change in clinical status during the delay.

As clinics and elective surgery were re-established, prioritization of the backlog of cases needed to be addressed. Telehealth practices were developed in the clinic and postoperative environment, and surgeons began to utilize videoconferencing technologies for postoperative visits to assess wounds and clinical course. Selected patients also had telehealth preoperative visits via video visit. A potential advantage of telehealth was the ability to evaluate the patient in their own home environment with family or caregivers present.

Many of the prior barriers for telehealth were removed by lifting of restrictive federal regulations and the allowance of billing for these services. Previous to COVID-19, these types of visits were not reimbursed or supported from hospital IT platforms. The urgent deregulation of these restrictions allowed expeditious response of hospital IT programs. Rapid training of large numbers of surgeons and physicians was necessary to adapt to this newly available outpatient care tool [39, 40].

32.3.2 COVID-19 and Social Disparities

There is a significant body of literature that indicates that there are significant disparities in outcomes in the US for trauma, EGS, and cancer surgery patients due to racial, social, and structural issues. It is also true that COVID-19 spread and outcomes are also affected by these same factors. Many comorbidities that lead to increased risk of COVID-19 complications and death, such as obesity, hypertension, diabetes, and chronic kidney disease, are more common in Black Americans and other groups. Overall, Black Americans have double the mortality of COVID-19 compared to Whites and Asians, and Black Americans aged 35–44 have 9 times the mortality from COVID-19 than their White peers [41]. The pandemic has placed a spotlight on these disparities. The data represents an overdue opportunity for surgeons to advocate to improve the access to care, strengthen our trauma and EGS systems, and remove barriers for these populations of patients.

32.3.3 Impact of Trauma Center Processes

The impact of the pandemic on the typical US trauma center was significant. Trauma Medical Directors and the ACS faculty had to adapt to finding and using PPE for all admissions, and using rapid SARS-CoV-2 testing when available, and prioritizing tests when there was limited test availability. Each facility required designation of at least one dedicated operating room for suspected and known COVID-19-positive surgical patients. OR, ED, and ICU rooms frequently required modification to control air flow, to generate negative pressure, and to create restricted access. ICUs had to be reorganized and redesignated for COVID-19 or non-COVID-19 cases [42]. Elective surgery was cancelled initially both to allow development of new processes and procedures and also to preserve PPE. However, increased demand pushed their reopening once these were created [43]. Staff, faculty, and residents all needed to learn proper use of PPE and how to perform procedures, including AGPs, safely [44]. Transferring suspect and known COVID-19 patients within the facility and designating spaces and corridors for their transport was another issue to be solved. In many locations, alternate ICU spaces had to be opened, such as in post-anesthesia care units or disused hospital wards [45].

Acute care surgery teams in some institutions have used their intensive care skills to relieve pulmonologists, sometimes to run additional ICUs. In other centers, they formed central line insertion teams, performed tracheostomies, or assisted with prone positioning. Assistance in providing family communications became a critical task as families and visitors were largely banned from the hospital. Multidisciplinary rounding on patients became more frequent during surges, and a larger in-house presence for surgical and critical care services was required. Telepresence and tele-critical care were used in some centers to avoid excess PPE use and room entries, especially in ICUs [46].

Leadership by surgeons and their teams was needed to manage fatigue. Lack of adequate PPE, fear of infection, frequent decontamination, donning and doffing of PPE, lack of usual pastimes, isolation from friends and families, and even being called a "hero" can take a significant emotional toll on HCWs [47, 48]. Burnout is a significant problem for surgical residents and surgeons dealing with this pandemic [49, 50]. Surgeons should anticipate these effects, be prepared to provide leadership, and demonstrate care and concern for their colleagues, trainees, and allies during the crises. In some cities, particularly in the northeast US early in the pandemic, volunteer, military, or federal HCWs were able to provide some relief to hospitals, but as more regions were affected, there were general shortages of many types of HCWs.

Other leadership skills needed by surgeons are those to negotiate with other departments and administration to ensure adequate staffing, space, testing, PPE, immunizations, and budget to maintain the trauma center and acute care surgery services. Support of the overall mission of the institution by surgeons must also be evident to maintain good relations with senior administration.

Many physicians not involved with their hospital's emergency management committee are surprised by the appearance and role of the Hospital Incident Command System (HICS), which is required by federal mandate and is delegated the responsibility for the hospital's specific response to an emergency. A better understanding of HICS and its responsibilities can be accomplished by taking online Federal Emergency Management Agency (FEMA) courses or the ACS Disaster Management and Emergency Preparedness (DMEP) course [51].

A concern about surges that threatened to overwhelm facilities with COVID-19 patients was whether resource allocation of ventilators, extracorporeal membrane oxygenation (ECMO), or other devices would be needed. Under a crisis standard of care, a triage process is proposed to determine which patients would achieve benefit and which patients would be excluded from being allowed to being placed on a ventilator [52, 53]. This triage process would have to apply to all patients in the hospital, not just COVID-19 patients, and would need to be performed in a standardized manner by a committee and not the bedside clinicians. Federal and state guidelines indicated how this crisis standard of care would be applied, but as of December 1, 2020, no facility has had yet to allocate ventilators under such as scheme. Concerns existed over the criteria used to for resource allocation, including whether disabled persons, aged persons, patients with cancer, and persons of color would be treated equitably [54, 55].

Education of surgical trainees was disrupted during the pandemic, sometimes unnecessarily. Medical students from many schools were initially banned from hospitals out of an abundance of caution, but eventually were returned to the wards. Medical students can be involved in COVID-19 patient care, including trauma and EGS care, if properly trained and equipped. Surgical residencies and fellowships were sometimes severely affected by the cessation of elective surgery [56]. Residency and fellowship interviews became virtual [57]. It is hoped that virtual learning, videoconferencing, social media, and telemedicine can replace some lost educational opportunities. Consideration of trainees' mental health is an issue and is an area where surgeon leadership is needed.

32.3.4 Trauma Systems Responses

Urban, Level 1 trauma centers are uniquely poised to be "command centers" for trauma care. It is essential trauma centers reach out to regional institutions by way of Trauma Medical Directors and Trauma Program Managers to provide resources and expertise, ensuring that regional trauma system's capacity is preserved. Level 1 trauma centers are also often burn centers and regional centers for EGS. The trauma center is a component of the trauma system, which itself has important interactions with the emergency medical system (EMS) and the public health system.

The trauma system is usually able to manage multiple casualty surges lasting a few hours. In some US states, the trauma system is also designated the disaster response system. However the COVID-19 pandemic is an event of broad geographic impact, lasting years, with multiple surges and that also provides direct risks to the HCWs themselves. Trauma systems are not specifically designed to manage pandemics alone. Instead, regional coordination of multiple hospitals is needed.

A Regional Medical Operations Center (RMOC) is a center that can provide situational awareness of hospital and EMS conditions, distribute patients, manage EMS resources, identify alternate care sites, ensure trauma and non-stroke emergencies are considered, provide consensus on crisis standards of care, and identify outbreaks in high-risk populations. The RMOC can coordinate the response of the emergency management (disaster) system, public health system, and acute care hospitals. The RMOC uses the framework of the EMS and trauma systems to operate. Formal agreements are made to insure collaboration, and representatives of all stakeholders are present physically or virtually. The RMOC has robust communications, including the Emergency Operations Center (EOC) for the region. It can monitor hospital capacity and EMS dispositions and distribute resources and patients across the system. The RMOCs in western Washington state and other areas have been successfully used to coordinate the health system's pandemic response [58, 59]. Unfortunately many parts of the USA lack such a well-integrated system resource as the RMOC.

32.3.5 Leadership and Advocacy for the Next Time

It is obvious that the health care system of the USA was not optimally prepared for a pandemic such as COVID-19. There was initially poor intelligence about the nature of SARS-CoV-2. Despite many states' stockpiles and the federal Strategic National Stockpile (SNS), there was a prolonged shortage of PPE and ventilators. COVID-19-positive patients were returned to their nursing homes, ill-advisedly. Many members of the public were reluctant to wear masks or perform social distancing. Messaging from Public Health and governmental authorities about how to protect oneself from COVID-19 was sometimes inconsistent. Some facilities were overwhelmed during surges with state or federal help arriving too late or not properly utilized. Many members of the public are now mistrustful of COVID-19 vaccines, which may limit participation. Surgical patients had prolonged delays in receiving care, leading to worsened outcomes, and vulnerable populations suffered disparately poor outcomes.

All these problems have been now been revealed, despite some prior efforts to prepare, plan, and stockpile for pandemic. Surgeons have an opportunity to lead advocacy efforts to ensure the next pandemic or disaster will be better managed by our healthcare system:

Nationally:
- We should demand the SNS is properly equipped to manage pandemics and mass trauma events, including adequate PPE and ventilators.
- There needs to be national trauma and emergency response system, which can be created by integrating military and civilian trauma systems to achieve zero

preventable deaths after injury, such as described by the National Academy of Medicine [60].
• Provide support to states and regions to create RMOCs.
• A system to rapidly increase manufacture PPE.
• Improve communication and education with the public to understand the nature of viruses and how to control pandemic spread.
• Provide consistent public health messaging before, during, and after pandemic.

Statewide:
• The state disaster stockpiles must be maintained to manage pandemics and mass trauma events, including adequate PPE and ventilators.
• Support for RMOCs to cover the state and coordinate disaster responses.
• Support for regional or hospital equipment caches for PPE and ventilators.

National professional organizations such as the American College of Surgeons and the American College of Physicians undertake significant advocacy efforts with state and federal governments. They can also provide advocacy training and opportunities to meet policymakers. Volunteer surgeons are a key component in advocacy for surgical patients. As surgeons are constituents and professionals who have worked on the front lines of this pandemic response, they have a credible message and can be effective in creating the needed changes in our health system for the next pandemic or disaster.

32.4 Conclusion

There were a number of lessons learned by acute care surgeons during the first year of the COVID-19 pandemic (Table 32.1). Challenges existed in providing both trauma, emergency, and elective surgery during the early pandemic due to mandated closures and inadequate supplies of PPE, ventilators, and tests. Acute care surgeons were challenged to provide surgical and critical care to COVID-19 patients despite these shortages and also supported their fellow pulmonary intensivists in the ICU. Lessons learned for the next time included issues in preparation, training, planning, provider wellness, burnout, surgical disparities, testing, PPE, operating rooms, cancellations of elective surgery, regional coordination, and information technology. Surgeons should be now ready to engage in advocacy efforts to ensure that the next pandemic can be better handled by the healthcare system.

Table 32.1 Lessons learned by acute care surgeons in COVID-19

Preparation:
- Surgeons will be involved considerably in response to pandemics.
- They must manage surgical complications of the pandemic disease.
- They must perform surgery on patients with active viral disease.
- They may need to assist pulmonary critical care teams by performing bedside procedures, or provide critical care for COVID-19 or non-COVID-19 patients.

Training:
- Acute care surgeons previously reported lower levels of pandemic personal preparedness compared to mass trauma; they should obtain training in disaster management that includes pandemics.
- Future hospital exercises and plans should incorporate lessons learned from COVID-19.

Planning:
- Surgeons must be involved in surge capacity planning. The American College of Surgeons trauma center verifications standards requires that a surgeon be a member of the hospital disaster (emergency management) committee.
- Surgeons should assist efforts to augment healthcare workforce contingency plans, including emergency credentialing of surgical personnel across states, retiree, volunteer, and military.

Provider wellness/burnout:
- Burnout, decreased wellness, and poor self-care were observed by surgeons and trainees during the pandemic.
- Surgeon wellness and self-care must be a priority for the profession and hospitals, a need reaffirmed by the COVID-19 pandemic.

Surgical disparities:
- The COVID-19 pandemic further exposed significant racial and social differences in disease prevalence, complications, and death.

Testing:
- Preoperative testing for SARS-CoV-2 is essential to maintaining adequate surgical services, including elective surgery.
- Rapid tests for SARS-CoV-2 significantly improve the ability to safely perform emergent surgical procedures.
- Employee/physician testing for SARS-CoV-2 should be mandatory for surgical personnel and should be performed on a regular basis, i.e., weekly.
- Some regions were able to create successful public-private.

PPE (personal protective equipment):
- Perioperative and surgical personnel must be given access to adequate PPE and training for appropriate PPE usage.
- Surgeons should be represented in decisions to allocate PPE resources within the hospital.

Operating rooms:
- The hospital should set aside at least one operating room for operating on COVID-19-positive and suspected cases.
- The COVID-19 operating room requires that the OR staff be educated in the safe performance of surgery on COVID-19-positive patients.

Cancellation of elective surgery:
- The decision in many regions to cancel elective surgery was made by public health officials, largely to maintain PPE stocks and reduce the number of persons entering hospitals.
- The cancellation of elective surgical cases during acute surges of COVID-19 admissions reduced consumption of PPE, personnel requirements, and permitted initiation of routine testing.
- However, cancellation of elective surgical cases also resulted in a backlog of cases and delays in surgery. This was associated with patients presenting with more advanced disease and worse outcomes.

(continued)

Table 32.1 (continued)

• Preparation for pandemics should include describing clear triggers for halting elective surgery and identifying when elective surgery can be restarted.
Regional coordination
• Some regions benefited from Regional Medical Operations Centers (RMOCs) which provided situational awareness of hospital and EMS conditions, distribute patients, manage EMS resources, identify alternate care sites, ensure trauma and non-stroke emergencies are considered, provide consensus on crisis standards of care, and identify outbreaks in high-risk populations.
Information technology:
• Telehealth use by surgeons and their patients expanded considerably during the pandemic including preoperative and postoperative virtual visits, although many patients were unable to participate.
Advocacy
• Surgeons and their professional societies should request that the Strategic National Stockpile performance be strengthened to be effective and efficient during a pandemic (e.g., expansion of ventilators and other durable medical equipment antibiotics, intravenous fluids, and other medicines to sustain critical care).
• Surgeons and their professional societies should request telehealth and payment reforms, including across state borders.
• The racial and social disparities further exposed by the pandemic require significant efforts to improve health equity.

References

1. Doucet J. Emergency preparedness: a survey of the AAST and American College of Surgeons Committee on trauma; unpublished.
2. Loeb M, McGeer A, Henry B, Ofner M, Rose D, Hlywka T, et al. SARS among critical care nurses, Toronto. Emerg Infect Dis. 2004;10(2):251–5.
3. Chou R, Dana T, Buckley DI, Selph S, Fu R, Totten AM. Epidemiology of and risk factors for coronavirus infection in health care workers: a living rapid review. Ann Intern Med. 2020;173(2):120–36.
4. Heinzerling A, Stuckey MJ, Scheuer T, Xu K, Perkins KM, Resseger H, et al. Transmission of COVID-19 to health care personnel during exposures to a hospitalized patient—Solano County, California, February 2020. MMWR Morb Mortal Wkly Rep. 2020;69(15):472–6.
5. Loozen CS, van Santvoort HC, van Duijvendijk P, Besselink MG, Gouma DJ, Nieuwenhuijzen GA, et al. Laparoscopic cholecystectomy versus percutaneous catheter drainage for acute cholecystitis in high risk patients (CHOCOLATE): multicentre randomised clinical trial. BMJ. 2018;363:k3965.
6. Gould CL, Alexander PDG, Allen CN, McGrath BA, Shelton CL. Protecting staff and patients during airway management in the COVID-19 pandemic: are intubation boxes safe? Br J Anaesth. 2020;125(3):e292–e3.
7. Begley JL, Lavery KE, Nickson CP, Brewster DJ. The aerosol box for intubation in coronavirus disease 2019 patients: an in-situ simulation crossover study. Anaesthesia. 2020;75(8):1014–21.
8. Fried EA, Zhou G, Shah R, Shin DW, Shah A, Katz D, et al. Barrier devices, intubation, and aerosol mitigation strategies: PPE in the time of COVID-19. Anesth Analg. 2021;132(1):38–45.
9. Kwak PE, Persky MJ, Angel L, Rafeq S, Amin MR. Tracheostomy in COVID-19 patients: why delay or avoid? Otolaryngol Head Neck Surg. 2020. https://doi.org/10.1177/0194599820953371.
10. Queen Elizabeth Hospital Birmingham COVID-19 airway team, et al. Safety and 30-day outcomes of tracheostomy for COVID-19: a prospective observational cohort study. Br J Anaesth. 2020;125(6):872–9.

11. Di Saverio S, Khan M, Pata F, Ietto G, De Simone B, Zani E, et al. Laparoscopy at all costs? Not now during COVID-19 outbreak and not for acute care surgery and emergency colorectal surgery: a practical algorithm from a hub tertiary teaching hospital in Northern Lombardy, Italy. J Trauma Acute Care Surg. 2020;88(6):715–8.
12. Aydin NE. Laparoscopic surgery for COVID-19 positive patients: a Dilemma. EndoNews, 26 May 2020.
13. Chadi SA, Guidolin K, Caycedo-Marulanda A, Sharkawy A, Spinelli A, Quereshy FA, et al. Current evidence for minimally invasive surgery during the COVID-19 pandemic and risk mitigation strategies: a narrative review. Ann Surg. 2020;272(2):e118–24.
14. Mintz Y, Arezzo A, Boni L, Baldari L, Cassinotti E, Brodie R, et al. The risk of COVID-19 transmission by laparoscopic smoke may be lower than for laparotomy: a narrative review. Surg Endosc. 2020;34(8):3298–305.
15. de Leeuw RA, Burger NB, Ceccaroni M, Zhang J, Tuynman J, Mabrouk M, et al. COVID-19 and laparoscopic surgery: scoping review of current literature and local expertise. JMIR Public Health Surveill. 2020;6(2):e18928.
16. Francis N, Dort J, Cho E, Feldman L, Keller D, Lim R, et al. SAGES and EAES recommendations for minimally invasive surgery during COVID-19 pandemic. Surg Endosc. 2020;34(6):2327–31.
17. Caputo KM, Byrick R, Chapman MG, Orser BJ, Orser BA. Intubation of SARS patients: infection and perspectives of healthcare workers. Can J Anaesth. 2006;53(2):122–9.
18. Zheng H, Li S, Sun R, Yang H, Chi X, Chen M, et al. Clinical experience with emergency endotracheal intubation in COVID-19 patients in the intensive care units: a single-centered, retrospective, descriptive study. Am J Transl Res. 2020;12(10):6655–64.
19. Chiu PWY, Ng SC, Inoue H, Reddy DN, Ling Hu E, Cho JY, et al. Practice of endoscopy during COVID-19 pandemic: position statements of the Asian Pacific Society for Digestive Endoscopy (APSDE-COVID statements). Gut. 2020;69(6):991–6.
20. Sultan S, Lim JK, Altayar O, Davitkov P, Feuerstein JD, Siddique SM, et al. AGA Rapid recommendations for gastrointestinal procedures during the COVID-19 pandemic. Gastroenterology. 2020;159(2):739–58.e4.
21. Tabah A, Ramanan M, Laupland KB, Buetti N, Cortegiani A, Mellinghoff J, et al. Personal protective equipment and intensive care unit healthcare worker safety in the COVID-19 era (PPE-SAFE): an international survey. J Crit Care. 2020;59:70–5.
22. Redd WD, Zhou JC, Hathorn KE, McCarty TR, Bazarbashi AN, Thompson CC, et al. Prevalence and characteristics of gastrointestinal symptoms in patients with severe acute respiratory syndrome coronavirus 2 infection in the United States: a multicenter cohort study. Gastroenterology. 2020;159(2):765–7.e2.
23. Sellevoll HB, Saeed U, Young VS, Sandbæk G, Gundersen K, Mala T. Acute abdomen as an early symptom of COVID-19. Tidsskr Nor Laegeforen. 2020;140(7):1–6.
24. Nahshon C, Bitterman A, Haddad R, Hazzan D, Lavie O. Hazardous postoperative outcomes of unexpected COVID-19 infected patients: a call for global consideration of sampling all asymptomatic patients before surgical treatment. World J Surg. 2020;44(8):2477–81.
25. Lei S, Jiang F, Su W, Chen C, Chen J, Mei W, et al. Clinical characteristics and outcomes of patients undergoing surgeries during the incubation period of COVID-19 infection. E Clin Med. 2020;21:100331.
26. De Simone B, Chouillard E, Di Saverio S, Pagani L, Sartelli M, Biffl WL, et al. Emergency surgery during the COVID-19 pandemic: what you need to know for practice. Ann R Coll Surg Engl. 2020;102(5):323–32.
27. COVIDSurg Collaborative. Mortality and pulmonary complications in patients undergoing surgery with perioperative SARS-CoV-2 infection: an international cohort study. Lancet. 2020;396(10243):27–38.
28. El Moheb M, Naar L, Christensen MA, Kapoen C, Maurer LR, Farhat M, et al. Gastrointestinal complications in critically ill patients with and without COVID-19. JAMA. 2020;324(18):1899–901.

29. Malas MB, Naazie IN, Elsayed N, Mathlouthi A, Marmor R, Clary B. Thromboembolism risk of COVID-19 is high and associated with a higher risk of mortality: a systematic review and meta-analysis. E Clin Med. 2020;29:100639.
30. Bankhead-Kendall B, Fong ZV, Kaafarani H, Parks J. A COVID-19 positive trauma patient with stab wound to the neck. Am Surg. 2020;86(6):562–4.
31. Basu A, Zinger T, Inglima K, Woo KM, Atie O, Yurasits L, et al. Performance of Abbott ID Now COVID-19 rapid nucleic acid amplification test using nasopharyngeal swabs transported in viral transport media and dry nasal swabs in a New York City Academic Institution. J Clin Microbiol. 2020;58(8):e01136–20.
32. Shrikhande SV, Pai PS, Bhandare MS, Bakshi G, Chaukar DA, Chaturvedi P, et al. Outcomes of elective major cancer surgery during COVID 19 at Tata Memorial Centre: implications for cancer care policy. Ann Surg. 2020;272(3):e249–52.
33. Sutherland M, McKenney M, Elkbuli A. Gun violence during COVID-19 pandemic: paradoxical trends in New York City, Chicago, Los Angeles and Baltimore. Am J Emerg Med. 2021;39:225–6.
34. Matthay ZA, Kornblith AE, Matthay EC, Sedaghati M, Peterson S, Boeck M, et al. The DISTANCE study: determining the impact of social distancing on trauma epidemiology during the COVID-19 epidemic-an interrupted time-series analysis. J Trauma Acute Care Surg. 2020.
35. Forrester JD, Liou R, Knowlton LM, Jou RM, Spain DA. Impact of shelter-in-place order for COVID-19 on trauma activations: Santa Clara County, California, March 2020. Trauma Surg Acute Care Open. 2020;5(1):e000505.
36. Kofman YB, Garfin DR. Home is not always a haven: the domestic violence crisis amid the COVID-19 pandemic. Psychol Trauma. 2020;12(S1):S199–s201.
37. Thomas EY, Anurudran A, Robb K, Burke TF. Spotlight on child abuse and neglect response in the time of COVID-19. Lancet Public Health. 2020;5(7):e371.
38. Cano-Valderrama O, Morales X, Ferrigni CJ, Martín-Antona E, Turrado V, García A, et al. Acute care surgery during the COVID-19 pandemic in Spain: changes in volume, causes and complications. A multicentre retrospective cohort study. Int J Surg. 2020;80:157–61.
39. Reeves JJ, Hollandsworth HM, Torriani FJ, Taplitz R, Abeles S, Tai-Seale M, et al. Rapid response to COVID-19: health informatics support for outbreak management in an academic health system. J Am Med Inform Assoc. 2020;27(6):853–9.
40. Meyer BC, Friedman LS, Payne K, Moore L, Cressler J, Holberg S, et al. Medical undistancing through telemedicine: a model enabling rapid telemedicine deployment in an Academic Health Center during the COVID-19 pandemic. Telemed J E Health. 2020.
41. Bassett MT, Chen JT, Krieger N. Variation in racial/ethnic disparities in COVID-19 mortality by age in the United States: a cross-sectional study. PLoS Med. 2020;17(10):e1003402.
42. Coleman JR, Burlew CC, Platnick KB, Campion E, Pieracci F, Lawless R, et al. Maintaining trauma care access during the COVID-19 pandemic: an urban, level-1 trauma center's experience. Ann Surg. 2020;272(2):e58–60.
43. Elizabeth Brindle M, Gawande A. Managing COVID-19 in surgical systems. Ann Surg. 2020;272(1):e1–2.
44. Heffernan DS, Evans HL, Huston JM, Claridge JA, Blake DP, May AK, et al. Surgical Infection Society Guidance for operative and peri-operative care of adult patients infected by the severe acute respiratory syndrome coronavirus-2 (SARS-CoV-2). Surg Infect (Larchmt). 2020;21(4):301–8.
45. Coimbra R, Edwards S, Kurihara H, Bass GA, Balogh ZJ, Tilsed J, et al. European Society of Trauma and Emergency Surgery (ESTES) recommendations for trauma and emergency surgery preparation during times of COVID-19 infection. Eur J Trauma Emerg Surg. 2020;46(3):505–10.
46. Subramanian S, Pamplin JC, Hravnak M, Hielsberg C, Riker R, Rincon F, et al. Tele-critical care: an update from the Society of Critical Care Medicine Tele-ICU Committee. Crit Care Med. 2020;48(4):553–61.
47. Davis KA, Kaplan LJ. Out of darkness. Ann Surg. 2020;272(3):e211–2.

48. Tatebe LC, Rajaram Siva N, Pekarek S, Liesen E, Wheeler A, Reese C, et al. Heroes in crisis: trauma centers should be screening for and intervening on posttraumatic stress in our emergency responders. J Trauma Acute Care Surg. 2020;89(1):132–9.
49. Coleman JR, Abdelsattar JM, Glocker RJ. COVID-19 pandemic and the lived experience of surgical residents, fellows, and early-career surgeons in the American College of Surgeons. J Am Coll Surg. 2020;232(2):119–135.e20.
50. Romanelli J, Gee D, Mellinger JD, Alseidi A, Bittner JG, Auyang E, et al. The COVID-19 reset: lessons from the pandemic on burnout and the practice of surgery. Surg Endosc. 2020;34(12):5201–7.
51. Committee on Trauma, American College of Surgeons. In: Doucet J, editor. Disaster management and emergency preparedness course manual. 2nd ed. Chicago: American College of Surgeons; 2017.
52. Institute of Medicine. Crisis standards of care: summary of a workshop series. Washington, DC: The National Academies Press; 2010.
53. University of California Critical Care Bioethics Working Group. Allocation of scarce critical resources under crisis standards of care. Oakland: University of California; 2020.
54. Cleveland Manchanda E, Couillard C, Sivashanker K. Inequity in crisis standards of care. N Engl J Med. 2020;383(4):e16.
55. Crisis Standards of Care Committee. Crisis standards of care: planning guidance for the COVID-19 pandemic: Executive Office of Health and Human Services: the Commonwealth of Massachusetts. 2020. Crisis Standards of Care Planning Guidance for ... - Mass.govwww.mass.gov › doc › download.
56. Dedeilia A, Sotiropoulos MG, Hanrahan JG, Janga D, Dedeilias P, Sideris M. Medical and surgical education challenges and innovations in the COVID-19 era: a systematic review. In Vivo. 2020;34(3 Suppl):1603–11.
57. Asmar S, Kulvatunyou N, Davis K, Joseph B. Virtual interviews for surgical critical care fellowships and acute care fellowships amid the COVID-19 pandemic: the show must still go on. J Trauma Acute Care Surg. 2020;89(4):e92–e4.
58. Mitchell SH, Bulger EM, Duber HC, Greninger AL, Ong TD, Morris SC, et al. Western Washington State COVID-19 experience: keys to flattening the curve and effective health system response. J Am Coll Surg. 2020;231(3):316–24.e1.
59. Capella J. Regional teamwork key to successful COVID-19 response. J Am Coll Surg. 2020;231(3):324–5.
60. Berwick DM, Downey AS, Cornett EA. A National Trauma Care System to achieve zero preventable deaths after injury: recommendations from a National Academies of Sciences, Engineering, and Medicine Report. JAMA. 2016;316(9):927–8.

Natural Disasters: Medical Management

33

Athanasios Kalogeropoulos and Anastasia Pikouli

33.1 Introduction

Natural disasters are major incidents caused by natural phenomena and are categorized mainly as geological, hydrological, meteorological, climatological, and biological disasters [1]. The amplitude of natural disasters has increased in recent years as well as their impact on morbidity and mortality [2]. Medical management of immediate and delayed injuries is of paramount importance in reducing reversible life-threatening causes. This chapter covers the medical management of the following natural disasters listed below (Fig. 33.1).

33.1.1 All Hazard Approach of Disaster Medical Management

Although there are a plethora of natural disasters with different characteristics, an all the hazard approach provides a valuable tool to medical disaster management. The Incident Command System (ICS) adopted by United Nations remains a flexible framework for efficient communication and effective coordination [4], which can be modified to meet the medical service's special needs (Fig. 33.2).

A. Kalogeropoulos (✉)
Orthopedic Surgery and Traumatology, Sonnenhof Hospital, Bern, Switzerland

NATO COE MILMEd, Budapest, Hungary

A. Pikouli
Third Department of Surgery, National and Kapodistrian University of Athens, Attikon University Hospital, Athens, Greece

© Springer Nature Switzerland AG 2021
E. Pikoulis, J. Doucet (eds.), *Emergency Medicine, Trauma and Disaster Management*, Hot Topics in Acute Care Surgery and Trauma,
https://doi.org/10.1007/978-3-030-34116-9_33

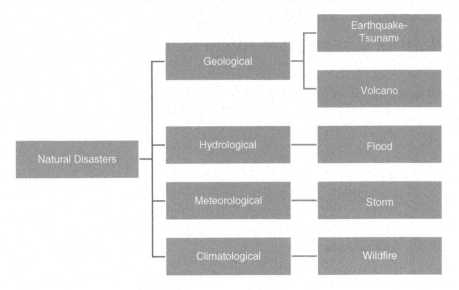

Fig. 33.1 Classification of natural disasters. (Modified from [3])

33.2   Disaster Management Medical Responders

Often in the management of natural disaster, more than one medical agency is included. Although the number of medical responders is progressively increasing, their setting remains the same. Governmental agencies, NGOs, national or international Red Cross, private sector, donors, academic institutions, the United Nations, and foreign states usually respond to disasters (Fig. 33.3).

33.3   Natural Disasters Medical Care

Although natural disasters have common characteristics that mandate a standard all hazard approach, they differ in their consequences in human health, requiring individualized medical response (Fig. 33.4).

33.4   Geological Disasters

33.4.1 Earthquakes

33.4.1.1   Introduction
Earthquakes are considered among the most disastrous natural phenomena. Approximately 500,000 earthquakes occur every yer, most of them in the Pacific Ring of Fire. During the last 20 years, more than one million deaths have been caused by earthquakes. Risk factors of their impact are the magnitude, the depth,

Fig. 33.2 Medical Service Incident Command System (ICS). (Modified from Mackway-Jones [5])

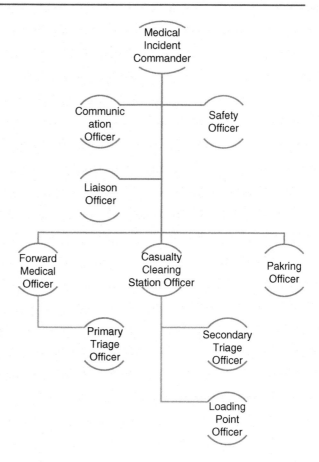

and their proximity to human habitat. Due to increasing urbanization and technological infrastructure, the number of casualties and deaths is raised to thousands [6]. Concomitant disasters are tsunamis, landslides, avalanches, fires, and floods. Hazards associated with earthquakes are collapse of buildings, falls, electrocution, smoke, dust, hypothermia, and prolonged entrapment.

33.4.1.2 Short-Term Management

The majority of patients seek medical care between 12 h and 3 days after the disaster and emergency departments reach their surge capacity within 24–48 h [7]. Children, the elderly, and the disabled are among those most affected [8]. The primary cause of injury is collapsed structures such as buildings, bridges, and infrastructure. The number of casualties depends on the severity of the injury, the duration of entrapment, and stamina until medical care is provided. Among other causes of injury are falling debris, flares, and smoke or dust inhalation. Collapsed buildings lead to immediate death or entrapment. Delayed extrication results in compartment syndrome as well as crush syndrome. Falling debris results in head and body injuries, impaled objects, massive bleeding, orthopedic, and soft tissue

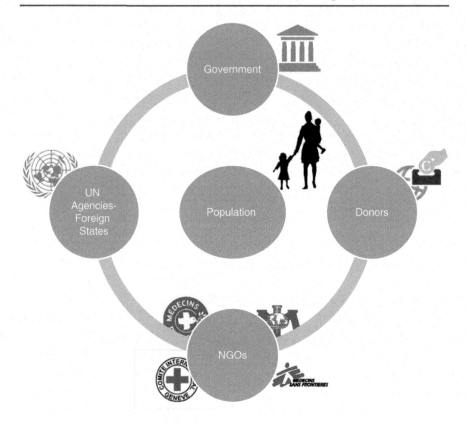

Fig. 33.3 Disaster management medical responders. Genuine

injuries. Destroyed electricity or gas networks may result in fire, which, in turn, causes burn injuries. A number of patients suffer from asphyxiation and pulmonary edema due to inhalation of smoke, dust, asbestos, or even burn inhalation. The loss of shelter makes patients vulnerable to hypothermia. The majority of patients sustain minor wounds, like superficial trauma, lacerations, sprains, and bruising, requiring out-patient care. A small percentage of casualties need hospitalization due to multiple fractures, head trauma, upper and lower limb injuries, internal wounds, crush syndrome, sepsis, and multiple organ dysfunction. Healthcare professionals need to provide effective pain and fracture management, perform a variety of surgical as well as medical interventions such as debridement of contaminated wounds, fasciotomy, or amputation in case of compartment syndrome, fluid administration, as well as renal dialysis to crash syndrome and rhabdomyolysis [9]. Rapid search and rescue is of paramount importance. When entrapment is prolonged, the death toll is increased due to delays in provision of lifesaving medical care. After 1–3 days death can result from myocardial infarctions and failure of medical technological infrastructure.

Fig. 33.4 Qualitative frequency of medical injuries based on disaster type. Green: High frequency, Yellow: Medium frequency, Red: Minor frequency. Genuine

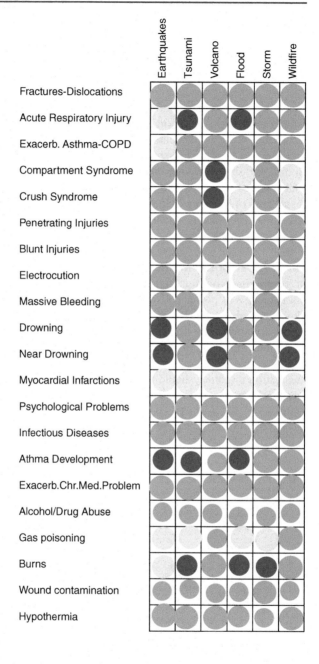

33.4.1.3 Long-Term Management

Post-disaster physiologic and psychological stress precipitates the deterioration of existing chronic conditions or provokes new illnesses. Existing research reveals an increase of BMI, serum lipid levels, smoking habits, and cessation of physical activity [10]. Among prevalent delayed post-disaster diseases are cardiovascular incidents, such as myocardial infarctions, heart failure, hypertension [11–13], as well as asthma and severe wheezing [14]. Poor glycemic control and abnormal HBA1c values are widely documented among survivors [15, 16]. Furthermore, basic survival needs are affected such as nutrition, sleep patterns, access to water, food, clothes, and shelter. Compromised hygiene conditions, ineffective refrigerators, and contaminated water supplies give rise to gastroenteritis and other infectious diseases. Loss of social networks may lead to depression and posttraumatic stress disorders. Delayed death is caused due to hypo-, hyperthermia, dehydration, crush syndrome, wound infection, and sepsis.

33.4.1.4 Hospital Medical Response

In the aftermath of an earthquake, hospital operation may be compromised. Fixed infrastructure of power and water supply may be disrupted, advanced equipment like renal dialysis devices, radiologic equipment, ventilators, blood analyzers, oxygen reservoirs may be destroyed and healthcare personnel may be injured. All these discontinue the function of specialized units at the emergency department, intensive care unit, and operation room at a moment when they are most needed. A basic medication inventory should include anesthetic, analgesic medications, respiratory management resources, hemodynamic management, and antibiotic prophylaxis (Table 33.1). In case of shortage, extra resources can be mobilized upon interhospital cooperation and private sector agreements in times of MCI [17].

Table 33.1 Essential resources for MCI response. (Modified from Rubinson et al. [17])

Number	Type	Drugs
1	Bronchodilators	Anticholinergic, beta-agonist
2	Crystalloids	0.9% NaCl, LR
3	Vasopressor	Upon hospital preference
4	Analgesics	Benzodiazapines
5	Analgesics	Opiods
6	Sedatives	Succinylcholine
7	Sedatives	Non depolarizing agents
8	Antibiotics	Guidelines of Infectious Disease Society of America or American Thoracic Society
9	Anticoagulant	Upon hospital preference
10	Hormone	Insulin
11	Hormone	Hydrocortisone/fludrocortisone

33.4.2 Tsunamis

33.4.2.1 Introduction
Tsunamis are giant waves, which are usually the result of earthquakes occurring in oceans with enormous human and social impact. Between 1700 and 2000, approximately 420,000 people were killed because of tsunamis and thousands others were injured or went missing. Vulnerable communities are those who lack defense infrastructure, resistant buildings, and evacuation lines based on early warning systems [18].

33.4.2.2 Short-Term Management
Most casualties suffer respiratory, orthopedic, and soft tissues injuries. Cases of drowning or near-drowning due to waves are common, followed by dislocation, fractures, lacerations and blunt injuries. Wound contamination from Clostridium tetani is due to flowing debris and low sanitation conditions [19]. Prompt identification, effective disinfection, wide debridement, delayed primary closure, fracture stabilization, follow-up controls, tetanus immunization, and wide spectrum antibiotic coverage are of paramount importance, since 67% of contaminated wounds were found to be infected within the first 24 h. Among commonly used antibiotics are third and fourth generation cephalosporins, quinolones, and aminoglycosides [20]. Medical management also relies on effective vertical and horizontal communication via various means such as runners, walkie-talkie, TETRA, Tannoy, satellite systems etc. Coordination among services is facilitated through common ICS protocols or pre-established response frameworks [21].

33.4.2.3 Long-Term Management
Compromised living conditions and loss of transportation and social network give rise to exacerbation of chronic diseases, spread of communicable diseases, and deterioration of psychological health [21]. Poor glycemic and blood pressure control, exacerbation of asthma, COPD, renal insufficiency, and alcohol and tobacco abuse have been documented among displaced people [15]. In transitional shelter, the close proximity of large numbers of people creates conditions conducive to the spread of influenza, malaria, and gastroenteritis outbreaks [22]. Psychological problems may develop among casualties, family members, or even rescuers, ranging from sleep deprivation, to changes in behavior, or even depression and PTSD. In the survivor's resting area (SRA), medical services can provide Psychological First Aid (PFA). Challenges may be presented by the management of dead bodies due to increased mortality, shortage of holding areas, difficulty in identification, and compromised transport.

33.4.2.4 Hospital Medical Response

In tsunamis, hospitals usually accept most casualties within the first 24–48 h after the disaster and should have the resources as well as the humanpower to operate autonomously for 48–72 h. Healthcare centers provide medical and nursing care as well as meet basic survival needs by providing shelter, nourishment, and hydration. Interdisciplinary drills should train personnel in mass casualty incidents in advance [23].

33.4.3 Volcanos

33.4.3.1 Introduction

Nowadays, nearly 1500 volcanos are considered to be active, affecting potentially 500 million people who reside close to them. Most active volcanoes are found on the Pacific Ring of Fire. During the last 300 years, 270,000 people lost their lives due to volcanic eruptions. Volcanic eruptions pose many hazards to humans, such as lava, pyroclastic flow (27% of volcanic fatalities), rocks, debris, tephra, gases, lahars (17%), and other concomitant threats like tsunamis (17%), earthquakes, and lighting [24].

33.4.3.2 Short-Term Management

Although lava looks apocalyptic, very few deaths are attributed to it. The majority of fatalities are due to pyroclastic flow, where a mass of hot gases, tephra, and debris travel up to 15 km, not always preceded by fierce eruptions. Hot pyroclastic flows of 600–900 Celsius if not lethal, still result in severe burns. Upon eruption, fragments travel with great speed, resulting in secondary blast injuries [25]. Ash clouds, usually containing tephra of less than 2 mm, are under investigation for causing acute silicosis (Fig. 33.5). However, causalities with asthma and bronchitis exacerbation is well documented, even lasting up to 3 weeks after high particle concentration is counted in the air [27]. The most common gas emission is water vapor followed by carbon and sulfur dioxide, carbon monoxide, hydrogen (chloride, fluoride, sulfide), helium, etc. Colorless and odorless carbon dioxide and monoxide increase after volcanic eruptions, resulting in respiratory distress, asphyxiation, and death, primarily affecting those found in low-lying places like parking areas and cellars. Hydrogen fluoride affects humans via respiration (irritant of respiratory tract) and via ingestion (livestock consumption). Fluorosis can be avoided by preventive measures. The "rotten egg" smell of hydrogen sulfide is a red flag for those living in low-lying places, resulting in eye irritation, pulmonary edema, and asphyxiation [28]. Volcanic lahar result from eruption, heavy rainfall, or earthquakes and may travel up to 50 km/h, destroying infrastructure potentially resistant to other disasters. There are documented cases were lahars happened

Fig. 33.5 Silicosis from volcanic ash [26]

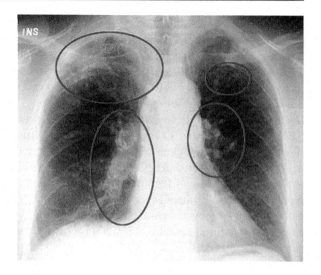

months after eruption by sudden breakout of formerly blocked volcanic deposits [25]. Volcanoes may cause concomitant threats like earthquakes and tsunamis when found underwater.

Since the majority of volcanic fatalities occur during the first 24 h, prompt medical care is important. Acute medical care consists of early transport to temporary evacuation sites in order to avoid pyroclastic flow, effective management of burn patients via adequate fluid administration, efficient wound care, and broad antibiotic coverage. Medical services should be prepared for mass casualty incidents and enable preexisting emergency operation plans. Respiratory care includes sufficient management of asthma and COPD exacerbations, early recognition of CO_2, CO-poisoning, oxygen administration, and the prompt use of hyperbaric chambers. Search and rescue personnel should evacuate people in low-lying areas [29]. Secondary orthopedic and soft tissue blast injuries should be splinted and management according to basic wound care principles. As in many disasters, provision should be taken for crush injuries, compartment syndrome, blunt head trauma, and amputations. Food and potable water should be checked for elevated fluoride levels in order to avoid fluorosis through ingestion.

33.4.3.3 Long-Term Management

Tephra fall and toxic gas concentrations may last for weeks or months, polluting air, water, and food supplies. Air pollution destabilizes chronic respiratory diseases. Compromised water and sewage systems lead to improper waste disposal, low sanitation conditions, poor vector control, and the spread of infectious diseases. Communicable diseases are commonly documented among disposed people in temporary evacuation centers. After the initial disaster, dead bodies may be exposed to weather conditions, posing a threat to public health. People with chronic respiratory problems are advised to stay indoors, wear masks, and use air-purification devices. Bottled water or water containers brought from other places solve the problem until the water system is repaired.

33.4.3.4   Hospital Medical Response

Healthcare providers deployed prehospitally should have access to N-100 or N-95 NIOSH respirators and CO-monitoring devices. Personal protective equipment should include glasses, gloves, boots, and hats. Hospitals close to volcanoes should have pre-established emergency operation plans and trained personnel in mass casualty incidents. In case of volcanic eruption, disruption of power and water supply should be expected, where generators should support medical activities for a minimum of 72 h. Prolonged tephra fall compromises air as well as land medical evacuation due to reduced visibility. Flexibility to overcome shortage of resources and personnel is imperative.

33.5   Hydrological Disasters

33.5.1 Floods

33.5.1.1   Introduction

Floods are usually caused by massive rainfall, deforestation, and melting of snow. They present the highest frequency (40%) and mortality among other disasters [30]. The affected population is located in lowlands, close to water reservoirs, or downhill from a dam. Most communities experience a flood within 6 h after heavy rainfall, provoked by sudden release of debris dam, known as flash floods.

33.5.1.2   Short-Term Management

Around 0.2–2% of casualties seek immediate medical aid. Causes of injury are flowing debris, crossing floodwater more than 6 in. by foot, or more than 2 ft by car. Injuries sustained from debris result in orthopedic and soft tissue trauma. There should be a high index of suspicion for cervical spine trauma and spine immobilization techniques should be undertaken. Wounds are assumed to be contaminated and should be treated with irrigation, disinfection, and closure by secondary healing. Patients in shock due to hypothermia should receive extensive resuscitation and rewarming efforts even for 40 min, since similar cases are documented with successful recovery after prolonged submersion in cold water [30]. Displaced animal (dogs, insects, snakes, arthropods) may pose a threat for bites [31]. The primary cause of death is drowning, associated mainly with vehicle entrapment. Bodies are recovered when flood waters recede. Near-drowning cases are very unusual due to limited access during the active phase. Unfortunately human loss is also documented among prehospital healthcare professionals [31].

33.5.1.3   Long-Term Management

Collapse of electrical network may hinder access for people with chronic illness to vital support devices (ventilators, dialysis machines, etc.) or may lead people to use fossil fuels for heating, which in turn increases the rate of carbon monoxide poisoning. The contaminated water supply and low hygiene conditions due to spread of debris and chemicals lead to infectious diseases and vector-borne illnesses (*E. coli*, Salmonella, Shigella, Hep. A virus, etc.) [32]. Humidity and mold in houses increase respiratory illnesses. Loss of property and loss of human support networks are identified as cause of mental health deterioration and alcohol and drug abuse [33].

33.5.1.4   Hospital Medical Response

Hospitals located in risk areas should develop disaster management plans, identify possible transport routes, evacuate their patients prior the disaster, store supplies (water, oxygen, food, generators, etc.) for 72 h autonomy, and establish alternative communication lines [34].

33.6   Meteorological Disasters

33.6.1 Storm

33.6.1.1   Introduction

Based on their location and strength, storms may be referred to as hurricanes, cyclones, and typhoons. They have been responsible for 1.9 million fatalities during last two centuries, raising the death toll up to 10,000 people per year [35]. Storms ranging from 100 to 2000 km in diameter with velocity up to 350 km/h create a hazardous threat to human communities. Storms are associated with primary hazards such as ferocious winds, flying debris, storm tides, and landslides. Secondary threats include fires and floods. Tertiary hazards consist of potable water, food shortage, and infectious diseases.

33.6.1.2   Short-Term Management

Strong winds and flying fragments result in lacerations, fractures, dislocations, concussions, and penetrating injuries. Medical care includes splinting, wound care, antibiotic coverage, tetanus immunization, and delayed primary closure. Storm tides and landslides have the highest death toll. Drowning occurs to persons trapped in buildings and vehicles or offshore on ships. In hilly areas, landslides destroy buildings and structures. Other causes of death are electrocution due to broken power lines and carbon monoxide poisoning due to indoor use of heaters [36].

33.6.1.3   Long-Term Management

After storms, wells, and other water deposits can be contaminated. The risk of cholera and diarrheal diseases outbreaks are imminent as a result of fecal-oral transmission [37]. Displaced populations are susceptible to depression, alcohol and drug abuse, and post-trauma stress disorder. In the short-term, sleep medication accompanied by effective psychotherapy have been proved to be beneficial.

33.6.1.4 Hospital Medical Response

Medical personnel deployed prehospitally in search and rescue operations are exposed to deleterious air participles such as dispersed chemicals from stored facilities, biological agents from sewage system failure, or mold from flooded facilities, or even asbestos and lead from collapsed buildings. Whereas prehospital, post-disaster injuries are caused by demolished structures, collapsed electric cables, and passing vehicles [38]. In anticipation of storms, hospitalized patients should be dismissed or transported to other facilities far away. Hospitals in affected areas should have active, preexisting emergency operation plans deploying sandbags against storm tides. Additional medical resources, foods, and water should be stored and protected from winds and floods. Generators should be fuelled and set in standby mode. Hospitals should be autonomous for 72 h. During a storm, a mass casualty influx of casualties is not expected in hospitals due to reduced outdoor circulation as well as temporarily ceased search and rescue operations. Hospital personnel may face fatigue due to prolonged shifts, sleep deprivation and mental stress, increasing the risk of injury, while hindering decision-making. Hospitals should mobilize resources to provide temporary shelter to non-medical displaced people, meeting their basic survival needs until the storm has ceased. Systems regulating temperature may be compromised, resulting in diagnostic device malfunction, threatening hospitalized patients' health or resulting in suboptimal staff performance [39]. Heating systems and air-conditioning devices should be deployed, in order to assure a comfortable working environment [40]. Air- conditioning devices should not be placed close to heating devices or generators, since that results in the accumulation of CO and potential poisoning [41]. Shutters in windows provide safety to staff as well as patients from flying debris and wind [42]. During disasters, resources packed in special supply carts can be deployed wherever there is need. These carts contain equipment for resuscitation, monitoring, and wound care [43].

33.7   Climatological Disasters

33.7.1 Wildfires

33.7.1.1   Introduction

Wildfires can be initiated by natural causes such as lightening, volcanoes, dry climate, or human causes such as arson, cigarettes, controlled burning, or power line arcs. Up to 90% of wildfires are attributed to human activity. Among documented hazards during a wildfire are thermal burns, smoke, dust, hazardous chemicals, falls, heat related illnesses, fatigue, cuts, electrocution, animal bites, unstable structures, and rhabdomyolysis [44].

33.7.1.2 Short-Term Management

Burns result from thermal injury, radiation, chemical exposure, and electrocution. In thermal burns, the first priority is to stop the burning process by extinguishing flames, removing smoldering clothes, and removing chemical substances. Prolonged exposure at the scene of wildfire exposes firefighters, healthcare professionals, volunteers, and other agencies to burns. Collapsed power lines remain a cause of electrocution. Smoke and dust containing ash and silica lead to inhalation injury, bronchial edema, bronchospasm, and pulmonary shunting. Carbon dioxide results in cellular hypoxia through the formation of carboxyhemoglobin, nausea, vomiting, headache, decreased level of consciousness, and death. Hydrogen cyanide poisoning leads to changes in the cellular level, altered levels of consciousness, neurotoxicity, seizures, and death. Strenuous and long working shifts, sleep deprivation, dehydration, and individual risk factors lead to heat exhaustion, cramps, and heat stroke. Medical personnel working outdoors during forest fires should be aware of bites from displaced wild animals, orthopedic injuries, as well as soft tissue injuries from collapsing buildings and falls from unstable structures [44].

Burn patient assessment should focus on the ABC approach. Management of airway includes high-flow oxygen, setting patients on a Semi-Fowler, or position of comfort, airway monitoring, prompt intubation for impending airway failure. Escharotomies for circumferential thoracic burns that compromise ventilatory function. Fluid administration with Ringer's Lactated via intravenous or intraosseous line. Burn Surface Area calculation can be based on rule of nines, rule of palms, or Lund-Browder chart. However BSA calculation seems inaccurate at the scene, since up to 62% of cases present inconsistencies among healthcare professionals [45], reducing the effectiveness of Parkland Formula. Mean arterial pressure and urine output are more reliable values for fluid resuscitation. Wound management prehospitally includes covering burns with dry, sterile dressings, whenever available. Analgesia is achieved with intravenous opiates. Evacuation to specialized burn centers should follow local protocols or American Burn Association referral criteria (Table 33.2) [46].

33.7.1.3 Long-Term Management

Ash and other air particicles remain on the ground for many weeks and months. Until the first rains wash the land, people with chronic respiratory problems are susceptible to asthma and COPD exacerbations. The elderly, children, smokers, and pregnant women are also vulnerable, even if exposure is at low air particle concentration and for short periods of time. Maternal stress affects birth weight and air pollution during pregnancy leads to development of asthma [47]. In the long run, burn patients are susceptible to hypothermia, dehydration, and contamination.

33.7.1.4 Hospital Medical Response

The majority of patients either die or survive with minor injuries. Few patients reach hospitals with major injuries [48]. Hospital patient management follows the same patient approach as prehospitally. Furthermore, more accurate TBSA calculations should be performed. Restrictive clothes and jewelry should be

Table 33.2 American Burn Association Burn Center Referral Criteria. http://ameriburn.org/wp-content/uploads/2017/05/burncenterreferralcriteria.pdf

Burn injuries that should be referred to a burn center include:

1. Partial thickness burns greater than 10% total body surface area (TBSA).
2. Burns that involve the face, hands, feet, genitalia, perineum, or major joints.
3. Third degree burns in any age group.
4. Electrical burns, including lightning injury.
5. Chemical burns.
6. Inhalation injury.
7. Burn injury in patients with preexisting medical disorders that could complicate management, prolong recovery, or affect mortality.
8. Any patient with burns and concomitant trauma (such as fractures) in which the burn injury poses the greatest risk of morbidity or mortality. In such cases, if the trauma poses the greater immediate risk, the patient may be initially stabilized in a trauma center before being transferred to a burn unit. Physician judgment will be necessary in such situations and should be in concert with the regional medical control plan and triage protocols.
9. Burned children in hospitals without qualified personnel or equipment for the care of children.
10. Burn injury in patients who will require special social, emotional, or rehabilitative intervention.

removed, avoiding potential compression and tissue ischemia. At the same time, casualties should be protected from hypothermia, resulting from compromised thermoregulation due to burn injuries [49]. If there is a suspicion of CO-poisoning, in addition to high-flow oxygenations, accessory laboratory tests should be ordered, and upon meeting inclusion criteria the use of hyperbaric chamber should be considered [50]. In the treatment of hydrogen cyanide poisoning, the administration of hydroxocobalamin remains the preferred choice of therapy [51]. The dispatch of medical personnel to the scene is under criticism, as it leads to injuries among healthcare personnel and delay of casualties to definitive treatment [52]. The transfer of local burn personnel to bigger overloaded burn centers is also counter-productive since the majority of burn patients may never reach a burn center, as they receive treatment by the receiving hospital [53]. However, it is advisable that an evaluation by a burn surgeon occurs within the first 24 h after a major incident. Burn ICU is expected to receive burn patients within an "intermediate" time of a burn disaster (6–120 h) through interhospital transfer [54]. Smoke and low visibility hinders medical evacuation and staff mobilization. Many healthcare providers may be not reach hospitals, since they decide to stay and protect their families. Photographic documentation of injuries at scene or in emergency department can speed up the preparation of operating theaters and ICU admittance. Burn patients need a multidisciplinary approach, since they will most likely need extensive surgery and ICU management [55].

33.8 Summary

Between 1990 and 2013, natural disasters affected 4.8 billion people around the world, causing 1.6 million deaths, 5.3 million injuries, while leaving 109 million people homeless [1]. Natural disasters are a part of human existence on earth and while human understanding over natural disasters increases, humans should continue to develop and incorporate preventive measures to palliate their disastrous impact on everyday life. Medical response is a health service's responsibility, but it is not limited to it. Communities and individuals should play an integral role through awareness, training, and mitigation.

References

1. EM-DAT. The OFDA/CRED International Disaster Database 2018. Brussels (Belgium): Catholic University of Louvain. http://www.emdat.be. Accessed 6 Jan 2019.
2. Reinhardt JD, Li J, Gosney J, et al. Disability and health-related rehabilitation in international disaster relief. Glob Health Action. 2011;4:7191.
3. Below R, Wirtz A, Guha-Sapir D. Disaster category classification and peril terminology for operational purposes. Brussels: Centre for Research on the Epidemiology of Disasters (CRED); 2009.
4. US Department of Homeland Security. National Incident Management System. 2008. https://www.fema.gov/pdf/emergency/nims/NIMS_core.pdf. Accessed 16 Dec 2018. Accessed 6 Jan 2019.
5. Mackway-Jones K. Major incident medical management and support the practical approach at the scene. 3rd ed. New York: Wiley-Blackwell; 2012.
6. Rosenberg M. Haiti death toll could reach 300,000: Preval Reuters 22 Feb 2010.
7. Al Khaldi KH. Earthquake: Ciottone's disaster medicine. Philadelphia: Elsevier; 2016. p. 572–4.
8. Liang N-J, Shih Y-T, Shih F-Y, et al. Disaster epidemiology and medical response in Chi-Chi earthquake in Taiwan. Ann Emerg Med. 2001;38:549–55.
9. Eknoyan G. The Armenian earthquake of 1988: a milestone in the evolution of nephrology advances in renal replacement and therapy. Adv Ren Replace Ther. 2003;10(2):87–92.
10. Tsubokura M, Takita M, Matsumura T, et al. Changes in metabolic profiles after the Great East Japan Earthquake: a retrospective observational study. BMC Public Health. 2013;13(1):267.
11. Furusawa T, Furusawa H, Eddie R, Tuni M, Pitakaka F, Aswani S. Communicable and non-communicable diseases in the Solomon Islands villages during recovery from a massive earthquake in April 2007. N Z Med J. 2011;124(1333):17–28.
12. Nakagawa I, Nakamura K, Oyama M, et al. Long-term effects of the Niigata-Chuetsu earthquake in Japan on acute myocardial infarction mortality: an analysis of death certificate data. Heart. 2009;95(24):2009–13.
13. Nakamura M, Tanaka F, Komi R, et al. Sustained increase in the incidence of acute decompensated heart failure after the 2011 Japan earthquake and tsunami. Am J Cardiol. 2016;118(9):1374–9.
14. Miyashita M, Kikuya M, Yamanaka C, et al. Eczema and asthma symptoms among schoolchildren in coastal and inland areas after the 2011 Great East Japan Earthquake: the ToMMo Child Health Study. Tohoku J Exp Med. 2015;237(4):297–305.
15. Fujihara K, Saito A, Heianza Y, et al. Impact of psychological stress caused by the Great East Japan Earthquake on glycemic control in patients with diabetes. Exp Clin Endocrinol Diabetes. 2012;120(9):560–3.

16. Leppold C, Tsubokura M, Ozaki A, et al. Sociodemographic patterning of long-term diabetes mellitus control following Japan's 3.11 triple disaster: a retrospective cohort study. BMJ Open. 2016;6(7):e011455.
17. Rubinson L, Nuzzo JB, Talmor DS, O'Toole T, Kramer BR, Inglesby TV. Augmentation of hospital critical care capacity after bioterrorist attacks or epidemics: recommendations of the Working Group on Emergency Mass Critical Care. Crit Care Med. 2005;33:2393–403.
18. Llewellyn M. Floods and tsunamis. Surg Clin North Am. 2006;86:557–78.
19. Edsander-Nord A. Wound complications from the tsunami disaster: a reminder of indications for delayed closure. Eur J Trauma Emerg Surg. 2008;34:457–64.
20. Doung-ngern P, Vatanaprasan T, Chungpaibulpatana J, Sitamanoch W, Netwong T, Sukhumkumpee S, et al. Infections and treatment of wounds in survivors of the 2004 Tsunami in Thailand. Int Wound J. 2009;6:347–54.
21. Saito T, Kunimitsu A. Public health response to the combined Great East Japan Earthquake, tsunami and nuclear power plant accident: perspective from the Ministry of Health, Labour and Welfare of Japan. Western Pac Surv Resp J. 2011;2:7–9.
22. Turner A, Pathirana S, Daley A, Gill PS. Sri Lankan tsunami refugees: a cross sectional study of the relationships between housing conditions and self reported health. BMC Int Health Hum Rights. 2009;9:16.
23. Wattanawaitunechai C, Peacock SJ, Jitpratoom P. Tsunami in Thailand disaster management in a district hospital. N Engl J Med. 2005;352:962–4.
24. European Space Agency. Volcanoes. 2009. http://www.esa.int/Our_Activities/Observing_the_Earth/Space_for_our_climate/Volcanoes. Accessed 6 Jan 2019.
25. Newhall CG, Fruchter JS. Volcanic activity: a review for health professionals. Am J Public Health. 1986;76(3 Suppl):10–24.
26. Gretchen W. Volcanic ash: more than just a science project. Geology and Human Health Topical Resources. 2012. https://serc.carleton.edu/details/images/37999.html. Accessed 6 Jan 2019.
27. Baxter PJ, Ing R, Falk H, Plikaytis B. Mount St. Helens eruptions: the acute respiratory effects of volcanic ash in a North American community. Arch Environ Health. 1983;38(3):138–43.
28. US Geological Survey. Volcanic gases and their effects. https://volcanoes.usgs.gov/vhp/gas.html. Accessed 6 Jan 2019.
29. Pan American Health Organization. Volcanoes: protecting the public's health. http://www.mona.uwi.edu/cardin/virtual_library/docs/1258/1258.pdf. Accessed 6 Jan 2019.
30. Noji E. Natural disaster management. In: Auerbach P, editor. Wilderness medicine: management of wilderness and environmental emergencies. 3rd ed. St Louis: Mosby; 1995. p. 644–63.
31. Centers for Disease Control and Prevention. Morbidity and mortality associated with Hurricane Floyd—North Carolina, September-October 1999. MMWR Morb Mortal Wkly Rep. 2000;49(23):518.
32. Alderman K, Turner L, Tong S. Floods and human health: a systematic review. Environ Int. 2012;47:37–47.
33. Du W, FitzGerald GJ, Clark M, Hou XY. Health impacts of floods. Prehosp Disaster Med. 2010;25(3):265–72.
34. Floyd K. Floods. In: Hogan D, Burstein J, editors. Disaster medicine. Philadelphia: Lippincott Williams & Wilkins; 2002. p. 187–93.
35. Adler RF. Estimating the benefit of TRMM tropical cyclone data in saving lives. In: American Meteorological Society, 15th conference on applied climatology, Savannah, GA, 20–24 June 2005.
36. Carmichael C, Neasman A, Rivera L, et al. Morbidity and mortality associated with Hurricane Floyd—North Carolina, September-October 1999. MMWR Morb Mortal Wkly Rep. 2000;49(17):369–72.
37. Waring SC, des Vignes-Kendrick M, Arafat RR, et al. Tropical Storm Allison rapid needs assessment—Houston, Texas, June 2001. MMWR Morb Mortal Wkly Rep. 2002;51(17):366–9.

38. National Institute for Occupational Safety and Health. Hurricane key messages for employers, workers, and volunteers. Centers for Disease Control and Prevention (U.S.). 2018. https://www.hsdl.org/?view&did=815992. Accessed 6 Jan 2019.
39. Rodriguez H, Aguirre BE. Hurricane Katrina and the healthcare infrastructure: a focus on disaster preparedness, response, and resiliency. Front Health Serv Manage. 2006;23:13–24.
40. Mahoney EJ, Biffl WL, Cioffi WG. Analytic review: mass-casualty incidents: how does an ICU prepare? J Intensive Care Med. 2008;23:219.
41. Tucker M, Eichold B, Lofgren JP, et al. Carbon monoxide poisonings after two major hurricanes—Alabama and Texas, August–October 2005. MMWR Morb Mortal Wkly Rep. 2006;55:236–9.
42. Bovender JO Jr, Carey B. A week we don't want to forget: lessons learned from Tulane. Front Health Serv Manage. 2006;23:3–12.
43. Lynn M, Gurr D, Memon A, Kaliff J. Management of conventional mass casualty incidents: ten commandments for hospital planning. J Burn Care Res. 2006;27:649–58.
44. Corey C, Dalsey L. Wildland fire fighting safety and health. NIOSH Science Blog. National Institute of Occupational Safety and Health. Archived on 13 July 2012. https://blogs.cdc.gov/niosh-science-blog/2012/07/13/wildlandfire/. Accessed 6 Jan 2019.
45. Giretzlehner M, Dirnberger J, Owen R, Haller HL, Lumenta DB, Kamolz LP. The determination of total burn surface area: how much difference? Burns. 2013;39:1107–13.
46. White CE, Renz EM. Advances in surgical care: management of severe burn injury. Crit Care Med. 2008;36(7 Suppl):S318–24.
47. O'Donnell MH, Behie AM. Effects of wildfire disaster exposure on male birth weight in an Australian population. Evolut Med Public Health. 2015;2015(1):344–54.
48. Cameron PA, Mitra B, Fitzgerald M, et al. Black Saturday: the immediate impact of the February 2009 bushfires in Victoria, Australia. Med J Aust. 2009;191:11–6.
49. Rowley-Conwy G. Management of major burns in the emergency department. Nurs Stand. 2013;27(33):66–8.
50. Buckley N, Juurlink D, Isbister G, Bennett M, Lavonas E. Hyperbaric oxygen for carbon monoxide poisoning. Cochrane Database Syst Rev. 2011;13(4):CD002041.
51. Hamel J. A review of acute cyanide poisoning with a treatment update. Crit Care Nurse. 2011;31(1):72–82.
52. Mackie D. Mass burn casualties: a rational approach to planning. Burns. 2002;28:403–4.
53. Dunbar J. The Rhode Island nightclub fire: the story from the perspective of an on-duty ED nurse. J Emerg Nurs. 2004;30:464–6.
54. Kearns RD, Conlon KM, Valenta AL, Lord GC, Cairns CB, Holmes JH, Johnson DD, Matherly AF, Sawyer D, Skarote MB, Siler SM, Helminiak RC, Cairns BA. Disaster planning: the basics of creating a burn mass casualty disaster plan for a burn center. J Burn Care Res. 2014;35:1–13.
55. O'Neill TB, Rawlins J, Rea S, Wood F. Complex chemical burns following a mass casualty chemical plant incident: how optimal planning and organisation can make a difference. Burns. 2012;38:713–8.

Natural Disasters: Mapping and Evaluating Incidents

34

Efthimis Lekkas, Emmanouil Andreadakis, Michalis Diakakis, Spyridon Mavroulis, and Varvara Antoniou

34.1 Introduction

A mostly demanding process in disaster management is resource allocation in space and time, while planning towards safety against all types of hazards, be they natural or man-made, technological or other. All efforts to protect life, property and the environment, in that order, especially during emergencies, need to be based on valid information about the stakes and their dynamic at any given time. One of the essential processes in logistics of planning and emergency action for natural disasters, is disaster and hazard mapping [1].

Mapping technologies have a significant role in disaster management [2] and have been used in a variety of hazard oriented contexts [3, 4] since as early as the late 1870s. Advances in computing and GIS have boosted the sector in recent decades [5, 6]. Zoning and microzonation are techniques used as the basis of geographic decision support systems that help outline spatially referenced safety guidelines and assign measures of risk mitigation, according to a rational prioritization based on a multi-criteria analysis. Multilayer data and multihazard/multirisk analyses are developed. In this context, thematic risk mapping is implemented from a local (e.g. municipality) to regional, national and global scale, leading to a continuous improvement of long term design of institutional measures and resource allocation, throughout global organizations, national governments and local authorities.

E. Lekkas (✉) · E. Andreadakis · M. Diakakis · S. Mavroulis · V. Antoniou
Department of Dynamic Tectonic Applied Geology, Faculty of Geology and Geoenvironment, National and Kapodistrian University of Athens, Athens, Greece
e-mail: elekkas@geol.uoa.gr

© Springer Nature Switzerland AG 2021
E. Pikoulis, J. Doucet (eds.), *Emergency Medicine, Trauma and Disaster Management*, Hot Topics in Acute Care Surgery and Trauma,
https://doi.org/10.1007/978-3-030-34116-9_34

Post-disaster mapping of phenomena and impacts is incorporated into the record of the affected area and risk is then reassessed, to be taken into account for the upgrade of safe planning and better designing. In the past, mapping disasters was generally a time consuming procedure, whose results were only available long after the response and recovery operations were completed. Recent advances in technologies have made it possible for disaster scene investigators to collect and analyze data and distribute critical information, depending on the conditions of the incident, in near real time or real time. This can be considered a breakthrough for disaster management, because it is now possible to provide to responders critical information during emergencies. These new capabilities upgrade not only resource allocation and operations design, but also the safety of operators and emergency responders themselves, allowing accurate outlining of crisis zones.

In recent years the field of UAV (Unmanned Aircraft Vehicles), RPAS (Remotely Piloted Aircraft Systems) or UAS (Unmanned Aircraft Systems), popularly known as drones, has seen a significant rise. It is not so long ago (2007) when satellite relayed UAV's (Unmanned Aircraft Vehicles) and live transmission of data worldwide was referred to as "a not too farfetched idea" by Scanlon [7]. Recent advances have made it possible to involve these tools into disaster mapping. As a result, an increasingly large number of applications are available. Humanitarian action, impact mapping, damage assessment in various cases are only a fragment of what is readily available by groups of responders and researchers. Urban damage assessment seems to be a field with great potential ([8–10]) for many different disaster types like earthquakes [11], cyclones, typhoons and hurricanes [12, 13], etc. A few more examples worth mentioning are use in humanitarian action in Haiti post-earthquake and post hurricane Sandy [14, 15], damage assessment and landslide mapping in the Amatrice earthquakes [16], flash flood magnitude assessment [17] and post-flood mapping after flash floods in Greece [18].

In the following cases we present three post-disaster mapping applications aided by the use of state of the art technologies and techniques. Aerial imagery, remote sensing, Unmanned Aircraft Systems, GIS, GPS and online platforms were the main categories of tools of the mapping inventory. Depending on the type and timing of the incident, these were deployed and used for mapping of effects, impacts, computations, visualization, presentation and distribution of data and results.

34.2   The Case of June 12, 2017 Lesvos (Northeastern Aegean Sea, Greece) Earthquake

On June 12, 2017, a shallow crustal strong earthquake with magnitude 6.3 occurred offshore, south of Lesvos (12:28 GMT), 35.8 km SSW of the capital of Lesvos Island, Mytilene, causing one fatality and severe structural damage in the SE part of the island [19]. The southeastern part of Lesvos Island suffered the most by the earthquake in its natural environment, building stock and infrastructure.

Building damage was observed in the southeastern part of Lesvos. Very heavy structural damage was limited in the traditional village of Vrissa [19]. Taking into account that Vrissa is located inland, further from the epicentre than other settlements with less damage, this village looks like an earthquake impact paradox. To interpret this paradox, a rapid field macroseismic reconnaissance was conducted performing not only classical methods of earthquake damage assessment (e.g. building-by-building inspection), but also modern and innovative techniques, which comprise the use of Unmanned Aerial Vehicles (UAV) and Geographic Information Systems (GIS) online applications as the basis of a rapid post-earthquake damage assessment, before any intervention was made in the settlement. Thus, all earthquake effects on the natural environment and the building stock of Vrissa were collected and saved with maximum accuracy for further processing and analysis.

34.2.1 UAS Deployment and Processing of Earthquake-Induced Damage

The UAS performed two flights designed for 3D modelling comprising scanning of the affected area along two sets of paths aligned perpendicular at a height of 90 m above ground in the research area (Fig. 34.1a). Moreover, real-time video streaming was provided through YouTube for all viewers interested and all agencies competent in civil protection and disaster management. The flight areas were overlapping so

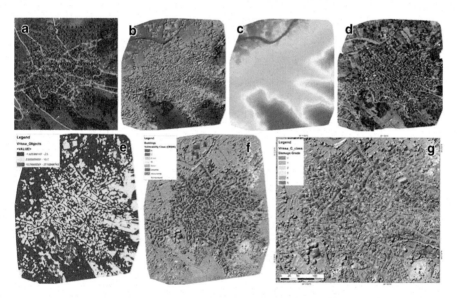

Fig. 34.1 (**a**) Camera positions during the flights of the DJI Phantom 4 Pro over Vrissa village, deployed on June 13th, the day following the 2017 Lesvos earthquake. (**b**) Digital Surface Model processed with Pix4D software. (**c**) Digital Terrain Model (processed with Pix4D Mapper Pro software). (**d**) Orthophotomap (orthomosaic) processed with Pix4D Mapper Pro. (**e**) Classified object raster into three categories (lower than building range: green, building range: yellow and higher than building range: red). (**f**) Final edit of building polygons, according to the EMS-98 vulnerability classes. (**g**) C class building damages in Vrissa over the DSM hillshade

that they would be intercalibrated. Four hundred forty images of Vrissa were acquired, and they were input for processing in the Pix4D Mapper Pro software. Processing in Pix4D software created a point cloud, a mosaic orthophotomap, a Digital Surface Model (Fig. 34.1b), a Digital Terrain Model (Fig. 34.1c) and a 3D model of the settlement (Fig. 34.1d). The difference between the two raster surfaces, DSM and DTM, is the recognized objects including trees, buildings, cars etc. The uniformity of Vrissa buildings, as the village is a traditional settlement, essentially enabled classification of objects into groups based on their shape and their height. After subtracting DTM from the DSM, the resulting raster contained only recognizable objects, which were then grouped into the three mentioned groups, and more specifically, building range between 2.5 and 10.7 m tall, shorter and taller (Fig. 34.1e). In order to refine and reassess damage grades, all objects above ground surface were isolated. Then, adjusting the histogram of the objects raster, large trees, poles, etc. were excluded, resulting in a raster containing all building surfaces and some of the trees, which were then converted to polygons in ArcGIS and finally edited manually. Damage assessment was re-run on final building polygons, applying field observations, but also editing errors of the field work, revisiting the site through the 3D model and with use of all footage available for any point on demand, in Pix4D. A review of damage grade and vulnerability class took place once more (Fig. 34.1f, g), using all 440 images. Once for every point of the model there is a number of images from different angles, field observations were actually supplemented by aerial observations.

34.2.2 Results from UAS

The resulting damage assessment is shown in Fig. 34.1g. This detail and spatial distribution allows for calculations of damage grade percentages and classification of areas with similar statistics of damage grade, and zonal application of the EMS-98 intensity scale in the area. Because the majority of buildings (>99%) belong to C Class, a map presenting damage grade of C class vulnerability buildings is shown (Fig. 34.1g). Most of the high grade damage is concentrated in the flat NW part of the village, consisting of loose alluvial sediments, along the terraces of the nearby river (visible at the north part of all maps).

34.3   The 2017 Mandra Flood

On November 15th 2017, a high-intensity convective storm reaching more than 280 mm in 8 h locally, hit the western part of the region of Attica in Greece, causing flash floods with catastrophic effects in the towns of Mandra and Nea Peramos and the tragic loss of 24 people. The study area is situated around the east and southeast foothills of Mt. Pateras. On its east side, the town of Mandra is situated on the western margin of the Thriassion plain within the catchment of Soures torrent and its main tributary (Agia Aikaterini). The river network flows eastward,

Fig. 34.2 Example of flood extent delineation based on UAV-captured imagery

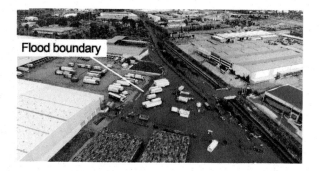

Flood boundary

reaching the Thriassion plain just downstream of the town of Mandra and turns south, towards the sea. High-resolution rainfall estimates from the X-band polari-metric radar of National Observatory of Athens were used to analyse the space-time dynamics of triggering rainfall, showing that the basin-average rainfall, was 153 and 194 mm total accumulation for Ag. Aikaterini and Soures catchment, respectively.

The research team carried out several flights of an Unmanned Aerial Vehicle (UAV) monitoring the ground situation during and after the flood. Using a combination of aerial and ground observations the team developed a detailed record of the physical characteristics of the flood along with impacts across the hit area. Evidence collected through this field investigation made possible an accurate delineation of flood extent, derived by digitizing the boundaries at the contrasting land surface/water boundary (Fig. 34.2).

Furthermore, the study used the slope-conveyance method [20] to estimate peak discharge. The research team surveyed to selected cross sections (one in Soures and one in Agia Aikaterini) and applied the Gauckler-Manning formula, using the uniform flow assumption. In these two locations a detailed Digital Surface Model (hereafter DSM), with a resolution of 2.7 cm, was created using the Structure from Motion technique (SfM) (Fig. 34.3) and imagery from a UAV. The detailed DSM was used to extract a cross section vertical to flow and calculate the cross sectional area as well as the wetted perimeter. To estimate the Manning n coefficient using the Arcement and Schneider [21] approach. Different checks were carried out to validate findings and reduce uncertainty [22]. Results showed that the flood caused inundation of a noteworthy extent (4.03 km²), in comparison with the catchment area of the two tributaries (35.84 km²) (Fig. 34.4). Floodwaters within the urban area moved along two axes of flow (one for each tributary), despite the lack of a formed riverbed and the complexity of the urban environment, following the local geomorphology.

Peak discharges in the two ungauged sections were estimated at 169.9 m³/s for Soures and 198.9 m³/s for Agia Aikaterini. To account for the uncertainty inherent in the discharge estimation [22], the research team provided a range of discharge values (141–203 m³/s for Soures and 157–257 m³/s for Agia Aikaterini), using minimum and maximum n coefficient calculations.

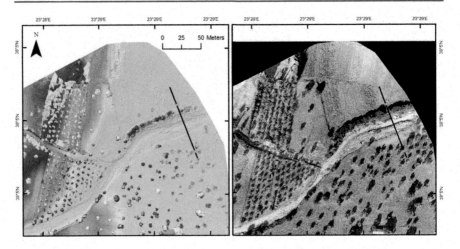

Fig. 34.3 Digital surface models (left) and orthophoto maps (right) of the Soures (up) and Agia Aikaterini (down) torrents at the locations of the studied cross sections. Green circles denote the flood marks (HWMs) identified from ground observations

Fig. 34.4 Maximum flood extent created around Mandra during the flood of 15 November 2017, illustrating critical culverts (*A, B, C*) that failed during the high water flow

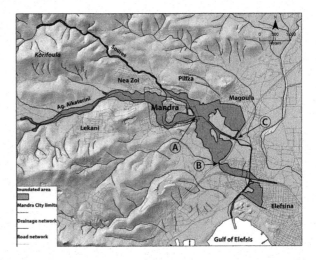

Unit peak discharge in both basins reached a value of approximately $10m^3/s/km^2$, close to the values reported for other extreme Mediterranean flash flood events. The collection of evidence testifies on the extremity of the event and further highlight the great potential of UAV sensors for the detailed mapping of similar hazards.

Particularly in the Eastern Mediterranean, recent inventories have shown the scarcity of information and observations regarding flash floods. Well-described events are rare and instrumentation usually sparse and inadequate despite the rich record of extreme storms and flash floods in the area. The combination of ground with aerial observation for post-flood mapping provides a useful tool for both estimating the extent of flooding and one of the most important physical characteristics (i.e. flood extent).

In the course of this survey, the UAV provided also (a) a faster overview of the flooded area in comparison with the traditional ground-based survey, (b) a rapid mapping of impacts (e.g. road closures and collapses, levee breaches, property damage assessment on a plot-by-plot or building-by-building basis), (c) an imagery from locations, where access was restricted or risky (e.g. in steep canyons), (d) maps of erosion and sediment deposition processes that were not possible from ground- and satellite-based observations (the latter due to time- and resolution-related issues), such as the mapping of sediment loads in the coastal area or the size of geomorphic effects (e.g. erosion of river banks). The survey highlighted also certain weaknesses inherent in the use of UAVs including restrictions in their use due to weather conditions, safety considerations, legal framework, licensing and permissions or battery use.

34.4   The 2016 Chios Island Fires

On July 25 and August 262,016 wildfires erupted in the south-western part of Chios Island (Aegean Sea, Greece). The first affected an area of approximately 47 km^2 and burned through almost 90% of olive groves and mastic trees, while the second broke out in a forested area a few kilometres to the north and affected approximately 6.6 km^2 of forest and farmland.

A research aiming at the post-fire landslide susceptibility (LS) mapping of both areas was conducted [23–25] using thematic layers in GIS environment and by analysing ten factors known to control landslide phenomena [26–28]:

(a) Morphological data, which derived from a 5 m-DEM model of the study areas provided: (a) the slope gradient, (b) the slope aspect (which affects water accumulation and soil moisture), (c) the curvature factor (which affects the acceleration or slowing of flow on a surface) and (d) the drainage network. For the drainage network a distance map was developed to represent the decrease in probability of mass movement phenomena as the distance from rivers increases.

(b) Lithological and geological data (including tectonic structures). The presence of scree, as well as of clastic formations found in some areas is an aggravating factor for landslide phenomena. Active faults form areas with intense morphology and zones with fragmented and unstable carbonate and clastic formations as well as unstable scree along which landslide phenomena can occur.

(c) Land cover derived from Worldview-2 satellite images before and after the fire events. Where the root systems are strong, the slopes have greater stability and thus the susceptibility to landslides phenomena is reduced. Severity was used instead of Land Cover for the post-fire susceptibility map.

(d) Soil thickness: Areas with increased soil cover thickness (>60 cm) are characterized by more favourable conditions for landslides phenomena along slopes.
Soil thickness was derived by field survey observations.

(e) Post-fire burn severity data was collected from field survey and satellite image
processing, road network from OpenStreetMap corrected using satellite
images and

(f) Annual rainfall data (as a factor that affects landslide occurrence) derived from
neighbouring meteorological stations.

(g) Road network: In areas with high geological heterogeneity and reduced coherence combined with inadequate technical works for hydraulic road protection,
roads can exacerbate the already disturbed balance and favour landslides
phenomena.

Post-fire landslide inventory was created after an extensive field survey,
enriched with data from pubic archives before the beginning of the rainfall period
(October 2016) and before the end of winter season (February 2017) together
with a map showing their distribution. Data classification of each factor according to its estimated LS followed, by using the reverse ranking method, where 1 is
the least susceptible and 10 is the most one. Each category was normalized to
100% and the final raster thematic maps of landslide controlling factors were
produced.

Finally, using numerical weight for each factor, which was assigned by the
Analytic Hierarchy Process [29] using Pairwise Comparison Method and according
to the weighted linear combination, a map was generated where each cell has a
certain post-fire LS index (LSI) value [30–33]. The higher the LSI value, the higher
the LS. This procedure was repeated twice, first using pre-fire land cover and secondly using the severity of the fire events.

The resulting maps, classified with natural breaks method, constitute the final
pre- and post-fire LS maps of the affected areas with five LS categories: very low,
low, moderate, high and very high. Comparison of these two final maps showed,
that forest fires that occurred did not affect the spatial distribution of areas of high
to very high risk of landslides susceptibility, but they burdened already existing ones
(Fig. 34.5). Also, the model created is considered to be well accepted as the high to
very high risk areas are identified with the positions of recorded landslide phenomena before and after the fires.

In the North fire-affected area landslide risk map, two major regions of high to
very high landslide susceptibility can be distinguished, one in the northern part and
one around Sidirounda settlement having an E-W direction. In these high slope
gradient areas, alternations of clastic formations and limestones occur, while existing road network have impacted slopes' stability. On the landslide risk map of the
South fire-affected area, two major high to very high landslide areas are identified,
one heading NE-SW and one N-S. In these areas, clastic formations, tectonic structures, high slope gradients and road network occur.

Both the model created and field survey have identified three main causes of
landslide phenomena: (a) the characteristics of lithologies involved, (b) the

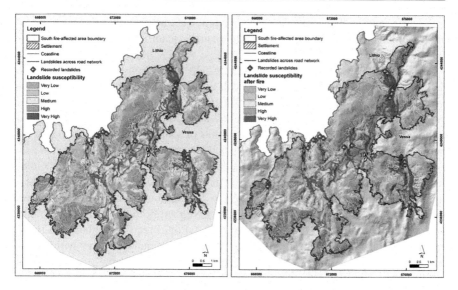

Fig. 34.5 Landslide susceptibility maps of South fire-affected area before (left) and after (right) the July 25 and August 262,016 wildfires

existence of an aquifer between the permeable carbonate formations and the relatively impermeable classical formations and (c) the high morphological gradients. Road network considered as triggering factor.

34.5   Conclusions

Results on the above cases, suggest that the systematic use of UAV-aided aerial mapping combined with ground observations in the investigation of a flash flood had important advantages. Firstly, the UAV allowed to capture imagery in a rapid way from an extensive area during flood flows despite that a large portion of it was inaccessible due to road closures. Especially for flash floods were inundation presents a rapid rise and withdrawal, it is virtually impossible for a field survey team to reach different parts of the inundated area and capture imagery during the flood. These capabilities can lead to obtaining very valuable information on flash flood events, as shown in this study and others (e.g. [17]), including videos with evidence on maximum water level and velocity [22]. In addition, combining UAV with the structure from motion technique provides detailed DSMs, suitable for measuring cross sectional areas on demand. These capabilities fit to the opportunistic approach of studying flash flood events in the sense that UAVs can rapidly collect information within the short time frame that these information is available (e.g. evidence on flow velocity), making UAVs a useful tool in flash flood event investigations.

Nevertheless, it has to be noted that the accuracy accompanying ground observations (for instance in capturing water level) cannot be substituted completely by aerial observations. Thus, based on the experience of this case study, UAV should be an additional source of evidence for a field survey team in the field, rather than a substitute for ground observations.

Finally, findings of this study suggest that UAV can be considered more suitable than other aerial photography sources such as manned aerial vehicles or satellites in the case of flash flood investigations. The reasons are that manned aerial vehicles take longer to prepare their flight plans and normally fly in higher altitudes than smaller and more agile UAVs. Given that flights of a large manned aircraft for these purposes is difficult to plan under emergency circumstances, especially when aerial search and rescue operations are underway, readily deployable and very low-flying UAVs have a better chance to capture the desired imagery in short timeframes. In higher altitudes sight may be severely limited by persistent cloud cover. Furthermore, vertically captured imagery from higher altitudes, is often unable to portray flood limits and water stage below vegetation canopy and other man-made covers. On the contrary, low-flying UAVs are able to capture imagery with a relatively small angle to the horizontal or even from multiple angles, reducing this problem. In addition, the rapid withdrawal of water may limit their captured material to only post-flood imagery, rather than picturing floodwaters during the flood. However, this disadvantage may not apply in all cases, as intense deposition of mud during the flood, may leave a clear trace even days after the withdrawal of flood waters.

Nevertheless, as shown in the third case from Chios, when it comes to extensive affected areas across several sq. kms, satellite imagery is irreplaceable, especially in cases such as wildfires (or large riverine floods), where multispectral imaging can rapidly outline and map the complete patchwork of severity and extension with reliable results.

References

1. Alexander DC. Natural disasters. London: Routledge; 1993. https://doi.org/10.1201/9780203746080.
2. Thomas D, Ertugay K, Kemec S. The role of geographic information systems/remote sensing in disaster management. In: Rodriguez H, Quarantelli EL, Dynes RR, editors. Handbook of disaster management. Newark: Springer; 2007.
3. Hodgson M, Cutter S. Mapping and the spatial analysis of hazardscapes. In: Cutter SL, editor. American hazardscapes: the regionalization of environmental risks and hazards. Washington, DC: Joseph Henry Press; 2001. p. 37–60.
4. Monmonier M. Cartographies of danger: mapping hazards in America. Chicago: The University of Chicago Press; 1997.
5. White GF. Human adjustment to floods: a geographical approach to the flood problems in the United States (Research paper no. 29), Chicago; 1945.
6. White GF. Natural hazards research. In: Chorley RJ, editor. Directions in geography. London: Methuen; 1973. p. 193–216.
7. Rodriguez H, Quarantelli EL, Dynes RR. Handbook of disaster research. Berlin: Springer; 2007.
8. Fernandez Galarreta J. Urban structural damage assessment using object-oriented analysis and semantic reasoning. Enschede: University of Twente; 2014. https://doi.org/10.5194/nhessd-2-5603-2014.

9. Fernandez Galarreta J, Kerle N, Gerke M. UAV-based urban structural damage assessment using object-based image analysis and semantic reasoning. Nat Hazard Earth Syst Sci. 2015;15(6):1087–101. https://doi.org/10.5194/nhess-15-1087-2015.

10. Palmer J. The potential use of unmanned aerial vehicles during on-site inspections. In: CTBT: Science and Technology; 2015.

11. Dong L, Shan J. A comprehensive review of earthquake-induced building damage detection with remote sensing techniques. ISPRS J Photogrammetry Remote Sens. 2013;84:85–99. https://doi.org/10.1016/j.isprsjprs.2013.06.011.

12. Alschner F, DuPlessis J, Soesilo D. Drones in humanitarian action—case study no. 9: using drone imagery for real-time information after Typhoon Haiyan in The Philippines. Geneva, Switzerland. 2013. https://drones.fsd.ch/en/case-study-no-9-using-drone-imagery-for-real-time-information-after-typhoon-haiyan-in-the-philippines/.

13. Meier P, Soesilo D. Drones in humanitarian action—case study no. 10: using drones for disaster damage assessments in Vanuatu. Geneva, Switzerland. 2015. https://drones.fsd.ch/en/case-study-no-10-monitoring-and-inspection-natural-disaster-i-acute-emergency-i-assessments/.

14. Lessard-Fontaine A, Alschner F, Soesilo D. Drones in humanitarian action—case study no. 6: rapid damage assessments of Tabarre and surrounding communities in Haiti following Hurricane Sandy. Geneva, Switzerland. 2016. https://drones.fsd.ch/en/case-study-no-6-mapping-rapid-damage-assessments-of-tabarre-and-surrounding-communities-in-haiti-following-hurricane-sandy/.

15. Lessard-Fontaine A, Alschner F, Soesilo D. Drones in humanitarian action—case study no 7: using high-resolution imagery to support the post-earthquake Census in Port-au-Prince, Haiti. Geneva, Switzerland. 2016. https://drones.fsd.ch/en/case-study-no-7-using-high-resolution-imagery-to-support-the-post-earthquake-census-in-port-au-prince-haiti/.

16. Zimmaro P, Stewart JP, Di Sarno, L, Durante MG, Simonelli AL, Penna A. Engineering reconnaissance of the 24 August 2016 Central Italy Earthquake. Version 2. 2016. https://doi.org/10.18118/G61S3Z.

17. Smith MW, Carrivick JL, Hooke J, Kirkby MJ. Reconstructing flash flood magnitudes using 'structure-from-motion': a rapid assessment tool. J Hydrol. 2014;519:1914–27.

18. Andreadakis E, Diakakis M, Nikolopoulos EI, Spyrou NI, Gogou ME, Katsetsiadou NK, Deligiannakis G, Georgakopoulos A, Zacharias A, Maria M, Lekkas E, Kalogiros J. Characteristics and impacts of the November 2017 catastrophic flash flood in Mandra, Greece. In: Geophysical research abstracts, vol. 20, EGU2018-12215, EGU General Assembly 2018, Viena, 8 April; 2018.

19. Papadimitriou P, Kassaras I, Kaviris G, Tselentis G-A, Voulgaris N, Lekkas E, Chouliaras G, Evangelidis C, Pavlou K, Kapetanidis V, Karakonstantis A, Kazantzidou-Firtinidou D, Fountoulakis I, Millas C, Spingos I, Aspiotis T, Moumoulidou A, Skourtsos E, Antoniou V, Andreadakis E, Mavroulis S, Kleanthi M. The 12th June 2017 Mw=6.3 Lesvos earthquake from detailed seismological observations. J Geodyn. 2018;115:23–42. https://doi.org/10.1016/j.jog.2018.01.009.

20. Gaume E, Borga M. Post-flood field investigations in upland catchments after major flash floods: proposal of a methodology and illustrations. J Flood Risk Manag. 2008;1(4):175–89.

21. Arcement GJ, Schneider VR. Guide for selecting manning's roughness coefficients for natural channels and floodplains. Water-supply paper 2339, U.S. Geological Survey; 1989.

22. Lumbroso D, Gaume E. Reducing the uncertainty in indirect estimates of extreme flash flood discharges. J Hydrol. 2012;414:16–30.

23. Aleotti P, Chowdhury R. Landslide hazard assessment: summary review and new perspectives. Bull Eng Geol Environ. 1999;58:21–44.

24. Guzzeti F, Carrarra A, Cardinali M, Reichenbach P. Landslide hazard evaluation: a review of current techniques and their application in a multiscale study, Central Italy. Geomorphology. 1999;31:181–216.

25. Hungr O. Some methods of landslide hazard intensity mapping (invited paper). In: Fell R, Cruden DM, editors. Proceedings of the landslide risk workshop. Rotterdam: A.A. Balkema; 1997. p. 215–26.

26. Gartner JE, Cannon SH, Bigio ER, Davis NK, McDonald C, Pierce KL, Rupert MG. Compilation of basin morphology, burn severity, soils and rock type, erosive response, debris-flow initiation process and event-triggering rainfall for 599 recently Burned Basins in the Western U.S. (USGS open-file report). Reston: US Geological Survey; 2006.
27. Iverson R. Landslide triggering by rain infiltration. Water Resour Res. 2000;36:1897–910.
28. Savage W, Baum R Instability of steep slopes, ch.4, p. 53–80. In: Jakob M, Hungr O, editors. Debris-flow hazards and related phenomena, 794 p. Berlin: Springer-Verlag; 2005.
29. Saaty TL. The analytical hierarchy process. New York: McGraw Hill; 1980, 350pp.
30. ESRI. ArcGIS desktop—ArcMap. 2016. http://desktop.arcgis.com/en/arcmap/.
31. Huabin W, Gangjun L, Weiya X, Gonghui W. GIS-based landslide hazard assessment: an overview. Prog Phys Geogr. 2005;29(4):548–67.
32. Ladas I, Fountoulis I, Mariolakos I. Using GIS and multicriteria decision analysis in landslide susceptibility mapping—a case study in Messinia prefecture area (SW Peloponnesus, Greece). Bull Geol Soc Greece. 2007;40(4):1973–85.
33. Ladas I, Fountoulis I, Mariolakos I. Large scale landslide susceptibility mapping using GIS based weighted linear combination and multicriteria decision analysis—a case study in northern Messinia (SW Peloponnesus, Greece). In: Proceedings of the 8th Panhellenic Congress of the Geographical Society of Greece, vol 1, pp. 99–108; 2007.

CBRNE and Decontamination

35

Bernd Domres, Yasmeen M. Taalab, and Norman Hecker

35.1 Introduction

CBRNE is an acronym for Chemical, Biological, Radiological, Nuclear, and high-yield Explosives. These agents hold the potential to initiate mass casualties and disaster and thus societal mass disruption. They are either deliberately or accidentally liberated during technological malfunctions, through the use of weapons of mass destruction, or terrorism [1, 2].

Weapons of mass destruction (WMD) are partially banned according to several international treaties and conventions; however a number of countries have not signed nor ratified them [3, 4].

Those treaties are:

1. Nuclear Non-Proliferation Treaty (NNPT)
2. Biological and Toxin Weapons Convention (BTWC)
3. Chemical Weapons Convention (CWP), etc. [3, 4]

CBRNE defense consists of mitigation, passive protection measures (e.g., personal protection garment, environment independent respiratory devices), contamination avoidance, detection, and decontamination. Decontamination is defined as removal or neutralization of CBRNE agents from the body surface to prevent further harm caused by continuous absorption following exposure [5–8].

B. Domres · N. Hecker (✉)
German Institute for Disaster Medicine and Emergency Medicine, Tübingen, Germany
e-mail: norman.hecker@disaster-medicine.com

Y. M. Taalab
Forensic Medicine and Clinical Toxicology Department, Faculty of Medicine, Mansoura University, Dakahlia Governate, Egypt

© Springer Nature Switzerland AG 2021
E. Pikoulis, J. Doucet (eds.), *Emergency Medicine, Trauma and Disaster Management*, Hot Topics in Acute Care Surgery and Trauma,
https://doi.org/10.1007/978-3-030-34116-9_35

463

35.2   Chemical Hazards

Toxic chemicals are chemicals that can pose a wide range of health hazards including irritation, sensitization, and carcinogenicity and furthermore are often associated with death, temporary incapacitation, or permanent harm to humans [9]. Additionally, they can induce other hazards such as fire, corrosion, and explosibility. In general, 11 million different chemicals are identified, and around 70,000 different chemicals are in use in modern-day industrial states. Every year, more than 600 million tons of these 70,000 chemicals are produced of which 10,000 agents are known to be toxic to both humans and the environment. Furthermore, since the year 1900, 70 agents were used as warfare and in terrorism [10–13]. Chemical weapons use toxic chemicals to induce intentional harm to humans during war. They were first used on a large scale during World War I, causing enormous casualties [14, 15]. They are prohibited by the Chemical Weapons Convention (CWC), which was signed in 1997. There are currently 193 states committed to the CWC [16]. The CWC specifies "allowed purposes" for toxic chemicals, such as for industrial or research usage [17–20]. Many toxic chemicals and precursors are "dual use," meaning they have permitted uses but could also be used as weapons [17]. For example, chlorine is used for water purification but can also be used as a choking agent [21–23]. The Organization for the Prohibition of Chemical Weapons (OPCW) monitors certain toxic chemicals and precursors to ensure that they are only used for "allowed purposes." Chemical warfare agents are categorized depending on their consequences [13].

35.2.1   Types of Chemical Toxins and Related Toxidromes

1. *Nerve agents* attack the victim's nervous system. Mostly caused by chemicals known as "organophosphates." Many common pesticides belong to this substance group. Examples of the nerve agents are however also sarin gas and Nowitschok, both causing cholinergic crisis, which have been used in terrorist attacks.
2. *Blister agents* also known as vesicants attack the skin of the victim resulting in blisters and skin burns. Mustard gas and lewisite are common blister agents and also known as corrosive toxins. Mustard gas, for example, was used during World War I.
3. *Blood agents* interfere with the blood oxygen-carrying capacity and its ability to deliver oxygen to organs. Therefore, they are so-called hemoglobin toxins resulting in knockdown syndrome due to suffocation and in the end disrupt the cellular oxygen delivery and/or utilization. Cyanide gases such as hydrogen cyanide (HCN) are the most common type of these agents.
4. *Choking/lung/pulmonary agents* are chemicals that attack the lungs causing them to fill with fluid. Chlorine gas and phosgene are typical choking agents and known as respiratory toxins resulting in inhalation or irritant gas syndromes.

5. *Incapacitating agents/riot control agents* usually irritate the skin, mucous membranes, airway passages, eyes, nose, lips, and mouth. Contact with these agents may cause vomiting or often intolerable pain, and they may lead to serious medical conditions. Their use is often permitted by law enforcement agencies to temporarily incapacitate individuals, but they are not originally designed to kill or cause permanent harm. For example, tear gas or pepper spray belongs to this group [24–26].

6. *Central nervous system (CNS)-acting agents* cause unclear thoughts or alter consciousness, with symptoms including paralysis and hallucinations. Examples include anesthetics. They may cause temporary incapacitation but can be fatal too [27–31].

7. *Herbicides* damage plants or crops [32]. The use of herbicides in warfare is prohibited [33]. However, herbicides are classed as chemical weapons if used for intentional harm to humans [10, 25].

8. *Toxins* are naturally occurring chemicals that can be classified as both biological and chemical weapons. For example, ricin and saxitoxin are listed in the CWC [9, 34]. To date, there have been two prosecutions under the Chemical Weapons Act 1996 for the production or purchase of chemical weapons, both involving ricin [35].

35.2.2 Special Aspects Regarding Chemical Agents in Terrorism and War

1. High toxicity (acute: LD50, LD75).
2. Ease of synthesis and dissemination.
3. Light availability.
4. Threat analysis and incident management may lack at first.
5. Release environment (wind, rain, snow, height, population density).
6. Antidote often lacking.
7. Decontamination (highly cost-intensive).
8. Risk perception and public preconception.

35.2.3 Modes of Delivery

Chemical weapons deploy the toxic chemicals [13] by different methods including explosion as in bombs or grenades, dispersal as in sprays, or contamination by gels or creams [36, 37]. The method of release is particularly dependent on the properties of the chemical, for example, its persistence (how quickly it disperses) [13]. Nonpersistent agents disperse quickly on release. They include volatile liquids that readily evaporate, such as sarin, and gases, such as chlorine [17]. While persistent agents, such as VX, are less volatile, they cause long-term contamination and retention [17]. "Binary weapons" are stored as two less toxic precursors that are mixed together when needed to form the toxic agent [13]. This reduces the risk of detection or unintended exposure. For example, some sarin munitions hold two precursors in separate compartments until deployment [10].

35.2.4 General Principles of Chemical Emergencies

The hot zone is the area of immediate contamination. Entry into a hot zone requires special equipment. It is imperative that the hot zone is isolated as soon as possible and entry is restricted, while threatened areas have to be evacuated. Chemical agents are especially likely to spread downwind, creating an additional risk area. Notably, dispersion dynamics of gases are such that "downwind" is rarely a straight line but more likely to be an expanding cone. Keep in mind that gases spread differently in the atmosphere during day and night. Meteorological conditions, population density, communication capabilities, the specifics of the agent involved, and the concentration released are factors that will define evacuation routes. The hot zone should be approached from an upwind direction by rescue forces. However this area is also the potential evacuation and treatment area.

35.2.5 Decontamination of Chemical Agents

Timely response is considered the most important factor. The most important and effective decontamination after any chemical exposure is done within the first 2 min. This is the "personal decontamination." Early action by the injured to decontaminate himself will make the difference between survival, or minimal injury, and death. Depending on the agent involved, simple means such as soap and water can save lives. Early administration of antidotes is also a life-saving measure. When clothes are contaminated, undressing them early on is furthermore an absolute must. However extreme care must be taken when undressing to avoid transferring chemicals. If necessary contaminated clothes are simply removed cutting them. During subsequent treatment, ensuring that the patient is decontaminated is also essential to avoid the risk of exposing medical staff [38]. Besides the "personal decontamination," "spot decontamination" by professional forces is considered the second most important measure. Eyes, nose, mouth, and face are usually decontaminated by normal saline solution, while other contaminated areas of the body are decontaminated by Na-hypochlorite. Wounds are addressed by hydrogen peroxide. The basic principle of spot decontamination is as follows: Rinse for 2 min, wipe by use of a sponge for 2 min, and then rinse for another 3 min.

The *sequence of measures* therefore is:

1. Personal decontamination
2. Rescue
3. Antidote
4. Registration
5. Undressing

6. Triage
7. Spot Decontamination
8. Wound dressing
9. Basic life support, antidote atropinization
10. Retriage, advanced life support
11. Hospital admission
12. Definite care

Example for a stock of antidotes:

Stock of antidotes		
Agent	Antidote	Dose
Alkyl phosphates	Atropine sulfate 1%	0.1 mg/kg body weight
	Obidoxime Toxogonin	750 mg/24 h
	Benzodiazepine	10–50 mg
Mustard	Na-thiosulfate	10–15 g
N-Lost		
HCN (+fire)	Na-thiosulfate	100 mg/kg body weight
	Flumicord spray	5 sprays/h
HCN (−fire)	4-DMAP	100 mg
	4-Dimethylaminophenol	

35.3 Biological Hazards

In general biological hazards have been part of human civilization since its very beginnings and have often decimated large parts of the global population. Basically they are known as epidemics, alas the outbreak of infectious diseases (e.g., bird virus influenza, cholera, HIV, measles, plague, tularemia, typhoid fever, and many more). Biological hazards, especially in our globalized world, have the potential to easily affect a large number of people within a short period of time. For example, traveling with modern technology, like plane, is faster than the typical incubation time of most agents. Also biological agents have been used regularly in warfare since ancient times. Just think of sieges when beleaguering troops used to catapult infected bodies over city walls, or contamination of fresh water reserves by cadavers.

35.3.1 Indications for Biologic Agents

1. An unusual temporal or geographic clustering of illness (e.g., persons who attended the same public event or gathering) or patients presenting with clinical signs and symptoms that suggest an infectious disease outbreak (e.g., patients presenting an unexplained febrile illness often imposing serious conditions like sepsis, pneumonia, respiratory failure)
2. An unusual age distribution for common diseases (e.g., an increase in what appears to be a chickenpox-like illness among adult patients, but which might be smallpox)

3. Many cases of acute flaccid paralysis with prominent bulbar palsies, suggestive of a release of botulinum toxin

35.3.2 Categorization of the Bioterrorism Agents/Diseases

Centers for Disease Control and Prevention (CDC) has categorized biological agents into groups according to:

1. Ease of dissemination and transmission
2. Potential for major public health impact
3. Potential for public panic and social disruption
4. Requirements for public health awareness and preparedness (diagnostic capacity, surveillance)

35.3.2.1 Category A
These are agents that can be easily disseminated or transmitted from person to person; they result in high mortality rates and have the potential for major public health impact and thus might cause public panic and social disruption.

Agents/Diseases
1. Anthrax (*Bacillus anthracis*)
2. Botulism (*Clostridium botulinum* toxin)
3. Plague (*Yersinia pestis*)
4. Smallpox (*Variola major*)
5. Tularemia (*Francisella tularensis*)
6. Viral hemorrhagic fevers, including filoviruses (Ebola, Marburg) or arenaviruses (Lassa, Machupo)

35.3.2.2 Category B
Second highest priority agents include those that are moderately easy to disseminate and usually result in moderate morbidity rates and low mortality rates. They require specific enhancements of CDC's diagnostic capacity and enhanced disease surveillance.

Agents/Diseases
1. Brucellosis (*Brucella* species)
2. Epsilon toxin of *Clostridium perfringens*
3. Food safety threats (*Salmonella* species, *Escherichia coli* O157:H7, *Shigella*)
4. Glanders (*Burkholderia mallei*)
5. Melioidosis (*Burkholderia pseudomallei*)
6. Psittacosis (*Chlamydia psittaci*)
7. Q fever (*Coxiella burnetii*)
8. Ricin toxin from *Ricinus communis* (castor beans)
9. Staphylococcal enterotoxin B

10. Typhus fever (*Rickettsia prowazekii*)
11. Viral encephalitis (alphaviruses, such as Eastern equine encephalitis, Venezuelan equine encephalitis, and Western equine encephalitis)
12. Water safety threats (*Vibrio cholerae, Cryptosporidium parvum*)

35.3.2.3 Category C
Third highest priority agents include emerging pathogens that could be engineered for mass dissemination in the future because of availability, ease of production, and dissemination. They hold the potential for high morbidity and mortality rates and major health impact.

Agents/Diseases
Emerging infectious diseases such as Nipah virus and Hantavirus.

35.3.3 An Alternative Classification Groups the Agents According to Their Impact

Agents of allergenic and toxic nature that form bioaerosols and are harmful for the respiratory tract, eyes, and/or skin of humans include viruses, bacteria, and fungi and their integral constituents' endotoxins, β-glucans, chitin, as well as plant particles, pollen, and protein sensitizers. Agents that cause infectious and parasitic diseases through one or more routes of transmission including disease vectors like insects and plants, direct or indirect physical contact (i.e., dermal exposure), air inhalation, and/or ingestion. Examples of agents belonging to this group include the zoonotic pathogens methicillin-resistant *Staphylococcus aureus* (MRSA), Coxiella burnetii (causative agent of Q fever), and Bacillus anthracis (anthrax) and the non-zoonotic bacterium *Legionella*.

35.3.4 The "Dirty Dozen" of Bioterrorism

Agent	Disease
Bacillus anthracis	Anthrax
Clostridium botulinum	Botulism
Brucella	Brucellosis
Yersinia pestis	Plague
Coxiella burnetii	Q fever
Ricin seed of castor oil plant	Lethal dose 22 μg/kg body weight
Variola major	Smallpox
Staphylococcus	Enterotoxin B
Fungi	Colonized with crops producing several toxins
Francisella tularensis	Tularaemia
Alphavirus EEE, WEE, VEE	Viral equine encephalitis
Filovirus and arenavirus	VHF, Ebola hemorrhagic fever, Lassa fever

Symptoms	Degree											
	1	2	3	4	5	6	7	8	9	10	11	12
Dermal symptoms												
Acral gangrene			+									
Ulcer	+		+									
Gastrointestinal symptoms												
Diarrhea	+	+		+	+			+	+	+		
Melena	+									+		
Neurological symptoms												
Ataxia								+				
Coma								+	+	+		
Diplopia	+							+				
Mydriasis	+											
Dysphagia	+											
Systemic symptoms												
Pancytopenia							+			+		
Uremia				+			+			+		

35.3.5 Biological Emergencies

Biological emergencies are those in which the microbes are released in the air causing illnesses and death. During biological emergencies, the decontamination procedures include all the universal safety precautions and procedures that are required to maintain sanitized environment in and around wards and especially diagnostic laboratories. External decontamination in such cases is to maintain sanitation and hygienic environment.

35.3.6 Standard Precautions for Biological Emergencies

During medical management of biological emergencies, the standard precautions to be followed by health workers include (a) hand wash after patient contact; (b)wearing gloves when touching blood, body fluids, secretions, excretions, and contaminated items; (c) wearing a mask and eye protection, or a face shield, during procedures likely to generate splashes or sprays of blood, body fluids, secretions, or excretions; (d) handling used patient care equipment and linen in a manner that prevents the transfer of microorganisms to people or equipment; and (e) care when handling sharp objects.

35.4   3. Radio-Nuclear Hazards

35.4.1 Types of Radiation

The types of radiation are:

- Alpha radiation, emitting a helium nucleus consisting of 2 protons + 2 neutrons.

- Beta radiation results from either transformation of a neutron into a proton of the atomic nucleus by the emission of a negative loaded electron or the transformation of a proton in a neutron by the emission of positive loaded electron with the result of production of beta-negative or beta-positive radiation.
- Gamma radiation, it is an electromagnetic radiation like X-rays, but with a much shorter wavelength and greater energy.

35.4.2 Effects of Radiation on Living Organisms

Alpha and beta radiation have the effect of ionizing elements; however the effect of alpha radiation is only dangerous for a few centimeters distance, while beta radiation is effective only for a few meters. Distance is the best protection in these cases. The greatest danger arises when they act as but internal radiation sources, e.g., when they are incorporated in the organism. The track of gamma radiation on the other hand is much longer, up to 3 km distance, and has much more energy involved. It can pass through solid materials. Radiation entering an organism displaces electrons from stable atoms with radicals being released. The two most significant radiosensitive organ systems in the body are the hematopoietic and the gastrointestinal systems. The relative sensitivity of an organ to direct radiation injury depends upon its component tissue sensitivities. Cellular effects of radiation, whether due to direct or indirect damage, are basically the same for the different kinds and dose of radiation. The simplest effect is cell death. Of course, then the cell is no longer present to reproduce and perform its primary function [39], thus posing the danger of (multi-)organ failure. Of course changes in cellular function at lower radiation doses than those that cause cell death may happen, too. These effects include delays in phases of the mitotic cycle, disrupted cell growth, permeability changes, and changes in motility [39–42]. In general, actively dividing cells are most sensitive to radiation. Radiosensitivity also tends to vary inversely with the degree of differentiation of the cell. The severe radiation sickness resulting from external irradiation and its consequent organ effects is a primary medical concern. When appropriate medical care is not provided, the median lethal dose of radiation, the LD50/60 (which will kill 50% of the exposed persons within a period of 60 days), is estimated to be 3.5 Gy. Contamination may happen externally or internally. External contamination will occur when contaminated areas are being entered without appropriate protection. The simple removal of outer clothing will, in most instances, effect a 90% reduction in the patient's contamination. Internal contamination will occur when radionuclide material is ingested and inhaled, or wounds get contaminated. The skin itself is impermeable to most radionuclides. Wounds and burns however also create a portal for contamination to bypass the epithelial barrier. All wounds must therefore be meticulously cleared and debrided, if they occur in a radiological environment. Any fluid in the wound may hide weak beta and alpha emission from detectors. Once a radionuclide is absorbed, it crosses capillary membrane through passive and active diffusion mechanisms, and then it is distributed throughout the body. The rate of distribution to each organ is related to organ metabolism, the ease of chemical transport, and the affinity of the radionuclide for chemicals within the organ. The liver, kidney, adipose tissue, and bone have higher capacities for binding radionuclides because of their high protein and lipid makeup. Within the respiratory tract, particles less than 5 μ in diameter may be deposited in the alveolar area. Larger particles will be cleared to the oropharynx by the mucociliary apparatus. Soluble particles will be either absorbed into the blood stream directly or pass through the lymphatic system. Insoluble particles, until cleared from the respiratory tract, will continue to irradiate surrounding tissues. In the alveoli, fibrosis and scarring are more likely to occur due to the localized inflammatory response [39, 40].

35.4.3 Whole-Body Radiation/Radiation Syndrome/ Radiation Illness

Dose (Gy)	Onset	Symptoms
>2	2 days	Hematopoietic syndrome, hemorrhage, and infection
>6	Hours	Severe gastrointestinal hemorrhage and death
>30	Minutes	Cardiovascular and central nervous system, fatal within 4 days

35.4.4 Comparable Levels of Radiation Exposure

Chest X-ray: 10 mrem
  CT abdomen: 1000 mrem
  Air travel Lima–Madrid: 4 mrem

35.4.5 Dosimetry

The transformation of an atomic nucleus is defined as disintegration and its measuring unit is 1 Becquerel (1 Bq) = 1 disintegration of one atom nucleus per second. The unit for the total absorbed doses of the body is Gray (Gy). The exposure of 4.5 Gy is the so-called lethal dose of radiation.

The equivalent dose of the biological effects on the body due to radiation is measured in Sievert (Sv), 1 Sv = 100 rem.

The annual natural radiation dose is 2.1 mSv = 210 rem, which is caused by terrestrial radiation and cosmic radiation. An annual dose of 250 mSv increases the risk of cancer by 1%, while the general risk to die of cancer is approximately 25%.

35.4.6 Acute Radiation Syndrome (ARS)

After exposure to ionizing radiation, the four early reacting organ systems (neurovascular (N), hematopoietic (H), cutaneous (C), and gastrointestinal (G) system) express different signs and symptoms. After very high doses, the prognosis of ARS depends mainly on the extent of damage to organs other than the bone marrow (e.g., lung, gastrointestinal tract, skin) with the risk of multiple organ failure as the maximal consequences. The METREPOL system of categorization uses a method of describing signs and symptoms and rating them with a degree of severity between 1 and 4. Zero is used when a given sign or symptom is absent, while four describes the maximal damage.

35.4.7 Considerations for Medical Assistance Teams' Personal Protection

1. Iodine protection of thyroid tissue
2. Special protection equipment
3. Full face respirator
4. Dosimeter

35.4.8 Considerations for Decontamination

1. Evacuation and rescue from the hot zone
2. Registration
3. Disrobing
4. Triage
5. First aid
6. Spot decontamination
7. Waterproof dressing of wounds
8. "External decontamination": using water, soap, H_2O_2, 0.5% Na hypochlorite, diethylenetriamine pentaacetate acid (DTAP)
9. "Internal decontamination": magnesium sulfate, chelate, alginate

35.5 Explosive Hazards

Explosives are intentionally used as military ordnances like bombs, grenades, land mines, and improvised explosive devices, or as commercial explosives, such as devices used during material extraction like in mineral mines. Furthermore explosions may occur unintentionally by a large variety of means.

35.5.1 Types of Blast Injuries

1. Primary blast injuries result directly from the effects of the abnormal ambient pressure generated during the blast wave. The magnitude of the energy resulting from the shockwave and the duration of the blast wave correlates with the risk of primary blast injury. The air around the blast is displaced by the wave of over-pressure resulting in high-velocity blast winds. Middle ear, lungs, and gastrointestinal tract are most susceptible to primary blast injuries. Resulting injuries encompass blast lungs, tympanic membrane rupture, abdominal hemorrhage and perforation, globe rupture, and traumatic brain injuries without physical signs of head injury.
2. Loose objects are displaced and form projectiles that have the potential to cause both blunt and penetrating injuries. These secondary blast injuries are the most common type of injuries following an explosion and encompass all thinkable types of injuries. Remember that wounds can be grossly contaminated, and delayed primary closure and tetanus vaccination might be needed.
3. Tertiary blast injuries are the result due to the impact of people being thrown against other structures when displaced by the blast wave or winds. These are usually blunt injuries but may include impalement. Typical for tertiary blast injuries are the crush syndrome with damage to the muscular system and subsequent release of myoglobin, urates, potassium, and phosphates which lead to oliguric renal failure and the compartment syndrome which results in decreased tissue perfusion and ischemia.
4. The quaternary (or miscellaneous) blast injuries include those injuries not attributable directly to the blast itself but which result from the effects of the blast. They may include burns; inhalational injury; contamination with chemical, biological, and radio-nuclear agents; as well as exacerbations of a chronic disease.

35.6 Protective Equipment

Dealing with CBRNE agents necessitate using personal protective equipment (PPE) that is originally designed to provide protection against injuries and illnesses effecting the respiratory system, skin, eyes, face, hands, feet, head, body, and hearing. These illnesses usually result from interaction with chemical, radiological, physical, electrical, mechanical, biological hazards and airborne particles. No single combination of protective equipment and clothing can protect against all hazards; however, achieving total individual protection requires an integrated approach.

In general, the personal protective equipment is divided into two major groups: respiratory protective devices and body surface protective equipment. Both groups have relatively complex additional internal division. Additional protective clothing which may be required to safely complete a task may include, but is not limited to, the following:

1. Environment independent respiration from contained pressurized air.
2. Whole-body water- and gas-proof protective garment, including the head, arms, and legs, is required in highly contaminated areas when there is a potential for encountering moisture or where excessive perspiration is likely to occur. For example, rainwear, plastic suits, veterinarians' gloves, canners gloves, waterproof boots, and latex gloves.
3. When it is anticipated that moisture and heat stress conditions are to be encountered, GORE-TEX suits should be used.
4. Canvas, cotton, or leather gloves should be worn as the outer pair of hand protection when working with duct tape.
5. Leather gloves should be worn as the outer pair of hand protection when working with sharp objects or heavy work that may penetrate rubber gloves during normal activities.
6. Rubber knee boots if working in areas with standing water.
7. Welders' coveralls if a rescuer is doing any cutting, grinding, or welding.
8. Helmet.
9. Two-way communication tool.
10. Autoinjector of antidotes.
11. GPS sensor.
12. Dosimeter.

35.6.1 Grading of Personal Protection Equipment

The primary protective mechanism against chem-bio agents is to protect the respiratory and contact protection of the skin. A properly fitted protective mask, when combined with an over garment, gloves, and boots, can provide excellent protection. The primary protective equipment to use against radiological agents are respiratory protection along with skin coverage, consisting of properly fitted protective mask combined with 100% cotton over garment, gloves, and boots. PPE should also be used in conjunction with other protective methods, including exposure control procedures and equipment. Several designs have been proposed to convey the levels of protection; however, some of the generally accepted designations for levels of protection are the following:

35.6.1.1 Level A
This consists of a SCBA or supplied-air respirator with an escape cylinder, in combination with a fully encapsulating chemical protective suit capable of maintaining a positive air pressure. The ensemble includes both outer and inner chemical-resistant gloves, chemical-resistant steel-toed boots, and two-way radio communications. It provides the highest level of protection for the skin, eyes, and the respiratory system. It also makes rapid and effective decontamination easier because the breathing apparatus is contained within the protective suit.

35.6.1.2 Level B
This has the same respiratory protection as Level A plus hooded chemical-resistant clothing, outer and inner chemical-resistant gloves, chemical-resistant steel-toed boots, and other, optional, items. It should be used when the highest level of respiratory protection is necessary, but a lesser level of skin protection is needed.

35.6.1.3 Level C
This is similar to Level B, except that a full- or half-face air-purifying respirator is worn, instead of the SCBA or "supplied-air" respirator. This should be used when:

1. The concentration and a type of an airborne substance is known
2. The criteria for using air-purifying respirators are met
3. The atmosphere is breathable

35.6.1.4 Level D
Protection is primarily a work uniform and is used for nuisance contamination only. It requires only coveralls and safety shoes/boots. Other PPE is based upon the situation (types of gloves, etc.). It should not be worn on any site where respiratory or skin hazards exist.

Keep in Mind
Personnel working under circumstances of protection level A are only able and allowed to work continuously for a short time, often only 30 min. Working under Level A conditions is mentally and physically demanding.

References

1. Malich G, et al. Chemical, biological, radiological or nuclear events: the humanitarian response framework of the International Committee of the Red Cross, vol 97, no. 899 Cambridge University Press Cambridge. 2015. 97(899): p. 647-661.
2. Be'eri E, et al. A chemical-biological-radio-nuclear (CBRN) filter can be added to the air-outflow port of a ventilator to protect a home ventilated patient from inhalation of toxic industrial compounds. Disaster Med Public Health Prep. 2018;12(6):739–43.
3. Gurr N, Cole B. The new face of terrorism: threats from weapons of mass destruction. London: IB Tauris; 2002.
4. Prockop LD. Weapons of mass destruction: overview of the CBRNEs (chemical, biological, radiological, nuclear, and explosives). J Neurol Sci. 2006;249(1):50–4.
5. Blacker SD, et al. Physiological responses of police officers during job simulations wearing chemical, biological, radiological and nuclear personal protective equipment. Ergonomics. 2013;56(1):137–47.
6. Cone DC, Koenig KL. Mass casualty triage in the chemical, biological, radiological, or nuclear environment. Eur J Med. 2005;12(6):287–302.
7. Knudson GB, et al. Nuclear, biological, and chemical combined injuries and countermeasures on the battlefield. Mil Med. 2002;167(Suppl 1):95–7.
8. Murphy RR, et al. Projected needs for robot-assisted chemical, biological, radiological, or nuclear (CBRN) incidents. In: 2012 IEEE international symposium on safety, security, and rescue robotics (SSRR). New York: IEEE; 2012.

9. UN, Convention on the prohibition of the development, production, stockpiling and Use of chemical weapons and on their destruction; 1997.
10. Evison D, Hinsley D, Rice PJB. Chemical weapons. Br Med J. 2002;324(7333):332–5.
11. Marshall VC. Major chemical hazards. Chichester: Ellis-Horwood; 1987.
12. Meulenbelt SE, Nieuwenhuizen MS. Non-state actors' pursuit of CBRN weapons: from motivation to potential humanitarian consequences, vol. 97, no. 899. Cambridge: Cambridge University Press; 2015. p. 831–58.
13. Shea DA. Chemical weapons: a summary report of characteristics and effects. Washington, DC: Congressional Research Service, Library of Congress; 2012.
14. Corps, U.S.A.C. A comparative study of world war casualties from gas and other weapons. Washington, DC: US Government Printing Office; 1928.
15. Prentiss AM. Chemicals in war. A treatise on chemical warfare. New York: McGraw-Hill; 1937.
16. Hendrikse J. A comprehensive review of the official OPCW proficiency test. In: Chemical weapons convention chemicals analysis: sample collection, preparation and analytical methods. Chichester: Wiley; 2005. p. 89–132.
17. Ganesan K, et al. Chemical warfare agents. J Pharm Bioallied Sci. 2010;2(3):166.
18. Robinson JPP. Difficulties facing the chemical weapons convention. Int Aff. 2008;84(2):223–39.
19. Vogel FJ. The chemical weapons convention: strategic implications for the United States. Carlisle, PA: Army War College; 1996.
20. Voigt K, Welzl GJ. Chemical databases: an overview of selected databases and evaluation methods. Online Inf Rev. 2002;26(3):172–92.
21. Clark RM, Sivaganesan M. Predicting chlorine residuals and formation of TTHMs in drinking water. J Environ Eng. 1998;124(12):1203–10.
22. Clark RM, Sivaganesan M. Predicting chlorine residuals in drinking water: second order model. J Water Resour Plan Manage. 2002;128(2):152–61.
23. Gopal K, et al. Chlorination byproducts, their toxicodynamics and removal from drinking water. J Hazar Mater. 2007;140(1-2):1–6.
24. Crowley M, "Drawing the line: regulation of 'wide area' riot control agent delivery mechanisms under the chemical weapons convention." Bradford Non-Lethal Weapons Research Project and Omega Research Foundation; 2013.
25. Mesilaakso M. Chemical weapons convention chemicals analysis: sample collection, preparation and analytical methods. Hoboken: Wiley; 2005.
26. Olajos EJ, Stopford W. Riot control agents: issues in toxicology, safety & health. Boca Raton: CRC Press; 2004.
27. Brennan RJ, et al. Chemical warfare agents: emergency medical and emergency public health issues. Ann Emerg Med. 1999;34(2):191–204.
28. Frank RG, Pollack HA. Addressing the fentanyl threat to public health. N Engl J Med. 2017;376(7):605–7.
29. Mathews RJ. Central nervous system-acting chemicals and the chemical weapons convention: a former scientific adviser's perspective. Pure Appl Chem. 2018;90(10):1559–75.
30. Rudd RA. Increases in drug and opioid-involved overdose deaths—United States, 2010–2015. MMWR Morb Mortal Wkly Rep. 2016;65(50-51):1445–52.
31. Sharp TW, et al. Medical preparedness for a terrorist incident involving chemical and biological agents during the 1996 Atlanta Olympic Games. Ann Emerg Med. 1998;32(2):214–23.
32. Stellman JM, Stellman SD. Agent Orange during the Vietnam War: the lingering issue of its civilian and military health impact. Washington, DC: American Public Health Association; 2018.
33. Aldrich GH. Customary International Humanitarian Law—an interpretation on behalf of the International Committee of the Red Cross. Br Year Book Int Law. 2006;76(1):503.
34. Balali-Mood M, Rice P, Matthews P, et al. Practical guide for the medical management of chemical warfare casulaties organisation for the prohibition of chemical weapons. The Hague, Netherlands; 2016.
35. Timperley CM, et al. Advice from the Scientific Advisory Board of the Organisation for the prohibition of chemical weapons on isotopically labelled chemicals and stereoisomers in relation to the chemical weapons convention. Pure Appl Chem. 2018;90(10):1647–70.

36. Meselson M. The problem of biological weapons. Bull Am Acad Arts Sci. 1999;52(5):46–58.
37. Metz S, Johnson DV. Asymmetry and US military strategy: definition, background, and strategic concepts. Carlisle, PA: Army War College Strategic Studies Institute; 2001.
38. Kumar V, et al. Chemical, biological, radiological, and nuclear decontamination: recent trends and future perspective. J Pharm Bioallied Sci. 2010;2(3):220.
39. Jarrett D. Medical management of radiological casualties handbook. Bethesda, MD: Armed Forces Radiobiology Research Institute; 1999.
40. Jarrett D, et al. Medical treatment of radiation injuries—current US status. Radiat Meas. 2007;42(6–7):1063–74.
41. Koenig KL, et al. Medical treatment of radiological casualties: current concepts. Ann Emerg Med. 2005;45(6):643–52.
42. Mettler FA Jr, Voelz GL. Major radiation exposure—what to expect and how to respond. N Engl J Med. 2002;346(20):1554–61.

Medical Care during Civil Unrest, Protests and Mass Demonstrations

36

Frederick Lough

Summary: Physicians, nurses, and hospital administrators need to prepare for the unexpected. Civil unrest, protests, and mass demonstrations are increasingly familiar worldwide events, stressing all aspects of society. Dedicated preparation by hospitals and healthcare workers is critical in order to save lives during these challenging events.

Introduction: Civil unrest, protests, and mass demonstrations are worldwide events, occur primarily in cities, and are increasing in frequency. They represent major challenges to local and national governments, fire and rescue resources, and healthcare leaders and organizations.

These events can be planned or occur spontaneously. The numbers of participants are unpredictable and can increase or decrease with time. Social media has a significant role in amplification of the number of individuals who are involved and in their behavior. The duration of the protests may be predictable or not. The location of the event may be limited or there may be multiple protests occurring simultaneously, and this too can change with time. Command and control of these events are dependent upon police and/or military resources, and these resources can be overwhelmed by circumstances. The response to the protests by police and military can also inflame and promulgate these situations.

Communication by police, fire and rescue, and healthcare leaders in dealing with these events is critical to limiting property damage and human injury. Dealing with the television and print media can also be a challenge.

There are many medical issues during mass demonstrations. They include security for the medical personnel, keeping accurate records of those treated, what was done, and the ultimate disposition of the patients. Use of physical space is also a major issue. An established hospital may be the treatment facility, or if not, other

F. Lough (✉)
Uniformed Services University of the Health Sciences, Bethesda, MD, USA
e-mail: frederick.lough@usuhs.edu

© Springer Nature Switzerland AG 2021
E. Pikoulis, J. Doucet (eds.), *Emergency Medicine, Trauma and Disaster Management*, Hot Topics in Acute Care Surgery and Trauma,
https://doi.org/10.1007/978-3-030-34116-9_36

479

buildings may need to be adapted to care for patients. Designation of triage areas, operating rooms, and ICU and extended care areas, as well as locations for the deceased also need careful consideration. Re-supply of medical units is an ongoing challenge as resources are consumed. Coordination of hospital assets, such as physicians and nurses, blood banks, pharmacy, and operating rooms, is critical. Other medical support available may include volunteers, street medics, fire and rescue personnel, police and military units, and fixed and flexible facilities. Crowd control agents, such as tear gas, have varying effects depending on atmospheric conditions and if the agents are used in a confined space [1, 2]. Patients exposed to these agents may have few symptoms, or they may be severely ill. Basic principles of triage and advanced trauma life support are fundamental to dealing with the casualties that can result from mass demonstrations. Flexibility, adaptability, and practice are the key to being able to deal effectively with these events.

36.1 Examples from the Recent Past

Detroit 1967: The Summer of 1967 saw riots across America. One of the worst riots occurred in Detroit, Michigan. This riot lasted 5 days, left 40 dead and 1500 wounded, and resulted in over $200 million dollars of damage. Detroit General Hospital dealt with 26 dead and 900 injured. The hospital was at full capacity when the riots began. This forced activation of the disaster plan, and discharging to home those patients who were well enough to leave. Physicians and nurses found it difficult to travel to and from the hospital for their shifts. Many of the protesters were arrested, but there was a shortage of handcuffs to control these individuals. Blood was also in short supply. The citizens of Detroit came forward to provide the needed life-saving blood. The staff worked long hours and were successful in limiting the loss of life. Recommendations that came from this period included rehearsing disaster plans, locking all doors except the receiving area, and not allowing visitors [3].

INDIA 1993: Bombay, India experienced violent communal rioting in January of 1993. Four hundred thirteen casualties were treated at the King Edward Memorial Hospital over 6 days. One hundred ninety four patients were admitted, and the numbers of patients, at times, overwhelmed the hospital. The casualties resulted from arson, violence, and gunfire. The injured were triaged into three categories, expectant, serious, and minimal. All patients were given temporary code names and registrations numbers. Detailed records of injuries and treatment rendered were maintained. Pattern of injuries were as follows, 93 limb, 61 head, 22 chest, 50 abdominal, and 43 multiple sites. Sixty-two major operations were performed and 99 minor procedures were required. Ninety-three percent were males and 51% were aged 21–30 years of age. The hospital was stressed economically by the number of operations, the use of antibiotics, and the in-hospital care required. Being prepared is critical to save lives. Preparation includes knowledge of the type of injuries, employing triage principles, having an efficient blood bank, and having a disaster management plan which is practiced and revised periodically. Also, during this riot, the hospital was isolated from the outside. Ambulances were used to bring hospital personnel to their duty stations. Feeding the staff was an issue, and the hospital kitchen was used to feed the physicians and nurses. Several violent episodes occurred in the hospital itself. Internal security was necessary. Registration of patients was challenging, as some arrived unconscious. It is recommended that pre-positioning bracelets with individual numbers be readily available. Preparation of casualty lists and dealing with the media were also problems. During this event, many relatives of the injured arrived at the hospital and had to be dealt with compassionately. Finally, dealing with the dead was challenging, and a coroner had to be positioned at the hospital. This episode demonstrated the myriad of challenges a hospital and the staff can face during mass protests [4].

Vancouver 2012: Riots can occur following normally innocuous events such as sporting contests. In 2012, following game 7 of the Stanley Cup Finals, rioting erupted in Vancouver which eventually resulted in 140 injured and 1 fatality. St. Paul's Hospital, the primary care facility, functioned well and was commended for their response to the riots [5].

Baltimore, Maryland, 2013–2015: Racial tensions and the deaths of African Americans while in police custody resulted in the outbreak of rioting in these cities. A common denominator included poverty and distrust between the local community and law enforcement. In the case of Baltimore, the response was led by the City Health Department and by the Fire and Police Department. Among the issues faced were the safety of the healthcare workers and assisting citizens in determining which hospitals and pharmacies were still functioning. The hospitals were successful in continuing to work and to avoid issues inside the facilities by skillful use of security personnel. The after-action analysis revealed that hospitals, during civil unrest, are largely on their own. Preparedness and stock piling of resources are critical to continue to function [6, 7].

Fire and Emergency Medical Response to Unrest: Healthcare leaders need to be aware of the techniques and measures that the Fire and Police personnel will take in dealing with mass demonstrations. Planning and interagency cooperation is critical and should be practiced. Emphasis should be placed on a unified command, clear communications, and frequent situational updates. Overhead observation and evaluation via helicopters and/or drones can be extremely helpful in assessing the situation and adapting to changes with time. Fires should be rapidly extinguished, debris such as trash and dumpsters should be moved from hospitals premises, and constructions sites should be secured. This will limit items that can be used to further destruction and injuries. Healthcare workers need to be aware of the various "weapons" that can be employed by both the protesters and those responding. Squirt guns can be used to spray ammonia, gasoline, and other chemicals. Molotov cocktails, a bottle filled with gasoline and thrown, are extremely dangerous. All loose items, rocks, bottles, etc. can be hurled resulting in injury. Riot control agents, collectively referred to a "tear gas," represent a group of compounds that are designed to be noxious and result in dispersing crowds. The human response to these agents is variable. Depending upon conditions such as wind, concentration and if the agent was used in a confined space patients can be only transiently affected or may be seriously ill. Physicians and nurses need to be aware of what agents are being used and the specific symptoms of severe exposure. Close cooperation between healthcare leaders and the fire and police responders is critical to minimizing human injury and property damage [8].

Lessons from Responders: The following is a brief list of the lessons learned from around the world in dealing with episodes of civil unrest, protests, and mass demonstrations.

1. Planning critical. No detail is too small to consider. Plans need to be practiced and revised.
2. Healthcare leaders need to coordinate with their local and national leaders to insure a coordinated response.
3. Communication channels need to be established well before rioting breaks out.
4. Healthcare leaders need to recognize that the police and fire resources can be rapidly exhausted and that hospitals may need to function totally on their own. This includes providing physical security for the patients, workers, and physical plant.
5. Leadership is fundamental to effectively dealing with mass demonstrations.
6. Information about the event and effective communication is critical to limiting damage and loss of life.
7. Preparing hospitals to function independently for 1–2 days is a common recommendation from events around the world.

36.2 Recommendations

1. For Individual Physicians and Nurses
   Prepare for the unexpected. Work with your hospital to develop a plan that provides guidance but is flexible. Know your area of responsibility, be able to function without everything you are used to. Develop a plan for rotation of your personnel that considers the limitations of hours worked and how performance deteriorates with exhaustion.
2. For Surgical and Emergency Teams
   Develop a plan to deal with many casualties, and practice and refine the plan to fit your individual situation. Ensure that all members of the team know their area of responsibility and can also fill other positions in case of absences of personnel.
3. For Hospitals
   Coordinate the development of an overall response plan. Work with local police and other authorities to insure the hospital's plan will work with the anticipated actions by police and fire. Insure that hospital personnel can arrive and leave the facility, that supplies can be brought in, and that the blood bank is prepared. Insure that there are appropriate measures to record arrival, treatment, and discharge of patients. Anticipate addressing the needs of families and of the media. Be cognizant of the potential benefits and possible problems of dealing with mass demonstrations in today's social media world.

Disclaimer The opinions or assertions contained herein are the private ones of the authors and are not to be construed as official or reflecting the views of the Department of Defense, the Uniformed Services University of the Health Sciences, or any other agency of the U.S. Government.

References

1. Facts about riot control agent interim document. Center for Disease Control and Prevention; 2013.
2. Riot control agent poisoning. Center for Disease Control and Prevention; 2015.
3. Stempniak M. Race riots overwhelmed Detroit hospitals back in 1967. Hospitals and Health Networks; 2016.
4. Dalvie SS, Pai PR, Shenoy SG, Bapat RD. Analytic data of January 1993 communal riot victims—KEM Hospital experience. J Postgrad Med. 1993;39(1):5–9.
5. St. Paul's Hospital worked with military like precision treating riot related injuries. Providence Health Care; 2012.
6. Hospital preparedness security paramount during the Baltimore riots. HC PRO Hospital Safety Center.
7. Wen LS, Warren KE, Shirli Tay BA, Khaldun JS, O'Neill DL, Farrow OD. Public health in the unrest: Baltimore's preparedness and response after Freddie Gray's Death. Am J Public Health. 2015;105(10):1957–059.
8. Vernon A, Fire/EMNS response to Civil Unrest Events. EMS WORLD. 2007. https://www.emsworld.com/article/10321832/fireems-response-civil-unrest-events.

Management of Combat Casualties

37

Kyle Remick and Eric Elster

> *"He who wishes to be a surgeon should go to war."*
>
> *—Hippocrates*

War provides significant opportunity to care for injured military personnel and civilians injured during the course of hostile action. Perhaps the only ultimate benefit of war is the massive amount of experience one can accumulate caring for the injured within a very short period of time. It has been said that a lifetime of experience can be gained in a short time during these unfortunate events.

Furthermore, war often provides scenarios that involve the care of multiple casualties with limited resources. One recent report from the US experience noted that one combat hospital in Iraq cared for 50 patients in 3 mass casualty events. During these events, there were 191 procedures performed equaling 3.8 procedures per casualty, and 76% of casualties required immediate surgery [1]. A report from another combat hospital in Iraq noted there were 26 days of mass casualty events over a 1-year deployment. During these events, 76% required immediate surgery [2]. These two experiences highlight the frequency of mass casualty incidents seen during war. In this sense, "disaster planning" for the battlefield is synonymous with preparedness for frequent mass casualty events.

It is thus essential for those deploying to war to care for the wounded to be prepared to deal with mass casualty events. One aspect is to be individually prepared to both deal with the chaos that occurs during these events and to be highly medically trained and ready. The other aspect of a successful response to mass casualty events is to ensure the trauma system of care is well organized and prepared to deal with

K. Remick (✉) · E. Elster
Department of Surgery, Uniformed Services University School of Medicine,
Bethesda, MD, USA
e-mail: kyle.remick@usuhs.edu

© Springer Nature Switzerland AG 2021
E. Pikoulis, J. Doucet (eds.), *Emergency Medicine, Trauma and Disaster Management*, Hot Topics in Acute Care Surgery and Trauma,
https://doi.org/10.1007/978-3-030-34116-9_37

the large influx of patients from mass casualty events. In the case of combat casualty care during war, the existing framework of the trauma system in often remote and austere locations with limited resources becomes of paramount importance. The goal of the chapter is to describe the organization of battlefield care that is optimally designed to deal with frequent mass casualty scenarios during war.

37.1 Organization of Combat Casualty Care

Unlike a civilian trauma system for optimal care of the injured patient, the organization of battlefield care must be structured but also fluid enough to move and adapt to changing battlefield locations and conditions. As part of the North Atlantic Treaty Organization (NATO), the US Military organizes battlefield care based on the agreed upon NATO convention [3]. Care on the battlefield is organized into defined roles of care.

37.1.1 Role 1

Role 1 care encompasses care from the point of injury (POI) through evacuation and until the patient reaches a defined battlefield trauma care facility. Over the past 25 years, battlefield trauma care has made exceptional advances based on the efforts of the Committee on Tactical Combat Casualty Care.

Tactical combat casualty care guidelines have redefined how we care for patients at the Role 1 on the battlefield [4]. During this phase both the casualty and the rest of the team are at ongoing risk of injury from gunfire and explosions. If medical providers were to rush the casualty at this point and provide full initial care, they would place themselves and other team members at risk of injury. Thus, the best initial action is to return fire until the enemy is suppressed meaning unable to inflict further injury. During this time, the only acceptable maneuvers are to attempt to move the patient out of immediate danger if possible and to stop obvious life-threatening bleeding. This is usually discussed in terms of placing a tourniquet on an injured extremity. This can be done by the patient themselves in some cases, and then the patient should also return fire if able. Alternatively, a nearby service member may also place a tourniquet if able to do so safely and without risk to self. A trained medic may also respond if there is little risk of injury to themselves. No further care is rendered during this phase of TCCC until the enemy is suppressed.

The next phase of TCCC is tactical field care. Trained medical personnel, commonly referred to as the "medic" may then render care when the firefight has ended. Medics must carry their medical equipment with them in a backpack; thus they have a limited amount of equipment to perform life-saving maneuvers at the POI. In general this entails continued efforts to halt life-threatening bleeding, the greatest cause of battlefield death. Bleeding wounds can be packed with hemostatic gauze, and tourniquets can be place to prevent life-threatening bleeding from the extremities. Injuries causing airway and breathing compromise can be treated. Fractures can be rapidly stabilized in order to prevent further bleeding and pain. If available and necessary, blood products can be infused preferably over other resuscitation fluids to maintain an acceptable blood pressure to sustain life. Pain control medications may be given. If there are multiple casualties, the medic must quickly assess all of the casualties and prioritize care based on injuries noted and resources available. Also important during this phase, the team leaders also play a pivotal role in that they must decide how and when the casualty or casualties will be evacuated. At times, the battlefield scenario may not permit immediate evacuation.

The last phase of TCCC is care during evacuation. Oftentimes, a single medic is faced with caring for multiple casualties until evacuation arrives and then during the movement of casualties to the next role of care. In recent conflicts, the US Military has had the luxury of immediate evacuation by medical evacuation helicopter, but this has been less true over the last several years of combat experience. Whether the patient is moved by vehicle or by air, the casualties must have ongoing re-evaluation of injuries and further treatment based on severity of injury. Furthermore, not all casualties may be able to be evacuated at one time and prioritization must occur.

Triage is a term that can be applied at this point. Triage is the prioritization of casualties based on injuries, chance of survival, and the availability of resources to save the most number of casualties. Triage occurs during TCCC but the concept will also apply at all roles of care on the battlefield. Unlike in most circumstances in civilian trauma and even in multiple casualty incidents in civilian trauma, difficult decisions on the battlefield must be made in order to do the greatest good for the greatest number. This translates into medical terms as attempting to save the casualties with the best chance of survival given limited resources to care for them. Not only is this a challenging decision based on the fact that life and death decisions must be made, but these must be made within the context of preserving the fighting force of the military unit for the ongoing mission. Ultimately, the medic on the scene must make the best decision based on resources and information available.

37.1.2 Role 2

NATO defines the Role 2 as the first battlefield facility. The type of facility is not as important as the personnel and trauma resources available, so this can be accomplished in a tent that can be moved to another location if needed or it can be provided in a building that has been occupied and set up to serve this purpose for a temporary or prolonged period of time. Often personnel are trained and equipped to provide a complete patient evaluation and with increased resources to care for the casualty. The Role 2 will usually have a physician, nurses, medics, and other specialists such as laboratory technicians and X-ray technicians who are trained to render advanced battlefield trauma care but usually not including surgical care. An organized approach to the evaluation and care of the trauma patient is performed to a standard such as taught in the American College of Surgeons Advanced Trauma Life Support course [5].

At this role of care, the patient is again evaluated first for immediately life-threatening injuries. Control of the airway with intubation, provision of ventilation for the non-breathing patient, decompression of tension pneumothorax or bleeding in the chest, and further control of visible life-threatening bleeding can be performed when necessary. Intravenous access for transfusion of blood products to increase blood pressure is often available. Adjunctive studies to identify other injuries and bleeding in the chest and abdomen using chest and pelvis X-rays and ultrasound examination of the abdomen for bleeding are often available. Pelvic bleeding can sometimes be controlled with a specially designed pelvic binder or a makeshift sheet wrapped around the pelvis tightly. The casualty can be warmed so as to prevent or reverse hypothermia which can contribute to further bleeding and shock. Further medications may also be given to slow life-threatening bleeding and to treat pain. The patient must be stabilized as best as possible with the resources available and prepared for further transport to a facility that has a surgical capability.

In the event of multiple casualties, the Role 2 may also become overwhelmed due to lack of personnel and resources. Many times these facilities will be capable of handling 2–4 patients at one time before becoming overwhelmed. If there are more casualties, a triage situation occurs. At the Role 2, there must be pre-planning for such an event. A mass casualty plan should be established in advance which includes a plan to surge all available medical personnel and resources available to render care to all casualties. When this is still not adequate, triage must occur just as at the Role 1.

The pre-planned and rehearsed mass casualty plan will include a plan for triage. A physician, nurse, or medic with experience preferably becomes the "triage officer." At a pre-designated location immediately outside the facility but in a safe place, the triage officer must quickly evaluate incoming casualties and prioritize them for care. The US Military uses the term "DIME" to describe the triage categories of "delayed," "immediate," "minimal," and "expectant." The most expedient way to perform the triage is to quickly survey all of the casualties taking about 5–10 s for each. If the casualty is awake and talking or is walking with apparent minimal injury, they are directed to a holding area that was pre-designated for minimal casualties. Those that appear to be lifeless or having catastrophic head injuries or with whole body disruptive injuries are categorized as expectant, meaning they are assessed as having little chance of survival even if all resources were dedicated to only their care. This is often a mentally challenging and frustrating situation and is best done by a medical provider with significant trauma experience. Of the remainder of casualties, those with immediately life-threatening injuries that may be saved with rapid intervention are the ones first moved into the Role 2 facility. Those with significant but lesser non-immediately life-threatening injures are moved to an area where they can be moved into the Role 2 after the immediate casualties are treated. Continuous re-evaluation of all of the casualties is essential to successful triage as some casualties often are found to have decompensated and need immediate treatment. The overarching goal of the triage officer is to ensure that the inside of the Role 2 facility is not overwhelmed with more casualties than beds available for care but to keep the lead medical provider inside the facility informed as to the ongoing situation in the triage area.

Simultaneously and if available, there should be one administrative medical officer in charge of calling for air or ground medical evacuation. It is of the utmost importance that after casualties are treated and stabilized within the Role 2 facility, they can be quickly evacuated out of the Role 2 facility so as to make room for the next patient in need of care.

Within the Role 2, a single medical officer, preferably the most experienced or the physician, should maintain positive awareness and control of the ongoing evaluation and interventions of all the casualties. This allows the medical officer to assist the nurses and medics with treatment decisions and to perform higher-level interventions when needed. After all the casualties are cared for and have been further evacuated, the Role 2 should conduct an immediate debrief of the scenario to assess for areas of improvement and to allow team members to express their thoughts and feelings regarding the event. Conducting this debrief facilitates improvement of the teams mass casualty plan and gives team members an opportunity to decompress after a usually stressful scenario involving life and death decisions and care. It is helpful to have a chaplain and/or psychologist available during this event and for team members who may struggle with the stress that can be difficult to deal with during these mass casualty scenarios.

37.1.3 Role 2: Surgical

Although not part of the NATO convention for battlefield care, the "Role 2—Surgical" nomenclature has become a familiar part of the US Military's battlefield organization. Commonly called a "surgical team," these units can be attached to a Role 2 for surgical augmentation or also have been used as stand-alone units on the battlefield.

The Role 2—Surgical will typically perform all the elements of the NATO Role 2 designation, but importantly, it will have the additional capability to perform immediate life-saving surgery. These units typically have a general trauma surgeon with or without an orthopedic trauma surgeon and an anesthesia provider. Additionally, they will have nurses and operating room technicians capable to assist in surgical care. Much like the Role 2, surgeons at the Role 2—Surgical must make difficult decisions regarding the prioritization of which casualties may benefit from immediate life-saving surgery first. In the mass casualty scenario, the physicians and surgeons must collaborate to determine which patients should be operated on first based on the number of operating room tables, number of surgeons, and number of anesthesia providers available. A typical surgical team may have two operating room tables.

Often, these units will also have a short-term post-operative or intensive care unit (ICU) section which can continue to perform critical care after the surgery is complete and until evacuation to the next level arrives. In general, the ICU section only has the personnel and equipment to hold a critically injured patient for 4–8 h but may also be augmented with personnel and resources to hold patients for longer periods of time.

37.1.4 Role 3

The largest and most robustly resourced facility on the battlefield is the Role 3 combat hospital. During the US experience in Iraq and Afghanistan, these combat hospitals had nearly all of the personnel and equipment that would be available at a civilian trauma center. The combat hospital will typically have an emergency room or resuscitation area staffed with emergency trained physicians, nurses, and medics able to provide initial life-saving interventions. There will be advanced adjunctive capabilities available such as X-ray, ultrasound, and even computed tomography. Their capacity will usually have four to ten emergency resuscitation beds with enough personnel to staff all of them simultaneously. There will normally be two to four operating rooms available with general and orthopedic trauma surgeons, anesthesiologists, operating room nurses and technicians, and often surgical subspecialists such as neurosurgeons, vascular surgeons, thoracic surgeons, head and neck surgeons, and plastic surgeons. As you may imagine, the configuration of these facilities may vary greatly from battlefield to battlefield. In a scenario where there has been ongoing conflict, these facilities may be built up over time and have capability much like a civilian trauma hospital. If the conflict is new and the Role 3 has just arrived, it may contain only the more basic elements. The overarching purpose of the Role 3 is to provide the final stabilization care within the actual battlefield prior to casualties being evacuated out of the combat zone and back to a standard trauma hospital in the home country or other partnered nation.

The Role 3 must also have a planned and rehearsed mass casualty plan as it must be prepared to receive casualties directly from the POI or may receive multiple casualties from multiple Role 2 facilities simultaneously. Although these facilities tend to have robust personnel and resources, they may still be overwhelmed during a larger mass casualty scenario. The same rules apply as to the Role 2 in that there must be a plan for triage should the number of casualties overwhelm the number of emergency beds or operating rooms available at any given time. Triage would occur using the same "DIME" system as described earlier, and personnel must know their roles and responsibilities within the triage plan as described earlier for the Role 2.

Also as in the case of the Role 2, the medical officers must have a plan to arrange for medical evacuation from the battlefield. Although the Role 3 typically has an ICU and holding bed capability, it still has the potential to be overwhelmed in large mass casualty scenarios. However the Role 3 generally has the ability to provide ongoing critical care and post-operative care for a significant number of patients. A typical robust Role 3 may have 4–10 ICU beds and anywhere from 10 to possibly hundreds of holding beds based on its configuration. In recent conflicts where the US Military has had air superiority, the ability to provide ICU care in the air with

"Critical Care Air Transport Teams" (CCATT) has allowed the Role 3 hospitals to minimize the number of general holding beds needed to 20–40.

37.2   Non-surgical Hemorrhage Control

Essential to saving lives on the battlefield is the ability to stop and prevent further hemorrhage as the highest priority. A review of deaths on the battlefield determined that of deaths in Afghanistan and Iraq between 2001 and 2011, 87% of combat casualties died in the pre-hospital environment. Of these, 24% were potentially survivable and 91% of those died from hemorrhage. Two-thirds of hemorrhage occurred in the torso where it could not be stopped without surgery. However, 19% were considered "junctional" meaning the injury was at the junction of the torso and the legs, arms, or neck. The remaining 13% died from extremity hemorrhage [6]. Thus, an awareness of basic non-surgical hemorrhage control interventions is key to combat casualty care and to successfully performing triage and treatment in mass casualty situations.

37.2.1 Extremity Hemorrhage

Bleeding extremity wounds can lead to death rapidly. Extremity bleeding can and should be stopped as rapidly as possible during initial treatment. Proper wound packing with a standard bandage or with cloth from a shirt if no formal medical bandage is available may be all that is required. The US Military has fielded a special dressing which is additionally impregnated with a substance which acts directly on injured tissues to halt bleeding. Should there be a traumatic amputation or near amputation or a wound from which bleeding cannot be controlled with packing, the use of a commercially available tourniquet device is warranted. In fact, on the battlefield, the TCCC recommended action for extremity bleeding is to place a tourniquet first and then re-evaluate the need for the tourniquet when there is no further threat of continued injuries from enemy fire.

37.2.2 Junctional Hemorrhage

Bleeding from the junctional regions as described above can be problematic in the pre-surgical environment as a tourniquet cannot be applied in these regions. Wound packing as described above can be attempted in particular with a hemostatic dressing. Recently, the US Military has fielded a "junctional tourniquet." There are several different brands of these devices that have been developed. The US Military sponsored the development of one device which wraps around the waist and has an air filled pressure chamber that will expand when insufflated, applying pressure directly deep into the junctional region. This cannot be used in the neck for obvious reasons.

37.2.3 Torso Hemorrhage

Bleeding that occurs within the chest and abdomen (known together as the torso) is often not obvious to the untrained nor visible to the eye. As noted above, two-thirds of potentially survivable injuries were the direct result of torso hemorrhage. Until recently, operative hemorrhage control was the only way to halt this bleeding.

In 2015, a balloon catheter specifically designed for ease of use in trauma received FDA approval in the US for the purpose of large vessel occlusion to prevent bleeding. This device is inserted through the groin into an appropriate point where its balloon is then inflated with fluid until the major artery no longer has blood flow beyond the balloon, thus halting the life-threatening bleeding from the injury site. However, this technology still requires a surgeon to be present immediately following this device's use or the device can cause serious adverse consequences that may cause critical illnesses and death as well. Another product was recently approved in the US for hemorrhage from junctional wounds or wounds with narrow wound tracks. It uses expandable foam sponges in a tube injected into the wound which then expand and apply pressure to halt bleeding. Finally, not yet approved for use but currently in a clinical trial is a rapidly expanding polymer foam that is injected into the abdomen and provides conforming pressure to halt or slow life-threatening intra-abdominal bleeding.

37.3   Damage Control Resuscitation

The term "damage control" was first used by the US Navy to describe the concept of rapid control of fire and flooding onboard a ship so that the ship could "survive" to complete its mission [7]. Essentially, the damaging event would be isolated and compartmentalized to prevent it from consuming the whole ship. The term was first applied to trauma care by Rotondo et al. in 1993 when they coined the term "damage control surgery" [8] which will be described in the subsequent section.

The term "damage control resuscitation" (DCR) was coined by two landmark articles by Hess et al. [9] and Holcomb et al. [10] in 2006–2007 and can be summarized by the title of the second article, "Damage control resuscitation: directly addressing the coagulopathy of trauma." These authors recognized that coagulopathy, or the pathophysiologic abnormality leading to a decreased ability for blood to clot, played a pivotal role in traumatic hemorrhage and one's ability to avoid death via reaching some sustainable equilibrium of blood pressure and clotting ability of blood. The simplistic way to understand this concept is that as blood pressure decreases due to hemorrhage, blood flow out of the injury site will slow to the point where the blood can actually clot so that one does not bleed to death. This equilibrium will not necessarily occur if coagulopathy continues to worsen.

Furthermore, there is a "triad of death" in which coagulopathy, hypothermia, and acidosis are all interrelated and a worsening of one may negatively influence the other two in a downward spiral towards death. In reality, the process is more complex than this, and today we have made much progress in understanding the pathophysiology of shock caused by injury. We now know that the injury itself causes a rapid change in the bodies clotting mechanism independent of the extent of hemorrhage and that extent of initial coagulopathy actually may predict outcome [11, 12]. Furthermore, there is evidence of genetic predisposition of response to injury, and one also has a unique phenotypic response to injury that affects care and outcomes [13].

It is important to understand the tenets of DCR in regard to personnel and resources available. DCR interventions in conjunction with hemorrhage control interventions at any role of care may be life saving for one or more casualties in order to sustain them until they can reach a surgical facility that provides definitive operative hemorrhage control. Some basic DCR interventions will be described to provide this familiarity. The US Department of Defense Joint Trauma System Clinical Practice Guideline for damage control resuscitation provides a reference for additional reading [14].

37.3.1 Permissive Hypotension

The goal of "permissive hypotension" is to ensure the casualty has an adequate blood pressure to sustain life prior to necessary surgical hemostasis. The goal systolic blood pressure should be 90 mmHg or if no blood pressure is available, one can judge adequate blood pressure if a casualty is awake and able to communicate. This technique should not be used if the casualty has a head injury which is worsened by a lower blood pressure. The concept of permissive hypotension has been shown to be of benefit prior to reaching a surgical facility since World War I [15–18].

37.3.2 Blood Products

The use of blood products in a casualty that is bleeding is preferred over the use of other crystalloid or colloid fluids for volume replacement to maintain blood pressure. When available, the use of packed red blood cells, plasma, and platelets should be used in a ratio close to 1:1:1. The concept of using blood early and at this ratio in a hypotensive casualty was first shown to provide a significant mortality benefit in severely injured at a deployed US combat hospital in Iraq in 2007 [19].

37.3.3 Massive Transfusion Protocol

It is important for the trauma team to have a massive transfusion protocol. When one or more casualties arrive that require immediate blood, this protocol is meant to describe how blood is delivered from the blood storage area to the patient. A reasonable goal that showed an independent mortality benefit is for blood to arrive and be transfused to the casualty within 10 min of arrival [20]. This protocol becomes even more important in the plan for a mass casualty scenario.

37.3.4 Tranexamic Acid

The use of tranexamic acid (TXA) in severely injured casualties showed a mortality benefit in a large European study [21] and at a UK Role 3 facility in Afghanistan [22]. TXA must be administered within 3 h of injury. TXA may assist in reversing coagulopathy by halting fibrinolysis that occurs acutely after injury.

37.3.5 Fresh Whole Blood

Over the past 50 years, blood banks in the US have separated blood into components in order to more efficiently use whole blood for specific types of medical diseases. This practice resulted in the use of packed red blood cells for combat casualties devoid of coagulation factors and platelets. Additionally standard protocols encouraged the use of crystalloid (salt-water type solution) for initial treatment of bleeding, and only those casualties who continued to be in shock would be given blood products. Only recently have we recognized that the use of crystalloid for severely injured bleeding combat casualties provided worse outcomes compared to using blood products early in their care. Furthermore, using a balanced blood product resuscitation as noted above was more beneficial when caring for bleeding casualties.

Even more recently, we have recognized that providing fresh whole blood in those severely injured casualties may have further benefit over balanced blood components. This was demonstrated at a combat hospital and a Role 2 surgical team [23, 24]. We also now recognize that whole blood (WB) may be cold-stored for up to 21 days and will maintain a greater hemostatic ability as compared to the balanced use of blood components [25]. Additionally, type-specific WB is not required. O type, low-titer (1:256) may be safely transfused [26]. The ability to cold-store whole blood and to use O type, low-titer has implications for mass casualty planning and caring for the severely injured.

Aside from the importance of understanding hemorrhage control and DCR from the perspective of caring for the individual casualty, it is equally important to understand this concept and the basics of these interventions as one that may be preparing for and responding to mass casualty events. In order to appropriately care for casualties on the battlefield at all roles of care from POI to Role 3, it is important to understand in terms of resources available during mass casualty scenarios and in terms of the prioritization of care of multiple casualties.

37.4 Damage Control Surgery

Surgeons, just as emergency and other physicians, nurses, ancillary staff, and administrators, need to be prepared and remain vigilant to care for the injured in disasters and mass casualty events. In his American Association for the Surgery of Trauma Fitts Lecture in 2006, Dr. Sten Lennquist urged trauma surgeons to participate in the leadership, planning, and management of disasters since the majority of events involve mechanical injuries [27]. Echoing this sentiment in the 2014 Scudder oration at the American College of Surgeons Annual Scientific Assembly, Dr. Bill Schwab emphasized the critical need for military and civilian surgeons to create strong military and civilian partnerships to ensure surgeons are prepared to provide optimal care for the injured both abroad and at home [28].

Just as in the pre-hospital environment, the key to a successful surgical response to any multi-casualty scenario is the delivery of the appropriate quantity of care to each individual casualty while controlling the use of resources based on the situation and flow of critical patients arriving from the event. Situational awareness of the event, hospital resources available and a knowledge of the regional emergency and trauma system are crucial. In most mass casualty or disaster events the surgical assets are critical and the deployment of these must be controlled to minimize death and disability.

Thus, the concept of "damage control surgery" or DCS is important to understand from the perspective of disaster planning. For example, those critically injured in the chest and abdomen from penetrating or blunt trauma have a high likelihood of death and many times the surgeon in the operating room is the only person who can provide life-saving hemorrhage control. One study of early trauma deaths at an urban trauma center noted that the patient with hypotension and a penetrating injury will require operative intervention within 19 min to provide a chance of survival. In fact, death from injury is highly dependent on mechanism of injury, body area injured, and time elapsed since injury occurred [29].

In the late 1980s, trauma surgeons in Philadelphia noted an increased use of semi-automatic pistols with an average of 2.7 wounds per person [30, 31]. Based on a paper by Stone et al. in 1983 describing abbreviated laparotomy with packing [32], they and others in the USA [33–35] recognized that the traditional surgical approach to abdominal trauma was no longer valid for treatment of these multiple handgun wounds. The traditional approach involved full and definitive repair of all viscera and vessels followed by abdominal closure during the initial operation. This strategy worked for a single wound and for a lower velocity penetrating abdominal injury with minimal collateral damage. However, this surgical strategy was not adequate for patients with multiple wounds and a downward spiraling physiology despite aggressive resuscitation with blood products. The decision to perform damage control must be made early in the patient's course in order to be successful and should take into account patient physiology, anatomy involved in injury, and mechanism of injury.

Damage control surgical principles may also be applied in disaster scenarios with multiple simultaneous casualties who require rapid control of hemorrhage and contamination. As noted previously, the recent US Military experience forced surgeons deployed to combat to manage multiple mass casualty events [1, 2]. Based on these experiences, these military surgeons realized additional challenges in combat impacted surgical decision-making, both for the individual patient on the operating room table and for simultaneous, multiple complex patients during ongoing mass casualty events at forward medical facilities. The challenge of additional factors that influenced decision-making required combat surgeons to have a broader situational awareness to include ongoing events on the local battlefield, trauma medical resources available at the medical facility, availability and timing of medical evacuation, and the location and capability of other trauma assets within the greater system of care on the battlefield.

Similar to this US Military combat surgical experience, during a civilian mass casualty event the correct response for an individual patient and for a group of patients will be based on maintaining a situational awareness. All surgeons must be directed, where appropriate to use damage control techniques for individual trauma patients. Implementing damage control techniques based on a situational awareness (and clinical need) to control bleeding and contamination promotes shorter operation times and allows surgical resources to be available to treat other critical patients. Constant communication with the hospital's incident command system leadership, the emergency medicine leadership who continue to receive patients, the critical care nurses and supervisors, and other ancillary personnel involved in trauma care is key to optimal use of a facility's resources during a disaster.

37.5 The Trauma System as the Foundation for a Successful Disaster Response

The origin of trauma systems in the US can be traced back to the National Highway Safety Act of 1966 (Public Law 89-564) mandating that "coordination, transportation, and communication are necessary to bring the injured person and definitive medical care together in the shortest practical time...." [36]. This has been a noble goal of both military trauma care and civilian trauma care since that time. The American College of Surgeons (ACS) established resource guidelines in 1976 by publication of "Optimal Resources for the Care of the Injured Patient" [37].

The benefit of trauma systems is decreased mortality. In a review of trauma system development in 1985, Cales and Trunkey found that the presence of trauma systems yielded improved outcomes over areas that did not have organized systems [38]. Other studies also demonstrated decreased mortality of 15–25% in designated trauma centers and trauma systems [39–42]. It was a reasonable assumption that providing a trauma system for the battlefield would decrease mortality just as an organized system of care did for civilian trauma in the United States.

Thus in 2004, a group of trauma surgeons recognized that the US Military needed a formal trauma system to effectively implement changes that would lead to optimal care for our wounded. Based on the public health model, all essential components for a trauma system of care were addressed in the system but adapted to the unique battlefield environment. These included (1) information systems collecting and analyzing data in real time to provide immediate feedback to the battlefield for best practices as well as to inform trauma research, (2) prevention efforts driven by real time analysis of morbidity and mortality, (3) education for trauma providers regarding best practice clinical guidelines and essential combat trauma skills, (4) leadership in battlefield trauma care with direct access to operational leadership in order to effectively inform and implement important changes, (5) pre-hospital integration with best practices of tactical combat casualty care applied to the battlefield, and (6) an emphasis on continuous performance improvement throughout the continuum of care from point of injury to hospital care at home [43].

The organized system of care provided by the JTS was superimposed on the NATO roles of care in Iraq and Afghanistan in order to ensure optimization of battlefield trauma resources to promote the "right patient, right place, right time, right care" [44]. Thus it also formed the basis for the response to mass casualties on the battlefield. The JTS, present and functioning on a daily basis for usual trauma care, was the essential foundation for a well-coordinated and successful response when a mass casualty event occurred in combat.

In regard to all-hazards disaster planning, the regional trauma system must be integrated into local and regional plans. There must be an assessment of the systems surge capacity based on most common or potential vulnerabilities in the region. Guided by this assessment, the disaster plan will best leverage all components of the established regional trauma system in the response to larger-scale casualty events. Mass casualty event preparedness and rehearsals should include all involved agencies in order to have an organized response to a chaotic situation. To paraphrase the JTS, including the usual trauma system of care in these rehearsals facilitates optimal use of system resources to ensure the right patient gets to the right care at the right time [37, 44].

37.6 Conclusion

War is an unfortunate reality. We can at least take advantage of these unfortunate situations by rapidly learning and assimilating lessons learned from war to improve the care for injured civilians. Furthermore, the recent US Military experience has demonstrated that an organized battlefield trauma system for combat casualty care likely saves lives. Lessons in the response to mass casualty incidents in war can inform how we prepare on the home front for natural disasters and intentional and unintentional civilian mass casualty events.

Disclaimer The opinions or assertions contained herein are the private ones of the authors and are not to be construed as official or reflecting the views of the Department of Defense, the Uniformed Services University of the Health Sciences, or any other agency of the US Government.

References

1. Propper BW, Rasmussen TE, Davidson SE, et al. Surgical response to multiple casualty incidents following single explosive events. Ann Surg. 2009;250:311–5.
2. Beekly AC, Martin MJ, Spinella PC, et al. Predicting resource needs for multiple and mass casualty events in combat: lessons learned from combat support hospital experience in Operation Iraqi Freedom. J Trauma. 2009;66:S129–37.

3. NATO logistics handbook. NATO headquarters, Belgium. 2007. https://www.nato.int/docu/logi-en/logist97.htm.
4. Tactical combat casualty care guidelines for all combatants. 2017. https://www.jsomonline.org/TCCC.html.
5. Advanced trauma life support student course manual. 9th ed. American College of Surgeons Committee on Trauma; 2012.
6. Eastridge BJ, Mabry RL, Seguin PG, et al. Death on the battlefield (2001-2011): implications for the future of combat casualty care. J Trauma. 2012;73(6):S431–7.
7. US Navy. Surface ship survivability. Navy War Publications 3-20.31. Washington, DC: Department of Defense; 1996.
8. Rotondo MF, Schwab CW, McGonigal MD, et al. "Damage control": an approach for improved survival in exsanguinating penetrating abdominal injury. J Trauma. 1993;35:375–83.
9. Hess JR, Holcomb JB, Hoyt DB. Damage control resuscitation: the need for specific blood to treat the coagulopathy of trauma. Transfusion. 2006;46(5):685–6.
10. Holcomb JB, Jenkins D, Rhee P, et al. Damage control resuscitation: directly addressing the coagulopathy of trauma. J Trauma. 2007;62:307–10.
11. Brohi K, Singh J, Heron M, Coats T. Acute traumatic coagulopathy. J Trauma. 2003;54:1127–30.
12. MacLeod JBA, Lynn M, McKenney MG, et al. Early coagulopathy predicts mortality in trauma. J Trauma. 2003;55:39–44.
13. Taylor JR III, Fox EE, Holcomb JB, et al. The hyperfibrinolytic phenotype is the most lethal and resource intense presentation of fibrinolysis in massive transfusion patients. J Trauma Acute Care Surg. 2018;84:25–30.
14. Damage Control Resuscitation (CPG ID:18). Joint trauma system clinical practice guideline. 2017. http://jts.amedd.army.mil/index.cfm/PI_CPGs/cpgs.
15. Cannon WB, Fraser J, Cowell EM. The preventive treatment of wound shock. JAMA. 1918;70:618.
16. Beecher HK. Preparation of battle casualties for surgery. Ann Surg. 1945;121(6):769–92.
17. Bickell WH, Wall MJ, Pepe PE, et al. Immediate versus delayed fluid resuscitation for hypotensive patients with penetrating torso injuries. NEJM. 1994;331(17):1105–9.
18. Duke MD, Guidry C, Guice J, et al. Restrictive fluid resuscitation in combination with damage control resuscitation: time for adaptation. J Trauma Acute Care Surg. 2012;73(3):674–8.
19. Borgman MA, Spinella PC, Perkins JG, et al. The ratio of blood products transfused affects mortality in patients receiving massive transfusions at a combat support hospital. J Trauma. 2007;63:805–13.
20. Cotton BA, Gunter OL, Isbell J, et al. Damage control hematology: the impact of a trauma exsanguination protocol on survival and blood product utilization. J Trauma. 2008;64:1177–83.
21. Crash-2 collaborators. Effects of tranexamic acid on death, vascular occlusive events, and blood transfusion in trauma patients, with significant hemorrhage (CRASH-2): a randomized, placebo-controlled trial. Lancet. 2010;59(6):612–24.
22. Morrison JJ, Dubose JJ, Rasmussen TE, Midwinter MJ. Military application of tranexamic acid in trauma emergency resuscitation (MATTERs) study. Ann Surg. 2012;147(2):113–9.
23. Spinella PC, Perkins JG, Grathwold KW, et al. Warm fresh whole blood is independently associated with improved survival for patients with combat-related traumatic injuries. J Trauma. 2009;66(4 Suppl):S69–76.
24. Nessen SC, Eastridge BJ, Cronk D, et al. Fresh whole blood use by forward surgical teams in Afghanistan is associated with improved survival compared to component therapy without platelets. Transfusion. 2013;53:107S–13S.
25. Pidcoke HF, McFaul SJ, Ramasubramanian AK, et al. Primary hemostatic capacity of whole blood: a comprehensive analysis of pathogen reduction and refrigeration effects over time. Transfusion. 2013;53:137S–49S.
26. Strandenes G, Berseus O, Cap AP, et al. Low titer group O whole blood in emergency situations. Shock. 2014;41(Suppl1):70–5.
27. Lennquist S. Management of major accidents and disasters: an important responsibility for the trauma surgeons. J Trauma. 2007;62:1321–9.

28. Schwab CW. Winds of war: enhancing civilian and military partnerships to assure readiness: white paper. J Am Coll Surg. 2015;221:235–54.
29. Remick KN, Schwab CW, Smith BP, et al. Defining the optimal time to the operating room may salvage early trauma deaths. J Trauma Acute Care Surg. 2014;76(5):1251–8.
30. Schwab CW. Violence: America's uncivil war—presidential address, sixth scientific assembly of the Eastern Association for the Surgery of Trauma. J Trauma. 1993;35:657–65.
31. McGonigal MD, Cole J, Schwab CW, et al. Urban firearm deaths: a five-year perspective. J Trauma. 1993;35:532–7.
32. Stone HH, Strom PR, Mullins RJ. Management of the major coagulopathy with onset during laparotomy. Ann Surg. 1983;197(5):532–5.
33. Burch JM, Ortiz VB, Richardson RJ, et al. Abbreviated laparotomy and planned reoperation for critically injured patients. Ann Surg. 1992;215(5):476–83.
34. Morris JA, Eddy VA, Blinman TA, et al. The staged celiotomy for trauma. J Trauma. 1993;217(5):576–86.
35. Talbot S, Trooskin SZ, Scalea T, et al. Packing and re-exploration for patients with non-hepatic trauma. J Trauma. 1992;33(1):121–5.
36. Mullins RJ. A historical perspective of trauma system development in the United States. J Trauma. 1999;47(3):S8–S14.
37. Resources for optimal care of the injured patient. American College of Surgeons Committee on Trauma; 2014.
38. Cales RH, Trunkey DD. Preventable trauma deaths. JAMA. 1985;254:1059–63.
39. Celso B, Tepas J, Langland-Orban B, Pracht E, Papa L, Lottenberg L, Flint L. A systematic review and meta-analysis comparing outcome of severely injured patients treated in trauma centers following the establishment of trauma systems. J Trauma. 2006;60:371–8.
40. MacKenzie EJ, Rivara FP, Jurkovich GJ, Nathens AB, Frey KP, Egleston BL, Salkever DS, Scharfstein DO. A national evaluation of the effect of trauma-center care on mortality. N Engl J Med. 2006;354:366–78.
41. Barringer ML, Thomason MH, Kilgo P, Spallone L. Improving outcomes in a regional trauma system: impact of a level III trauma center. Am J Surg. 2006;192:685–9.
42. Nathens AB, Jurkovich GJ, Maier RV, Grossman DC, MacKenzie EJ, Moore M, Rivara FP. Relationship between trauma center volume and outcomes. JAMA. 2001;285:1164–71.
43. Eastridge BJ, Jenkins D, Flaherty S, Schiller H, Holcomb JB. Trauma system development in a theater of war: experiences from operation Iraqi Freedom and Operation Enduring Freedom. J Trauma. 2006;61:1366–73.
44. Bailey J, Spott MA, Costanzo GP, Dunne JR, Dorlac W, Eastridge B. Joint trauma system: development, conceptual framework, and optimal elements. San Antonio: U.S. Department of Defense, U.S. Army Institute for Surgical Research; 2012.

Incidents Caused by Terrorism

38

Morgan P. McMonagle

38.1 Historical Background

The word *terrorism* is thought to have evolved from the Latin word *tersere*, later becoming *terrere* (later translation to *terrible*). It became a more commonly used term in the European vernacular during the Reign of Terror (*La Terreur*) 1793–1794, which saw mass state-sponsored violence and executions (usually in public) by guillotine by the French authorities. It is ironic to note that the origins of the word originated from acts of violence perpetrated by a government against its own people, rather than the other way around!

38.2 Definition of Terrorism

Terrorism is broadly considered any act of violence or the threat of violence that instils terror or fear in people or a population. Although there is no single internationally recognised and accepted definition of terrorism, the United Nations Security Council Resolution 1566 (2004) describes an act of terror as *any criminal acts, including against civilians, committed with the intent to cause death or serious bodily injury, or taking of hostages, with the purpose to provoke a state of terror in the general public or in a group of persons, intimidate a population or compel a government or an international organization to do or to abstain from doing any act, which constitute offences within the scope of and as defined in the international conventions and protocols relating to terrorism, are under no circumstances justifiable by considerations of a political, philosophical ideological, racial, ethnic, religious or other similar nature.*

M. P. McMonagle (✉)
St. Mary's Hospital, London, UK

© Springer Nature Switzerland AG 2021
E. Pikoulis, J. Doucet (eds.), *Emergency Medicine, Trauma and Disaster Management*, Hot Topics in Acute Care Surgery and Trauma,
https://doi.org/10.1007/978-3-030-34116-9_38

Despite the rather cumbersome description above and the lack of agreement internationally as to what constitutes an act of terrorism, there are commonalities amongst the various legal definitions used across various jurisdictions around the world. Terrorism may be defined as *the premeditated and calculated use of violence (or threat of violence) against civilians (non-combatant targets) by subnational or clandestine groups in order to attain ideologic goals.* These goals may be numerous and ill-defined but are typically categorised within one or more of the following: political, economic, religious, ideologic or social. The tactics used by terrorists and their associated organisations are typically designed to coerce or intimidate society at large with the potential for far-reaching repercussions (including financial and economic).

38.3 Goals of Terrorist Activity

1. Casualty generation
2. Emergency and hospital service overwhelmed
3. Property destruction
4. Social panic
5. Economic uncertainty

38.4 Techniques and Tactics of Terrorist Incidents

The **mode** is the methodology or mechanism of delivery of an attack (limited only by the imagination of the terrorist), usually to the public, its infrastructure or other significant target (e.g. military, industry, internet, etc.). This may be carried out by a *group of individuals* (e.g. London Bridge Attack, June 2017) or a *lone individual (lone-wolf)* attack (e.g. Westminster Bridge attack, March 2017). Either way, the attacker(s) may act on a sole basis (i.e. acting alone) or on behalf of a wider group (e.g. IRA, ISIS), where the attack has been planned and orchestrated by a larger organisation (as opposed to the attacker idealising such a group without their direct involvement).

An attack may be across *numerous locations* (Paris attacks, London Tube attacks 07/07/2005) simultaneously in time and space or in close succession or may occur at a *single geographical location* (e.g. Bataclan attack, Paris, 2015, Orlando nightclub, FL, USA, Las Vegas, NV, USA, 2017). Attacks once started may be *stationary*, occurring only at a single site (e.g. bomb at single location such as Manchester Arena, UK, 2017), or *moving* (e.g. Paris attacks, London Bridge, London tube), where the attacker(s) or attacking body is in motion during the incident, making the target potentially more difficult for the security forces to contain, with heightened social panic.

An attack may come with a *warning* to security (or other) forces or *without warning* (surprise attack/*coup de main*). Surprise attacks generally are associated with a greater number of deaths and injuries in addition to the greater level of fear and uncertainty with the possibility of further attacks (real or imagined).

Mode/Mechanism of Attack Once known, this will help to determine the threat at scene (and subsequently hospital management), and the potential nature of the expected injuries that may present. Typical mechanisms include:

- Marauding attack
- Shooting
- Bomb blast
- Vehicular
- Hijacking/kidnapping
- Poisoning
- CBRNE
  - Chemical
  - Biological
  - Radioactive
  - Nuclear
  - Explosive

Marauding Terrorist Attack Anecdotal evidence suggests that the most rapidly growing mode and most prevalent terrorist threat in current times is a *marauding terrorist attack* (MTA). In an MTA, the attacker(s) is mobile (non-contained) and aims to cause as much damage, violence and fear as possible, in a short space of time and typically over a smaller area (i.e. often on foot). It may occur in the form of multiple terrorists acting across multiple locations with a multitude of weapons (London Bridge Attack (2017), Paris terrorist attack (2015)) or as a single 'lone-wolf' in a more confined (but still mobile) environment until the treat is neutralised. Weaponry may be sophisticated such as guns or more rudimentary (but easily and readily available) such a knife, swords, blunt instruments modified sharp objects (MSO) or weaponised vehicles (i.e. the use of a vehicle to cause injury). The use of a weaponised vehicle will obviously potentially increase the area covered during an attack in addition to the volume and severity of injuries as demonstrated in the Westminster Bridge (2017) and Nice (2016) terrorist attacks.

Shootings and Blast Shootings in a terrorist event are more often associated with small (concealable) arms, which in the western world are typically low velocity handguns with a lower energy displacement (e.g. 9 mm handgun). However, higher-energy weapons have been used (e.g. Las Vegas (2017), Bataclan, Paris (2015)) which will generate a greater number of casualties (rapidly fired rounds with more accuracy) and fatalities (higher-energy dump after striking the target). More sophisticated groups may use explosives as the mode of choice if the expertise and facilities are available (e.g. IRA in the 1970s and 1980s), but most urban bomb blasts associated with terrorism are rudimentary home-made devices. Although not typically of comparable high energy blast power or range, these can be very destructive to life, limb and property if close to the epicentre of the blast. In addition, the destructive effects are greater if detonated within a confined space (e.g. London bombings (2005), Madrid Bombings (2004)) due to the ricochet effect of the blast wave within the closed space which retards the blast energy decay, thereby prolonging its effects. However, the commonest cause of death after a blast is building collapse.

Hijackings and Kidnappings Although more popular in the 1970s and 1980s as an act of terror, hijackings and kidnappings (including aeroplanes) were used where the principal aim was to generate high media attention and public fear, often for a ransom (e.g. release of political prisoners, etc.). The hijacking of aeroplanes has become less common since the 9/11 attacks in New York and Washington (2001), where the planes were also used as a weapon against people, property and the economy, probably due to greater awareness and stricter security control at airports and other urban environments.

CBRNE This is a broad classification encompassing chemical, biological, radioactive, nuclear or explosive, with a resurgence seen in recent times in the UK, possibly by Russian dissidents (e.g. novichok used against Sergei and Yulia Skripal (UK, 2018)). Generally, (explosions excepted), it covers various poisonings, which may be targeted at an individual (or group) or may be large-scale industrial (i.e. chemical or nuclear plant targeted). The chemical poison of choice may be liquid (e.g. novichok) or in gaseous form (e.g. Sarin, Tokyo 1998). Other poisons include biological (e.g. anthrax, used in numerous 'letter attacks') or even nuclear (Polonium-210 used against Alexander Litvinenko (London, 2006)). It is generally not unknown what types or how much 'illegal' agents are available to terrorist organisations throughout the world, especially since the fall of the old (but previously very powerful) Eastern Block as many of these agents have originated from laboratories in Russia and other parts of Asia.

38.5 Managing a Terrorist Incident: Preparedness

Although similarities exist in the response to any large-scale incident or disaster, there are several additional considerations unique to the terrorist attack both pre-hospital and in-hospital. After a mass terrorist event, the following must be considered:

- Security (local, regional and national).
- Mass casualty incident (over time and space).
- Blast injury more likely (± confined space).
- Penetrating injury more likely (GSW, knife wounds).
- Variety of mechanisms of injury possible (e.g. blunt from car followed by penetrating from knife wound).
- Attackers are often very determined and additionally violent. This is often fuelled by a misplaced idealism and a willingness to die in carrying out their attack (e.g. suicide bomber, 9/11 attacks in NYC, 7/7 attacks in London)).
- Uncertainty and fear.
- Media, political and public expectations.

38.6   Health Service Response to a Terrorist Incident

The first official co-ordinated response to a terrorist event is typically by the civilian security forces (i.e. police) who may have been informed by a member of the public. Once a response is mounted, the police (or others) will often notify ambulance control and/or any other responders (e.g. fire service, etc.) as required, including an armed security response. It must be decided early in the event, if possible, by one of these responding organisations whether or not to declare a mass incident or not.

Any 'high-threat' response system plan involves a complex cross-interaction between all emergency responders: police, fire & rescue, ambulance, pre-hospital medical care and the hospital(s). The responding hospital (ideally a Major (Level 1) Trauma Centre) becomes the central point of activity outside of the incident scene itself, as most people (whether genuine patients or not) will flow towards this focal point (including relatives, media and other members of the public) after a disaster. Thus, the incident plan should be built around the hospital as a fixed central point within the plan. The major incident plan (MIP) is constructed so that the whole healthcare system responds *in unison* and in a pre-planned way. Many MIP models have been described, which are often more sophisticated at certain 'hot spots' (where a high threat level remains) around the world. Regardless, the plan must be pre-planned, involving all relevant stakeholders, in writing with regular (annual or biannual) practice runs. There should also be structures in place for quality improvement (QI), risk assessment and appropriate feedback and updates. This will ensure a more streamlined response from all responders during a high threat mass incident. Thus, the response becomes a well-integrated multidisciplinary operation with effective leadership, including at the command level. A well-publicised plan, including a gap analysis and hazard vulnerability assessment (HVA), is made available to all agencies and hospitals involved in the response. Not only does this aid in ensuring an effective response to an incident in real-time, but it also ensures that individuals and agencies are used more effectively, maximising strengths whilst minimising wastage.

Declaring a Mass Disaster Although no one definition for all eventualities exists, a disaster is typically one where a large-scale response from the health service (and/or other services) is required or one where the number or types of casualties is likely to rapidly overwhelm the system. The number of victims required to declare a mass incident response varies between jurisdictions and is often arbitrary. Often it is the type and severity of injuries encountered (e.g. multiple penetrating, blast, chemical, etc.) that determines the magnitude of the response required, rather than the absolute numbers of victims. In most urban environments, the ambulance service, *via* ambulance control, are the first to declare the incident, as they begin to triage the wounded. However, other 'on-scene' organisations (e.g. police, fire service or other pre-hospital groups) should also have authority to trigger the mass disaster plan for a region. Ideally, this is co-ordinated through a *central command* (ideally a centralised office responsible for such events), but if one does not exist, then ambulance control (or other emergency operator) will suffice. This 'trigger' will ensure that the proper pre-hospital care providers are notified (with optimal numbers) and all hospitals in the area that respond to trauma and disasters are also directly notified so that they may prepare. Each hospital then has the role of triggering their own MIP as a result of the pre-hospital declaration and/or information from central command.

Casualty Generation This includes both the **total numbers** *injured* and *killed*, which in turn is dependent on the *lethality* of the incident. This lethality is reflected by the proportion who have died on scene. The top three most common causes of death after trauma are traumatic brain injury (TBI), exsanguinating haemorrhage and severe chest injury. This is also true in the disaster environment (esp. blast), but generally with more polytrauma (hence higher mortality rates). Most victims of a major terrorist event either die at scene or suffer relatively minor injuries (i.e. most are walking wounded). As a general rule, after a large-scale incident, the number of wounded requiring hospital treatment averages about 10–20% of the total numbers dead on scene and most of these will be walking wounded.

However, the on-scene survivors have far better outcomes when rapid care is given, even the critically injured. This serves only as a general guide but may aid the health service to prepare for the predicted 'fall-out' after an incident, with regard to numbers of patients expected. Although the lethality has a profound effect (esp. the 'perceived threat') on society, it is the total number of severely injured that will overwhelm the health service at all levels. This crippling effect may happen very quickly as resources are rapidly used up pre-hospital and at hospital level (esp. manpower). For example, a single severely injured person will typically require a minimum of two rescuers/pre-hospital care providers and a transport vehicle (e.g. ambulance) followed by a multitude of in-hospital resources including a whole resuscitation team, doctors, nurses and blood/medications. In addition, the subgroup in need of emergency surgery are often very challenging with multi-system severe injuries, high blood transfusion requirements in need of damage control surgery. The required surgical input is often multi-disciplinary including trauma surgery, orthopaedics and plastic, general and neurosurgery. Injuries amongst survivors are predominated by soft tissue musculoskeletal trauma, especially lower limb. Most survivors with TBI are non-critical.

38.7   Pre-hospital Response

One of the recognised factors that may itigate against the on-scene mortality (where deaths are not immediate) is the timely availability of medical resources within the disaster zone itself. An on-scene medical presence in a sophisticated trauma system allows for immediate life-saving techniques to be applied (e.g. haemorrhage control) followed by rapid triage and transportation to a major trauma centre. Thus, the rate-limiting step in the pre-hospital environment are twofold: (1) getting a pre-hospital response rapidly to the injured and (2) getting the injured out safely and quickly.

Getting a Pre-hospital Response to the Injured The optimal response may be obstructed by the fact that the scene may not yet have been declared 'safe' (i.e. when the scene is deemed secure and the risk of further events is negligible), but the need for on-going casualty care is ongoing. This is especially true in the pre-hospital environment, where there may still be a risk of further terrorist incidents. Therefore, the police (and other security responders, depending on the type of incident) will have overall authority until such a time as the scene is neutralised and declared 'safe' for others to enter. This may mean that healthcare personnel (or indeed civilian first responders) will have a to work *in parallel* with the security response, keeping in mind that healthcare workers may be hindered by an ongoing incident and/or commands of the police service, including but not limited to refusal of entry to the scene. Always remain cognisant, especially in the pre-hospital environment, that there is potentially a live and ongoing, active terrorist threat! A scene (including a potential attacker) must be declared 'safe' and the attacker declared 'neutralised' (from weapons such as chemical, explosive devices or any other weapons that may injure a responder). This is primarily the responsibility of the police (and/or other authority), but all personnel have this responsibility in an ongoing and dynamic manner, including when a patient is brought to the hospital, who may be a potential attacker.

Getting the Injured Out Safely and Rapidly Patients may be examined in the standard 30-s sieve (simple triage and treatment (START)) on scene. This is to identify the most life-threatening injuries rapidly that can be managed by simple means followed by (or in parallel with) rapid transportation to the MTC. However, as security is also a priority, the walking wounded should be removed en masse from the scene, by security, then accounted for and processed in a safe area, well outside the 'hot zone' of the incident. Any wounded who cannot stand and walk should be triaged rapidly without wasting further time or resources on futile care (i.e. those likely to die very soon). Under-triage occurs when a patient is assigned a 'delayed' critical level of injury when in fact a more urgent level is required, which could manifest as a preventable death, whilst over-triage is the over-assignment of victims to 'immediate' or 'urgent' care when they should be labelled 'delayed'. This latter scenario may rapidly use up limited resources (including manpower) whilst neglecting more urgent cases. Therefore, both under-triage and over-triage must be kept to a minimum, keeping in mind that triage is an ongoing and dynamic process and patients may be moved up or down the triage ladder depending on the evolving injuries and physiology over time. The standard approach to triage in a mass incident for the non-walkers is to perform a chin-lift (to assess breathing) followed by a pulse check (to assess circulation). However, this is neither sensitive nor specific in a mass casualty incident where there is a potential for an ongoing threat. Most likely, after major trauma, patients will either have a pulse or not and will either be unconscious or not. If a patient does not have a pulse after severe trauma, then they are declared dead. Those that do have evidence of circulatory life should be rapidly removed from the scene to an environment where higher level care may be rendered. We would advocate keeping pre-hospital interventions to a minimum (haemorrhage control, O_2, iv-line, splinting) as shorter pre-hospital times after trauma are associated with better outcomes. In addition, clearing the scene has a security benefit, especially if there is a potential for a reprise attack. Any patients declared dead ideally should be left as such as it is also a declared crime scene requiring further forensic examination. Furthermore, moving the dead at this time will unnecessarily use up resources.

38.8   Hospital Response

Surge Capacity This describes the tolerance or potential capacity that a hospital or department has to accommodate the surge (sudden increase) in acute admissions at a time of crisis. Typically, a hospital should have a surge capacity of about 10% at any one time (i.e. no more than 90% of hospital beds should be occupied on a normal working schedule). This is dependent on numerous factors, including physical bed space, availability of additional nursing and medical staff to meet the demands of a surge. Typically, a crisis event is impossible to predict and thus the normal volume of working staff cannot accommodate the surge for any prolonged length of time. Additional staffing and their needs should also be factored into the MIP. If bed occupancy is at or near 100%, then efforts are needed to create additional space by re-arranging admissions, cancelling other admissions and discharging patients (or transferring to another institution) if safe to do so.

The hospital response must plan for the following:

1. Security
2. Operation response
   (a) Gold Command
   (b) Silver command
   (c) Bronze command
3. Media
4. Politics and public opinion

The most important concept here is that of *hospital preparedness*. The hospital response follows a similar format to any major trauma or mass incident, but with additional security concerns. Each hospital (esp. the MTC) must have its own MIP (ideally one that has been co-ordinated with the wider regional MIP). Once a mass disaster has been declared by one of the responsible pre-hospital agencies, the responsible officer at the hospital (e.g. medical director) in turn activates the hospitals MIP. As a backup, the trauma team leader (TTL) or consultant in emergency medicine on duty may also declare this (as contacted through the major trauma phone or emergency hospital phone) in the event where the medical director (or his deputy) cannot be reached. In addition, in the event where a major disaster has not yet been declared, but where, based on events known or the probability of a need for escalation in service delivery, a hospital alone may initiate a major incident plan for itself, independent of the pre-hospital declaration. Of course, the hospital cannot declare this for another healthcare facility, as this is a stand-alone independent declaration and thus under such circumstances, the regional co-ordinator must be involved.

The MIP must be rehearsed and rehearsed often, so that all participants (management, medical, nursing and ancillary staff) are familiar with it, preferably with annual or biannual drill exercises. Other rehearsals may include tabletop exercises, workshops and online professional education courses, which are updated regularly.

The MIP should be scrutinised on a regular basis (e.g. annual or every 2 years) and especially after an attack (or other major event) with quality improvement feedback. In addition, the use of quick reference 'action cards' are used in many jurisdictions, as a quick reminder to all individuals involved in a response, what their role is and how to carry it out (especially if someone has not taken part in a drill exercise but is on duty). This prescribed pathway for an individual will help to manage any scenario, at a time when the likelihood of confusion is much higher.

38.9   Security Response

There are numerous facets to the security response, which, may include drafting in additional staff not currently rostered. The prime security issues include:

- Crowd control (incl. media)
- Staff identification
- Hospital entry and exit points
- The perpetrator(s)

Hospital security must immediately cordon off the hospital surrounds, especially the entry points (depending on the time of day, but typically includes the emergency department entry and the main entrance to the building). Large crowds of people may arrive at the hospital and thus should be kept away, unless they are arriving for immediate medical attention. Usually the police will assist with this, as the crowds will be in a public area also. Any potential patients arriving should be triaged at the door and a rapid decision made whether they require attention at that hospital or whether transfer out (including by private transportation) is preferable. Crowd control also includes media control at the cordoned off area, but most professional journalists are already familiar with this and will follow instructions and respect the exclusion zone around the hospital.

As part of the MIP, an en mass 'call out' to staff will occur. It is imperative that each staff member has their hospital identification checked by security upon arrival, as only essential staff should arrive, in addition to ensuring no other member of the public, media or indeed potential terrorist group has access to the hospital. All other hospital ingress and egress points must be secured to prevent anyone else gaining access to the building.

As with the pre-hospital response, it is imperative that any presumed perpetrator or member of the attack group who has been brought to the hospital is 'sanitised' before entering the building and 'declared safe'. Ideally, this should take pace in the pre-hospital environment (and before transportation by ambulance) to ensure there are no other weapons on the person (including explosives or chemical agents). This is a complex role and will involve the armed police response (or other law enforcement specialist group), but all persons coming in to contact with the alleged attacker have a duty of care to themselves and others.

In addition, there will likely be a large security presence (police, counter-terrorism forces, armed response units) present in the ED (and other areas of the hospital), who will be heavily armed. It is important not to allow this to become a distraction during treatment and resuscitation, including during treatment of a potential suspect. It is best to work with these services, whose job is to protect in addition to collect forensic evidence. Ideally, the senior incident commander and bronze commander (see below) will liaise directly with the senior police officer/detective present, so that the trauma bay does not become unworkable. This is especially true if treating a potential suspect, or even if a suspect has been declared dead. If possible and available, treat a suspect in a separate area, or unannounced in a separate trauma bay. This is important for security. Allow the security presence during management, but you may politely ask them to step back if management is being hindered. This is not the time to start an argument with the police! If a suspect has been declared dead, then ideally, for operational and security reasons, move the body to a separate area of the department, away from the main activity, the public and any media present. This will free up a trauma bay in addition to removing the forensic evidence and attention away.

38.10 Operational Response

The hospital MIP is a hierarchical and tiered **command and control** response: *gold*, *silver* and *bronze*. Each has a unique but interdependent role.

Gold Commander There is only one, single gold commander, who is responsible for the hospital groups strategic response during the crisis. He/she delegates tactical decisions to the silver (and occasionally bronze) commanders. The role is primarily strategic and managerial. They also interact with all other stakeholders at gold level involved in the response, including ambulance, police and fire services (i.e. director level interactions with partner organisations). They are supported by a *gold command team* (other managerial and senior clinical decision makers) in the *command room* and do not necessarily need to visit the response site (unless this is strategically desirable).

Silver Commander The silver commander is responsible for co-ordinating a single hospital (or site's) tactical response to the incident and is supported by the silver command team. Each hospital involved has a separate silver commander, but the gold commander may be responsible for several hospitals if they fall under the same management structure.

Bronze Commander There are numerous bronze commanders (i.e. managers of an individual team or department), responsible for the operational response to the incident. Once an MIP is declared, each bronze commander must begin to reorganise their respective teams/departments in accordance with the plan until such a time as the incident has been declared 'stood down'. For example, bronze commanders will ensure the safe transfer or rearrangement of patients within the emergency department (including timely discharge where appropriate), the cancellation/postponement of surgery (as long as this is safe to do) and the reorganisation/discharge of patients from critical areas of the hospital (e.g. ICU/HDU, trauma ward, acute care ward, etc.) to prepare for the surge of acutely injured patients.

Staff Roles Staff are categorised depending on the situational requirements. This is a dynamic categorisation and will change as the incident unfolds or matures over a few hours. *Red* are those essential to the response, which includes the various commanders, in addition to emergency staff (ED, surgery, critical care, anaesthetics, etc.). *Amber* staff are those who have an important role but are not required immediately. They often arrive in after the call went out and may include orthopaedics, plastics, and other health care workers, including those providing relief to other red staff. *Green* staff are those not immediately required in the response, but have an important role to play as the response develops, including cleaning, catering, etc. They may not form part of the normal on-call roster in the hospital, but instead arrive in as part of their ethical duty to the crisis.

As staff arrive, once they have passed the security check, they should be directed to a rendezvous point. This will vary between hospitals (e.g. front lobby). I have found that the recovery bay in the operating suite is an excellent muster point. This is typically a large room that can accommodate larger groups of people in one area, making it easier then to account for staff and then further direct them as required. In addition, during an MIP, the recovery bay is cleared as required to make room for post-operative patients. Thus, there is often available space in the recovery room for a number of hours as the incident matures.

38.11 Departmental Roles

The operational hospital response is a co-ordinated effort between all departments (led by their respective Bronze Commanders): emergency department, trauma and emergency surgery teams, anaesthetics, operating rooms, intensive care unit and the trauma ward staff.

Emergency Department The emergency department (ED) is a principle hub of activity after a terrorist event and is the principle point of arrival, triage and treatment. However, there is a 'chain of hubs' interconnected including radiology suite, theatres, critical care unit and the trauma ward. Within the ED, the trauma/resuscitation bay will be the principle site of clinical activity. A single bronze commander is responsible for the trauma resuscitation room, supported by a TTL and trauma team dedicated to each bay. A separate senior clinician (also bronze commander) acts as triage officer. It is unlikely that this person will alter the pre-hospital triage label (if one has taken place), but it is important that on arrival each patient is quickly assessed (re-triaged if appropriate) and then appointed to a trauma bay for full assessment and treatment. In addition, clerical support documents their arrival and appoints a unique identification number (for investigations, blood transfusion and treatment, as required). It is also imperative, that all documentation occurs in a contemporaneous fashion and on paper (rather than computer). The triage officer may triage up or down, but once triaged and appointed to a trauma bay, the trauma team manages them as per any major trauma, but in a more rapid, often abbreviated fashion to quickly identify those patients who require immediate emergency surgery (e.g. laparotomy for haemorrhage control) or those who are haemodynamically stable enough for further radiological investigations (and/or step down to an observation bed outside of the trauma bay whilst waiting further assessment). This enables efficient throughput of the trauma bay and to clear it in a progressive fashion to allow for the arrival of the next surge of patients. As part of the ED response, the blood bank (hospital and regionally (as required)) are informed in addition to activating the massive transfusion pathway. Radiographers are present (i.e. without being specifically summoned) to perform trauma series X-rays.

Trauma and Emergency Surgery Teams Rapid, focussed assessments are required. As the hospital will become overwhelmed very quickly, an attempt to identify the most immediately life-threatening injuries is made, which may involve going straight to the operating suite for emergency surgery (laparotomy, pelvic packing, thoracotomy, etc.) without further investigations (i.e. if non-compressible haemorrhage is suspected). All surgeons must be experienced in the concept and practice of damage control surgery and rapid haemorrhage control, as this is more likely to be required in a mass casualty situation (i.e. abbreviated surgery to ensure efficient use of theatre space and time in addition to the higher likelihood of severe injuries and major bleeding). Once identified, the patient is transferred directly to the operating suite with the appropriate anaesthetic staff for immediate exploratory surgery. A senior bronze commander surgeon should remain in the operating suite and act as co-ordinator with anaesthetics, theatre staff and ICU as patients are transferred in and out. They guide the operating team to the correct operating suite for surgery in addition to being responsible for clearing the post-operative recovery bay and for cancelling any surgeries that are not yet under way. This is done in consultation with the anaesthetic bronze commander in theatres. On occasion, it may not be possible to cancel an operation (e.g. another emergency operation, not related to the incident is under way or about to start). As a general rule, if surgery has not started (i.e. no first cut) begun and it is safe to postpone in the context of a major incident, then the bronze commanders from surgery and anaesthetics have a duty to postpone it.

Anaesthetics There needs to be an anaesthetic presence in the trauma bay and theatres, depending on the jurisdiction (i.e. in some countries/hospitals, the ED staff will intubate and manage the airway), but an anaesthetist/anaesthesiologist may be required to intubate if the airway is very challenging. However, regardless of the normal protocol for airway management, if emergency surgery is required, then anaesthesia will lead on the delivery of the anaesthetic and ventilation during surgery. As discussed above, there should be an anaesthetic bronze commander in the operating suite, responsible for delegating staff to each theatre required in addition to postponing surgery in conjunction with surgical bronze for non-essential patients.

Operating Rooms As discussed above, any surgeries that have not started should be postponed pending an update on the 'surge' requirements. It is often difficult to decide whether to proceed with surgery when the patient has already been anaesthetised and prepared, and this is often a judgement call on a case-by-case basis. We would recommend that all day cases are suspended if the operation has not begun. More complex or sicker patients that have already been anaesthetised (especially emergency surgery) should probably proceed. Day cases should be discharged (if safe to do so) and all other operations put on hold pending an update from the clinical director. The post-operative recovery room should be 'cleared' as soon as possible to make way for a potential surge in emergency surgery cases, if it is safe to do so. This rearrangement of theatres is a combined effort of the bronze commanders in surgery, anaesthetics and theatre nursing.

Intensive Care Unit The bronze commander in ICU will rapidly round (with appropriate staff and bed management) on the patients currently in the ICU/HDU/ other critical care area to identify those who may be able to be extubated or 'stepped down' to a lower level of care to make way for the potential surge of more severely injured patients (as long as it is safe). Bed/nursing management will have contemporaneous records of where the potential step-down beds are and whether there are empty critical care beds currently and if they can be safely staffed, in addition to identifying those patients who may be safely transferred out to another facility.

Trauma (and Other) Ward Any patients identified for potential discharge should be reassessed and the discharge fast tracked where possible to make room for additional patients (e.g. those stepping down from ICU or those in need of in-hospital care, but not critical care). These patients may need to be transferred to a discharge lounge, pending further review and paperwork and follow-up plans. Any ongoing physiotherapy or rehabilitation may need to be organised at home or in the community earlier than previously expected or patients brought back early for a needs assessment.

Bed Management Bed management must identify all available beds and potential discharges and communicate/co-ordinate with the medical director, director of nursing and trauma teams to ensure there is efficient throughput for patients. In addition, it is important that any patients discharged early to meet the surge capacity have appropriate paperwork and follow-up organised so that mistakes are not made.

38.12 Media, Politics and Public Opinion

An additional consideration for all healthcare providers in a major terrorist incident, which may become intrusive, is the public's insatiable requirement for information and updates as the incident unfolds. This may be requested by the security forces to update regional management and ultimately the political powers, regionally and nationally in an attempt to assuage the wave of panic that often spreads after such a major security incident. In addition, the media (who are the most powerful tool in spreading and controlling news) will have a presence at the site of the incident and at the hospital. They will need information as the situation develops about the attack and it is better to involve them responsibly to avoid misinformation, fake news or other causes of public anxiety. In general, all comments to the media should go through the hospital's media office, once approved by the Gold Command, CEO of the hospital and the senior management team. All other staff should refrain from commenting or making any statement (unless authorised to do so), especially comments regarding patient treatment or identification, including images. Any other behaviour is inappropriate, potentially destructive to the operational process, including the legal investigation and may also be deemed potentially illegal or a dereliction of a doctor's (or other healthcare professional) duty of proper care. Careful and responsible comments to the media (via the hospital's media office) are also important to avoid a large crowd surge of uninjured on-lookers arriving at the hospital (including those with vigilante aims) in addition to preventing making the hospital a target by other members of the terrorist organisation. This is particularly important when an incident is across a densely populated region (e.g. London, Paris), where it may be appropriate not to disclose the prime hospital receiving the most severely injured or where any members of the terrorist group responsible may be receiving treatment. This has very sound operation and security reasons behind it.

38.13 Ethical Dilemmas

Remember, both the victims of the attack and the suspected attackers themselves may need care. Although it is easy for emotion to get in the way of rendering health care to an injured (who by their own act of violence have become a victim) suspect, we would always advocate treating all patients with the same level of ethics and moral judgement as any patient whilst leaving the course of justice to the police investigation and judicial system afterwards. It is neither the correct time nor our role as healthcare providers to apportion blame or make any other assertions about the incident or potential perpetrators. In addition, we may get it wrong as by definition, at this stage they are only a suspect! However, if an individual member of the terrorist group (or a suspected member) is being actively treated, ensure security personnel are present and engaged. Often it will not be released to the media or public if or where a suspect is being treated (even if deceased) for operational and security purposes whilst an incident unfolds. Maintain the highest level of ethics in addition to the highest level of medical care at all times at all patients!

Bibliography

1. Fine J. Political and philological origins of the term 'terrorism' from the ancient near east to our times. Middle East Stud. 2010;46:271–88.
2. https://www.un.org/counterterrorism/ctitf/en/sres1566-2004.
3. Chuhan R, Conti BM, Keene D. Marauding terrorist attack (MTA): prehospital considerations. Emeg Med J. 2018;35:389–95.
4. Hirsch M, Carli P, Nizard R, Riou B, Baroudjin B, Baubet T, Chhor V, Chollet-Xemard C, Dantchev N, Fleury N, Fontaine JP, Yordanov Y, Raphael M, Paugam Burtz C, Lafont A. The medical response to multisite terrorist attacks in Paris. Lancet. 2015;386:2535–8.
5. Carli P, Pons F, Levraut J, Millet B, Tourtier JP, Ludes B, Lafont A, Riou B. The French emergency medical services after the Paris and Nice terrorist attacks: what have we learnt? Lancet. 2017;390:2735–8.
6. Lockey DJ. The shootings in Oslo and Utoya island July 22, 2011: lessons for the International EMS community. Scand J Trauma Resusc Emerg Med. 2012;20:4.

7. Gaarder C, Jorgensen J, Kolstadbraaten KM, Isaksen KS, Skattum J, Rimstad R, Gundem T, Holtan A, Walloe A, Pillgram-Larsen J, Naess PA. The twin terrorist attacks in Norway on July 22, 2011: the trauma center response. J Trauma Acute Crea Surg. 2012;73:269–75.

8. Brandrud AS, Bretthauer M, Brattebo G, Pedersen MJB, Hapnes K, Bjorge T, Nyen B, Strauman L, Schreiner A, Moller K, Helljeen GS, Bergli M, Nelson E, Morgan TS, Hjortdahl P. Local emergency medical response after a terrorist attack in Norway: a qualitative study. BMJ Qual Saf. 2017;26:806–16.

9. Federal Bureau of Investigation Counterterrorism Division. Terrorism 2002—2005. https://www.fbi.gov/file-repository/stats-services-publications-terrorism-2002-2005-terror02_05.pdf.

10. Broad WJ. Sowing death: a special report; how Japan germ terror alerted world. The New York Times, 26th May 1998

11. Takahashi H, Keim P, Kaufmann AF, Keys C, Smith KL, Taniguchi K, Inouye S, Kurata T. Bacillus anthracis incident, Kameido, Tokyo, 1993. Emerg Infect Dis. 2004;10:117–20.

12. Hilmas CJ, Smart JK, Hill BA. Chapter 2. History of chemical warfare: an American perspective. In: Medical aspects of chemical warfare. Washington, DC: Office of the Surgeon General at TMM Publications; 2008.

13. Dembek ZF. Chapter 2. The history and threat of biological weapons and bioterrorism. In: Joseph H, McIsaac II, editors. Hospital preparation for bioterror: a medical and biomedical systems approach. New York: Elsevier/Academic Press; 2006.

14. Allison G. Nuclear terrorism: the ultimate preventable catastrophe. New York: Henry Holt and Company; 2005.

15. Peleg K, Jaffe DH, the Israel Trauma Group. Are injuries from terror and war similar? A comparison study of civilians and soldiers. Ann Surg. 2010;252:363–9.

16. Aharonson-Daniel L, Waisman Y, Dannon YL, Peleg K, Members of the Israel Trauma Group. Epidemiology of terror-related versus non-terror related traumatic injury in children. Pediatrics. 2003;112:e280–4.

17. Frykberg ER. Medical management of disasters and mass casualties from terrorist bombings: how can we cope? J Trauma. 2002;53:201–12.

18. Khorram-Manesh A. Europe on fire; medical management of terror attacks—new era and new considerations. Bull Emerg Trauma. 2016;4:183–5.

19. Wang DW, Liu Y, Jiang MM. Review on emergency medical response against terrorist attack. Mil Med Res. 2014;1:1–4.

20. Goralnick E, Van Trimpont F, Carli P. Preparing for the next terrorism attack: lessons from Paris, Brussels and Boston. JAMA Surg. 2017;152(5):419–20.

21. Turner CD, Lockey DJ, Rehn M. Pre-hospital management of mass casualty civilian shootings: a systematic literature review. Crit Care. 2016;20:362–74.

22. Veatch RM. Disaster preparedness and triage: justice and the common good. Mt Sinai J Med. 2005;72:236–41.

23. Caldicott DGE, Edwards NA, Tingey D, Bonnin R. Medical response to a terrorist attack and weapons of mass destruction. Emerg Med. 2002;14:230–9.

24. Aylwin CJ, Konig TC, Brennan NW, Shirley PJ, Davies G, Walsh MS, Brohi K. Reduction in critical mortality in urban mass casualty incidents: analysis of triage, surge and resource use after the London bombings on July 7, 2005. Lancet. 2006;368:2219–25.

25. Hick JL, Hanfling D, Evans B, Greenberg S, Alson R, McKinney S, Minson M. Health and medical response to active shooter and bombing events. Washington, DC: National Academy of Medicine; 2016.

26. Craigie RJ, Farrelly PJ, Santos R, Smith SR, Pollard JS, Jones DJ. Manchester arena bombing: lessons learnt from a mass casualty incident. BMJ Mil Health. 2020;166:72–5.

27. Merin O, Sonkin R, Titzhak A, Frenkel H, Leiba A, Schwarz AD, Jaffe E. Terrorist stabbings—distinctive characteristics and how to prepare for them. J Emerg Med. 2017;53:451–7.

28. Merin O, Goldberg S, Steinberg A. Treating terrorists and victims: a moral dilemma. Lancet. 2015;385:1289.

The Role of the Crowds in Managing Disasters: Toward a Bottom-Up Participatory Approach

Korinna-Zoi Karamagkioli, Vassileios Tokakis, Anastasia Pikouli, and Evika Karamagioli

39.1 Introduction

The advent of both natural and manmade disasters is increasingly highlighting the role of citizens (ranging from spontaneous volunteers and first responders to emergent entities and communities of civic action) as inevitable and potentially valuable resource in their management.

Although for a long period of time they were treated with mistrust regarding their effectiveness and efficiency as part of the managing disaster process, collaborative schemes with citizens in individual but also community format is more and more getting ground.

The advancement of mobile and social technologies (i.e., social media, virtual platforms for community building), by facilitating citizens interactions and bottom-up communication in the sense of reporting information, self-organizing, and volunteering and thus responding to disasters outside of traditional emergency management structures, has empowered this phenomenon [1].

However this new reality characterized by a spontaneous and many times autonomous participation of informal communities and individuals from the first moment

K.-Z. Karamagkioli
Clinical Psychiatry SpR, NHS, CNWL, Imperian, London, UK

V. Tokakis
"Global Heath—Disaster Medicine", National and Kapodistrian University of Athens, Athens, Greece

A. Pikouli
Third Department of Surgery, National and Kapodistrian University of Athens, Attikon University Hospital, Athens, Greece

E. Karamagioli (✉)
"Global Heath—Disaster Medicine", Media Faculty, National and Kapodistrian University of Athens, Athens, Greece

© Springer Nature Switzerland AG 2021
E. Pikoulis, J. Doucet (eds.), *Emergency Medicine, Trauma and Disaster Management*, Hot Topics in Acute Care Surgery and Trauma,
https://doi.org/10.1007/978-3-030-34116-9_39

a catastrophic event arises has raised a lot of controversies and concerns from a public policy perspective.

Taking into consideration the fact that dealing with disasters needs planning, training, and advanced skills for staff and stakeholders involved in emergency medicine and disaster management under the 4C mechanism, Command, Control, Coordination, and Communication, there were a lot of arguments in favor of a centralized, top-down approach that expects all volunteers to conform to emergency management organization and procedures.

The fear of panic, looting, and other forms of antisocial or exploitative behavior or event passivity in disaster setting was the main argument against directly involving individuals and emergency entities as part of the emergency response mechanisms.

International literature and research however supports that such behavioral patterns, are not typical. The reality shows that spontaneous entities and individuals acting under that same cause in an informal way become more unified, cohesive, and altruistic in such events and are eager to offer their services in any way they can [2].

The scope of the chapter is to present this phenomenon and discuss why and how emergency managers and public authorities should not neglect this reality of bottom-up emergent social structures composed by spontaneous volunteers and first responders to emergent communities of civic action that act and react in disasters.

39.2 Individuals and Informal Communities as Key Disaster Response Stakeholders

One of the main issues that need to be taken into consideration during the disaster preparedness and recovery phases independently the type of disaster (natural or manmade) is the fact that individuals and self-organized entities most of the times are mobilized even before the formal mechanisms, and there are many examples documented all around the world that they have become an important resource for emergency response efforts [3].

Tasks ranging from search and rescue, prehospital injured management, and psychological first aid support are indicative activities that we have seen being performed by spontaneous volunteers and first responders as well as emergent entities and communities of civic action long before emergency managers, civil protection officials, decision-makers, disaster planners, and humanitarian agencies arrive on the spot. Additionally collecting, transporting, and distributing relief supplies and clothing and providing food and drink to victims and emergency workers are indicative activities.

Most importantly there are numerous cases that live testimonies from the disaster field via social media or other internet platform have guided emergency response planning and are even considered as proper legal information and material (i.e., during legal action by Greek prosecutors investigating the deaths of more than 100 persons due to the wildfires in July 2018 in the area of Mati in Greece).

But who are those individuals that act individually and/or gather in informal entities? There profile is not unanimous, but their common characteristic is the spontaneity and their will to contribute and most of all the catastrophic event that acts a triggering mechanism for their mobilization. There is a great variation depending of the type and the scale of the disaster, the country of reference, and the sociopolitical and economic context. Actually we are talking most of the times about people without appropriate training or specific technical and non-technical (soft) skills related to disaster management.

39.3 Individuals and Informal Communities: Burden or Powerful Tool for the Emergency Response Systems?

Disaster preparedness, management, and recovery independent of the type of disaster and the density require coordination, planning, and execution by skilled and trained personnel and experts. Interprofessional collaboration and clearly defined and allocated roles among all agencies involved are paramount. Under this context the intensity and scale of spontaneous acting by individuals and informal communities can present significant coordination, integration, communication, logistical, and health and safety challenges and burden to the emergency managers.

Most of the times individuals have very limited or inexistent field experience. Additionally there is a lot of uncertainty about the legal liability of volunteer responders (i.e., the case of floods in 2018 in a suburban area near Athens in Greece where several volunteers rushed to help and were injured or as in the case of wildfires in the suburb of Mati the same year were killed). Also they are not familiar with top-down decision-making processes and service delivery methods and/or due to the informal character of the entities that they form they suffer from inexistent communication mechanisms and channels with emergency managers. They either put themselves at risk of injury or obstruct the formal emergency response effort, and most of the times, they require extra resources so as to be managed [3].

As a result, many if not most of the times especially in the first hours after the disaster occurs are underutilized or even rejected [4, 5].

However, the reality is that the social capital composed by all these individuals acting independently or in the framework of emergent communities is usually renewed and enhanced, easily accessible, inexhaustible, free, and abundant during disasters [6]. They are there to stay, and many times they have a power that public authorities cannot neglect at need to cope with (i.e., during terrorist attacks in Belgium in 2015, the national police had to request for silence across social media).

39.4 Toward an Inclusive Bottom-Up Model for Individuals and Informal Communities Mobilization During Disasters Management and Recovery

According the recent literature when a disaster strikes, community members are the main actors in emergency management, and they have to be involved as active participants and key stakeholders of the emergency management process although historically this was the role of first responders and governmental agencies [7, 8].

This inclusive bottom-up approach of emergency management supports and argues in favor of the development of resilient and sustainable mechanism where multiple stakeholders (e.g., residents, community leaders, government) work together to strengthen capacities and build community resilience [9, 10].

Given that disasters will always be a reality, spontaneous actions and reactions will also be a repeated pattern that cannot be neglected or be bypassed or be 100% controlled, and therefore developing strategies for not only ensuring but also promoting the community involvement in disaster preparedness and mainly response should be in the top of public health and national security agenda.

Community members are a natural support system with many advantages. They have the essential local knowledge and support networks to take collective action, improve system response capabilities, and generate relevant data to mitigate adverse health impacts [11].

The way forward seems therefore to introduce in the 4C mechanism, Command, Control, Coordination, and Communication, an additional C+ for the crowd in the sense of spontaneous volunteers and first responders as well as emergent entities and communities of civic action so as to include their needs, capacities, and resources. The argument in favor of such introduction could be that if the goal of disaster response and recovery is to make an affected community functional, then members of that community must be included in the process that concerns and affects them.

39.5 Conclusion

As the crowd (ranging from spontaneous volunteers and first responders to emergent entities and communities of civic action) is inevitably involved in disaster management and relief, emergency managers and public authorities should not neglect this reality of emergent social structures and should introduce and coordinate participatory response mechanisms and processes that encourage bottom up synergies.

References

1. Clark M. Spontaneous volunteers: community participation in disaster response and recovery. Ottawa: The Conference Board of Canada; 2016.
2. Eyre A. Literature and best practice review and assessment: identifying people's needs in major emergencies and best practice in humanitarian response. London: UK Department for Culture, Media and Sport; 2006, 112 pages.
3. Twigg J, Mosel I. Emergent entities and spontaneous volunteers in urban disaster response. Environ Urban. 2017;29(2):443–58.
4. Scanlon J. Putting it all together: integrating ordinary people into emergency response. Int J Mass Emerg Disasters. 2014;32(1):43–63.
5. Whittaker J. A review of informal volunteerism in emergencies and disasters: definitions, opportunities and challenges. Int J Disaster Risk Reduct. 2015;13:358–68.
6. Dynes R. Community social capital as the primary basis for resilience. Preliminary paper 344. University of Delawere. Disaster Research Centre; 2005.
7. Chari R, Petrun Sayers EL, Amiri S, et al. Enhancing community preparedness: an inventory and analysis of disaster citizen science activities. BMC Public Health. 2019;19:1356.
8. Gursky EA, Bice G. Assessing a decade of public health preparedness: progress on the precipice? Biosecur Bioterror. 2012;10:55–65.
9. Federal Emergency Management Agency. A whole community approach to emergency management: principles, themes, and pathways for action. Washington, DC: FEMA; 2012.
10. Moreno J. The role of communities in coping with natural disasters: lessons from the 2010 Chile Earthquake and Tsunami. Procedia Eng. 2018;212:1040–5.
11. Haklay M. Citizen science and volunteered geographic information—overview and typology of participation. In: Sui DZ, Elwood S, Goodchild MF, editors. Crowdsourcing geographic knowledge: volunteered geographic information (VGI) in theory and practice. Berlin: Springer; 2013. p. 105–22.

Part IV

After the Disaster

Infectious Diseases Outbreaks Following Natural Disasters: Risk Assessment, Prevention, and Control

40

Eleni Kakalou and Costas Tsiamis

40.1 Summary

Infectious diseases outbreaks pose a threat following natural disasters, but they are generally rare especially in developed countries. The impact of disasters such as flooding, tropical cyclones, tornadoes, earthquakes, tsunamis, landslides, and volcanic eruptions on populations is directly linked to many factors. Those include disease endemicity, presence of vectors, environmental conditions, the robustness of health services and infrastructure, poverty, inequality, political stability, and the overall vulnerability of communities. The magnitude of the occurring event, the underlying vulnerability of affected communities, and the resulting population displacement play a vital role to whether outbreaks become major concerns of the response. Events with great impact can overwhelm even developed countries; however overall capacity for rapid containment is directly linked to previous local capabilities and endemic conditions.

Diseases can be waterborne, airborne, foodborne, vector-borne or due to various exposures such as direct wound contamination and person-to-person transmission. Disasters create conditions for unusual exposures of the affected population such as inhalation of dust, near drowning or exposure of wounds to contaminated water and debris, water contamination by sewage or other contaminants, and crowded living conditions in temporary shelters with sub-standard hygienic conditions. What's more, population displacement can interrupt ongoing treatments such

E. Kakalou (✉)
Global Health-Disaster Medicine, School of Medicine, National and Kapodistrian University of Athens (NKUA), Athens, Greece

C. Tsiamis
Department of Public and Integrated Health, School of Health Sciences, University of Thessaly, Volos, Greece
e-mail: ktsiamis@uth.gr

© Springer Nature Switzerland AG 2021
E. Pikoulis, J. Doucet (eds.), *Emergency Medicine, Trauma and Disaster Management*, Hot Topics in Acute Care Surgery and Trauma,
https://doi.org/10.1007/978-3-030-34116-9_40

as for tuberculosis (TB) and place extra burden on surveillance systems or health infrastructures that remain functional after a disaster.

Based on observational data from previous natural disasters, acute respiratory infections (ARIs), diarrhea, and skin or wound infections are the most common health problems among survivors and affected populations. Epidemics of measles, diarrheal diseases such as *E. coli* or norovirus gastroenteritis, cholera, hepatitis A and E, leptospirosis, tetanus, skin infections (mycoses), meningitis, malaria, and dengue fever have been described depending on previous vaccination coverage, local infrastructure, and economic conditions prevailing before the occurrence of the natural disaster event. Outbreaks following natural disasters have ranged from relatively limited events after major disasters in developed countries such as Japan or the USA up to emblematic epidemics like cholera in Haiti following the 2010 earthquake that mobilized worldwide response efforts.

The misconception that dead bodies after a disaster pose a serious threat to public health is widely held. In reality, corpses linked to the disaster itself do not pose any such risk. The presence of dead bodies in a disaster zone can cause emotional, cultural, and religious stress to communities, but they are not linked to infectious diseases outbreaks.

Anthropogenic climate change is aggravating extreme weather events leading to natural disasters that are becoming more frequent. Even in the best-case scenario of limiting global warming to the 1.5 °C goal of the Paris Agreement, hundreds of millions of people are expected to be affected. In this environment, preparedness and comprehensive frameworks for recovery of public health and disease surveillance systems following natural disasters are essential components of the overall response, especially when it comes to preventing outbreaks of infectious diseases and mitigating their possible impact on the affected population.

40.2   Infectious Diseases and Transmission Mechanisms

The impact phase of the disaster lasts up to 4 days following the event. During this phase immediate extrication of victims and timely treatment are essential. Trauma, hypothermia, heat stroke, and dehydration are the main drivers of morbidity and mortality during this phase. The period up to 4 weeks after a disaster can be characterized by the occurrence of airborne, waterborne and foodborne illnesses among the population. Respiratory infections of viral (*influenza, respiratory syncytial virus-RSV, adenovirus*), bacterial (such as *pertussis, Strep pneumoniae, Mycobacterium tuberculosis, Mycoplasma pneumoniae, Legionella*) and other diseases transmitted by the respiratory route such as measles, meningitis, and varicella can occur [1, 2]. Water- and foodborne infections such as cholera, hepatitis A and E, bacterial dysentery, salmonella, typhoid, paratyphoid, giardiasis, and other parasitosis as well as leptospirosis are of concern. Tetanus and wound or skin infections also appear during this phase.

The recovery phase begins after 4 weeks when diseases with longer incubation periods or vector-borne can occur. Leishmaniasis, leptospirosis, malaria, dengue, yellow fever, viral encephalitis, and TB can become a concern depending on the social and environmental conditions prevailing. Chronic diseases can also pose a serious problem especially if a significant percentage of the health facilities and infrastructure have been seriously impacted [3–5].

40.2.1 Waterborne and/or Foodborne: Personal Hygiene

Personal hygiene, availability of safe potable water, sewage, and disposal systems can be greatly affected and compromised following natural disasters. Conditions of crowding in temporary shelters along with the abovementioned challenges further aggravate the risks of person-to-person transmission of infectious diseases. Waterborne diseases include diarrheal diseases such as dysentery caused by enterotoxigenic *Escherichia coli*, *Salmonella typhi* or *paratyphi*, hepatitis A or E, leptospirosis and cholera. Contaminated food can also play an important role in the transmission of such diseases. Diarrheal diseases have affected communities following flooding or hurricanes in West Africa, Sudan, Mozambique, Bangladesh, and Nepal [6].

Outbreaks of hepatitis A and E have been described following the tsunami in Indonesia. Leptospirosis has been described following typhoons in Taiwan, China, and India. Diarrheal diseases are known drivers of mortality in disaster and camp settings especially in developing countries. Polluted water sources by fecal contamination, shared water containers and cooking pots, and contaminated and unsafe food have been implicated for outbreaks in disaster settings. When safe water is not accessible in adequate quantities and hygienic materials such as soap, disinfectants, and fuel for boiling water are scarce, risks for potential outbreaks are raised. Several months after the earthquake in Haiti in 2010, a cholera outbreak with a high case fatality rate (CFR: 6.4%) occurred. Vibrio cholerae had been imported to a susceptible population amidst preexisting poor living and sanitary conditions that fueled its rapid escalation [7].

Leptospirosis is spread through contamination of water, food, and soil with the urine of infected rodents. Human transmission happens through contact with nonintact skin or mucous membranes. Viral hepatitis A and E are common in areas where preexisting waste, sewage disposal and sanitation are generally poor. Viral hepatitis is usually self-limited, but in rare cases it can result in fulminant liver failure. Pregnant women and immunocompromised people are highly susceptible to severe disease with high mortality (up to 20–25%). Hepatitis E has only recently been introduced into Africa from Asia, and as a result adults lack immunity to the disease.

40.2.2 Airborne/Droplet Spread

Acute Respiratory Infections (ARIs) are among the most common reasons of morbidity and mortality following disasters. Children under the age of 5 are particularly affected, and particularly coupled with underlying malnutrition, they can account for up to 20% of all deaths in this age group in developing countries. Overcrowding conditions especially in cold weather are causal factors for pneumonia that carries a high risk of death in this age group. Elderly people and those with underlying chronic diseases are also highly susceptible. Studies after various disasters have described prevalence of ARIs from 14% in Iran during the Bam earthquake in 2003 up to 30% after the El Salvador one in 2001. Even in developed countries such as Japan and USA, epidemics of influenza or norovirus diarrheal diseases have spread by air droplet and person-to-person transmission in crowded conditions.

Near drowning can cause "aspiration pneumonia" due to salt water contaminated with soil in disasters characterized by flooding, hurricanes, and tsunamis. "Tsunami Lung" is a type of pneumonia with cavitary lung disease and possible brain abscess, occurring up to weeks following near drowning. It is a polymicrobial pneumonia described in survivors of the 2004 tsunami in Indonesia. The main pathogens identified were *Aeromonas hydrophila*, *Pseudomonas aeruginosa*, *Nocardia*, *Pseudallescheria boydii*, *Burkholderia pseudomallei*, and *Streptococcus* spp.

Following landslides, volcano eruptions, tornadoes, hurricanes, earthquakes, and sandstorms, the population can be exposed to rare fungal diseases. Spores can be displaced from their routine habitats resulting in their increased concentration in the environment in water, soil, and air causing lung disease or wound contamination (*Coccidioidomycosis* spp., *Aspergillus* spp., *Mucorales* spp., *Fusarium* spp., *Candida* spp., *Penicillium* spp., etc.). Such cases have been described in California counties in 1977 and 1994, after Katrina Hurricane in 2005 as well as a Tornado in 2011 in Missouri [8].

Measles epidemics have also been described after disasters such as in Pakistan earthquake in 2005 or in camps following the tsunami in Indonesia in Banda Aceh in 2004. The risk for an outbreak and its severity depend on preexisting vaccination coverage, underlying malnutrition, and access to timely and high-quality medical care. Prioritization of mass vaccination very early after a disaster that results in population displacement, especially for those under the age of 15, has the potential to greatly reduce risk of an outbreak and adverse outcomes.

Meningitis by *Neisseria meningitidis* is an important cause for morbidity and mortality among pediatric populations in Africa and Asia. However, outbreaks have been described quite rarely such as after the 2005 earthquake in Pakistan and the 2004 tsunami in Indonesia.

TB remains a concern during population displacement. Following disasters crowded shelters and camps are possible foci for local transmission. Interruption of treatment for already diagnosed patients due to difficult access to services can put patients and their communities at risk.

40.2.3 Vector-Borne (Malaria, Dengue Fever)

Stagnant waters after disasters can facilitate the proliferation of mosquitoes and, coupled with large numbers of displaced people sleeping in sub-standard shelters or in tents without the necessary protection measures, can lead to outbreaks of vector-borne diseases. As result outbreaks of malaria, dengue, Japanese encephalitis and yellow fever can occur. Such outbreaks have been described after flooding in Bolivia in 2007 (dengue) or a hurricane in Haiti in 1966 (malaria). Malaria mortality can be very high in areas of high endemicity receiving populations from areas of low endemicity who lack immunity and are highly susceptible [9, 10].

40.2.4 Contamination of Wounded Injuries and Skin

Tetanus can be a very severe problem among non-vaccinated people following disasters due to resulting trauma either during the event or shortly after in the effort to extricate survivors, help people, or move debris around. Tetanus cases with high fatality rate have been recorded during the 2004 tsunami in Indonesia and the 2005 earthquake in Pakistan [11].

Exposure of wounds to water and soil following disasters (floods, tsunamis, hurricanes, tornados) can cause common, necrotizing and fungal soft tissue infections and even severe fatal sepsis [12]. Cutaneous mucormycosis cases have been described after a tornado that hit Missouri in USA in 2011.

40.2.5 Sexually Transmitted Infections and Sexual Violence (STIs and SV)

Sexually transmitted infections and sexual violence can become an issue of concern during protracted population displacement. Prevention measures as well as access to appropriate medical care must be included in the design of the recovery phase response.

40.3   Prevention and Control Measures

40.3.1 Dead Bodies and Myths

Great misunderstandings occur around the mistaken belief that following natural disasters, epidemics are expected to occur with certainty. This belief is linked to the presumed potential of dead corpses to cause significant disease transmission. However, this is not the case as corpses are linked to the impact of the disaster itself and belong to generally healthy people that have perished instantly or shortly after the event due to mainly traumatic causes. Basic precautions for those handling corpses aiming at protection from bodily fluids with the use of gloves and adequate protective clothing as well as hand hygiene and use of body bags are essential. Equipment and vehicles used must be disinfected. However, except in case of death due to cholera, shigellosis, or hemorrhagic fevers, bodies do not need special handling. It is recommended to apply burial ensuring that the lower level of graves is higher than the water table level to protect water sources.

40.3.2 Site Planning

Site planning should take into account issues of environmental safety, weather protection, sanitation, avoidance of overcrowding, access to basic services, and proper disposal of waste and sewage. Protection from flooding and stagnant waters offer prevention of vector-borne diseases as well as diseases transmitted by the oral-fecal route. Insecticide-treated nets (ITNs), bedding, and clothing are important for the prevention of vector-borne diseases and especially malaria. Protection from criminality and especially sexual violence must be incorporated into site planning. Adequate lighting, placement of toilets, sanitation facilities, washing and cooking areas, and the presence of security services are essential components of proper site planning.

40.3.3 Food, Water Supply, Sanitation (WASH)

Ensuring safe water supply at a minimum of 20 L per person per day as well as adequate facilities and materials for personal hygiene according to the SPHERE STANDARDS are crucial elements of a successful response.

40.3.4 Vector Control

Preexisting vector control activities can suffer after a major disaster as staff and infrastructure can be impacted or diverted to other perceived as more pressing needs by the authorities. What's more, the conditions following a disaster could call for not only continuation but even expansion of such activities to protect the population.

40.3.5 Vaccination

Vaccination coverage before the disaster hits, is a critical determinant of the risk for future outbreaks. Rapid mass measles vaccination must be undertaken within 72 h and not later than a week among the susceptible population, and provision of vitamin A in children 6–59 months of age can reduce complications and mortality. Rapid vaccination for meningococcal diseases is also a priority. Pneumococcal polyvalent vaccine, hepatitis A, and possibly tetanus are among the main vaccines to be offered.

40.3.6 Health Promotion

Health promotion activities are critical to ensure that the population has the means to use the resources and services offered and incorporate them into their daily routine and activities. Creating an appropriate health-seeking behavior following a disaster is essential for protection from infectious diseases outbreaks. Sanitation, vaccination, and early access to diagnostic services and medical care are key factors for the protection of affected communities, especially when important risk factors exist that cannot be minimized or greatly reduced due to practical, financial, social, and cultural barriers.

40.3.7 Surveillance

Disease surveillance systems and early warning systems are essential for the detection and rapid response to potential clusters of disease in order to avert large scale outbreaks. However, surveillance systems are heavily dependent on technology and tools, especially in developed countries, which are the first to collapse following a disaster. For this reason, preparedness and application of credible, simple, and flexible surveillance systems adapted to local context and capacities are crucial at every post disaster phase. This is even more important during the first weeks when infrastructure could be damaged and not restored yet.

40.3.8 Disease Management

Finally, ensuring that services for management of diseases are accessible and adequate during all phases of the disaster response is very important for the reduction of morbidity and mortality and certainly a key priority. Good quality of medical care is essential, and there is need to continually adapt to the changing conditions as the response moves from the impact to the recovery phase of the disaster. Longer-term operational plans must be drawn. Chronic disease sufferers such as patients with diabetes, heart disease, and neurologic and psychiatric illness and of course HIV and TB patients on ongoing treatment must be located and swiftly linked to care. Models of care for chronic diseases must be adapted to the new reality post-disaster.

40.4   Case Studies

Below the reader can go through a short presentation of clusters of infectious diseases or outbreaks following disasters. The presentation of key facts for each event can facilitate the understanding of all drivers of possible outbreaks in natural disasters and the magnitude of their impact on the affected communities.

Impact of river flooding on groundwater quality in India, 2015–2016 [13]
- In 2015, after the flooding of the Adyar River in Chennai, India, water was tested for major ions, trace metals, bacterial population and other pathogens concentrations.
- Total bacterial count (TBC) in groundwater was high in most affected locations.

- *Escherichia coli* and *Enterobacter aerogenes* concentrations were high in four affected areas.
- *Staphylococcus epidermidis* concentrations were high in both affected and non-affected areas.
- *Shigella*, *Streptococcus*, and *Salmonella* strains (*S. flexneri*, *S. pyogenes*, and *S. typhi*) concentrations were also high in the affected areas.
- *Vibrio cholerae* was detected only in the affected areas.
- The concentrations and dynamics of TBC, coliforms, and pathogens were considered to be the result of the heavy rainfall.
- Low temperatures, high soil humidity, neutral or alkaline soil pH, and the presence of organic carbon enhanced the survival of these microorganisms in soil along with groundwater after the floods.

Serratia spp. in Katmandu, 2015 [14]
- In 2015, two massive earthquakes struck upon Katmandu.
- After the earthquakes, in a neonatal intensive care unit cases of blood stream infections of *Serratia* spp. (six cases of *Serratia rubidaea* and five of *Serratia marcescens*) were detected.
- Whole genome sequencing confirmed the blood stream infections.
- All patients were severely ill and one patient died.
- The identification of the source of the outbreak was unsuccessful.
- According to the speculation of the physicians, the deficits in hygienic behavior in combination with the lack of standard infection control, after the earthquakes, contributed to this unusual outbreak.

Cholera in Germany, 1892 [15]
- In 1892 a cholera outbreak occured in the port city of Hamburg.
- Days before the outbreak, the level of Elba River was low due to an extreme heat wave. The river water was pushed back upstream and the water supplies were contaminated.
- The total number of patients had reached 17,000 and 8,600 had died.

Leptospirosis in Fiji islands, 2012 [16]
- Extreme flood events in Western Fiji caused the largest outbreak of leptospirosis recorded in the South Pacific, with 1217 total suspected cases.
- 83% of the cases occurred within 6 weeks of the flood events.
- The transmission appeared to occur during or immediately after the floods.
- Genotyping studies suggest that multiple animal reservoirs were implicated in the outbreak.

Leptospirosis in Philippines, 2009 [17]
- After a typhoon in September 2009, an outbreak of leptospirosis occurred in Metro Manila, the Philippines. A total of 471 cases met clinical criteria for leptospirosis and 51 died.
- All patients received antimicrobial therapy. The 51 patients died of acute respiratory distress syndrome and acute renal failure.

Rotavirus in Solomon Islands, 2014 [18]
- In 2014, in Honiara, a tropical depression caused rainfall, ten times the mean weekly rainfall.
- Flooding on the area of Solomon Islands precipitated an epidemic of diarrhea.
- The outbreak spread to the unaffected by flooding regions.
- During the outbreak, six of nine provinces in the Solomon Islands reported diarrhea outbreaks.
- The epidemic caused more than 6,000 cases and 27 deaths.
- Illness and deaths caused by rotaviruses primarily affect the <5 years age group.
- Rotavirus was identified in 38% of case-patients.

Hepatitis A in India, 2013 [19]
- In 2013, the Himalayan Tsunami affected the Himalayan and Sub-Himalayan region of Uttarakhand.
- After the devastating Tsunami, an outbreak of possible hepatitis A infection (HAV) was reported among children <10 years of age in a flood rescue camp with very poor hygienic conditions.
- Among the 28 samples tested, 25 (89.3%) were found positive for anti-HAV IgG and IgM antibodies.
- Twenty-three of the samples (92%) were confirmed as positive for Hepatitis A serology by anti-HAV IgM-ELISA.
- Mild clinical symptoms were observed, and no mortality due to the infection was reported.
- All the eight water samples collected from the nearby water sources were found affected by fecal contamination and with a concentration of >180 thermotolerant coliforms/100 ml of water.
- The hygienic conditions in the camp were very poor and of sub-standard quality.

***Cryptosporidium hominis* in Germany, 2013** [20]
- In 2013, the river Haale (Saale) overflowed and damaged the sewage systems.
- 24 cases of cryptosporidiosis were notified to the surveillance system in the city of Halle.
- Stool specimens were tested by microscopy and PCR, and *Cryptosporidium* DNA was sequenced.
- Samples from public water system, swimming pools, and river Saale were examined for *Cryptosporidium* oocysts by microscopy and PCR.
- Oocysts were detected in samples from the river, two local lakes, and three public swimming pools by microscopy, but not in the public water supply.
- Overall, 167 cases were detected, and 24% of them were classified as secondary cases.

Norovirus in USA, 2005 [21]
- Hurricane Katrina struck the Gulf Coast in 2005.
- An estimated 240,000 persons, mostly from Louisiana, were evacuated to Texas.
- An estimated 24,000 evacuees were sheltered temporarily at facilities in Reliant Park, a sports and convention complex.

- Approximately 6,500 of the estimated 24,000 evacuees visited the Reliant Park medical clinic, and 1,169 persons reported symptoms of acute gastroenteritis.
- No deaths were reported.
- Norovirus was confirmed in 22 specimens.

Influenza A (H3N2) in Japan, 2011 [22]
- A mega-earthquake (magnitude 9.0) struck Japan in 2011.
- A large-scale tsunami that followed the earthquake devastated many coastal areas.
- 105 confirmed cases were detected.
- The cases occurred in patients aged 15–64 years, who were likely to have engaged in search and rescue activities.
- No deaths were reported in this outbreak.

Malaria in Costa Rica [23]
- In 1991, a 7.4 magnitude earthquake struck Costa Rica.
- After the earthquake, the region was affected by floods.
- 13 months after the events, a survey was held by the Costa Rican Ministry of Health's malaria control program.
- Some areas experienced increases in the incidence of malaria as high as 1,600% and 4,700% above the average monthly rate for the pre-earthquake period.
- The changes in human behavior such as increased exposure to mosquitoes while sleeping outside and a temporary pause in malaria control activities were the main causal mechanisms behind this increase.

Tetanus in Indonesia, 2006 [24]
- The earthquake struck Indonesia in the region of Yogyakarta.
- 26 patients with tetanus were admitted to 8 hospitals following the earthquakes.
- 8 of the 26 patients died.
- According to the statistical results, it was shown that the distance and type of hospital were significant predictors of death.

Cutaneous leishmaniasis in Iran, 2003 [25]
- Two mild earthquakes struck the rural town of Zarindasht in the southern Iranian in 2003.
- The annual incidence of cutaneous leishmaniasis increased from 58.6 detected cases/100,000 in the 12 months before the earthquakes to 864 detected cases/100,000 in the following 12 months.
- About half (50.4%) of the detected skin lesions were on the face.
- Most (89.7%) of the skin lesions were caused by *Leishmania major.*

References

1. Shimouchi A, Kobayashi N, Nogata Y, Urakawa M, Ishkawa N. The influence of the Great East Japan Earthquake on tuberculosis control in Japan. Western Pac Surveill Response J. 2015;6(4):30.

2. Iwata O, Oki T, Ishiki A, Shimanuki M, Fuchimukai T, Chosa T, et al. Infection surveillance after a natural disaster: lessons learnt from the Great East Japan Earthquake of 2011. Bull World Health Organ. 2013;91:784–9.
3. Lemonick DL. Epidemics after natural disasters. Am J Clin Med. 2011;8(3):144–52.
4. Koudio IK, Aljunid S, Kamigaki T, Hammad K, Oshitani H. Infectious diseases following natural diseases: prevention and control measures. Expert Rev Anti Infect Ther. 2012;10(1):95–104.
5. Fitter DL, Delson BD, Guillaume FD, Schaad AW, Moffet DB, Poncelet JL, et al. Applying a new framework for public health systems recovery following emergencies and disasters the example of Haiti following a major earthquake and cholera outbreak. Am J Trop Med Hyg. 2017;97(Suppl 4):4–11.
6. Marahatta SB. Control of the outbreak of disease aftermath earthquake: an overview. Nepal J Epidemiol. 2015;5(2):468–9.
7. Summer SA, Turner EL, Thielman NM. Association between earthquake events and cholera outbreaks: a cross-country 15-year longitudinal analysis. Prehosp Disaster Med. 2013;28(6):567–72.
8. Hernandez H, Martinez LR. Relationship of environmental disturbances and the infectious potential of fungi. Microbiology. 2018;164:233–41.
9. Hsieh YH. Ascertaining the impact of catastrophic events on dengue outbreak: the 2014 gas explosions in Kaohsiung, Taiwan. PLoS One. 2017;12(5):e0177422.
10. Feng J, Xia Z, Zhang L, Cheng S, Wang R. Risk assessment of malaria prevalence in Ludian, Yongshan, and Jinggu counties, Yunnan Province, after 2014 earthquake disaster. Am J Trop Med Hyg. 2016;94(3):674–8.
11. Pascapurnama DN, Murakami A, Chagan-Yasutan H, Hattori T, Sasaki T, Egawa S. Prevention of tetanus outbreak following natural disaster in Indonesia: lessons learned from previous disasters. Review. Tohoku J Exp Med. 2016;238:219–27.
12. Kawano T, Hasegawa K, Watase H, Morita H, Yamamura O. Infectious disease frequency among evacuees at shelters after the great eastern Japan earthquake and tsunami: a retrospective study. Disaster Med Public Health Prep. 2018;8(1):58–64.
13. Gowrisankar G. Chemical, microbial and antibiotic susceptibility analyses of groundwater after a major flood event in Chennai. Sci Data. 2017;4:170135.
14. Karkey A, et al. Outbreaks of Serratia marcescens and Serratia rubidaea bacteremia in a Central Kathmandu hospital following the 2015 earthquakes. Trans R Soc Trop Med Hyg. 2018;112(10):467–72.
15. Hays JN. Epidemics and pandemics: their impacts on human history. CA: ABC-Clio; 2005. p. 321–9.
16. Togami E, et al. A large leptospirosis outbreak following successive severe floods in Fiji, 2012. Am J Trop Med Hyg. 2018;99(4):849–51.
17. Al-Shere A, et al. Outbreak of leptospirosis after flood, the Philippines, 2009. Emerg Infect Dis. 2012;18(1):91–4.
18. Jones FK, et al. Increased rotavirus prevalence in diarrheal outbreak precipitated by localized flooding, Solomon Islands, 2014. Emerg Infect Dis. 2016;22(5):875–9.
19. Pal S, et al. An outbreak of hepatitis A virus among children in a flood rescue camp: a post-disaster catastrophe. Indian J Med Microbiol. 2016;34(2):233–6.
20. Getler M, et al. Outbreak of *Cryptosporidium hominis* following river flooding in the city of Halle (Saale), Germany, August 2013. BMC Infect Dis. 2015;15:88.
21. Centers for Disease Control and Prevention (CDC). Norovirus outbreak among evacuees from hurricane Katrina–Houston, Texas, September 2005. MMWR Morb Mortal Wkly Rep. 2005;54(40):1016–8.
22. Kamagaki T. Investigation of an influenza A (H3N2) outbreak in evacuation centres following the Great East Japan earthquake, 2011. BMC Public Health. 2014;14:34.
23. Sáenz R, Bissell RA, Paniagua F. Post-disaster malaria in Costa Rica. Prehosp Disaster Med. 1995;10(3):154–60.
24. Sutiono AB, Qiantori A, Suwa H, Ohta T. Characteristic tetanus infection in disaster-affected areas: case study of the Yogyakarta earthquakes in Indonesia. BMC Res Notes. 2009;2:34.
25. Fakoorziba M, et al. Post-earthquake outbreak of cutaneous leishmaniasis in a rural region of southern Iran. Ann Trop Med Parasitol. 2011;105(3):217–24.

Basic Management of Dead Disaster Victims

41

Dimitrios Papakonstantinou, Pavlos Patapis,
Nikos Machairas, and Evangelos Misiakos

41.1 Introduction and Purpose

Large-scale disasters unavoidably leave tens of hundreds or even thousands of dead victims in their wake, and therefore managing the dead is a core component of the disaster response in such situations. Recent experiences with hurricane "Mitch" in Central America (1998), the 2004 tsunami that struck Southeast Asia, and the massive earthquake that hit Haiti in 2010, among many others, demonstrate that the chaos ensuing in the aftermath of massive disasters might overwhelm local authorities with subsequent mishandling of fatalities [1, 2]. Hence, being familiar with the basic practices of managing the dead beforehand has the potential of making an enormous difference. The aim of this chapter to equip the reader with the procedural knowledge required to handle dead disaster victims, on a basic level.

41.2 Why Managing the Dead Matters

Although searching for survivors and ensuring their timely evacuation from a potentially hazardous environment is of utmost importance in the first phase of an organized disaster response, proper handling of the dead in the subsequent phases should not be underemphasized for a variety of reasons.

Firstly, the retrieval, identification, and dignified disposal of dead bodies help ease the psychological burden on the living and the local community as a whole [3, 4]. The families of the dead should be allowed to grieve their dead according to their

D. Papakonstantinou (✉) · P. Patapis · N. Machairas · E. Misiakos
Third Department of Surgery, University General Hospital "Attikon", National and
Kapodistrian University of Athens, Athens, Greece

© Springer Nature Switzerland AG 2021
E. Pikoulis, J. Doucet (eds.), *Emergency Medicine, Trauma and Disaster
Management*, Hot Topics in Acute Care Surgery and Trauma,
https://doi.org/10.1007/978-3-030-34116-9_41

own religious and cultural practices so as to come to terms with their loss thus setting in motion the process of disaster recovery.

Secondly, rapid retrieval of dead bodies ensures that survivors and bystanders are not exposed to the sight and smell of dead bodies, an experience which can admittedly be distressing and further scar the stricken populace [4].

Lastly, prompt disposal of dead bodies following a disaster ensures that the public does not panic over contagious diseases or possible contamination of water and/ or food sources owing to decaying cadavers. The public health risk is considered to be miniscule [5], even in mass casualty situations, and can most often be attributed to infectious diseases such as Hepatitis B or C, HIV, and tuberculosis, diseases often already prevalent in the affected population. However, public belief that dead bodies cause diseases holds strong, especially in many developing countries, and this may inadvertently lead to adoption of unacceptable and hastily devised methods of body disposal such as mass burials, which may cause even more hardships to an already bereaved society.

Proper management of dead victims follows three steps: retrieval, identification, and disposal. Local and international authorities as well as humanitarian organizations should be involved in organizing the above process and take care of material and logistic requirements. Extreme diligence is required to make certain that the recovery process is as smooth as possible with no mishaps or complications.

41.3 Coordinating the Response

Management of dead disaster victims, as mentioned above, is a multistep process that starts with the search and retrieval, body identification, transfer to a mortuary facility, and finally delivery of the body to family members so that they may enact its proper disposal according to social and cultural norms. Coordination of the various institutions involved in this process is of exceeding importance to avoid misplacement of available resources. To that end, a public administrative office such as the Ministry of Interior Affairs, the Ministry of Health, the Attorney General's Office, or any other public institution specified by local law should undertake the task of coordinating government agencies and appropriately distribute the tasks of body recovery, identification, and burial arrangements. In those cases in which the local law fails to specify a coordinating institution to assume leadership in massive disaster situations, a committee should be assembled by the government's initiative. It is important to state that hospitals and caregivers should be exempted from this role, as their priorities lie in managing the living.

In general, civil agencies such as law enforcement agencies, military branches, fire departments, paramedic agencies, as well as municipal authorities should always be involved in the disaster response as the above public organizations usually employ skilled personnel that can adapt quickly to the responsibilities of dead disaster victim management [6, 7]. Humanitarian organizations and volunteers can be of special importance in resource-poor countries. A schematic representation for the hierarchical structure described herein is provided in Table 41.1.

Table 41.1 Schematic representation of the structure of a coordinated disaster response in regards to dead disaster victim management

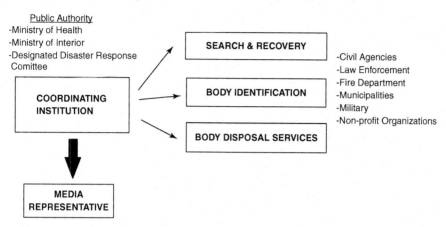

Once a proper hierarchy is established, a plan should promptly be devised and circulated widely on a local, regional, and national level. All authorities involved in managing the cadavers should be made familiar with the plan in order to further subdivide responsibilities and avoid duplicate efforts. Nevertheless, this does not mean that the involved personnel needs to be informed about all the intricacies and components of the action plan, for example, identification and body retrieval personnel does not to be informed about the methods of body disposal or the mortuary service does not need to be informed about the recovery operations, as this may cause confusion and delays.

Emphasis should be given on the continued communication of the involved agencies with the community. Communication with local and national media should provide the public information about the extent and the type of the disaster. This should ideally be done by a spokesperson with experience in media handling. This person is to be designated by the leading institution and provide precise, realistic, and credible information in order to leave no room for misinterpretation and rumors.

41.4   Body Search and Recovery

Search for dead bodies should begin as soon as possible, after the living are rescued and taken care of. Delays in the recovery process lead to exposure of the cadavers to the devastating environmental effects of a massive disaster aftermath. It is obvious that prolonged exposure to the elements may hinder future efforts of body identification due to distortion of key facial or body features [6–8].

The first step in the process of body search and recovery is locating where the bodies are. Survivors found on the scene of the disaster or reports from the teams of first responders usually provide information on the location of the dead bodies. Based on this information, organized search parties and specialized recovery teams arriving on the scene can be directed towards possible points of interest. Special care should be taken to avoid entering a hazardous environment such as a burning building or an exposed high voltage power line without proper precautions. This might endanger recovery personnel and perhaps even lead to even more, needless, loss of life.

Teams involved in this phase of disaster response should be allocated basic equipment for carrying human remains (body bags, stretchers, and gurneys) as well as tools useful for illumination and for performing basic recovery tasks such as digging and clearing debris. When a corpse is located, it should be individually placed on the ground. Piling bodies or human remains is an unacceptable practice on the field. At this point, it is very important that the recovery personnel photograph the cadaver in order to procure material useful in the identification process, before decomposition settles in. Pictures of the entire length of the body, the face, any and all distinguishing features (i.e., tattoos, marks, scars) and pictures of worn clothing items are appropriate.

Subsequently, body metrics and data should be recorded. Data of interest is the gender, estimated height and body, hair color and length, skin color, and probable age. A body tag with a unique ID should then be placed on the corpse, and afterwards all photographs and information collected should be filed under the same ID to avoid confusion or misplacement of important data.

After body documentation is completed, the corpse should be put in a body bag, if available. Then, extraction of the body from the scene of the disaster follows. This is greatly facilitated by the availability of stretchers; however a two-person technique in which each person supports opposite parts of the body may also be employed. Evacuation points should be designated in advance to avoid confusion in the field.

In general, mass casualty situations rarely provide the time for a preliminary autopsy on the scene. Moreover, lack of specialized resources limits its effectiveness. Provided that a meticulous and systematic documentation process as mentioned above is implemented, field autopsies should not be considered mandatory. In cases of manmade disasters, forensic information should be collected before body extraction, under the guidance and supervision of local law enforcement authorities.

41.5   The Process of Body Identification

Identification of dead victims heavily relies on the proper recovery of the bodies, adequate collection of data concerning the bodies, matching the information with lists of missing persons, and finally acquiring visual confirmation from the families of the dead. Evidently, the best time frame for visual identification is before decomposition starts affecting the body and altering its key features. Furthermore, injuries, dirt, or mutilations may lower the chances of a successful visual confirmation of identity. Additionally, grief-stricken and stressed family members might be unable or reluctant to identify the dead body as their loved one. It is in all these circumstances that forensic experts are called upon to apply specialized identification techniques to supplement any visual confirmation.

The primary assessment in unidentifiable bodies is to verify basic aspects of identity such as sex, race, age, height, weight, hair color, and any birthmarks. These preliminary assessments are especially helpful in mass casualty situations in order to rule out or rule in a positive identification, and even though absolute identity cannot be established using these criteria, shortlists can be created and pave the way for a more concentrated and effective application of other, resource heavy methods [9].

Radiology studies have a limited role in the body identification process and can only be used as an adjunct [6]. Plain films can be obtained and inspected for previous bone injuries or deformities that correspond with the past medical history of a missing person. Perhaps of greater importance are dental radiographs which when superimposed to a presumed victim previous films can yield extremely valuable information regarding the body's identity.

The most scientifically acclaimed method of body identification is the method of DNA identification. Since the introduction of the polymerase chain reaction (PCR) technique in the early 1990s, DNA identification kits have become so widespread that are currently used in a myriad of forensic laboratories. Bodily fluids or tissues can be sampled from a dead victim and be processed so that nuclear genetic material is analyzed and profiled. This can be subsequently matched to a sample drawn from presumed victim's personal belongings in order to obtain a positive genetic fingerprint match. The most frequently utilized forensic methods for DNA profiling rely on short tandem repeats (STR) profiling or single-nucleotide polymorphisms (SNP) markers [10]. The technical intricacies of DNA sample procurement and analysis are beyond the scope of this chapter; however, it must be stressed that even this technique is not entirely foolproof, as extensive research on the topic confirms. Consequently, combining multiple methods of identification (fingerprint comparison, DNA forensics, photographs, dental records, and visual confirmation) is appropriate for matching a dead body to a presumed dead or missing victim [11, 12].

41.6 Proper Body Storage and Disposal

The purpose of a structured dead body disposal plan is twofold ensuring proper disposal of human remains in a time efficient and sanitary fashion as well as making sure the families of the victims get the emotional closure they deserve by performing the funeral rites that their cultural and religious customs dictate.

The first step in taking care of the remains of dead disaster victims is to make certain that acceptable storage conditions are available. The best way to store cadavers is in individual plastic and waterproof body bags, each assigned with a unique ID tag, as stated above, which are to be kept preferably in a refrigerated environment. When such conditions cannot be met due to strained resources, then temporary burial can be contemplated. In that case, individual graves can be used for a small number of casualties, while trench graves in which bodies are to be placed in a side by side manner can be dug for larger numbers of deceased. Detailed maps and records of the burial locations are to be kept in order to facilitate future exhumation of the bodies once arrangements have been made for their final disposal. If temporary burial is not possible, bodies can be stored in any building that provides shelter from the heat and the sun, albeit only for a short period of time [6].

The purpose of body storage is that they may be delivered in a decent condition to their family members. Afterwards, final disposal can take place in accordance to the family's wishes usually by burial, although cremation is an acceptable practice in many countries. When the remains are handed over, a paper trail should be left in place so as to avoid future confusion as to where the body ends up and ensure its traceability. Burial sites should be chosen well away from sources of drinking water, and prevailing religious practices (i.e., heads facing toward Mecca) should be kept in mind. If cremation is chosen, then it should be performed by specialists in state-accredited centers to ensure proper disposal of the remains.

41.7 Conclusion

Mass casualty disasters have been a scourge on mankind since the very early years of humanity, as surfaced evidence from the Minoan volcanic eruption of Thera (circa 1600 BCE) that wiped and entire civilization from existence proves and common experience shows that they will keep occurring periodically and unpredictably causing grief and distress to human communities. Preparedness for such events is therefore important and can make an enormous difference on the impact disasters have on society. The core of any and every disaster response plan is centered on rescuing and caring for the survivors, and indeed this should be the priority in any case. However, one should bear in mind that those unlucky ones to suffer catastrophic wounds that end their life still retain their identity as a human being. It is thus necessary to include these victims in every disaster plan so that their dignity is upheld for the sake of them, their families, and the society in general. The present chapter by no means provides a comprehensive guide to managing the dead bodies but instead outlines the basic principles pertaining to recovering the dead, storing the cadavers, and handling their final disposal. Hopefully, efforts made by international humanitarian organizations such as the Red Cross and the World Health Organization will establish guidelines addressing these issues so that future catastrophes are dealt with in a more methodical and efficacious way, in the years to come.

References

1. Morgan OW, Sribanditmongkol P, Perera C, Sulasmi Y, Van Alphen D, Sondorp E. Mass fatality management following the South Asian tsunami disaster: case studies in Thailand, Indonesia, and Sri Lanka. PLoS Med. 2006;3(6):e195. https://doi.org/10.1371/journal.pmed.0030195.
2. Sumathipala A, Siribaddana S, Perera C. Management of dead bodies as a component of psychosocial interventions after the tsunami: a view from Sri Lanka. Int Rev Psychiatry. 2006;18(3):249–57. https://doi.org/10.1080/09540260600656100.

3. Bezabh YH, Abebe SM, Fanta T, Tadese A, Tulu M. Prevalence and associated factors of post-traumatic stress disorder among emergency responders of Addis Ababa Fire and Emergency Control and Prevention Service Authority, Ethiopia: institution-based, cross-sectional study. BMJ Open. 2018;8(7):e020705. https://doi.org/10.1136/bmjopen-2017-020705.
4. Everly G, Perrin P, Everly G. Psychological issues in escape, rescue, and survival in the wake of disaster. Ment Health. 2008;12:21–30.
5. Goyet D. Epidemics caused by dead bodies: a disaster myth that does not want to die. Rev Panam Salud Pública. 2004;15(5):297–9.
6. Ellingham S, Cordner S, Tidball-Binz M. Revised practical guidance for first responders managing the dead after disasters. Int Rev Red Cross. 2017;98(902):647–69. https://doi.org/10.1017/S1816383117000248.
7. Management of dead bodies in disaster situations. (PAHO disaster manuals and guidelines on disaster series, no. 5). Washington: Pan American Health Organization; 2004.
8. International Federation of Red Cross and Red Crescent Societies. Management of dead bodies after disasters: a field manual for first responders. 2016, p 78. Retrieved from https://www.ifrc.org/Global/Publications/communications/0880_002_Management-of-dead-bodies_8.pdf.
9. Ziętkiewicz E, Witt M, Daca P, Zebracka-Gala J, Goniewicz M, Jarząb B, Witt M. Current genetic methodologies in the identification of disaster victims and in forensic analysis. J Appl Genet. 2012;53(1):41–60. https://doi.org/10.1007/s13353-011-0068-7.
10. Manjunath BC, Chandrashekar BR, Mahesh M, Vatchala Rani RM. DNA profiling and forensic dentistry--a review of the recent concepts and trends. J Forensic Legal Med. 2011;18(5):191–7. https://doi.org/10.1016/j.jflm.2011.02.005.
11. Butler JM. The future of forensic DNA analysis. Philos Trans R Soc Lond Ser B Biol Sci. 2015;370(1674):20140252. https://doi.org/10.1098/rstb.2014.0252.
12. Brough AL, Morgan B, Rutty GN. The basics of disaster victim identification. J Forensic Radiol Imaging. 2015;3(1):29–37. https://doi.org/10.1016/j.jofri.2015.01.002.

Disaster-Induced Psychological Trauma: Supporting Survivors and Responders

42

Anna Polemikou

> *You are more than a survivor. You have been transformed.*
>
> —*Eleanor Brownn*

42.1 Introduction

Throughout the twentieth century, the psychological impact of stress, adversity, and trauma has constituted a perennial topic of interest for mental healthcare professionals. Several studies, journal publications, and discourses on the impact of experiences of overwhelming proportions on mental health have repeatedly affirmed the painful imprint of extreme anxiety on the human psyche. Initially coined as *physioneurosis* by A. Kardiner, who published the first comprehensive investigation on combat-related psychological sequelae (1941; cited in [1]), and later referred to as *combat fatigue*, a more cohesive picture of clinical phenomena tracing what is nowadays known as posttraumatic stress disorder began to emerge, peaking upon the return of survivors, prisoners and veterans of World War II and the Vietnam and Korean Wars.

Eventually, these unclassified psychological manifestations were drawn together so as to feature within the taxonomies of popular and reputable classification and reference systems, such as the *Diagnostic and Statistical Manual of Mental Disorders* (DSM), produced by the American Psychiatric Association, and the Classification of Mental and Behavioral Disorders (ICD) by the World Health Organization (WHO). Nonetheless, the condition continued to be largely undermined as "transient" and "situational" for several decades, whereas patients were frequently misdiagnosed as psychotic or schizophrenic, leading to subsequent revisions and incremental adjustments and specifications in the following editions of the DSM and the ICD, regarding the clinical features that constitute accurate, actual, and/or differential diagnoses.

A. Polemikou (✉)
Department of Medicine, Athens University, Athens, Greece
e-mail: apolemikou@aegean.gr

© Springer Nature Switzerland AG 2021
E. Pikoulis, J. Doucet (eds.), *Emergency Medicine, Trauma and Disaster Management*, Hot Topics in Acute Care Surgery and Trauma,
https://doi.org/10.1007/978-3-030-34116-9_42

Nowadays, we approach disturbances arising from major crises or catastrophic events via interdisciplinary means, which focus on a person's subjective experience of the stressor, adversity, and/or trauma and its effect on regulatory structures of cognition and affect and behavioral functions. As we aspire to devise more comprehensive diagnostic models and criteria, destigmatization ensues, access to psychological support is facilitated and encouraged, and prevention and recovery for those afflicted becomes more efficient.

The focus of the present chapter is twofold. Firstly, to present the growing body of scientific evidence regarding the psychological costs of life-threatening incidents on survivors and disaster response employees. Secondly, it offers a set of guidelines on prevention and intervention, which are likely to inhibit the permanence of negative mental health outcomes and to reinstate the status of those affected into full functionality as soon as possible following the event. However, before we proceed with the clinical features of crisis-related disorders, let me first introduce a concept that is centrally positioned in disaster-induced psychological manifestations: psychological trauma.

42.2 Defining Psychological Trauma

Psychological trauma involves witnessing and responding to an actual or perceived threat [2] to the security/integrity of the self or others that exceeds one's ability to cope or integrate the emotions involved in that experience. The initiating event may not necessarily implicate physical harm, but may result in overwhelming emotions of intense fear or helplessness in response to heightened or repeated disturbance. Psychological trauma is the "normal" reaction to an "abnormal" situation and makes sense in the context of fear-based or anxiety-provoking circumstances. Although often triggered by objective stressors, with sufficient impact to produce significant emotional reactions, being traumatized by an event remains a subjective experience [3, 4], often escalating into physical/medical symptoms, alongside the main psychological manifestations. It is positively associated with feelings of powerlessness and insecurity and can be triggered by (1) one-time extraordinary stressful events, such as natural or man-made disasters, violent crimes, the sudden death of a loved one, a painful breakup from a significant relationship, etc., or by (2) the persistent recurrence of anxiety-provoking incidents, such as living in a crime-ridden neighborhood, experiencing a life-threatening illness, being the recipient of humiliating and disappointing behavior (i.e., workplace bullying), etc.

Likewise, for disaster workers, professional trauma may result from responding to and witnessing a critical one-time event or from absorbing ongoing, relentless stress, which in a sense is inherent in occupational groups involved in rescue operations [5]. Unique to this population is the "line of duty" constellation of traumatic experiences, which includes an array of incidents such as heavy physical activity, personal injury or the death of a crew companion, as well as potential post-incident services (i.e., after action review (AAR), the term applied to describe the reviewing process that takes place at the aftermath of an operation). The personal and public cost of mental health impairments of occupational groups affected by disasters is incredibly taxing, not only in financial resources but also in terms of a decline in work performance. The fear that a responder's emotional dysregulation may negatively affect the quality of care provided to the general population, or may let down his/her colleagues, often contributes to secrecy and stigma regarding mental health impairments. Hence, it should be emphasized that engaging in appropriate self-care practices is an important aspect of well-being for rescue employees. At the same time, it is important to remove oneself from the stereotype of stoicism and invincibility that is so prominent in the culture of first responders and to be compassionately vigilant and encouraging toward fellow co-workers who might also require support.

Finally, in the event of a preexisting disorder or predisposition to mental illness, a traumatizing event is likely to either exacerbate symptomatology or precipitate the onset of a disorder, introducing the possibility of comorbidity between various mental conditions.

42.3   Trauma- and Stressor-Related Disorders

On May 18, 2013, the American Psychiatric Association released the latest revision of its *Diagnostic and Statistical Manual of Mental Disorders*. As a result, a new diagnostic category was introduced with the publication of the fifth edition (DSM-5); Trauma- and Stressor-Related Disorders were proposed, which explicitly list a close encounter with an event of great distress as a diagnostic criterion for posttraumatic stress disorder (PTSD). The classification criteria for PTSD were once again updated and further specified, so as to include symptoms which apply to children aged 6 years and younger, as well as a dissociative subtype of PTSD, with the addition of Acute Stress Disorder following exposure to death or violence. The taxonomy includes some of the following: intrusion symptoms (i.e., recurrent, involuntary, and distressing memories, dreams, flashbacks of the event); marked physiological reactions; avoidance of triggering situations; alterations in cognition, affect, and arousal; etc. Moreover, the DSM specifies the existence of co-occurring dissociative symptoms by the presence of manifestations of depersonalization (i.e., mental detachment) and derealization (a dreamlike distortion of reality and consciousness).

Of course, that is not to say that all survivors are destined to develop eventual or lasting mental health conditions, nor that everyone will experience distress with the same intensity, or even exhibit the same clinical manifestations. There is a great deal of individual variability [6] and just as many protective factors that may contribute to one's resilience against reaching a critical level of maladjustment. Historically, academic interest on traumatic stress has focused on the subjective differences in an individual's perception and appraisal of stressful events [4]. The meaning-making narrative and the personal meaning production that ensues, in accordance to one's subjective experience [7], is increasingly being found at the heart of accumulated published thought, proposed as a potential protective mechanism [8–11]. A person's attempt to engage in a narrative discourse, through which he or she may construe meaning when none is readily evident, constitutes a promising avenue of future exploration.

42.4 Professional Personnel Involved in Rescue Operations: Who Helps the Helpers?

As reviewed above, the recent inclusion of Trauma- and Stressor-Related Disorders in DSM-5 [2] sets the actual or threatened peritraumatic event as a diagnostic premise for membership in the aforementioned clinical taxonomy. This means that the event itself serves as a diagnostic criterion for this cluster of disorders. In light of this information, how does mental health or illness sit within the broader context of occupational stressors typically experienced by disaster-exposed employees? In essence, the two are inseparable: professional help providers are always present throughout the unfolding of disastrous events. Whether prior to the incident, during the uncertainty of a developing outcome, or at the aftermath of a life-threatening episode, emergency responders are in close proximity to the scenes of terror, witnessing the aversive details, and in a constant state of insecurity, chronic stress, ambiguity, and alarmed preparedness or readiness to respond [12].

The knowledge that an event of great distress, adversity, and trauma can have a profound effect on one's psychological functioning is hardly a new discovery in the field of clinical psychology and psychiatry. However well documented, research on psychological impact has primarily focused on the immediate victims/survivors of the traumatic incident, at the detriment of professional helpers, who often become the "hidden victims" in need of help themselves [5, 6, 13, 14]. Manifestations of trauma reside in a multitude of diagnostic labels: including anxiety and stress disorders, somatoform disorders, brief psychosis, personality disorders, etc. [15]. Negative health outcomes, such as posttraumatic stress disorder, dissociation, death anxiety, depression, substance abuse and dependence, are particularly common among disaster employees [16–18], which inversely relates to the amount of scholarly attention that has conventionally been attributed to this specific population.

Within the different occupational groups affected by disasters (e.g., search and rescue responders, police officers, firefighters, military personnel, emergency healthcare professionals, humanitarian relief workers, etc.), some—more so than others—share certain commonalities in their cultures. These include similar psychological defense mechanisms, mostly pertaining to dissociative or altered states of consciousness (often integral to PTSD symptomatology) such as stoicism, depersonalization and derealization [3, 17, 19].

It is plausible to postulate that those who systematically assist during the search, rescue, and recovery phases of an emergency operation are exceptionally susceptible to developing variable expressions of clinical distress and negative health outcomes compared to other occupations [20]. Whether in the form of acute, short-term, or persistent manifestations of psychopathology, there is no denying that their deep immersion in the critical and aversive aspects of a catastrophe carries adverse mental health reactions, often confirmed by the high rates of suicidal ideation and/ or behaviors encountered in responder personnel [5, 16]. Nonetheless, as it emerges, exposure to critical incidents is a necessary but insufficient condition for the manifestation of trauma-related disorders. It seems that various risk factors may mediate a traumatic event and the onset of PTSD. Career-initiated exposure to stressors may not necessarily relate to PTSD in a causal fashion, but may appear to be significant predictors of PTSD symptoms, which leads to the final section of this chapter: How does one address early mental health intervention, in order to provide ample support to the affected populations?

42.5 Best Practice Guidelines to Psychological Support

In the wake of a disaster, attending to the basic needs of affected individuals is of utmost importance and priority. While the crisis scene is being evacuated and the wounded are offered medical care, providing a safe environment, assessing for ongoing threats, moving those affected to secure premises as fast as possible, and enhancing survival by offering nourishment, shelter and medication, are all crucial aspects of effective psychological support immediately after the incident. The main focus after a disaster is to protect and preserve life, property and the environment. An outline of the guidelines proposed by the National Institute of Mental Health [21] is provided in Table 42.1, most of which can be implemented by mental health personnel or by other occupational groups alike.

Early mental health intervention heavily relies on mobilizing and establishing a social support network, by reconnecting families, fostering communication between established community structures, and providing accurate information, risk communication, education, and training to existing services and organizations, so that they can contribute to the community thread of social resilience.

42.6 The Six-Stage Model of Crisis Intervention

Despite the complexity of crisis situations, an intervention model that combines immediacy and efficiency in its application constitutes a useful asset for protection response professionals. The six-stage intervention model proposed by Gilliland (1982 [22]) facilitates this aim and can be applied by different groups of professionals, as well as volunteers, carers, parents, or teachers in the context of psychological support provision, irrespective of their level of specialization. The six-stage model focuses on the conditions surrounding the crisis; it is action-oriented and its success relies upon the initiative of those who apply it. Simultaneously, instead of requiring a mechanistic application, it embraces a philosophy of flexibility toward the flow of events and the reformation of perceptions as new developments unfold. Each of the proposed six steps lays the foundation for reinstating a sense of control and restoring the affected individual's basic coping skills. Needless to say, the model requires an overall assessment of the situation on behalf of the helper.

Table 42.1 Steps to addressing early mental health intervention according to the guidelines recommended by the NIMH ([21], September 2)

(1) Basic needs (safety, security, survival)
    Food and shelter
    Orientation
    Connection with social supports
(2) Psychological first aid
    Protect survivors from further harm
    Reduce physiological arousal
    Mobilize support for those who are most distressed
    Keep families together and facilitate reunion with loved ones
    Provide information, foster communication and education
    Use effective risk communication techniques
(3) Needs assessment
    Current status of recovery environment; how well are needs addressed
    Assess additional interventions needed (group, population, individual level)
(4) Monitoring the rescue and recovery environment
    Observe and listen to those most affected
    Monitor environment for past and ongoing threats (i.e., stressors, toxins)
    Monitor services that are being provided
    Monitor media coverage and rumors
(5) Outreach and information dissemination
    "Walking around therapy"[a]
    Using established community structures
    Websites, social media
    Media interviews, releases, programs
    Communication with family, friends, community
(6) Technical assistance, consultation, and training
    Provision to mental health professionals, responders, leaders, organizations
    Improve capacity to re-establish and safeguard community structure
(7) Fostering resilience/recovery
    Social interactions
    Coping skills training
    Risk assessment skills training
    Educate on stress response, traumatic/risk, (ab)normal functioning, service availability
    Group and family interventions
    Fostering natural social support
    Assisting the bereaved
(8) Triage/clinical assessment
    Identify the vulnerable, high-risk individuals, and groups
    Emergency hospitalization
(9) Treatment
    Symptom reduction/amelioration; re-establish functioning via: psychotherapy (individual, family, group), pharmacotherapy, spiritual support, etc.

[a]Ensuring service availability informally through one's presence at common gathering places and aid stations

The first three steps, (1) defining the problem, (2) ensuring client safety, and (3) providing support, are mostly based on active listening rather than action. The final three steps, (4) examining alternatives, (5) making plans, and (6) obtaining commitment toward positive action, are mostly behavior-oriented, even though a responder never gives up active listening throughout the whole process.

The model unfolds in a linear, sequential presentation. However, in actuality, moving between these steps is not uncommon and should be expected, depending on situational changes and occasional regressions. Some steps are sustained throughout as background operations (e.g., Step 2), whereas the last steps (4, 5, and 6) which emphasize active involvement follow each other and combine as a whole to function together in a more systemic fashion.

Step 1: Defining the Problem. The first step in mental health intervention is to determine the exact problem from the viewpoint of the person experiencing it. This stage constitutes a valuable part of the process, in that it initiates and establishes a connection of mutual understanding between the responder and the affected individual. Experiential listening proves to be important during this stage: asking open-ended questions and exhibiting empathy, genuineness, and positive regard.

Step 2: Ensuring Client Safety. Prioritizing the issue of security is always important in crisis intervention. Assessing the mental health risks that the client is currently facing, with the intent to reduce suffering or the likelihood of self-harm, must remain at the forefront of the counselor's list of concerns and priorities. The security parameter is just as important as the crisis worker's initial evaluation, listening skills, and strategies of action; anyone called upon to intervene in critical situations is urged to embrace safety as a natural extension of his thinking and behavior.

Step 3: Providing Support. Once the client is physically safe and the problem has been adequately defined, the next step for the crisis worker is to make his/her approval and validation of the client evident. It is not enough to assume that whoever appeals for and receives help should automatically feel that they are being given value and personal care. Verbal statements such as "this is where you will always find someone who cares" communicate acceptance, attribute value and confirm the feeling that the person being supported is accepted and cared for positively and unconditionally by those who are there to assist.

Step 4: Examining Alternatives. Once basic physical and emotional needs have been met, crisis intervention turns toward an aspect that is often neglected: exploring the wide range of appropriate options available to the person experiencing the crisis. Traumatic events often immobilize one's initiative, hinder any vantage point, and obstruct one's ability to consider options and solutions at their disposal. An effective crisis worker is able not only to recognize, but will also be able to reassure the client of the existence of many alternatives. He or she may encourage and facilitate this process, by presenting information, pointing out choices that may be more preferable than others, and assisting the individual in arriving at his/her own solutions of dealing with the problem. In attempting to identify alternatives, one can move along the following steps based on (a) situational supports, (b) coping mechanisms, and (c) positive and constructive thinking patterns. Establishing a support network of people who care can be a great source of help, and the quest of embedding people in a web of social relationships should be considered. Retrieving from resources or response mechanisms that might prove to be helpful in overcoming the current crisis is another avenue for exploration. Finally, engaging in thinking patterns that might provide new insights toward solving the problem, and might reduce anxiety and distress, is also a preferable choice.

Although the availability of possible courses of action may seem limitless to the effective counselor, it is important to present a manageable number of objective and achievable choices. Disaster-exposed individuals are immersed in psychological overload, and too many choices can easily overwhelm them. It is, thus, preferable to be selective with option availability and keep them realistic, within the context of the situation.

Step 5: Making Plans. The fifth step flows naturally from Step 4, whereby the outcome depends on ensuring that the plans remain realistic and reachable, so that the client doesn't feel disempowered and intimidated. Therefore, plans must focus on the systematic solutions and should correspond to the person's ability to follow the course of action to completion. A key aspect of Step 5 is to encourage plans that emerge in collaboration, so that the client recognizes his/her contribution in shaping them. The basic component of planning a course of action is not to deprive the client of power, independence, or dignity. Appropriate collaboration does not entail making decisions on behalf of the client or imposing one's own opinion; rather, it focuses on positive reinforcement and support, which may take on many forms, such as working on relaxation techniques together, in order to restore the client's faith in his own abilities. The main aim is to regain a sense of control and to progressively restore autonomy, so that those receiving help need not depend on the provision of support for an indefinite period of time.

Step 6: Obtaining Commitment. The sixth and final step arises directly from Step 5 and is easy to follow, provided all the previous helpful steps have been implemented correctly. This stage seeks to obtain a confirmation of the client's sincere and appropriate commitment to the intervention. Backing up an action plan with a proper commitment can be as simple as requesting a summarizing statement, such as "Now that we covered what you plan to do the next time you… (i.e., get angry with someone), briefly tell me what you will do to ensure that you won't lose your temper, and what you will do to ensure that you prevent this feeling from escalating into another crisis." A written commitment may help the already psychologically compromised client keep focus of the intermediate steps without getting further overwhelmed, and both crisis worker and client will be able to trace the progress of the. Skills such as basic active listening are just as important at this stage, as are all the steps that come before (i.e., assessment, security, and support).

We hope that the interventions presented in the current chapter will be of assistance to mental health specialists and other occupational groups involved in crisis intervention. These sets of guidelines are designed to provide relief to those affected by means of planning ahead, monitoring and applying humanitarian comfort. At the same time, they are aimed towards the professional who is committed to his/her own self-care, as well as members of the wider community of responders and rescue workers who are commited to perserving their own psychological well-being.

References

1. Ozer E, Best S, Lipsey T, Weiss D. Predictors of posttraumatic stress disorder and symptoms in adults: a meta-analysis. Psychol Bull. 2003;129(1):52–73.
2. American Psychiatric Association. Diagnostic and statistical manual of mental disorders: DSM-5. 5th ed. Author: Washington, DC; 2013.
3. Adler-Tapia R. Early mental health intervention for first responders/protective service workers including firefighters and emergency medical services (EMS) professionals. In: Luber M, editor. Implementing EMDR early mental health interventions for man-made and natural disasters: models, scripted protocols and summary sheets. New York: Springer Publishing Company; 2013.
4. Kilpatrick FP. Problems of perception in extreme situations. Hum Organ. 1957;16(2):20–2.
5. Kleim B, Westphal M. Mental health in first responders: a review and recommendation for prevention and intervention strategies. Traumatology. 2011;17(4):17–24.
6. Raphael B, Singh B, Bradbury L, Lambert F. Who helps the helpers? The effects of a disaster on the rescue workers. Omega (Westport). 1983;14(1):9–20.
7. Park CL. Meaning making in the context of disasters. J Clin Psychol. 2016;72(12):1234–46.
8. Bonanno GA. Meaning making, adversity, and regulatory flexibility. Memory. 2013;21(1):150–6.
9. Meng WC, Dillon D. Meaning making model: inner purpose, goals, and religiosity/spirituality partially predict acceptance strategies and volunteerism behaviours. Int J Existent Psychol Psychother. 2014;5(1):105–23.
10. Wong PTP. Existential positive psychology. Int J Existent Psychol Psychother. 2016;6(1):7. Retrieved from http://journal.existentialpsychology.org/index.php/ExPsy/article/view/179.
11. Wong PTP, Wong LCJ. A meaning-centered approach to building youth resilience. In: The human quest for meaning: theories, research, and applications. New York: Routledge; 2013. p. 585–618.
12. Pedersen MJB, Gjerland A, Rund BR, Ekeberg Ø, Skogstad L. Emergency preparedness and role clarity among rescue workers during the terror attacks in Norway July 22, 2011. PLoS One. 2016;11(6):1–12.
13. Brooks SK, Dunn R, Amlôt R, Rubin GJ, Greenberg N. Social and occupational factors associated with psychological wellbeing among occupational groups affected by disaster: a systematic review. J Ment Health. 2017;26(4):373–84.
14. Fullerton CS, McCarrol JE, Ursano RJ, Wright KM. Psychological responses of rescue workers: firefighters and trauma. Am J Orthopsychiatry. 1992;62(3):371–8.
15. Arnold L, Pinkston A. Other-being: traumatic stress and dissociation in existential therapy. Int J Existent Psychol Psychother. 2014;5(1):96–104.
16. Gulliver SB, Pennington ML, Leto F, Cammarata C, Ostiguy W, Zavodny C, et al. In the wake of suicide: developing guidelines for suicide postvention in fire service. Death Stud. 2016;40(2):121–8.
17. Polemikou A, Vantarakis S. Death anxiety and spiritual intelligence as predictors of dissociative posttraumatic stress disorder in Greek first responders: a moderation model. Spiritual Clin Pract. 2019;6(3):182–93.
18. Stein DJ, Koenen KC, Friedman MJ, Hill E, McLaughlin KA, Petukhova M, et al. Dissociation in posttraumatic stress disorder: evidence from the world mental health surveys. Biol Psychiatry. 2013;73(4):302–12.
19. Lanius RA. Trauma-related dissociation and altered states of consciousness: a call for clinical, treatment, and neuroscience research. Eur J Psychotraumatol. 2015;6:1–9.

20. Kaplan JB, Bergman AL, Christopher M, Bowen S, Hunsinger M. Role of resilience in mindfulness training for first responders. Mindfulness. 2017;8(5):1373–80.
21. National Institute of Mental Health. Mental health and mass violence. Evidence based early psychological intervention for victims/survivors of mass violence: a workshop to reach consensus on best practices. Washington, DC: Government Printing Office; 2002. Retrieved from https://www.nimh.nih.gov/index.shtml.
22. James KJ, Gilliland BE. Crisis intervention strategies. 7th ed. Pacific Grove, PA: Brook/Cole; 2013.

Psychological Support in Times of Crisis and Natural Disasters

43

Aikaterini Lampropoulou, Chryse Hatzichristou, and Spyros Tadaros

43.1 Understanding Crisis, Traumatic Events, and Trauma

Crisis, traumatic events, and trauma are often used interchangeably, although they are not quite the same terms. Crisis is defined as a temporary situation of distress and disorganization where the person's current resources and coping mechanisms are insufficient [1]. Crises could include a serious health condition, assault, physical injury, accident, death, suicide, robbery, homicide, or rape. These events affect a person itself and/or his/her family, but there are also events that affect a broader group or groups of people. These include natural disasters (i.e., fire, earthquakes, flood), nuclear accidents, epidemic diseases, war, riots, terrorism, etc. While a crisis can result in negative outcomes, it also may have the potential for quite positive results depending on several factors at a personal, family, or social level [1].

The fifth edition of the American Psychiatric Association's *Diagnostic and Statistical Manual of Mental Disorders (DSM-5)* defines a traumatic event as an event experienced, witnessed, or confronted by a person that involves either actual or threatened death, or serious injury, or a threat to the physical integrity of self or others. There are many developmental, neurobiological, and environmental factors that have an impact on the way a person perceives a difficult event. In order to determine whether a person perceives an event as traumatic or not and to understand the severity of the reactions, his/her unique filter of information processing should be taken into consideration [2].

According to the American Psychological Association, trauma is an emotional response to a very serious event like an accident, rape, or natural disaster. Trauma is evoked when the individual experiences or perceives one or more events or situations as being physically or emotionally harmful or life-threatening and having a

A. Lampropoulou · C. Hatzichristou · S. Tadaros (✉)
National and Kapodistrian University of Athens, Athens, Greece
e-mail: hatzichr@psych.uoa.gr; sgtan@psych.uoa.gr

© Springer Nature Switzerland AG 2021
E. Pikoulis, J. Doucet (eds.), *Emergency Medicine, Trauma and Disaster Management*, Hot Topics in Acute Care Surgery and Trauma,
https://doi.org/10.1007/978-3-030-34116-9_43

lasting adverse effect on everyday life or function and on physical, mental, social, emotional, or spiritual well-being and management capacity [2, 3].

Various types of trauma are identified in the relevant literature with different and distinct characteristics. One of these is the *single incident* trauma which mainly occurs as a result of isolated events. On the other hand, *complex trauma* is usually interpersonal and involves "being or feeling" trapped; it has more severe and persistent consequences which tend to be cumulative [4].

Another type of trauma is the *primary trauma* that refers to the consequences of the direct exposure to a traumatic event, while *secondary* or *vicarious trauma* refers to the emotional and behavioral symptoms that occur as a result of internalizing the trauma experienced by someone else. People at risk for secondary trauma may include friends, family, and acquaintances of the victim, people who have simply heard about the trauma or crisis, and people who help victims, such as paramedics, rescue team members, medical staff, firemen, or emergency responders [5].

Sanctuary trauma refers to the trauma experienced by people who although they expect to be in a protective and supportive environment, they find themselves encountering a hostile environment which causes them greater trauma (e.g., Vietnam War veterans) [6].

The National Institute of Mental Health, USA, defines *childhood trauma* as the experience of an event by a child that is emotionally painful or distressful, which often results in lasting mental and physical effects. If a child perceives the event as threatening, there is an increased possibility that the child will be severely affected. These perceptions are influenced by (a) the type of the event itself, (b) the exposure to the event, (c) relations with the victims, (d) adult responses to trauma, and (e) a variety of individuals/personal vulnerabilities [7].

43.2   Symptoms and Reactions

The consequences of a crisis and natural disaster exposure include emotional, cognitive, behavioral, and physical reactions. Some of the potential symptoms can be (a) *emotional reactions*, i.e., intense emotion and reactivity (intense anxiety, anger, shock), numbness (detachment, denial, disbelief), depression, nightmares, and re-experience of trauma by thoughts and memories which further intensifies a sense of not having control, and (b) *physical reactions*, i.e., aches and pains, trouble sleeping, eating disorders, drug and alcohol abuse, weakness and fatigue, heart palpitations, profuse sweating and chills, susceptibility to illnesses, and easily startled by noises and/or unexpected touch [8].

Post-traumatic stress disorder (PTSD) is a disorder with various psychological and somatic symptoms that appears as a result of a person's exposure (either by experiencing or by witnessing) to a traumatic event. According to *DSM-5*, PTSD is included in a newly developed category called "Trauma- and Stressor-Related Disorders." Diagnostic criteria include one of the following: the person had (a) direct experience of the traumatic event, (b) witnessed the traumatic event in person,

(c) learned that the traumatic event occurred to a person close to him/her, or (d) experienced first-hand repeated or extreme exposure to aversive details of the traumatic event.

Additional criteria for the diagnosis of PTSD include duration of symptoms, consequences, and exclusion of substance abuse or medical conditions. The main types of the symptoms of the disorder according to DSM-5 are living the trauma again and again through uncontrolled and unpleasant memories, flashbacks, and nightmares, apathy, or avoidance of anything that could remind the person of the trauma and increased stimulation (e.g., sleeping and concentrating problems, feeling nervous, and being easily aggravated and distempered). PTSD is a serious disorder since it can have severe impact to a person's functioning at a social, family, and/or professional level. It should be noted that these symptoms may appear years after the event and can affect people at any age [9, 10].

In comparison to adults' symptoms, children's responses have a basic difference; they are mediated through an entity which is not complete but rather still evolving in all levels, and who is usually living within a protective context like the family [11]. There are few studies of the long-term psychological effects of children being exposed to traumatic events. Most findings indicate that girls are more likely to manifest anxiety symptoms after exposure and to subsequently experience increased anxiety and mood symptoms, while boys may manifest more disruption in their behavior [12].

A number of authors have noted that older children are more vulnerable than younger children in relation to the psychological effects of trauma [13]. The younger child's psychological response resonates with the parental response as they have less cognitive capacity to independently evaluate the dangers. However, in general, children's psychological response to trauma is related to parental responses. It should be noted that due to the developmental risks, it is important to identify the children that are considered more vulnerable the soonest possible after a traumatic event [14].

Several symptoms can be noticed in children after crisis exposure, which are usually common for all ages like increased anxiety and/or psychosomatic symptoms. Preschool children may exhibit temper tantrums, insecure attachment, and repeated representation/expression of the traumatic events to which they have been exposed through play or may avoid playing with other peer children. In latency, some of the symptoms include emotional numbness, loss of interest and reduced ability to concentrate in school, reduced school performance, school avoidance, withdrawal, or phobias that something bad will happen. In adolescence, some symptoms may include negative mood, feelings of guilt, shame, helplessness, disruptive behavior, vengeance phantasies, changes in the way of thinking about the world, difficulty in interacting with others, and falling back to past experiences [12, 14].

Some helpful guidelines for caregivers in order to support people who have experienced a crisis or a traumatic event include recognition of personal feelings and understanding that they are a normal reaction to an abnormal situation, talking about the experience but in a person's own time and pace, connecting to others and accepting support, engaging in physical activity, and involving with meaningful and important things [14, 15]. It is also important to provide support without judgment, to listen with understanding and empathy, to respect the others' needs and provide time and space, and to reinforce feeling of safety and focus on taking advantage of the difficult situation for resilience enhancement and growth [16, 17]. Especially for children, it is important to give them time and reassure them that they are safe and to enhance peer activities and focus on building their resilience and copying strategies [18].

43.3 Intervention

The next step after the occurrence of a crisis or a natural disaster is intervention in order to deal with the consequences of the difficult situation. Interventions require needs identification in order to identify specific areas of concern and develop effective practices. These can be implemented at an individual, or system, level (family, schools, community, institutions, organizations). The target groups can include victims, friends, family, people who have heard, and people who have helped. The phases of intervention include (a) *prevention* that can be either enhancing resilience of individuals and systems or developing a model of crisis intervention (a plan) so that schools, communities, and countries can be prepared to act immediately and effectively; (b) *on-site intervention* that involves the immediate actions taken at the actual moment of the event, when it is on its peak; and (c) *post-crisis intervention* that includes all the actions taken to help individuals and systems return to their equilibrium and deal with the consequences of the events after the event [19].

Resilience enhancement is basic for any intervention. Resilience refers to positive adaptation under difficult and adverse circumstances and the ability to recover when dealing with life contingencies [20]. In particular, resilience is defined as "The capacity of individuals to navigate their ways to resources that sustain well-being; The capacity of individuals' physical and social ecologies to provide those resources; and The capacity of individuals and their families and communities to negotiate culturally meaningful ways to share resources" [21, p. 1].

Resilience is a concept usually related to risk and protective factors since any intervention for resilience enhancement should aim at both reducing risk factors and increasing protective factors at individual and system levels. Risk factors are characteristics of individuals and/or systems that are associated with an increase in health risks such as poverty, violence, health problems, substance abuse, etc. Protective factors are characteristics of individuals and systems, associated with a reduction in the vulnerability to adversities such as sense of humor, intelligence, high neighborhood quality, caring relationships, good public health care, access to emergency services, etc. [20, 22].

There is a need to differentiate between crisis and trauma intervention. Crisis intervention offers the prompt and immediate help to people facing the adversity in order to return to stability. It refers to the short-term, immediate, intensive, and brief professional assistance after a traumatic experience. The goal is to help individuals cope and return to a previous level of physical or emotional functioning and establish equilibrium preventing the development of a serious long-term disability [23].

Most people have just temporary difficulties after a traumatic event, and usually they recover and adjust well. Intervention during the initial stages of the event usually aims at providing psychological first aid to people affected, focusing on providing humane, supportive, and practical help. According to the National Child Traumatic Stress Network (https://www.nctsn.org/), psychological first aid is an evidence-informed modular approach for assisting people in the immediate aftermath of disaster and terrorism in order to reduce initial distress and to foster short- and long-term adaptive functioning.

Psychological first aid in cases of natural disasters is also critical for people who are the first to respond and arrive on a scene for immediate help (e.g., rescue workers, police officers, firefighters, humanitarian relief workers, etc.) [24]. A model of psychological first aid has been suggested that focuses on basic domains such as education, peer support, speedy recovery, mental health accessibility, and a continuum of care [15, 25].

In relation to PTSD, specific psychological interventions include the following: psychological debriefing interventions, including critical incident stress debriefing (CISD) and critical incident stress management (CISM), psychological first aid (PFA), trauma-focused cognitive behavioral therapy (CBT), cognitive restructuring therapy, cognitive processing therapy, exposure-based therapies, coping skills therapy (including stress inoculation therapy), psychoeducation, normalization, and eye movement desensitization and reprocessing (EMDR). These therapies are designed to prevent the onset of PTSD and development of trauma-related stress symptoms soon after exposure to a traumatic event [26].

Schools can play a decisive role in supporting children after a crisis. Trauma-informed schools and trauma-informed practices are essential in order to be prepared to deal with the devastating effects of a traumatic event. To that end, several models have been used for training and crisis prevention and intervention in school settings such as (a) the NOVA model of crisis intervention focusing on the provision of immediate emergency consultation crisis intervention services with additional follow-up during a limited period of time; (b) the BASIC Ph Coping Model that stresses six modalities/channels that facilitate coping and resilience, beliefs, affect, social, functioning, imagination, cognition, and physiology, while it places emphasis on the importance of the language an individual uses to tell his/her story [27]; and (c) the PREPaRE model for school-based crisis prevention and intervention that has been developed by the National Association of School Psychologists, USA, and is designed to help schools meet the needs of students, staff, and families having as a primary goal to build crisis management capacity at the local level [1, 28].

A multilevel model for crisis preparedness and intervention has been proposed and developed in the Greek educational system based on a multidimensional conceptual framework and empirical findings at an international and national level [14, 29]. The model consists of several domains including development of a synthetic conceptual framework, education and training, intervention, publications, and collaboration/partnerships. Several evidence-based intervention programs have been developed within the context of the model and implemented in schools after the emergence of several crises and natural disasters in Greece such as earthquakes, wildfire, the economic recession, or the recent refugee crisis [14, 30].

The experience of a crisis, a natural disaster, or a traumatic event can be an overwhelming experience that can affect people indiscriminately and in all ages. Although a significant number of people will experience some kind of symptoms during a short- or long-term period after the incident, most people will remain resilient and manage to recover. There will be, however, a small number of people that will develop mental health difficulties such as PTSD and will require professional assistance. The availability of effective social support and the sensitization of caregivers in order to be able to provide the appropriate support and assist people in need to seek help can play a decisive role for those affected by such events. The development of a crisis preparedness and intervention model is critical for dealing effectively with such events. Such models are vital not only at a community/state level but also at a school level where early interventions, in particular, have the potential to build and enhance people's and systems' resilience and prepare people to deal with situations that are not a matter of "if" but a matter of "when" they will occur.

References

1. Brock S. WS2: PREPaRE: crisis intervention & recovery: the roles of the school-based mental health professional. 2nd ed. Bethesda, MD: National Association of School Psychologists; 2011.
2. Cowan K, Rossen C. Responding to the unthinkable. School Crisis Response and Recovery. 2013;95(4):8–12.
3. Substance Abuse and Mental Health Services Administration: SAMHSA's Concept of trauma and guidance for a trauma-informed approach. HHS Publication No. (SMA). Rockville, MD: Substance Abuse and Mental Health Services Administration; 2014.
4. Cohena J, Mannarino A, Kliethermes M, Murray L. Trauma-focused CBT for youth with complex trauma. Child Abuse Negl. 2012;36(6):528–41.
5. Hydon S, Wong M, Langley AK, Stein BD, Kataoka SH. Preventing secondary traumatic stress in educators. Child and Adolescent Psychiatric Clinics of North America. 2015;24(2):319–33.
6. Bloom S, Farragher B. Restoring sanctuary: A new operating system for trauma-informed systems of care. Oxford: UK: Oxford University Press; 2013.
7. National Association of School Psychologists. Trauma: Brief facts and tips. 2015; Available on line at https://www.nasponline.org/resources-andpublications/resources-and-podcasts/school-climate-safety-and-crisis/mental-health-resources/trauma.
8. Roberts AR. An overview of crisis theory and intervention model. In: Yeager K, Roberts AR, editors. Crisis intervention handbook: assessment, treatment, and research. 4th ed. New York, NY: Oxford University Press; 2015. p. 288–316.
9. American Psychiatric Association (APA). Diagnostic and statistical manual of mental disorders. 5th ed. Washington, DC: American Psychiatric Association; 2013.
10. Pai A, Suris AM, North CS. Posttraumatic Stress Disorder in the *DSM-5*: Controversy, change, and conceptual considerations. Behavioral Sciences. 2017;7(1):7.
11. Essays UK. Children's psychological responses to. Trauma. 2013; Retrieved from . https://www.ukessays.com/essays/psychology/childrens-psychological-responses-1081.php?vref=1

12. Kaplow JB, Layne CM, Pynoos RS, Cohen J, Lieberman A. DSM-V diagnostic criteria for bereavement-related disorders in children and adolescents: developmental considerations. Psychiatry. 2012;75:243–66.
13. De Bellis MD, Zisk A. The biological effects of childhood trauma. Child Adolesc Psychiatr Clin N Am. 2014;23(2):185–222.
14. Hatzichristou C, editor. Διαχείριση κρίσεων στη σχολική κοινότητα [Crisis management in the school community]. Athens: ΤΥΠΩΘΗΤΩ; 2012.
15. Kelly CM, Jorm AF, Kitchener BA. Development of mental health first aid guidelines on how a member of the public can support a person affected by a traumatic event: a Delphi study. BMC Psychiatry. 2010;10:49.
16. Bisson JI, Collings I. Disaster management. In: Guthrie E, Rao S, Temple M, editors. Seminars in liaison psychiatry. London, UK: Royal College of Psychiatrists; 2012. p. 253–64.
17. Harvard Medical School. Anxiety and stress disorders: a guide to managing panic attacks, phobias, PTSD, OCD, social anxiety disorder, and related conditions, Specialhealth report. USA: Harvard Health Publishing; 2018.
18. NASP School Safety and Crisis Response Committee. Recovery from large-scale crises: guidelines for school administrators and crisis teams. Bethesda, MD: National Association of School Psychologists; 2018.
19. Kanel K. A guide to crisis intervention. Stamford, CT: Cengage Learning Solutions; 2015.
20. Masten AA, Barnes A. Resilience in children: developmental perspectives. Children. 2018;5(7):98.
21. Resilience Research Centre. The resilience research centre adult resilience measure (RRC-ARM: research). Canada: School of Social Work, Dalhousie University; 2016.
22. Ungar M. The social ecology of resilience: addressing contextual and cultural ambiguity of a nascent construct. Am J Orthopsychiatry. 2011;81(1):1–17.
23. Lasiuk G, Hegadoren K, Austin W. Trauma- and stress-related disorders, crisis and response to disaster. In: Austin W, Boyd MA, editors. Psychiatric and mental health nursing for Canadian practice. 3rd ed. Philadelphia, PA: Wolters Kluwer; 2015. p. 288–316.
24. Dieltjens T, Moonens I, Praet KV, Buck ED, Vandekerckhove P. A systematic literature search on psychological first aid: lack of evidence to develop guidelines. PLoS One. 2014;9(12):1–13.
25. Castellano C, Plionis E. Comparative analysis of three crisis intervention models applied to law enforcement first responders during 9/11 and Hurricane Katrina. Brief Treat Crisis Interv. 2006;6(4):326–36.
26. Gartlehner G, Forneris C, Brownley K, Gaynes B, Sonis J, Coker-Schwimmer E, Jonas D, Greenblatt A, Wilkins T, Woodell C, Lohr K. Interventions for the prevention of posttraumatic stress disorder (PTSD) in adults after exposure to psychological trauma. AHRQ Comparative Effectiveness Reviews. Report No.: 13-EHC062-EF. Rockville, MD: Agency for Healthcare Research and Quality; 2013.
27. Berger R, Lahad M. A Safe Place: ways in which nature, play and creativity can help children cope with stress and crisis - establishing the kindergartenas a safe haven where children can develop resiliency. Early Child Develop Care. 2009;180(7).
28. Brock SE, Nickerson AB, Reeves MAL, Conolly CN, Jimerson SR, Pesce RC, Lazzaro BR. School crisis prevention and intervention: the PREPaRE model. 2nd ed. Bethesda, MD: National Association of School Psychologists; 2016.
29. Hatzichristou C, Issari P, Lykitsakou K, Lampropoulou A, Dimitropoulou P. The development of a multi-level model for crisis prevention and intervention in the Greek educational system. Sch Psychol Int. 2011;32(5):464–83.
30. Hatzichristou C. Συμβουλευτική στη Σχολική Κοινότητα [Counseling and consultation in the school community]. Athens: Gutenberg; 2014.

Part V

Evaluation, Ethical Issues, Education and Research

Errors of Disaster Health Management: Health Care System Errors, Prehospital and Hospital Emergency Medical Service

44

George Charalambous

44.1 Introduction

Emergency departments (ED) are characterized of a multitude of challenges and constraints that frequently lead to diagnostic errors and serious implications for patient care and safety, mainly due to the large number of patients, variety in pathology, shift work, and distractions [1]. Therefore, EDs are unevenly susceptible to errors, most of which are often preventable.

Especially during disasters, large inflows of patients may lead to increased incidence of medical errors and ultimately to poor patient outcomes. Managing a crisis is an inherently complex task and demanding challenge, even for well-prepared and organized health facilities; thus the systematic implementation of proactive measures can facilitate timely and robust hospital-based reactions [2]. Effective emergency medicine may significantly impact the outcomes of managing complicated and unexpected events. These types of situations, frequently occurring in EDs, call for effective planning on preventing all possibly preventable errors and mitigating the accompanying risks. Timely multisectoral cooperation among all health professions and effective contingency plans, as well as readiness to respond promptly, are critical factors for the provision of qualitative and patient-safe services [3, 4].

The aim of this chapter is to map and conceptualize this error framework and recommend strategies for reducing them, especially in the emergency department.

G. Charalambous (✉)
Emergency Department, Hippocratio General Hospital, Athens, Greece

44.2 Factors Contributing to Avoidable/Potentially Avoidable Errors in an Emergency Department

An annual size of 250,000 deaths per year in the USA occurs due to medical errors [5] mostly due to improper information processing by doctors rather than due to lack of the adequate knowledge or information itself. As noted by the authors of the former study, "… It's critical that we understand how and why these errors happen so that we can start to work to prevent them …."

Even though EDs radically differentiate from the clinical environment of an inpatient ward, doctors tend to succumb to contiguous types of errors to those made in hospitalized patients, mainly attributed to information processing errors, lack of proper verification of the information accumulated, and misjudgment of the impact of a finding that frequently leads to a wrong diagnosis; in fact, patients with abdominal complaints (representing one of the most frequently reported complaints of ED visitors of high diagnostic uncertainty) may be especially prone to those errors.

The first research data focusing on errors in emergency medicine emerged in the international literature in 1999 [6], while, in 2000, a conference in Error in Emergency Medicine sponsored by the Society for Academic Emergency Medicine (SAEM) set the ground for defining, identifying, and measuring the errors in emergency medicine [7]. The vast majority of the previously published studies [8–12] concentrated on highlighting the outcomes of hospitalized patients and, thus, disregarded the portion and types of error attributed to dealing with the patients while visiting and receiving treatment in an ED. According to their findings, substantial rates of preventable errors occurred in the ED which led to permanent disability or death, mainly due to misdiagnosis caused by physicians' training deficits and an extensive patient workload accompanied by restricted time per patient. These suggest that the combination of cognitive errors and poor clinical decisions is critical for patient safety. In fact, figures could have be even higher in the cases of patients discharged from the ED without being hospitalized by integrating systematic feedback mechanisms in order to identify what went wrong. Unfortunately, data from European countries regarding missed diagnosis and diagnostic errors in the ED are scarce, and most of the studies are limited in Anglo-Saxon countries [1].

Factors that increase the possibility of preventable errors occurring in an ED are often associated with the ED's singular operating characteristics, i.e., high diagnostic uncertainty, decision density, acute levels of activity, distractions, abbreviated and interrupted care, time limitations, shift work, lack of information and ground for productive teamwork [6].

In particular, as patients are not known to the ED medical and nursing personnel, substantial gaps in continuity of care are usually observed. Along with the relatively limited time span committed per patient, the patients' medical history is frequently not taken into consideration in its entirety—historical and diagnostic information is rather limited—therefore leading to diagnostic errors and/or missed diagnoses. Also, the large number of decisions that doctors must make during a shift in an ED, the complex cognitive background that the doctor must draw up, and the diagnostic uncertainty that the common patient complaints entail (e.g., weakness, chest or abdominal pain, etc.) demand for effective differential diagnosis seem to cause many cognitive errors and high error prevalence. This decision density and cognitive load are additionally burdened with the extended number of physical, diagnostic, and laboratory tests performed in an ED and the need to act quickly and interpret their findings in precision.

Moreover, ED's constant calling for frequent interruptions and distractions has a negative impact on the clinical decision-making process, while the phenomena of overcrowding, prolonged waiting times, and lack of human and medical resources compromise the diagnostic accuracy. As teamwork spirit constitutes one of the most desirable features for excellent ED performance and can vastly affect the decision-making process, when it is compromised by limited resource availability, the quality of both decision-making and the care provided by the team may ultimately decline.

Finally, shift work and the lack of timely and reliable feedback among emergency department physicians, physicians from other specialties, nurses, and other staff involved in patient care lead to disruption of care and increase the chance of error by impairing physicians' performance and cognitive and diagnostic skills.

44.3   Identification and Measurement of Error Using the Joint Commission Taxonomy

As the exact nature and extent of ED error is relatively complex to be defined [6], it is crucial that errors in emergency medicine and EDs are properly identified, measured, and monitored and also reporting and feedback mechanisms are developed and incorporated in the decision- and policy-making process [13].

One of the most coherent and widely accepted systems for identifying and classifying patient safety events that are potentially related to errors in different healthcare settings is the Joint Commission on Accreditation of Healthcare Organizations (JCAHO) Patient Safety Event Taxonomy [14] (see Fig. 44.1).

The primary elements comprising this taxonomy are the following:

1. *Impact*: The "Impact" element reflects the outcomes of errors that constitute failures and impairments for patient safety issues, by distinguishing between medical (psychological or physical) and nonmedical (legal, social, or economic) effects.
2. *Type*: The "Type" element reflects the processes of what went wrong mainly with regard to communication, patient management, and clinical performance issues.
3. *Domain*: The "Domain" element reflects the setting features when an event of endangering patients' safety occurred, including health professionals and patients' characteristics involved.
4. *Cause*: The "Cause" element reflects the contributing factors to errors and its adverse events by distinguishing between system setbacks (e.g., lack of information, inadequate staffing levels, unsuitable physical environment, organizational omissions, etc.) and human failures referring to issues such as communication problems, patient assessment, continuity of care, etc.

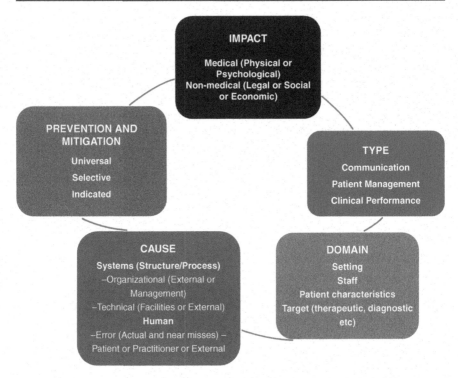

Fig. 44.1 The Joint Commission on Accreditation of Healthcare Organizations (JCAHO) Patient Safety Event Taxonomy. (*Source*: Adjustment by the author, from Chang et al. [14])

5. *Prevention and Mitigation*: The "Prevention and Mitigation" element reflects the suggested strategies to minimize errors and their adverse events by distinguishing between universal, selective, and indicated preventive and reparative measures.

According to the finding of studies conducted based on the classification of the errors as described in the Joint Commission on Accreditation of Healthcare Organizations (JCAHO) Patient Safety Event Taxonomy, the most common areas of emergency care where the highest numbers of errors are often reported are the areas of diagnosis and treatment, administrative procedures and documentation, administration of medication, communication and information processing, and finally the area of environmental characteristics of an ED [14–16]:

• *Diagnosis and treatment* involve types of errors such as omissions of essential procedures, inappropriate or untimely therapeutic interventions, complications of an appropriate treatment, radiologic and laboratory misinterpretations, knowledge deficits, delays in starting correct treatment (due to misinterpretation of clinical signs), "human" failure such as "rule-based" errors, etc.

- *Administrative procedures* involve types of errors such as errors in patient registrations (lost paperwork, misfiled and/or mislabeled patient records, etc.), inappropriate admission/discharge procedures, identification problems due to miscommunication, etc.
- *Administration of medication* involves types of errors such as inappropriate medications and incorrect doses ordered leading to medical reactions, prescriptions carried out incorrectly, incorrect storage of medications, etc.
- *Documentation* involves types of errors such as inappropriate and/or incorrect documentation (inaccurate and/or incomplete charting, documenting in wrong patient's chart, etc.).
- *Communication and information processing* involve types of errors such as inaccurate medical history reporting, inappropriate use of damage control techniques, incomplete/inaccurate information from external departments, miscommunication among ED staff and between ED staff and patients, misidentification of patients, communication errors, etc.
- *Environmental characteristics* involve types of errors such as misplacement of equipment, lacks/shortages of equipment and/or medication because of unavailability, inadequate checking of equipment, malfunctioning equipment (e.g., ventilator malfunction), etc.

However, a significant lower number of errors is reported in the areas of emergency stabilization and triage, while the majority of the reported errors embedded *adverse events of low risk* (e.g., misplaced paperwork, incorrect documentation, etc.), and only a low percentage showcased *adverse events of higher risk* (e.g., incorrect performance of resuscitative procedures and administration of incorrect medication) [13].

44.4 Strategies for Reducing Errors in the Emergency Department

Following the identification and measurement of error in the emergency department, it is crucial that for these errors to be avoided, as much as possible, mitigation strategies should be adjusted in the clinical practice and the working environment of an ED [7, 16].

Simplification, standardization, and establishment of issues of, firstly, safe staff levels; secondly, safe working standard hours; and thirdly, safe timelines for standard procedures should hold high places in the priority procedure agenda. This way, errors will be minimized, and the quality and safety of the provided health services in EDs will be enhanced. For example, the standardization of the framework for administering thrombolytic therapy has resulted in remarkable improvements in diminishing potentially serious or life-threatening implications for patients with heart attack, stroke, and pulmonary embolism [17]. The establishment of standards can set the boundaries for recognizing when potential safety calamities may occur and the processes to deal with them effectively. Time schedules for the proper working and resting times should be safeguarded at least for standard procedures; for example, short-term actions could include standardization of fixed time lapses between shifts and specific turnaround after night shift. Also, information systems can definitely increase safety monitoring and standardization of procedures and facilitate proper information processing in order to minimize errors [7].

Errors in medication prescription and administration represent events of high occurrence in emergency departments. Therefore, a stepwise process for mitigating these errors should be developed so as to face inefficiencies throughout the medication-use process in the ED, including processes for standardizing medication use, use of bar-coding systems, proper education schemes, monitoring and reporting mechanisms, dispensing systems, etc. [18]. Also, since the execution of laboratory and radiology tests explicitly affects the level of quality and the effectiveness of the ED services provided, as they are unquestionably correlated with the diagnosis and the accompanying decision-making process for treating a patient, as well as the smooth workflow of an ED, strategies should focus on the efficient cooperation between the two domains.

Moreover, as interruptions of health professionals in an ED are rather usual, a working balance between minimizing distractions and preserving awareness must be adopted. Also, attention should be paid toward eliminating physical factors that contribute to overworking and job dissatisfaction, while conflict resolution techniques based on multidisciplinary approaches for the staff, patients, and their families should be put in effect in order to achieve effective teamwork among caregivers and decrease certain types of errors that are caused due to miscommunication.

Finally, strong managerial skills and consistency in aims are required from an ED manager and from all the interconnected commanding levels in order to ensure sustainability in systematically reducing preventable errors. A major part toward this accomplishment can be held by targeted training and educational efforts for all medical and nursing personnel, especially customized to meet the needs of effectively safeguarding safety guidelines and protocols.

44.5 Conclusions

Errors in emergency medicine and mainly diagnostic errors and/or missed diagnoses reflect significantly on the quality of services provided in an ED and jeopardize patients' care and safety. Error prevalence, root systemic, and human factors affecting its occurrence and increase must be systematically monitored and measured so as to reduce their impact to the minimum. In order to mitigate the implications of the errors occurring in the EDs, cognitive, behavioral, and organizational issues must be well understood and taken into consideration by all practitioners in an emergency room so as to put in effect preventive and reparative measures in order to eliminate these types of errors.

These strategies presuppose an effective teamwork process among the staff that should be continually reinforced by the establishment of quality assurance guidelines and standard procedures related to the identification, measurement, and monitoring of errors. Educational interventions must be implemented and integrated in the clinical practice, addressing the training needs that all staff involved in the ED present, regarding the importance to tackle the frequency and acuity of the errors that occur in the ED and can be potentially avoided.

Therefore, it is imperative that policy-makers and hospital and emergency department managers proceed to proactive planning so as to effectively respond to complex and unpredictable situations and prevent often avoidable errors that occur at times of crises.

References

1. Moonen PJ, Mercelina L, Boer W, Fret T. Diagnostic error in the Emergency Department: follow up of patients with minor trauma in the outpatient clinic. Scand J Trauma Resusc Emerg Med. 2017;25(1):13.
2. WHO. World Health Organization – Regional Office for Europe. Hospital emergency response checklist. An all-hazards tool for hospital administrators and emergency managers Supported by The European Commission Together for Health. January 2010. https://doi.org/10.13140/2.1.3047.6160.
3. Mohammed Alraga S. An investigation into Disaster Health Management in Saudi Arabia. J Hosp Med Manag. 2017;03(02) https://doi.org/10.4172/2471-9781.100037.
4. Peleg K. Disaster and emergency medicine – a conceptual introduction. Front Public Health. 2013;1 https://doi.org/10.3389/fpubh.2013.00044.
5. De Gruyter. Medical errors in the emergency room: understanding why: 250,000 deaths per year are caused by medical error. ScienceDaily, 28 July 2018. www.sciencedaily.com/releases/2018/07/180728084100.htm.
6. Croskerry P, Sinclair D. Emergency medicine: a practice prone to error? CJEM. 2001;3(04):271–6. https://doi.org/10.1017/s1481803500005765.
7. Vincent C, Simon R, Sutcliffe K, Adams JG, Biros MH, Wears RL. Errors conference executive summary. Acad Emerg Med. 2000;7(11):1180–2. https://doi.org/10.1111/j.1553-2712.2000.tb00461.x.
8. Brennan TA, Leape LL, Laird NM, Hebert L, Localio AR, Lawthers AG, et al. Incidence of adverse events and negligence in hospitalized patients: results of the Harvard Medical Practice Study I. N Engl J Med. 1991;324(6):370–6.
9. Gawande AA, Thomas EJ, Zinner MJ, Brennan TA. The incidence and nature of surgical adverse events in Colorado and Utah in 1992. Surgery. 1999;126(1):66–75.
10. Ogilvie RI, Ruedy J. Adverse drug reactions during hospitalization. Can Med Assoc J. 1967;97(24):1450.
11. Schimmel EM. The hazards of hospitalization. Ann Intern Med. 1964;60(1):100–10.
12. Wilson RM, Runciman WB, Gibberd RW, Harrison BT, Newby L, Hamilton JD. The quality in Australian health care study. Med J Aust. 1995;163(9):458–71.
13. Fordyce J, Blank FS, Pekow P, Smithline HA, Ritter G, Gehlbach S, et al. Errors in a busy emergency department. Ann Emerg Med. 2003;42(3):324–33.
14. Chang A, Schyve Paul M, Croteau Richard J, O'Leary Dennis S, Loeb Jerod M. The JCAHO patient safety event taxonomy: a standardized terminology and classification schema for near misses and adverse events. Int J Qual Health Care. 2005;17(2):95–105. https://doi.org/10.1093/intqhc/mzi021.
15. Montmany S, Pallisera A, Rebasa P, Campos A, Colilles C, Luna A, Navarro S. Preventable deaths and potentially preventable deaths. What are our errors? Injury. 2016;47(3):669–73. https://doi.org/10.1016/j.injury.2015.11.028.

16. Vioque SM, Kim PK, McMaster J, Gallagher J, Allen SR, Holena DN, et al. Classifying errors in preventable and potentially preventable trauma deaths: a 9-year review using the Joint Commission's standardized methodology. Am J Surg. 2014;208(2):187–94. https://doi.org/10.1016/j.amjsurg.2014.02.006.
17. Society for Vascular Surgery, (2018). Thrombolytic therapy. Retrieved from https://vascular.org/patient-resources/vascular-treatments/thrombolytic-therapy.
18. Weant KA, Bailey AM, Baker SN. Strategies for reducing medication errors in the emergency department. Open Access Emerg Med. 2014;6:45.

Current Ethical Dilemmas and Code of Conduct in Disasters

45

Boris E. Sakakushev

In every phase of their development, disaster management strategies are dependent on ethical attitudes and approaches, which arise from complex dilemmas, requiring definite codes of conduct. Exploring appropriate responses to these intriguing challenges, one should be aware of both basic and specific ethics knowledge (Fig. 45.1) to understand the motivation for certain reaction and the mode of action based on relevant ethical principles.

Fig. 45.1 Complex dilemmas requiring specific approaches to disaster management

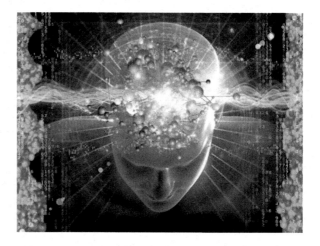

B. E. Sakakushev (✉)
RIMU/Research Institute of Medical University/ Plovdiv, Medical University Plovdiv/ University Hospital St George Plovdiv, Plovdiv, Bulgaria

© Springer Nature Switzerland AG 2021
E. Pikoulis, J. Doucet (eds.), *Emergency Medicine, Trauma and Disaster Management*, Hot Topics in Acute Care Surgery and Trauma,
https://doi.org/10.1007/978-3-030-34116-9_45

45.1   Ethical Principles

Ethical principles applied prior to disaster are prevention measures, good quality healthy environment, education, training and awareness, participation—public input at national and local level—freedom of expression, and access to justice [1]. Ethical principles applied during disasters should be based on humanitarian assistance, information and participation during disasters, compulsory evacuation of populations, respect of dignity and persons, emergency assistance for the most vulnerable persons, measures to safeguard and rehabilitate the environment, strengthening resilience to the effects of disasters, and protection of economic, social, cultural, civil, and political rights [1].

The principles of internal displacement adopted by the United Nations Commission and the General Assembly are aimed to protect all internally displaced persons in internal conflict situations, natural disasters, and other situations of forced displacement.

The principle of impartiality states: "It makes no discrimination based upon nationality, race, religious beliefs, class, or political opinions." The American Red Cross, as a member of the International Red Cross and Red Crescent Movement, adheres to the fundamental principles of the International Red Cross and Red Crescent Movement [2].

Joint responsibility constitutes the shared responsibility between governments, communities, businesses, and individuals. Civil laws must assure nondiscrimination principles of the law, which require equal access for, and prohibit discrimination against, people with disabilities in all aspects of emergency planning, response, and recovery [3].

Solidarity requires "deliberate and freely chosen unity among certain groups or populations." "When referring to health care, solidarity means the obligation to share the financial risks of illness and handicap with others not necessarily of one's own social group."

Currently, ethics is very relevant to society because it includes social responsibility and requires governance. Ethics is important and versatile; it contains basic human values of compassion, empathy, and respect for dignity of others. "Ethics is not about what is – but what should be."

45.2   History of Ethics

Ethical statements date from Ancient Greece: "Do good work consider end use" (Aristotle) and Renaissance: "Evaluate both ends and means" (Kant).

According to Aristotle (384–322) (Fig. 45.2), the moralist states: my life view is superior; other views are inferior; I have the answers; I need no other authority. The ethicist claims: my life view is based on reflection; I evaluate life views; I have questions; I respect others.

Fig. 45.2 Aristotle
(384–322) School
of Athens

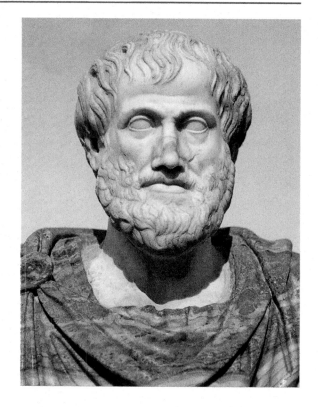

There are many ethical directives for the practice of medicine throughout centuries up to the present time, the oldest one being the oath of Hippocrates [4] (Fig. 45.3).

45.3   General Ethics

Moral philosophy and ethics are defined as "the achievement of wisdom and choosing actions that are beneficial and acceptable in the long term or sustainable" and "determining rights and wrongs, selecting actions to achieve good results, and evaluating motives" [5].

Ethical relativism defining the basic principles and theories of ethics states that morality varies between people and societies according to their cultural norms and universal or objective moral theories, formulating the fundamental principles—substantive and procedural—invariant throughout time and space [6]. The substantive principles are equity and solidarity, individual liberty, privacy, duty to provide care, trust, protection of the public from harm, proportionality, reciprocity, and

Fig. 45.3 Oath of
Hippocrates, fourth BC

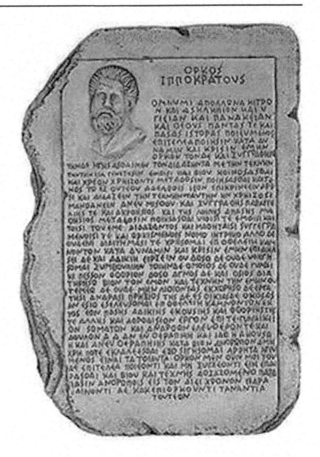

stewardship. The procedural principles are openness, transparency, reasonability, inclusiveness, responsiveness, and accountability [7].

There are four basic forms of ethics: metaethics (what is good?), normative ethics (what should we do?), applied ethics (ethics in work and lives), and descriptive ethics (morals people follow).

Symmetrical ethics claims to do to others what you want them to do to you, as well as if you demand from others, demand from yourself (even more). The idea is to see yourself as the others, or transmitting empathy. Asymmetrical ethics demonstrates domination of a party in resources, knowledge, and power. Compliance of ethics is applied in laws, standards, guidelines, and morals, where the "compliance officer follows a standard," ensuring that the organization "does no wrongs" but is difficult [8]. Positive ethics is when it is contributing positively to the society, organization, profession, or environment. Code of ethics is the application of ethics to a profession or discipline like engineering, medicine, law, journalism, psychology, etc.

There are three aspects of a disaster on man—physical, emotional, and spiritual. The specific mental health stressors are self or family member injury, life threat fear and panic during an event, relocation, peri-traumatic responses, and horror separation from family and property damage or financial loss. Persons with disabilities may experience personal vulnerability as well as protective factors. They may suffer systemic vulnerability or protective factors across environments and ecologies. Disaster response practices intend to diminish risk factors.

45.4 Disaster Preparedness

One of the core concepts of disaster preparedness is to have straightforward plans and protocols that staff are familiar with and can automatically follow [9].

Disaster preparedness depends on money, manpower and materials, evaluation from past experience, location of disaster, communication, information and warning system, coordination and response mechanisms, public education programs, national and international relations, keeping stock of foods and drugs, etc. (Fig. 45.4).

The challenge of disaster preparedness is how we give the best care possible under the worst possible circumstances. Lessons learned from disastrous past incidents could improve preparedness relying on better understanding and expertise [10].

One of the core concepts of disaster preparedness is to have straightforward plans and protocols that staff are familiar with and can automatically follow [9].

Fig. 45.4 Preparing for disaster/crisis standards of care ("CSC")—a piece of the puzzle

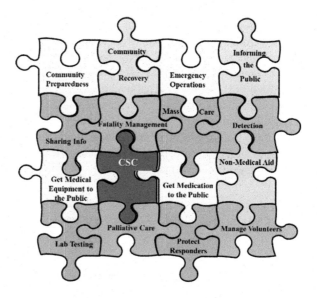

The International Preparedness and Response to Emergencies and Disasters (IPRED) shares insights and lessons learned from diverse types of emergencies and disasters, facilitates educational programs, and shares knowledge on improving emergency preparedness and networking between various parties [11].

Investments in preparedness and prevention (mitigation) will yield sustainable results, rather than spending money on relief after a disaster because most disasters are predictable, especially in their seasonality and the disaster-prone areas, which are vulnerable.

45.5   Disaster Response

Disaster response includes measures taken in anticipation of, during and immediately after, a disaster to ensure that the effects are minimized. The respoce activities include post-disaster safety assessments, rapid safety assessments, detailed safety assessments, other building damage assessments, inspections and other code-related functions in the aftermath of a disaster. Reviewing legal and organizational regulations, developing health-care related guidelines, and disaster recovery plans, establishing on-call ethics committees as well as adequate in-service training of health-care workers for ethical competence are among the most critical steps [12]. This is achieved by implementing the disaster management plan, usually by the rescue team, setting up medical camps and mobilizing resources for epidemiologic surveillance and disease control, and providing adequate shelter and sanitary facilities. Disaster response involves working with different people, performing different procedures, solving different problems, using different resources for routine emergencies, and establishing different priorities for action than for routine emergencies [9].

The cardinal virtues of disaster response are prudence, courage, justice, stewardship, vigilance, self-effacing charity, and communications. Professional ethics is the accepted principles or moral codes that conform to the accepted standards of that profession [13]. People affected by a disaster may not be capable of responding to human rights violations, so it is the first responders who must be cognizant of their responsibility to protect the victims' dignity and rights. Ethical treatment of survivors entails a crucial blend of knowledge about ethnic culture, religious beliefs, and human rights. A strong awareness of ethical principles is merely a beginning step to well-informed decision-making in disaster situations [14].

Fig. 45.5 Prof. Donald Trunkey, MD, 3R rule

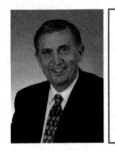

The 3R rule

"Get the Right patient

to the Right place

at the Right time…"

Fig. 45.6 Time intervals
for adequate medical aid

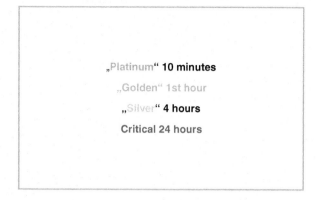

„Platinum" **10 minutes**

„Golden" 1st hour

„Silver" **4 hours**

Critical 24 hours

The disaster ethics in the early response phase are those of non-maleficence, beneficence, justice, and the respect for autonomy. Reaching the disaster site as quickly as possible is the most crucial step, where it is appropriate to generally apply the 3R rule triage principle (Fig. 45.5).

In the early response phase, the triage, as the second most important step, is considered as critical in the distribution of limited medical resources, where the highest priority should be given to the principles of beneficence and justice. The mass casualties approach follows the principle of decision making for saving more lives. It is the "triage" principle, not life support. Disaster triage is the process of allocating treatment and evacuation priorities to patients based on the severity of their injuries [9]. Triage is a form of rationing care delivery. Rationing delivery of care is justified only in situations in which the amount of resources available is less than "adequate" (first and foremost, insufficient to meet the critical requirements) [15]. World Medical Association's statement on medical ethics in the event of disasters says that in selecting the patients, the physician should consider only their medical status and should exclude any other consideration based on nonmedical criteria [16]. Triage and ethics in MCI unite on saving more lives, where selecting and referring only the "red"-coded patients is a rule without exceptions, which has proved its effectiveness through practice and research. Similar triage color-coded approach of timing of response can be generally used (Fig. 45.6). "Public health institutions should act in a timely manner on the information they have within the resources and the mandate given to them by the public" [17].

45.6   Disaster Ethics Management

In disaster medicine management, one must not only follow principles of triage, life support, and on-time emergency treatment, but also go along with ethical issues. Being aware of disaster impact causing versatile negative disaster effects, like deaths, disability, disease, psychological problems, food shortage, socioeconomic losses, and shortage of water, drugs, and medical supplies, one must take fast, but optimal, decisions, working under pressure. Practically, having 20 critically ill victims at open field, one has to "triage" all of them as fast as possible (15–20 s), giving them chance for life. One even may become rude, speak loud, cry to hear you, or obey your orders. Here, ethical issues are not obligatory—one does not select children, pregnant, or disabled. All have the priority of the "red" code. The first one is the closest one. The second is next to him. One cannot afford spending time on observing all the 20 injured.

It is exactly like in surgery teaching and learning—acquiring and implementing knowledge, skills, and attitudes. Discussions on triage decisions with respect to the victim's age, gender, social status, ethnic origin, or profession (e.g., health workers) also conflict with the basic right to live at the individual level and justice principle, in general. "Ideological issues must not eclipse the humanistic priorities embodied in ethical rules" [18].

Ethical approach to allocation of scarce resources and triage should be based on fairness, transparency, consistency, proportionality, accountability, and a duty to attempt to obtain best outcome for the greatest number of patients with available resources—it does not mean to save the most lives, because a comfortable death may be a good outcome [19].

The traditional "trans-vertical" triage advocates with scarce resources to provide the maximum benefit to the population, even if it means that individual victims, who can be saved under other circumstances, are sacrificed for the greater good. The "longitudinal" triage necessitates sacrificing victims now, for the benefit of future victims. In mass casualty medicine, the clinical paradigm is replaced by the rescue paradigm in which it is necessary to save lives and minimize aggregate morbidity [20]. Questions of where consideration for the individual ends and the rights of the majority begin remain valid ones in the face of limited resources [21].

Disaster management concerns ethical dilemmas like the impact of a terror act on decision-making concerning triage of casualties (Fig. 45.7). There the decisions

Fig. 45.7 The 11.09 attack

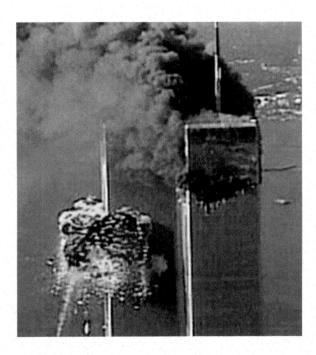

must not discriminate terrorists, although the situation is highly emotional, where attackers and victims are treated simultaneously on-site [22]. Biohazards can be considered in certain circumstances as mass casualty incidents; therefore, exportation of hazards constitutes both ethical and legal issues.

For daily triage decisions, a new model of resource allocation, known as accountability for reasonableness, claims that resource allocation should proceed on the basis of relevant criteria that are public, that decision-making be accountable, and that an appeals process exists in cases of conflict [23]. Health-care organizations can deploy a triage and scarce resource allocation team to oversee and guide ethically challenging clinical decision-making during a crisis period. The goal is to help health-care organizations and clinicians balance public health responsibilities and their duty to individual patients during emergencies in as equitable and humane a manner as possible [24]. To understand whether disaster triage, as currently advocated and practiced in the western world, is actually ethical, we should clarify whether resources truly are limited, whether specific numbers should dictate disaster response, and whether triage decisions should be based on age or social worth [25, 26].

The social contract states: "Government has an obligation, to prepare citizens for survival in second states of nature caused by disaster. Such preparation requires implementation through public policy" (John Locke). These rights are presumed in the US Declaration of Independence and protected by the first ten amendments of the constitution [27].

Local, national, and global documents which can be related to ethics envisage the current paradigms of ethics in disaster management [28].

45.7 Ethical Codes of Conduct in Disasters

Professional codes of ethics act as follows: "Professions governed by Codes of Ethics approved by their members are functioning on the assumption that these codes will not be violated in practice" [27]. Ethical dilemmas and codes of conduct include announcing bad news under pressure to patient (if conscious), to relatives, friends, and media (Fig. 45.8).

Fig. 45.8 Announcing bad news to relatives

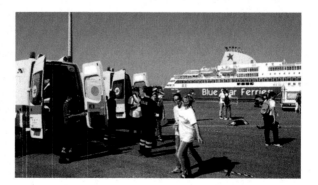

The code of conduct for International Red Cross and Red Crescent Movement and NGOs in disaster relief was drawn up in 1992 by the Steering Committee for Humanitarian Response (SCHR) to set ethical standards for organizations involved in humanitarian work [29]. In 1994, the SCHR adopted the code and made the signing of it a condition for membership in the alliance.

Disasters vary considerably with respect to their time, place, and extent; therefore, ethical questions may not always have "one-size-fits-all" answers. On the other hand, embedding ethical values and principles in every aspect of health care is of vital importance. Reviewing legal and organizational regulations, developing health-care-related guidelines and disaster recovery plans, and establishing on-call ethics committees, as well as adequate in-service training of health-care workers for ethical competence, are among the most critical steps. It is only by making efforts before disasters, that ethical challenges can be minimized in disaster responses [30]. The Japan disaster mental health guidelines provide a comprehensive description on what to do and say in times of disaster. With dissemination and use of guidelines, local mental health systems can be improved and will be better prepared ahead of future disasters [31].

Quality assurance of emergency response teams should be based on specified standards, which will methodologically improve the successful response to different types of emergency scenarios, regardless of their variable components [32]. Defining specified standards prior to the emergency response will methodologically enable improvement of the successful response to different types of emergency scenarios, regardless of their variable components [32, 33]. The standard of care is a case- and time-specific analytical process in medical decision-making, reflecting a clinical benchmark of acceptable quality medical care [34].

The Delphi technique can be used for reaching consensus of data, comprising process, structure, and outcome indicators, identified as essential for recording indicators essential for data reporting from the response of major incidents, and can serve as a base for a generally acceptable national register [35].

Responsible for ethical information in disasters are the local emergency management command centers, including police, fire, EMS, public health agencies and departments, bioethics committees, physician, and nursing education teams. The leader in MCI acting under pressure must address the team in brief, precise, encouraging, positive, and definite manner. The complexity of acquiring informed consent while conducting studies in disaster medicine should be widely reviewed and weighed in light of the importance for expanding the science of disaster management [36].

The code of professional ethics for rehabilitation counselors includes primary responsibility, proper diagnosis of mental disorders, and respect for confidentiality and adaptation to work environment. They should maintain roles and relationships, appropriate termination, referral and transfer of services based on competences like preparation and response, cultural diversity, advocacy and accessibility, scientific basis for intervention, technique/procedure/modality skills, and finally—yet importantly—monitor effectiveness. Strategies to maximize care concerning space are putting patient beds in hallways, conference rooms and tents. Using operating rooms only for urgent cases; supplying/sterilizing and reusing disposable equipment;

limiting drugs/vaccines/ventilators to patients are other activities needed. Other recource dependent intiatives include prioritizing comfort care for patients who will die (and staff), having nurses provide some care that doctors usually would provide, and having family members help with feeding and other basic patient tasks.

In the rehabilitation phase, one must act in accordance with the main problems and needs—water supply, food safety, basic sanitation and personal hygiene, as well as vector control.

Recovering from disaster activities to support emergency-affected areas in reconstruction of the physical infrastructure and restoration of economic and emotional well-being is performed.

45.8   Education and Training in Disaster Ethics

Education and training are especially important in understanding, implementing, and disseminating of knowledge and skills in disaster medicine ethics (Figs. 45.9 and 45.10) [37].

Fig. 45.9 Disaster conferences and congresses

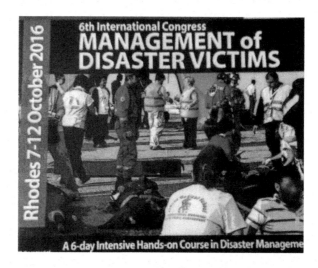

Fig. 45.10 Disaster simulation exercises

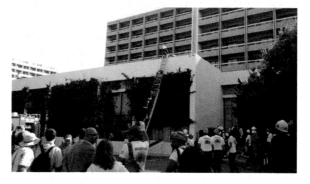

45.9 Research in Disaster Ethics

The future direction in meeting goals in legislation and recommendations is developing ethical guidelines. These require legislative task force, state committee, ethics board, studies, and regulations with resolutions and considerations. The considerations for developing ethical guidelines comprise of resource owner; recognizable voice; big city and budget disaster allocation; public and research activities like discussions, presentations, and conferences; ethics research and analysis center; and state agencies.

In light of the importance for expanding the science of disaster management, the complexity of acquiring informed consent while conducting studies in the realm of disaster medicine should be widely reviewed and weighed [36].

Research ethics should take the format of an iterative evolving and constructive learning process, with a time of reflection and critical debate [38]. Potential need for nonstandard ethics review procedures for MCI settings is to ensure appropriate dissemination of disaster research results among researchers, to share information, and to develop projects to evaluate how well the ethical issues are addressed in the research. Particular attention should be given to assessing participants' perceptions of how ethics is addressed in specific projects [39].

Guidelines on research in disaster must balance the need for scientific evidence and the need to protect research subjects from possible harm from the research itself. Some guidelines emphasized the strong ethical mandate to do research in disaster settings "to prevent further death and illness in present or future disasters" [40], with some suggesting it might be unethical not to do such research [41].

Guidelines do not provide specific methods for evaluating risks and benefits [39]. One possible approach was applying the minimal risk requirement suggested in three guidelines: for research in refugee populations [42] and in clinical research [43]. Justice in selection of participants means "making political and ethical choices about which voices are heard and whose knowledge counts" [44].

Research participants should be chosen on scientific reasons and not on any other reason, like accessibility, cost, gender, or malleability [43]. Ethics in disaster medicine should be based on evidence (Fig. 45.11) [44].

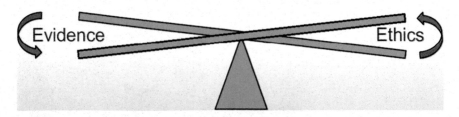

Fig. 45.11 The dual imperative in disaster research ethics [44]

The benchmarks of ethical research stand on eight pillars [45–47]:

1. Collaborative partnership
2. Social value
3. Scientific validity
4. Fair selection of study population
5. Favorable risk-benefit ratio
6. Independent review
7. Informed consent
8. Respect for recruited participants and study communities [45–47].

45.10 Future

The future objectives before ethics in disaster medicine are encourage and consolidate knowledge networks; mobilize and train disaster volunteers—army, police firemen, scouts and guides, civil defense, and guards—and build capacity and learn from best practices.

The future directions are:

- Anticipatory governance—simulation exercises and scenario analysis
- Knowledge systems and coping practices
- Living with risk—community-based disaster risk management
- Inclusive, participatory, gender-sensitive, child-friendly, eco-friendly, and disabled-friendly disaster management
- Technology-driven but people owned
- Knowledge management—documentation and dissemination of good practices
- Public-private partnership

What to expect? Dr. Simon Day of the University College London and Dr. Steven Ward from the University of California predict that the Cumbre Vieja volcano on the Canary Islands will erupt and create the largest tsunami in recorded history (Fig. 45.12). Pete Riley, a scientist at Predictive Science, after analyzing solar storm records from the past 50 years, concluded that there is a 12% chance of a major solar storm hitting Earth in the next 10 years (Fig. 45.13).

Policy makers have important evidence-based data to be used in making crucial decisions regarding allocation of health funds in trauma systems, which have shown to be fundamental in determining injury outcomes in severe and critical traffic casualties. Thus, the crucial role of the trauma system needs to be better acknowledged and funded appropriately [48]. The tragic terrorist attacks seen worldwide have proven that no one is immune from terror. Trauma and disaster management training should be a must in medical students' curriculum to provide them skills with an emphasis on practical training and assessment in this field [49].

Fig. 45.12 Largest
tsunami ever,
Caribbean, unknown

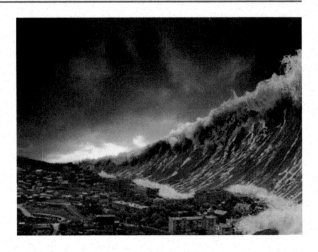

Fig. 45.13 Major solar
storm, 2015–2025

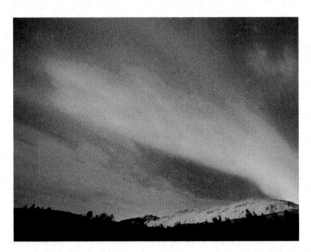

In managing ethics in disasters, specific knowledge, skills, training, and teamwork are necessary to face the ethical dilemmas and implement the appropriate
codes of conduct alongside with some simple moral human concerns like honesty,
sincerity, sympathy, and trust.

"In nothing do men more nearly approach the gods than in giving health to men"
(Cicero) (Fig. 45.14).

Fig. 45.14 Cicero

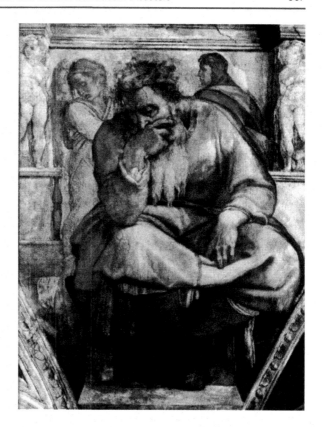

References

1. Prieur M. Ethical principles on disaster risk reduction and people's resilience. European and Mediterranean Major Hazards Agreement (EUR-OPA). 2012. http://www.coe.int/t/dg4/majorhazards/ressources/pub/Ethical-Principles-Publication_EN.pdf.
2. Steering Committee for Humanitarian Response. http://en.wikipedia.org/wiki/.
3. FEMA. http://www.fema.gov/iv-non-dscrimination-principles-law/.
4. Edelstein L. The Hippocratic oath: text, translation, and interpretation. Baltimore: Johns Hopkins Press; 1943.
5. Sternberg J, editor. Wisdom: its nature, origins, and development. Cambridge: Cambridge University Press; 2003. ISBN-10: 0521367182.
6. Etkin D, Davis I. The search for principles of disaster management. Working draft paper, May 30, 2007, 28 pages. Forms of ethics.
7. Ross U, et al.. Stand on guard for thee ethical considerations in preparedness planning for pandemic influenza. A report of the University of Toronto Joint Centre for Bioethics Pandemic Influenza Working Group. 2005.
8. The Ethics & Compliance Officer Association (ECOA). December 2010. www.theecoa.org.
9. Wong D. Managing mass casualty events is just the application of normal activity on a grander scale for the emergency health services. Or is it? J Emerg Prim Health Care. 2011;9(1):990448.

10. Jahangiri K, et al. Pattern and nature of Neyshabur train explosion blast injuries. World J Emerg Surg. 2018;13:3. https://doi.org/10.1186/s13017-018-0164-7.
11. Adini B, Ohana A, Furman E, Ringel R, Golan Y, Fleshler E, Keren U, Reisner S. Learning lessons in emergency management: the 4th international conference on healthcare system preparedness and response to emergencies and disasters. Disaster Mil Med. 2016;2(1)
12. Karadag C, Hakan A. Ethical dilemmas in disaster medicine. Iran Red Crescent Med J. 2012;14(10):1–11.
13. Karadag C, Hakan K. Ethical dilemmas in disaster medicine. Iran Red Crescent Med J. 2012;14(10):602–12.
14. Varghese S. Cultural, ethical, and spiritual implications of natural disasters from the survivors' perspective. Crit Care Nurs Clin North Am. 2010;22(4):515–22.
15. Domres B, Koch M, Manger A, Becker H. Ethics and triage. Prehosp Disast Med. 2001;16(1):53–8.
16. World Medical Association. Statement on medical ethics in the event of disasters. Updated version. WMA General Assembly, South Africa. 2006. http://www.wma.net/en/30publications/10policies/d7/index.html/.
17. Principles of the ethical practice of public health, version 2.2 © 2002 Public Health Leadership Society.
18. Halpern P, Larkin G. Ethical issues in the provision of emergency medical care in multiple casualty incidents and disasters. In: Ciottone G, editor. Disaster medicine. 3rd ed. Philadelphia: Elsevier Mosby; 2006.
19. Statement on Disaster and Mass Casualty Management. The following statement was developed by the College's Ad Hoc Committee on Disaster and Mass Casualty Management of the Committee on Trauma, and was approved by the Board of Regents at its June 2003 meeting.
20. Singh S. Book review of "The Ethics of Coercion in Mass Casualty Medicine" by Griffin Trotter MD, PhD. Philos Ethics Humanit Med. 2007;2(1):20.
21. Hawryluck L. Ethics review: position papers and policies – are they really helpful to front-line ICU teams? Crit Care. 2006;10(6):242.
22. Edwards D, McMene L, Stapley S, Patel H, Clasper J. 40 years of terrorist bombings-a meta-analysis of the casualty and injury profile. Injury. 2016;47:646–52.
23. Daniels N, Sabin J. Setting limits fairly: can we learn to share medical resources? Oxford: Oxford University Press; 2002.
24. Kuschner W, Pollard J, Ezeji-Okoye S. Ethical triage and scarce resource allocation during public health emergencies: tenets and procedures. Hosp Top. 2007;85(3):16–25.
25. Sztajnkrycer M, Madsen B, Alejandro Báez A. Unstable ethical plateaus and disaster triage. Emerg Med Clin North Am. 2006;24(3):749–68.
26. Holt G. Making difficult ethical decisions in patient care during natural disasters and other mass casualty events. Otolaryngol Head Neck Surg. 2008;139(2):181–6.
27. Zack N. Ethics for disaster, series: studies in social, political, and legal philosophy. Lanham: Maryland Rowman & Littlefield Publishers; 2009.
28. Health Disaster Management: Guidelines for evaluation and research in the "Utstein Style". Chapter 8: Ethical issues. Prehosp Disast Med. 2002;17(Suppl 3):128–43.
29. American College of Medical Quality, policy 3. http://www.acmq.org/policies/policies3and4.pdf/.
30. Suzuki Y, Fukasawa M, Nakajima S, Narisawa T, Kim Y. Development of disaster mental health guidelines through the Delphi process in Japan. Int J Ment Heal Syst. 2012;6(1):7.
31. Rådestad M, Jirwe M, Castrén M, Svensson L, Gryth D, Rüter A. Essential key indicators for disaster medical response suggested to be included in a national uniform protocol for documentation of major incidents: a Delphi study. Scand J Trauma Resusc Emerg Med. 2013;21(1):68.
32. Leaning J, Guha-Sapir D. Natural disasters, armed conflict, and public health. N Engl J Med. 2013;369:1836–42.
33. Gardemann J, Wilp T. The Humanitarian Charter and minimum standards in humanitarian response are applicable in German refugee facilities. Bundesgesundheitsblatt, Gesundheitsforschung, Gesundheitsschutz. 2016;59(5):556–60.

34. Geale SK. The ethics of disaster management. Disaster Prev Manag. 2012;21(4):445–62.
35. Hick J, Hanfling D, Cantrill S. Allocating scarce resources in disasters: emergency department principles. Ann Emerg Med. 2012;59(3):177–87.
36. Frith L, Appleton R, Iyer A, Messahel S, Hickey H, Gamble C. Doing challenging research studies in a patient-centred way: a qualitative study to inform a randomized controlled trial in the paediatric emergency care setting. BMJ Open. 2014;4:e0050.
37. Tambo E. Non-conventional humanitarian interventions on Ebola outbreak crisis in West Africa: health, ethics and legal implications. Infect Dis Poverty. 2014;3(1):42.
38. Schopper D, Dawson A, Upshur R, Ahmad A, Jesani A, Ravinetto R, Segelid M, Sheel S, Singh J. Innovations in research ethics governance in humanitarian settings. BMC Med Ethics. 2015;16:10.
39. Mezinska S, Kakuk P, Mijaljica G, Waligóra M, O'Mathúna D. Research in disaster settings: a systematic qualitative review of ethical guidelines. BMC Med Ethics. 2016;17(1)
40. Jennings B, Arras J. Ethical guidance for public health emergency preparedness and response: highlighting ethics and values in a vital public health service. Ctr Dis Control Prev. 2008;
41. Indian Council of Medical Research. ICMR's ethical guidelines for biomedical research on human participants. 2006. http://icmr.nic.in/ethical_guidelines.
42. Leaning J. Ethics of research in refugee populations. Lancet. 2001;357(9266):1432–3.
43. Sumathipala A, Jafarey A, De Castro L, Ahmad A, Marcer D. Ethical issues in post-disaster clinical interventions and research: a developing world perspective. Key findings from a drafting and consensus generation meeting of the Working Group on Disaster Research and Ethics (WGDRE) 2007. Asian Bioeth Rev. 2010;2:124–42.
44. O'Mathúna DP. The dual imperative in disaster research ethics. In: Iphofen R, Tolich M, editors. SAGE handbook of qualitative research ethics. London: SAGE; 2018.
45. Emanuel E, Wendler D, Grady C. What makes clinical research ethical in developing countries? The benchmarks of ethical research. J Infect Dis. 2004;189(5):930–7.
46. O'Mathuna DP. Research ethics in the context of humanitarian emergencies. J Evid Based Med. 2015;8(1):31–5.
47. WADEM Webinar: O'Mathъna DP. Disaster research ethics: developing evidence ethically. 2017. https://wadem.org/resources/webinar/.
48. Goldman S, Siman-Tov M, Bahouth H, et al. The contribution of the Israeli trauma system to the survival of road traffic casualties. Traffic Inj Prev. 2015;16(4):368–73. https://doi.org/1 0.1080/15389588.2014.940458.
49. Rivkind A, Faroja M, Mintz Y. Combating terror: a new paradigm in student trauma education. J Trauma Acute Care Surg. 2015;78(2):415–21.

The Importance of Education and Training in Disaster Management: An Overview

46

46.1 Introduction

46.1.1 Disaster Management and Emergency Medicine: Requirements

Advancements in technology and industrialization increase the rate of natural and man-made disasters [1]. The international disaster database reports in 2017 globally 318 disasters, 136 in Asia, 93 in Americas, 42 in Africa, 39 in Europe, and 8 in Oceania with 9503 deaths altogether (see Table 46.1). This number was much lower if compared to the average 68,302 deaths per year from 2007 to 2016. The majority of human losses in 2017 was due to weather-related disasters especially by floods [2].

Table 46.1 shows a classification of disasters, as published by Huntington.

Education in preparedness of an emergency event has to involve knowing the contact persons and institutions in a disastrous event. The hierarchy often is complex, since many people are involved with different designated duties. The department staff should know about the triage process, basic incident command system, isolation, and personal protective equipment application [4].

46.1.2 Staff and Stakeholders Involved in Emergency Medicine and Disaster Management

When considering the staff, which is involved in emergency medicine and disaster management, the administrative staff, the medical doctors, as well as the nurses

A. Exadaktylos (✉)
Department of Emergency Medicine, Inselspital, Bern University Hospital, University of Bern, Bern, Switzerland
e-mail: Aristomenis.Exadaktylos@insel.ch

© Springer Nature Switzerland AG 2021
E. Pikoulis, J. Doucet (eds.), *Emergency Medicine, Trauma and Disaster Management*, Hot Topics in Acute Care Surgery and Trauma,
https://doi.org/10.1007/978-3-030-34116-9_46

Table 46.1 Type of disasters from Huntington and Gavagan [3]

Natural	Accidents	Intentional acts of violence
Meteorological (e.g., hurricane, blizzard, heat/cold wave)	Transportation (e.g., airplane, bus, train)	Bombing
Geological (e.g., earthquake, volcanic eruption, flood)	Structural (e.g., building or bridge collapse)	Shooting
Other (e.g., fire, explosion, disease outbreak)	Nuclear (e.g., radioactive waste release, meltdown)	Nuclear/radiological (e.g., fissile bomb, "dirty" bomb, or other types of radiological poisoning)
	Agricultural or industrial (e.g., hazardous chemical or biological spill or other exposure, fire, explosion)	Biological agent: • Bacteria (e.g., anthrax, cholera, plague, tularemia Q fever) • Virus (e.g., smallpox, Venezuelan equine encephalitis, viral hemorrhagic fevers) • Toxin (e.g., botulinum, staphylococcal enterotoxin B)
		Chemical agent: • Nerve agent (e.g., sarin, insecticides, pesticides) • Blister agent (e.g., lewisite, mustard) • Precursors (e.g., chlorosoman, chlorosarin) • Choking agents (e.g., phosgene, chlorine) • Blood agents (e.g., hydrogen cyanide, cyanogen chloride) • Riot control agents (e.g., tearing agents, vomiting agents)

should be taken into account [5] they have to work together and should be aware of the disaster plan, their roles, and the needed actions.

46.1.3 Recommendations for Interdisciplinary and Interprofessional Training

Several countries have emergency guidelines and plans in place. The curriculum guideline for physicians of the American Academy of Family Physicians covers, for example, the medical knowledge, patient care, and systems-based practice areas [3] (see Table 46.2).

The WHO [6] states that in situations of humanitarian crisis and conflict, a well-planned emergency response is essential. In order for health workers to able to coordinate the delivery of care when emergency situations arise, they need an interprofessional education. This leads to the mobilization of resources and secures that expertise within the health system, and broader community is available. The

Table 46.2 Example of the curriculum recommendation of the American Academy of Family Physicians for the United States; from Huntington and Gavagan [3]

Medical knowledge	Patient care	Systems-based practice
A basic understanding of the primary importance of safety in disaster responses, including personal protective equipment, decontamination, and site security	An understanding of the principles of triage and the ability to effectively perform triage in a disaster setting	A basic knowledge of the National Incident Management System (NIMS) and the Incident Command System (ICS), including its application to the planning, coordination, and execution of disaster responses
	The clinical competence to provide effective care in a setting of extremely limited resources	An understanding of psychological first aid and earing for responders

same is valid for epidemics and pandemics, where individuals who are used to work in a collaborative practice team can enhance a region's capacity to respond to such security issues. The WHO also states that in the event of a global epidemic or natural disaster, this collaboration is the only way to manage the crisis [6].

46.2   Methods: Search Strategy for Publications

Open-access references which dealt with educational needs for stakeholders and doctors in emergency medicine and disaster were searched for in PubMed and Google Scholar. Keywords were disaster medicine, emergency medicine, education, training, effectiveness of outcome, and a combination of those words. Only open-access references were chosen due to cost reasons and since the target audience is based on emerging countries.

46.3   Results: Overview on Studies Measuring Training Effectiveness on the Outcome During Disaster

There are only little studies available showing the training effect of staff on disaster outcome. Most studies deal with training needs to be prepared for disaster. Most of the studies are also not open-access publications; hence, the base of this article is quite limited.

In 2006, Bartley et al. conducted a survey of senior medical, nursing, and administrative staffs that were felt to be likely put into a position of responsibility during a disastrous event in Australia [5]. The survey asked whether the facility had a plan for a disastrous event, if the organization had decontamination equipment, and if the staff was prepared to decontaminate patients. It also had questions if they knew where to assemble in the case of a disaster and if the participants of the study felt that they were personally prepared for a disastrous event in their organization. Thirty-two percent of the respondents answered that they were not personally prepared for a disastrous event [5]. Seventy-five percent of the respondents even said that their organization—170 hospitals— was not prepared.

Medical directors and department chairs of 135 academic emergency medicine departments of the United States took part in a survey asking for command and control, the development of a written plan (which included surveillance and detection), triage and patient flow, personnel, supplies and infrastructure, and communications. The conclusion of the study is that there are significant deficits in preparedness for pandemic influenza and other disease outbreaks, which appear to be related in part to the size of the emergency departments. Bigger departments seemed to be better prepared [7].

Also a recent study in Italy found a poor knowledge base of basic hospital disaster planning concepts by Italian emergency department physicians-on-duty. The authors come to the conclusion that authorities should enhance staff disaster preparedness education, training, and follow-up. This shall ensure that disaster plans are known to all who have the responsibility for disaster risk reduction and management capacity [8].

In 2018, van Loenhout et al. summarized priorities for hospitals in zones at high risk of tropical cyclones. They found that the accessibility to the hospital has to be guaranteed, that the capacity for urgent obstetric needs should be foreseen in countries where fertility is high and should be taken into account during a disaster, that the most common diseases after the cyclone Haiyan were gastroenteritis and pneumonia, and that hospitals should be prepared to treat large numbers of patients with these diseases and incorporate this into their disaster plans. Also a higher risk of admission by children and elderly should be taken considerably [9].

Orach et al. [10] assessed in Uganda the district disaster team's performance, roles, and experiences following a training. They found that the most frequently applied capabilities for the management of disasters were provision of emergency healthcare services and response management. After the training, the following skills should be perceived: response to epidemics, disaster management planning, hazards and vulnerability analysis, and principles of disaster planning. The activities most frequently implemented following disaster management teams training were conducting planning meetings for disasters, refinement of plans, and dissemination of skills gained. The district teams found the main challenges in inadequacy of finance and logistics as well as lack of commitment by key partners toward disaster preparedness and response [10].

In Canada, undergraduate students from emergency medicine-related programs followed an 8-week online course, which was highly interactive including videos, a discussion forum, an online board game, and the opportunity to participate in a high-fidelity disaster simulation with professional staff. The learning aim was to gain interprofessional competency. A study performed with those students indicates that the course supported the participants in getting knowledge of disaster management content and also enhanced awareness of the interdisciplinary team [11].

46.4   Discussion

46.4.1 Current Situation

Preparedness for disasters means to ensure that the resources, necessary for responding effectively in the event of a disaster, arc in place. The staff involved in the disaster has to know how to use those resources. This includes the planning processes and implementing disaster plans, stocking resources necessary for effective response in case of disaster, and ensuring that the staff has the right skills and competencies for effective performance of disaster-related tasks. This also includes safety trainings when a disaster occurs, such as training on protective actions during earthquake or flood, toxic and hazardous materials spill, or terrorist attacks. It also should enable to take protective actions for property, disaster damage and disruption and the ability to engage in post-disaster restoration and early recovery activities [12]. Most of the participants in the abovementioned studies felt unprepared for such situations, and they also thought that their whole organization was unprepared.

46.4.2 Desired Improvements

There is a lack of knowledge in regard to response to disaster situations, which leads to an inefficiency of the system and chaos once an emergency situation occurs [1]. The WHO recommends putting programs in place which contain interprofessional education so that the systems can work more efficiently [6]. It provides health workers with the kind of skills which are needed for the coordination of care delivery in emergency situations [6].

Seyedin et al. conclude that more workshops, annual training courses, and maneuvers which are based on the evaluated needs can help to be better prepared for disaster. Also a continuous education curriculum for nurses should be taken into place with fields as bioterrorism agents, use of personal protective equipment, epidemiological and psychological first aid, disaster management processes, mass causalities management, and command systems. Moreover, a formal curriculum in mass casualty and disaster management for improvement of knowledge and skills in all nurses was found to be important [1]. The curriculum could follow a blended learning approach, with learning by highly interactive online trainings, classroom trainings given by experienced senior staff, and also learning in simulated emergency situations and disasters. This can be enhanced by international exchange of emergency staff during disaster.

Also training plans need to be on the one hand individualized on the regions according to the main kind of disaster which can occur and the expected diseases caused by the disaster as well as on the administrative structure in case of an emergency event, and on the other hand, there also have to be internationally harmonized plans in place covering medical knowledge, patient care, and systems-based practice. Also unexpected disaster should be covered.

The administrative structure as well as the steps to follow in case of a disaster easily could be trained and evaluated by online courses, which could be part of a yearly curriculum. Also theoretical medical knowledge and safety instruction can be part of an online curriculum with regular repetitions, followed by simulated practice situations.

Trainings have to be reinforced for the whole staff on a regular basis in order that everyone knows what to do and with which kind of patients and challenges to deal with in case of an emergency.

However, Huntington et al. [3] reviewed the literature on evidence for training effectiveness in family medicine on the following competencies: general disaster medicine, training on standards of the National Incident Management System of the United States (NIMS/ICS), safety training, triage training, training for clinical competence, and psychological first aid training. They found limited evidence due also to the lack of studies.

46.5 Conclusions for Educational Needs and Trainings

The abovementioned studies come to the conclusion that especially trainings on communication and interprofessional trainings on collaborative competences have to be further established in order to avoid chaos once a disaster occurs. Interdisciplinary training and training on the structures during a disaster are key. Interprofessional training leads to a better understanding of each team member's duties. Online courses and computer simulations as well as classroom training can help to enhance the capability and the mutual understanding of the different stakeholders.

Also a harmonization of current recommendations into global guidelines could help to have globally prepared staff which can act in every country in case of emergency, regardless of where the education took place.

References

1. Seyedin H, Abbasi Dolatabadi Z, Rajabifard F. Emergency nurses' requirements for disaster preparedness. Trauma Mon. 2015;20(4):e29033. https://doi.org/10.5812/traumamon.29033.
2. EM-DAT. (2018). The international disaster database. Retrieved from https://www.emdat.be/index.php.
3. Huntington MK, Gavagan TF. Disaster medicine training in family medicine: a review of the evidence. Fam Med. 2011;43(1):13–20.
4. Garbutt SJ, Peltier JW, Fitzpatrick JJ. Evaluation of an instrument to measure nurses' familiarity with emergency preparedness. Mil Med. 2008;173(11):1073–7.
5. Bartley BH, Stella JB, Walsh LD. What a disaster?! Assessing utility of simulated disaster exercise and educational process for improving hospital preparedness. Prehosp Disaster Med. 2006;21(4):249–55.
6. WHO. Framework for action on interprofessional education & collaborative practice. 2010. WHO (2010) WHO/HRH/HPN/10.3.

7. Morton MJ, Kirsch TD, Rothman RE, Byerly MM, Hsieh YH, McManus JG, Kelen GD. Pandemic influenza and major disease outbreak preparedness in US emergency departments: a survey of medical directors and department chairs. Am J Disaster Med. 2009;4(4):199–206.

8. Paganini M, Borrelli F, Cattani J, Ragazzoni L, Djalali A, Carenzo L, et al. Assessment of disaster preparedness among emergency departments in Italian hospitals: a cautious warning for disaster risk reduction and management capacity. Scand J Trauma Resusc Emerg Med. 2016;24(1):101. https://doi.org/10.1186/s13049-016-0292-6.

9. van Loenhout JAF, Gil Cuesta J, Abello JE, Isiderio JM, de Lara-Banquesio ML, Guha-Sapir D. The impact of Typhoon Haiyan on admissions in two hospitals in Eastern Visayas, Philippines. PLoS One. 2018;13(1):e0191516. https://doi.org/10.1371/journal.pone.0191516.

10. Orach CG, Mayega RW, Woboya V, William B. Performance of district disaster management teams after undergoing an operational level planners' training in Uganda. East Afr J Public Health. 2013;10(2):459–68.

11. Atack L, Parker K, Rocchi M, Maher J, Dryden T. The impact of an online interprofessional course in disaster management competency and attitude towards interprofessional learning. J Interprof Care. 2009;23(6):586–98. https://doi.org/10.3109/13561820902886238.

12. Tang R. Evaluation of hospital preparedness for public health emergencies in Sichuan (China). Brisbane: Bachelor of Public Health, Queensland University of Technology; 2015.

The Value of Training: Debriefing

47

Monika Brodmann Maeder

47.1 Introduction

Education in disaster management plays a crucial role in disaster preparedness. The goal of all efforts is to overcome the consequences of natural and man-made disasters worldwide [1]. As the management of disasters or mass casualties involves many different professionals and agencies, it is important to define tasks and responsibilities of the involved team members and to find good educational methods in order to improve their collaboration. In the last decades, the international community has taken large efforts to define core competencies in disaster management [2, 3]. Today, many national and international programs in disaster management exist [4]. The curricula cover all aspects of disaster management and are either integrated in universities or high schools with mostly achieving master levels or certificates in European countries [4]. The Association of American Medical Colleges defined disaster medicine as the core content of their curricula, but it is not regularly implemented [5]. Many examples of integrating education in disaster preparedness in their curricula stem from nurse education [6, 7]. But besides healthcare professionals, many other professions are involved in disaster management [8]. Collaboration and coordination within these multiprofessional and multidisciplinary ad hoc teams is probably the most important but also the most challenging part to prepare these teams for their possible future humanitarian work in disaster management [9]. Disaster management is teamwork under rapidly changing, dynamic, and often unsafe conditions. Competencies for this challenging work always cover knowledge and skills emanating from the basic profession but also many so-called nontechnical

M. Brodmann Maeder (✉)
Department of Emergency Medicine, Inselspital, Bern University Hospital and University of Bern, Bern, Switzerland

Institute of Mountain Emergency Medicine, EURAC Research, Bolzano, Italy
e-mail: monika.brodmannmaeder@insel.ch; monika.brodmannmaeder@siwf.ch

© Springer Nature Switzerland AG 2021
E. Pikoulis, J. Doucet (eds.), *Emergency Medicine, Trauma and Disaster Management*, Hot Topics in Acute Care Surgery and Trauma,
https://doi.org/10.1007/978-3-030-34116-9_47

skills (NTS). These NTS or CRM (crisis or crew resource management) skills are superordinate qualities that enable team members from different disciplines and professions to effectively collaborate even under the most complex and confusing situation of a medical emergency [10]. This is even truer for disasters where oftentimes many people with different professions but also cultural background gather and have to collaborate.

47.2 Core Competencies for Disaster Management

Defining core competencies for disaster management is challenging, as they must not only cover task- or profession-related competencies but also cross-disciplinary competencies [2]. Walsh et al. described a meticulous process using surveys and expert working group meetings in order to define core competencies for disaster medicine and public health [3]. They defined 11 core competencies and 35 subcompetencies for disaster medicine and public health that should be applied to all persons involved in disaster planning or response. Many of them cover aspects of team collaboration and NTS like knowing his or her role in a group, demonstrating situational awareness, and communication or management and leadership skills. Collaboration and coordination cannot be trained in a classroom or during a lecture: Interactivity is of utmost importance, and therefore the need for interactive learning methods with the provision of feedback is high.

47.3 Adult Learning in Disaster Medicine

Competency is defined as an observable ability of a health professional, integrating multiple components such as knowledge, skills, and attitudes [11]. Competency-based (medical) education is an outcome-based approach to the design, implementation, assessment, and evaluation of medical education programs, using an organizing framework of defined competencies [11]. Acquiring new knowledge can be reached by reading books, by memorizing and rehearsing, or by listening to a lecture. Although the amount of new knowledge, that we get from classic lectures, is very limited and just about 5% of the content, Ingrassia et al. found that the prevailing teaching method in education and training initiatives for crisis management in the European Union were lectures with 84% [4]. New educational methods try to avoid knowledge transfer via ex-cathedra teaching and use interactive presentations as the first step to make presentations more profitable for the learners. Acquiring new skills or psychomotor capabilities usually requires an introduction by showing the task, followed by many repetitions by the learner and supervision and feedback on the performance by an experienced instructor. Attitude usually covers behavioral and social aspects of interacting with other individuals, and with the help of special teaching methods like simulation or learning in small groups, like PBL (problem-based learning), this important part of competency can be enhanced [11]. Disaster medicine is a highly dynamic, interprofessional domain that requires highly competent professionals. They must have appropriate individual knowledge, a broad spectrum of technical and nontechnical skills, and excellent personal abilities, which enable them to collaborate as a team.

47.4 Nontechnical Skills and CRM

In newer literature, the expressions non-technical skills (NTS) and crew/crisis resource management (CRM) are frequently used to define these special competencies that enable teams or so-called action teams to work together in highly dynamic situations [12, 13]. The expression nontechnical skills covers a whole set of different observable behaviors that improve group performance [14]. CRM can be characterized as "the ability to implement the know-how, what needs to be done, into effective team action, even under the most adverse and confusing situation of a medical emergency" [15]. This meets very well the situation of a mass casualty or disaster. NTS and CRM might differ in details, but the focus in both structures is on aspects of coordination, communication, and collaboration in a team attributable to individuals working with other team members. Publications showed that training teams in nontechnical skills could not only improve team performance and reduce error rates but also most importantly had a positive financial outcome [16].

47.5 Interprofessional Collaboration

Many teams are composed of members of different professions, with their individual cultural imprint and socialization. This situation can be a threat to efficient teamwork and deteriorate team performance considerably. Today, the challenges of interprofessional collaboration are recognized and addressed—even the World Health Organization published a famous statement on how to overcome these difficulties [17]. Some of the key elements to overcome the challenges of collaborating in teams with different "professionals" are transparency, clarity on the role of the different team members, and again high-quality nontechnical skills. These competencies need to be developed and trained, because "teams are not born, they are made." For this preparation, we need to develop high-quality teaching moments where teams can learn to work together.

47.6 Simulation for MCI Disaster Management

Simulation is a technique to replace or amplify real experiences with guided experiences, often immersive in nature, that evoke or replicate substantial aspects of the real world in a fully interactive fashion [11]. Within the simulation as educational method, we can differentiate between manikin simulation,

simulation with standardized or simulated patients (so-called SPs), hybrid simulation—a mix between SP and manikin simulation—and virtual reality [12, 13]. For many years, CPR drills were the prevailing simulation scenarios used for emergency and other healthcare teams. Hence, in the last one or two decades, simulation has evolved into a highly specialized educational method with meticulous structures and sophisticated training for instructors. The size of these scenarios differs substantially: They range from a 1:1 scenario with a standardized patient and a healthcare professional up to full-scale MCI simulations with several hundred participants either as simulated patients or as professionals who must deal with the situation. The method chosen depends on the learning objectives, which must be defined beforehand. If communication skills are the focus, it makes sense to use a SP. Multiple trauma management on the other hand is usually the domain of manikin simulations, where invasive procedure like thoracotomies or intubations can be trained. Hybrid simulation is a promising tool where an SP acts as the patient and has, e.g., an artificial arm where the trainee should put an IV line.

47.6.1 Core Elements of Simulation

Simulating relevant and almost real events can be threatening for participants and even harmful unless rules are defined and followed by faculty members and participants. If the faculty ignores to address these issues transparently and vigorously, the learning experience can lose its power and even become harmful. They include:

- Confidentiality and social safety: Participants must be reassured that nothing what is said and done during a simulation scenario or the debriefing will be carried outside. This is especially important if the training takes place in an institution where participants and faculty members know each other or even work together. Simulation for team training is a teaching method and should not be used as qualifier and assessment of either an individual trainee or team performance. Confidentiality is an important point if the simulation scenario is videotaped. The faculty should state that the videotapes are exclusively used as support for the debriefing and will be destroyed afterward.
- Respect and positive regard: Simulation is not reality. The art of simulation is to create a relevant learning experience for the participants, but it can never be real. This situation can be challenging for participants who have difficulties of accepting these limitations: Their performance during a simulation scenario might not correspond with their competencies during daily work. The faculty must clarify this beforehand, and participants are asked to deal with this situation by showing respect and positive regard for their teammates.
- Constructive feedback: Feedback is a strong learning instrument that allows deep learning. In order to take most of the profit from feedback, it must be timely, specific, short, and concise, and it should focus on observed behavior and on the issue, not the person.

47.7   Simulation as Teaching Method

47.7.1 Scenario Development for Disaster Simulation

Developing simulation scenarios consists of several steps: The first step is to define the characteristics of the learners and a meticulous needs assessment for the participants but also a general needs assessment. Defining adequate learning objectives is the most crucial but also the challenging part of the development of a simulation scenario, and it should integrate objectives related to knowledge, skills, and CRM aspects. If we have participants with different professional background, we should take care that we define profession-specific learning goals for all team members and common CRM goals that define team collaboration and performance. These learning objectives are not only important for the scenario development, but they are also the cornerstones of every debriefing. According to the learning goals, we will decide on the simulation method and the "history" which will be given to the learners. The last step is the assessment: Do we want to have the participants' feedback on the course or program? The question behind every assessment should be whether the training has not only met the defined learning objectives but also the participants' needs and expectations.

47.7.2 Faculty Development: From Teacher to Facilitator

Simulation events very much depend on the competencies of the faculty members: Teachers or instructors always act as role models for their learners [18]. Working as faculty member for simulation events therefore is very challenging, bearing in mind all the prerequisites that we defined as core elements of simulation. Persons who want to be involved in simulation education should carefully be selected and supervised during their first involvements. They must show a special commitment in order to facilitate simulations. They should be defined instructors, stressing their task of conveying content to their learners, or even better facilitators: Facilitating implies a very strong role to make use of the existing experience in the group and integrating these competencies into the simulation session. Even for experienced simulation, facilitators or educators should regularly receive feedback on their performance in order to maintain their teaching competencies [19], either through peer coaching or by using existing tools like the Debriefing Assessment for Simulation in Healthcare (DASH) [20, 21].

47.7.3 The Process of Simulation Scenarios: Briefing, Scenario, and Debriefing

Every simulation scenario starts with a briefing of the involved participants. A faculty member explains the setting, defines the "players" and the observers, and appoints faculty members who will support the team during the scenario. The learners have time to discuss their roles and responsibilities during the scenario. They might also agree on the tasks during the first minutes. The scenario itself starts after the briefing and stops either after a defined duration or if the faculty decides to end it.

47.7.4 Debriefing

The debriefing is the centerpiece of every simulation scenario. Debriefing has very diverse definitions and meanings, ranging from questioning a person after a completed mission or undertaking to special methods attempting to lessen or prevent psychological damage in crisis victims. In connection with simulation as educational tool, debriefing is "a facilitated conversation after such things as critical events and simulations in which participants analyze their actions, thought processes, emotional states, and other information to improve performance in future situations" [21, 22]. Usually, a faculty member facilitates the debriefing, but other methods like peer debriefing can be used [23]. Videotapes of the scenario can help to show the team that has been active in the scenario a special situation. Still, the use of this technology is discussed controversially, and its effectiveness has been challenged [24, 25]. Debriefing is a form of formative assessment and largely depends on the participants' abilities to reflect their performance in a simulation scenario but also their clinical practice. Rudolph et al. propose a four-step model of debriefing.

47.7.4.1 Step 1: Emotions
The first step allows learners to express their emotions during the scenario, using the "flashlight" method: The facilitator asks the performing team members one after the other to state their first impression in one sentence. This gives the facilitator a good impression of what were the most troubling topics.

47.7.4.2 Step 2: Analysis
This is the more structured and often facilitator-centered part of the debriefing. A very simple method to start an analysis is to ask what went well and what could be improved in the scenario (instead of stating what went wrong!), avoiding blaming of persons and using the rules of constructive feedback: The analysis should be concrete, be constructive, and focus on the issue. For more intimate and small groups, many very sophisticated methods like the "A&I" (Advocacy and Inquiry) or the PEARLS method help to define performance gaps, to investigate the reasons for the gap and try to "close" the observed gap [22, 26]. However, the larger the group, the more simple should the instrument be. In this phase, facilitators should revise the learning objectives and possibly actively add topics that had not yet come as discussion points.

47.7.4.3 Step 3: Summary
The ending phase of a debriefing should allow all learners to highlight the lessons learned. This can either be done by a facilitator or even better by one or more

learners. The end should be another "round" of one-sentence statement, facilitated by the question: "What do you as individual take home from this scenario?" or "What was your personal "pearl" in this scenario? This allows collecting and sharing different views.

47.8 Summary

Preparing teams for disaster management is multifaceted and includes special educational efforts: Oftentimes, teams are assembled on the spot under very dynamic and uncontrollable situations. The team members have different cultural and professional background and bring different competencies into the team. Educational efforts must be aware of these challenges and define special training opportunities to improve the competencies of the individuals but also the teams. Core competencies in disaster medicine cover topics like communication, situational awareness, role clarity, leadership, or decision-making. These attitudes can be found in the so-called nontechnical skills. Simulation offers a wide spectrum of different interactive learning tools that can enhance not only these competencies but also deep individual learning. The quality of this instrument largely depends on the simulation scenario but even more on the competency of the faculty to facilitate the process of briefing, simulation, and debriefing. Respect, social safety, and providing constructive feedback are crucial elements in order to improve team performance during the educational event. Well-designed teaching moments can help to better prepare teams for the unpreparable mass casualties and disasters.

References

1. Kunz N, Reiner G, Gold S. Investing in disaster management capabilities versus pre-positioning inventory: a new approach to disaster preparedness. Int J Prod Econ. 2014;157:261–72.
2. Gallardo AR, Djalali A, Foletti M, Ragazzoni L, Della Corte F, Lupescu O, et al. Core competencies in disaster management and humanitarian assistance: a systematic review. Disaster Med Public Health Prep. 2015;9(4):430–9.
3. Walsh L, Subbarao I, Gebbie K, Schor KW, Lyznicki J, Strauss-Riggs K, et al. Core competencies for disaster medicine and public health. Disaster Med Public Health Prep. 2012;6(1):44–52.
4. Ingrassia PL, Foletti M, Djalali A, Scarone P, Ragazzoni L, Della Corte F, et al. Education and training initiatives for crisis management in the European Union: a web-based analysis of available programs. Prehosp Disaster Med. 2014;29(2):115–26.
5. Smith J, Levy MJ, Hsu EB, Levy JL. Disaster curricula in medical education: pilot survey. Prehosp Disaster Med. 2012;27(5):492–4.
6. Chapman K, Arbon P. Are nurses ready?: disaster preparedness in the acute setting. Australas Emerg Nurs J. 2008;11(3):135–44.
7. Jose MM, Dufrene C. Educational competencies and technologies for disaster preparedness in undergraduate nursing education: an integrative review. Nurse Educ Today. 2014;34(4):543–51.
8. Burkle FM. The development of multidisciplinary core competencies: the first step in the professionalization of disaster medicine and public health preparedness on a global scale. Disaster Med Public Health Prep. 2012;6(1):10–2.

9. Bradt DA, Drummond CM. Professionalization of disaster medicine—an appraisal of criterion-referenced qualifications. Prehosp Disaster Med. 2007;22(5):360–8.
10. Gaba DM, Fish KJ, Howard SK. Crisis management in anesthesiology. New York: Churchill Livingston; 1994.
11. Østergaard D, Dieckmann P, Lippert A. Simulation and CRM. Best Pract Res Clin Anaesthesiol. 2011;25(2):239–49.
12. Flin R, Maran N. Basic concepts for crew resource management and non-technical skills. Best Pract Res Clin Anaesthesiol. 2015;29(1):27–39.
13. Manser T. Teamwork and patient safety in dynamic domains of healthcare: a review of the literature. Acta Anaesthesiol Scand. 2009;53(2):143–51.
14. Fletcher G, Flin R, McGeorge P, Glavin R. Anaesthetists' non-technical skills (ANTS): evaluation of a behavioural marker system. Br J Anaesth. 2003;90(5):580–8.
15. Howard SK, Gaba DM, Fish KJ, Yang G, Sarnquist FH. Anesthesia crisis resource management training: teaching anesthesiologists to handle critical incidents. Aviat Space Environ Med. 1992;63(9):763–70.
16. Moffatt-Bruce SD, Hefner JL, Mekhjian H, McAlearney JS, Latimer T, Ellison C, et al. What is the return on investment for implementation of a crew resource management program at an academic medical center? Am J Med Qual. 2017;32(1):5–11.
17. World Health Organization. Framework for action on interprofessional education and collaborative practice. http://www.who.int/hrh/resources/framework_action/en/. Accessed 26 Mar 2015.
18. Reuler JB, Nardone DA. Role modeling in medical education. West J Med. 1994;160(4):335–7.
19. Cheng A, Grant V, Dieckmann P, Arora S, Robinson T, Eppich W. Faculty development for simulation programs: five issues for the future of debriefing training. Simul Healthc. 2015;10(4):217–22.
20. Cheng A, Grant V, Huffman J, Burgess G, Szyld D, Robinson T, et al. Coaching the Debriefer: peer coaching to improve debriefing quality in simulation programs. Simul Healthc. 2017;12(5):319–25.
21. Brett-Fleegler M, Rudolph J, Eppich W, Monuteaux M, Fleegler E, Cheng A, et al. Debriefing assessment for simulation in healthcare: development and psychometric properties. Simul Healthc. 2012;7(5):288–94.
22. Rudolph JW, Simon R, Raemer DB, Eppich WJ. Debriefing as formative assessment: closing performance gaps in medical education. Acad Emerg Med. 2008;15(11):1010–6.
23. Doherty-Restrepo J, Odai M, Harris M, Yam T, Potteiger K, Montalvo A. Students' perception of peer and faculty debriefing facilitators following simulation- based education. J Allied Health. 2018;47(2):107–12.
24. Jacobs PJ. Using high-fidelity simulation and video-assisted debriefing to enhance obstetrical hemorrhage mock code training. J Nurses Prof Dev. 2017;33(5):234–9.
25. Grant JS, Dawkins D, Molhook L, Keltner NL, Vance DE. Comparing the effectiveness of video-assisted oral debriefing and oral debriefing alone on behaviors by undergraduate nursing students during high-fidelity simulation. Nurse Educ Pract. 2014;14(5):479–84.
26. Rudolph JW, Simon R, Dufresne RL, Raemer DB. There's no such thing as "nonjudgmental" debriefing: a theory and method for debriefing with good judgment. Simul Healthc. 2006;1(1):49–55.

Medical Education: Modern Methods and Alternative Methods to Animal Procedures

48

Apostolos Papalois and Maria-Anna Tsoutsou

48.1 Continuing Medical Education: Continuing Professional Development

The continuing advancement of medical and veterinary science, in combination with the inevitable internationalization and population transfer, has led to an urgent need for production of highly qualified doctors. Nowadays, new graduate doctors have a high level of theoretical knowledge; however, this is not sufficient. There is a need for professionals who can work independently from the very first day to any hospital or institution in the European Union (or in another continent). Furthermore, it is a well-established fact that there is one thing that a junior doctor needs to know: He/she has to know how to learn. Living with the belief of continuous learning, in the progress of his/her specialty and afterward, he/she will be able to adopt a personal tactic of continuous learning that will enable him/her to gain the current knowledge and experience. To sum up, he/she will be capable of treating his/her patients the best possible way [1].

Continuing medical education (CME) is a process of continuous and lifelong training and represents an integral part of a wider concept: continuing professional development (CPD). CPD includes not only the principles of continuous improvement of abilities and clinical skills but also the cultivation, the lifestyle, and the communication between the patients and the society.

The rapid development of medical science, as well as the overwhelming demands of a modern society, necessitates the constantly redefinement of medical knowledge and skills. The institutional enforcement of CME is of a great significance in order to accomplish quality control of the medical community. It should also be a requirement for the effective operation of the healthcare system.

A. Papalois (✉) · M.-A. Tsoutsou
Experimental, Educational and Research Center ELPEN, Pikermi, Greece

© Springer Nature Switzerland AG 2021
E. Pikoulis, J. Doucet (eds.), *Emergency Medicine, Trauma and Disaster Management*, Hot Topics in Acute Care Surgery and Trauma,
https://doi.org/10.1007/978-3-030-34116-9_48

Lifelong medical education guarantees the quality of services and preserves the prestige of the medical community.

The CME was a general concept by the end of the decade of the 1980s. In the early 1990s, it was discussed by competent health authorities until it became official in 1993 with the revised Dublin Regulation where the definition and the aim were presented. The Dublin Regulation states the following [1]:

- The CME is a moral obligation and a personal responsibility of each doctor.
- The primary goal is to provide the maximum medical care in the general population.
- The term CME refers to the continuous renewal and the enrichment of medical knowledge and techniques.
- Every doctor is entitled to CME and should be encouraged to exercise this right.

On October 28, 1994, the European Union of Medical Specialists (UEMS) assumes a formal and substantive role as a coordinating scientific body of the CME in Europe and establishes a body responsible for its implementation and organization at national and pan-European level. CME should be:

- Credible
- Valid
- Comparable
- Widespread
- Quantifiable in a grading scale (credits)

48.2 Contemporary Medical Training Methods

In modern methods of medical education, the following categories are included:

- Training using animal models
- Training using digital projections
- Training using cadaver tissues
- Training manikins-electronic simulators
- Training using three-dimensional structures
- Participation in surgery
- Training using alternative methods
- Combination of the above [2–5]

In any case, the presence of experienced and trained instructors, clear curriculum, and appropriate training laboratories is demanded [6–8].

Training with the use of *animal models* (mainly pigs and rats) is the most widespread, since they widely simulate human responses. However, a proper design is required in order to follow the principles of the 3Rs (replacement, refinement, reduction). Moreover, the existence of fully organized laboratories is essential (Directive 2010/63/EU). *Digital projections* are constantly gaining ground and are particularly useful to younger doctors. They have many advantages as they are low cost, they can be easily repeated, and they offer great room for discussion. But in any case, they are just a pre-stage of a more advanced education. Recently, in courses of trauma surgery in emergency medicine, it is followed virtual scenario viewer trauma with actors in video viewing. This view is paused at crucial points when difficult decision must be made. As a result, the trainer and the trainees have the opportunity to discuss the possible solutions based on the vital signs and other parameters. Seminars that use *cadaver tissues* have an important advantage that we should take into account during their evaluation: the accurate human anatomy. For instance, the hand surgery training, the neurosurgery, and the otolaryngology benefit greatly by using cadaver tissues. However, the extensive use is neither recommended nor be encouraged, unless it is absolutely necessary. Furthermore, the existence of fully organized laboratories and the compliance with the proper legislation are essential again. In the future, training with use of *manikins- electronic simulators* will have a great development because it offers great potential. Training manikins have the ability to execute a large number of interventions and manipulations. Additionally, they can respond to changes in physiology and pathophysiology, and they have a one-time purchase cost. This purchase cost may be high, but the maintenance cost is something manageable. In addition, any mistakes during the training by the trainees as part of their training work in their benefit. The same mistake in an animal model would cause harm. The *three-dimensional models* are relatively new technology and are the evolution of the well-known "training boxes" and "pelvic trainers" of laparoscopic surgery. The main difference is that they are more advanced as they feature vessel flow, hemostasis, as well as injury caused by wrong handling, replacing the use of animals with an animal organ (e.g., liver-kidney). Despite the fact that in our time, their use is not notably widespread, it is anticipated to become more popular in the future inside hospitals or in organized labs. A well-known and profound training method is the *participation in operating rooms*. If not possible, however, the use of modern digital projections in modern operating rooms is essential, and its educational element is indispensable for junior as well as for advanced/professional doctors. *Alternative* training methods should not be underestimated as they will be a major part of medical education in the future. They are also low cost and follow the principles of the 3Rs. For instance, in the Royal College of Surgeons, practice in wound cleansing is performed with the use of a piece of meat purchased from a store. Abdominal wall closure techniques training is made with the use of a box. The stitching is done with the use of simple material. Beneath this material, an inflated balloon is placed. Inaccurate placement of the stitching leads to popping the balloon. For the placement of microsurgery stitches (8-0, 9-0, 10-0, or 11-0), a piece of surgical glove can be used, instead of living tissue. For intraosseous infusion in infants or toddlers, a chicken's femur purchased from the store can be used. Finally, the simple manikins are an important aid (e.g., intubation, cardiopulmonary resuscitation, etc.).

48.3   Conclusion

The major development of medical and veterinary science over the years, in combination with the continuing technological achievements, renders the continuing education and training (lifelong learning) the keystone of security in the execution of their profession. Modern and alternative training methods contribute toward the successful completion of these goals.

References

1. European Union of Medical Specialists. 2008. επίσημη ιστοσελίδα (www.uems.net).
2. Alexakis N. Surgical education and training with the use of animal models. Hellenic and international experience. In: Proceedings of the first Panhellenic seminar for experimental biomedical research, Athens, 11–14 December, 2007, p 96.
3. Aufses AH. Residency training programmes then and now. Surgery Mt Sinai J Med. 1989;56(5):367–9.
4. Porter RW. Surgical training and education. J Am Coll Surg. 1996;183(5):499–505.
5. Sawyers JL. Presidential address. Graduate surgical education. Am Surg. 1981;47(1):1–5.
6. Gomes MPSF, Davies BL. Computer-assisted TURP training and monitoring, Lecture notes in computer science. Berlin: Springer; 2004. 1935/2000: eh 393.
7. Griffen WO. Back to the future. Curr Surg. 1986;43(5):372–6.
8. Pieper SD, Laub DR, Rosen JM. A finite-element facial model for simulating plastic surgery. Plast Reconstr Surg. 1995;96(5):1100–5.

Leadership and Management in Disasters–Command, Control, Coordination, Communication

49

Efstratios (Steve) Photiou

49.1 Introduction

Leadership is a universal issue, given that it is required in almost every complex operation or activity.

Leadership is the highest form of the art of inluencing people. Practically, it is the process of:

(a) Influencing others to understand and agree what needs to be done and how it can be done effectively.
(b) Facilitating individual and collective efforts to accomplish the shared objectives.

Leadership differs from management; leadership sets policy and grand strategy, while management is the process of directing a group for a precise scope.

Leadership is operated by management through the 4C mechanism: command, control, coordination, and communication. If one of these four elements lacks, no strategy or tactics can be carried out effectively.

Command, control, coordination, and communication is performed through the Incident Command System (ICS).

Every incident or disaster should be managed by an incident commander.

E. (S.) Photiou (✉)
Emergency Department, San Valentino Hospital, AULSS 2 "Marca Trevigiana", Montebelluna (TV), Italy

© Springer Nature Switzerland AG 2021
E. Pikoulis, J. Doucet (eds.), *Emergency Medicine, Trauma and Disaster Management*, Hot Topics in Acute Care Surgery and Trauma,
https://doi.org/10.1007/978-3-030-34116-9_49

49.2   Leadership and Management

Nowadays, much is said about leadership. Actually, from highly hierarchized settings (military, for instance) to the financial world, leadership is being imported to many other situations which, for their complexity, need to be "governed." This may be especially important in settings where numerous stakeholders are involved.

Sometimes, the barriers between leadership and management may not be clear to many people. Leadership differs from management: leadership sets policy and grand strategy, while management is the process of directing a group for a precise scope.

Leadership is the process of:

(a) Influencing people to understand and agree what must be done and how it can be done.
(b) Facilitating efforts (individual and collective) and mentoring collaborators to accomplish the objectives enounced by the leader.

Leadership: key characteristics:

- Sets the organization's strategic direction, level of ambition, broad objectives, and long-term goals
- Does not handle details (avoids micromanagement)
- Sets the plan
- Shares it with the collaborators and inspires them to follow it
- Establishes principles
- Empowers and mentors the team to lead them to their goals
- Promotes engagement in new endeavors
- Exercises long-term, high-level focus

Effective leadership requires specific *skills*:

- Knowledge
- Experience
- Flexibility
- Intelligence: Information collection and elaboration
- Communication
- Networking
- Teambuilding
- Delegating
- Decision-making
- Sensemaking
- Listening/learning
- Planning
- Improvising
- Educating/training
- Situational awareness
- Accountability

Ideally, leadership must inspire the group toward a common endeavor, improvement, and change. Thus, it is often called "inspirational leadership," because it stimulates and creates purpose for collaborators and excitement and momentum for change. Individuals strive toward a future vision by embodying the organization's values and policy. Moreover, they become proactive: able to work up solutions and prone to "run a mile more."

In fact, inspirational leadership (the highest form of leadership) encompasses:

- Clear goals
- Clear objectives
- Shared purpose
- Motivational support

The *inspirational leadership's 16 core competencies* are the following:

1. Vision and vision-sharing
2. Passion and commitment
3. Compassion
4. Flexibility and adaptability
5. Analysis and synthesis
6. Understanding and insight
7. In-depth knowledge
8. Self-awareness and situational awareness
9. Strategic outlook
10. Decisiveness and accountability
11. Drive to change
12. Empowering, mentoring, and coaching
13. Teamworking
14. Proneness to engage
15. Art of communication
16. Art of building resonant relationships

In order to build positive (resonant) relationships, a leader should count on *Aristotle's four cardinal virtues*:

- *Fortitude* (courage): to push toward innovation
- *Prudence* (mindfulness): to be reflective prior to action
- *Temperance*: to control one's emotions
- *Justice*: to be fair

What is *visionary leadership?*

- Creating an idea
- Sharing the idea or strategy
- Setting clear focus
- Consultation vs consensus
- Delegating to the right people

- Knowledge of processes: "go and see how it works" (similarly to "Gemba walks")
- "Learn by whom knows best"
- Imagination
- Innovation

What is *persuasive leadership*? It is the style of leadership that makes people feel "part of the team" and enhances teamworking. In certain moments, a real leader might become aware that *something does not work* properly, especially if some signs become evident:

- Flattery
- No "bad news"
- Half truths
- Stagnation

The real leader will consider this moment as an opportunity to make a new start out of the problem:

- Challenge oneself by self-assessment
- Demonstrate courage and the ability of being able to face the problem
- Listen and discuss

In order to enhance leadership capability, the leader should take time to reflect. Self-reflection can help the leader to better understand leadership style, gaps, and flaws, thus becoming able to improve leadership skills.

49.3 Leadership: Facts

As already stated, leadership is the highest form of the art of dealing with people. Some people are gifted: they possess innate charisma and social intelligence, a sort of personal "something magic" creating an aura of popularity. Naturally, not everyone is born with this "something magic," but who possesses it has an advantage in expressing leadership. Anyhow, leadership can be learned and cultivated by highly committed people.

In order to become leaders, persons need to be "exposed": to have the chance to emerge and express themselves. This chance may be offered by being summoned (to assume responsibilities), by the course of events, or by being "in the right place at the right moment." The momentum of exposure is not always foreseeable.

Leaders are facilitators of their team members' success.

They ensure that their collaborators:

- Have their necessities sorted in order to be successfully productive
- Are well trained
- Have minimal obstacles in their path way
- Are acknowledged for good performance
- Are coached

49.3.1 Who Can Be the Leader?

Anyone in the team who:

- Has a particular talent or is highly committed
- Is creative
- Has an idea
- Thinks "out of the box"
- Has experience in a certain aspect of the project that can prove useful to the manager and team

49.4   Management

Management is the process of directing a group for a precise scope.

Managers are in charge of, or responsible for, something. Management is limited-scale executing on specific areas within responsibilities, while focus is kept on sectorial or minor systems or fields.

Which are the manager's *tasks*?

- "Apply the strategy, perform the tactics"
- Enforcement of the organization's policies
- Direction and monitoring of the team to achieve its specific goals
- Work by objectives
- Short-range perspective
- Short-term focus
- Attention to the details (micromanagement)
- Eye on results
- Acceptance and maintenance of the status quo
- Does what is needed to accomplish the plan
- Containment of risks for the organization

49.4.1 Who Can Be a Manager?

Managers are usually appointed to a position of command. Sometimes, they progress from technical proficiency to supervisory roles.

What is needed in order to become a manager?

- Knowledge
- Proficiency developed through training or experience
- Ability
- Authority
- Respect
- Clear perspectives

- Situational awareness
- Teamworking
- Flexibility in performing tactics
- Clear communication methods

With good leadership and poor management, an organization will have the goals, inspiration, and plan to succeed, but no one to execute the plan.

With good management and poor leadership, an organization will be able to execute anything, but without an overall strategy.

Leaders and managers should create and enhance teamworking:

- Buildup and maintenance of trustworthy relationships
- Collaboration with others, being part of a team
- Sharing all relevant information with others
- Seeking others; inputs
- Free expression of one's opinion (learn to listen)
- Assuming the role of teamleader (in their respective fields)
- Resolving conflict among team members

49.5 Leadership During Crisis

No one can predict when and how a disaster will strike, nor its evolution.

Commanders must be able to make decisions and to delegate, under time pressure.

The goal of emergency management is "…to devise policy and to implement programs that will reduce vulnerability, limit the loss of life and property, protect the environment, and improve multi-organizational coordination in disasters" [1].

During a major crisis, a complex event, or a disaster, the challenge for a leader is to deal with the uncertainties and threats deriving from them. A successful leader is the person who must fare with problems and try to bring things back to normality. On the opposite, unsuccessful leadership will exacerbate the impact of catastrophes.

What should a leader do in case of disaster? One should engage collaborators within the organization, as well as external stakeholders, to act collectively as a team, toward a common scope, given that disaster response is the result of teamworking among different, often disparate, public and private actors.

It must be kept in mind that major disasters may provoke, depending on the magnitude of the event, dismay and uncertainty: practically, disaster is the reign of chaos. It is impossible to anticipate when and how a disaster will strike, as well as to foresee its evolution. Therefore, it is paramount to deal with (possible) disasters beforehand while, in case of disaster, chaos must be managed. Naturally, experience in managing routine emergencies will help facing disasters. Though, leadership needs to be understood across all phases of comprehensive emergency management (i.e., mitigation, preparedness, response, recovery) [2]. According to the "disaster cycle," preparedness against disasters starts prior to the event and goes through it to recovery:

- Mitigation: reduce risks
- Preparedness: training (all hazard approach)
- Response: manage crisis
- Recovery: reevaluate, lessons learned

Complex, highly hierarchized systems, like the military, healthcare systems, and financial institutes, need to be effectively governed.

This can be achieved through *command and control* or, to be more precise, the 4C: *command, control, coordination,* and *communication.*

49.5.1 Command

Command is the exercise of direction by a commander over assigned forces or elements in the accomplishment of a mission:

- Personnel
- Equipment
- Communications
- Facilities
- Procedures
- Stakeholders

The elements of command are:

- Situational awareness
- Roles
- Establishment of the initial conditions
- Continuing assessment
- Intelligence
- Allocation of resources

49.5.2 Control

- Determine if efforts are on track
- Follow evolution
- Make adjustments

49.5.3 Coordination (of Multiple Stakeholders)

Coordination is a mechanism to ensure:

- That the incident is handled appropriately
- Teamworking
- Fine-tuning

Coordination is fueled by information flow.
Optimal levels of coordination:

- Unity of command: an individual has only one superior to whom he is directly responsible (accountability; clear line of supervision)
- Unity of effort: all parties collaborate
- Focus upon the same agreed objectives (MoU)
- Working together to achieve them (teamworking)
- Established chain of command: line of authority

49.5.4 Communication

A good leader must be an excellent communicator.
A leader must possess:

- Critical communication skills
- Ability to receive and distribute effectively information
- Assure that information was understood

The leader, through communication, must be able to:

- Give work assignments
- Request support or additional resource
- Report progress of assigned tasks
- Assure free information flow in- and outward
- Impose mutual intelligibility (common language and common terminology)
- Inform collaborators
- Give instructions
- Update (SitReps)
- Discuss options
- Inform stakeholders
- Inform media
- Inform public

The leader may be involved in communicating with the public who, in case of disaster, is the ultimate stakeholder, by performing *crisis and emergency risk communication (CERC)*.
The key questions to answer are the 5Ws:

- Who?
- What?
- When?
- Where?
- Why?

That comes to some clear messages to communicate the following:

- What is the hazard?
- What damage can it do?
- How will the community be affected?
- How complicated is the situation?
- Can it be averted?
- What can be done?

Sound communication should be:

- Timely
- Accurate
- Simple
- Understandable
- Credible
- Consistent
- Empathetic
- Competent
- Expert
- Honest
- Open
- Accountable
- Committed

49.6   Leadership and Management in Disasters

Disasters, by definition, provoke a failure of normal healthcare provision, caused by direct damage to healthcare facilities and/or by the large influx of disaster victims, thus overwhelming their existing healthcare capacity.

During a disaster, healthcare organizations must shift their activity and levels of care from ordinary to disaster mode: from "everything for all" to "highest possible level of care for the ones likely to survive." Moreover, they must "return to normal" as soon as possible (disaster dismissal).

It must be kept in mind that healthcare systems and hospitals are deemed parameters of social stability, because the public is aware that, in case of need, they can seek help there. On the other hand, hospitals are high-reliability organizations (HRO), given that low chances of error exist, due to interdisciplinary teamworking and cross-controls.

In case of disaster, leadership and management is applied through command and control (4C) which is performed through the Incident Command System (ICS) or Hospital Emergency Incident Command System (HEICS) by the Incident Commander (IC).

ICS is a model for command structure designed to manage chaos; and disaster is actually chaos.

The system was created in the 1970s in order to manage and coordinate multiple agencies involved in large incidents. Nowadays, ICS is applied in various responses, like prehospital or inhospital disaster, firefighting, police action, military operations, etc.

The ICS is:

1. A *standardized approach to 4C* through a definitive determination of common hierarchy.

   The main purpose of ICS is:
   - To manage chaos
   - To get a plan working
   - To help the various stakeholders work together in a coordinated and systematic approach
2. A *tool* (*not* a complete disaster plan) that:
   - Allows a structured, coordinated organizational approach of hospital disaster management
   - Allows multiple departments within the hospital to work together for a common objective
   - Provides instructions for tasks that differ from everyday activities
3. A *disaster management strategy*:
   - Standardized organization and procedures
   - Modular, scalable system
   - Manageable span of control
   - Procedures for establishing command and handover

The ICS *basic units of structure* are:

(a) Incident commander
(b) Section chiefs
(c) Directors
(d) Unit leaders
(e) Officers

The ICS helps ensure full *utilization* of *incident resources* by:

- Establishing predesignated incident facilities
- Maintaining a manageable span of control
- Implementing resource management practices
- Ensuring integrated communications
- Mutual intelligibility (common language)
- Course of action (prioritization)
- Maintaining surge capacity
- Applying the emergency plan

The *functionality* of a disaster plan encompasses:

- The level of medical ambition (LoMA): an action of policy-making
- The level of training on the plan
- The plan's updates
- The personnel's "disaster education" level

The leader's five steps in facing a crisis are the following:

1. Express organization's policy and direction (doctrine)
2. Establish incident objectives (level of ambition)
3. Select strategy
4. Technical direction (tactics)
5. Achieve goal

As the incident grows, general staff positions (modular organization) are activated in the ICS.

Concepts

- Unity of command: each person reports to only one supervisor
- Chain of command (orderly line of progression from IC to resource)
- Manageable span of control (manages expansion and contraction of the organization; ideal range is 1:5)

The 12 principles:

1. Five primary management functions (aforementioned)
2. Established transfer of control and command
3. Single or unified command
4. Unity and chain of Command
5. Management by objectives
6. Comprehensive resource management
7. Consolidated action plans
8. Manageable span of control
9. Modular organization
10. Personal accountability
11. Common terminology (intelligibility)
12. Integrated communications

The 16-step ICS response:

- Assumes and announces command (and exercises control, coordination, and communication): "the one-man's law"
- Gathers information
- Assesses situation

- Identifies and sets perimeters (hot/inner/outer)
- Establishes command post (safe)
- Assigns safety officer and staging officer (supplies)
- Identifies and establishes liaisons with all stakeholders
- Identifies resources
- Establishes plan (strategy/tactics/objectives)
- Establishes level of ambition
- Coordinates operations
- Promotes teamworking
- Activates preexisting MoU
- Requests additional resources
- *As the incident grows*, general staff positions are activated

The *first qualified responder* to arrive on a scene *becomes the incident commander* (IC):

1. The initial IC is initially responsible for all duties
2. The IC recruits staff as needed
3. Positions are added to the organizational structure only when needed
4. IC develops middle managers as needed
5. The initial IC is responsible for the organization until authority is delegated to another person
6. The IC may not necessarily be one single person
7. The IC is usually assisted by three command staff members (liaison officer, safety officer, and information officer)

The "should-be":

- Every incident must have an IC
- IC is the only mandatory position within the ICS
- The IC maintains overall responsibility for the incident
- The IC accomplishes functions from the Incident Command Post (ICP, EOC)
- ICP should be placed in a reasonably close but safe position
- Positions in command staff are added according to needs
- Each position may have assistants if necessary
- Large incidents should be managed *piecemeal* and by objectives

Standard operating procedures (SOPs):

1. Policy for activation of the plan
2. Policy for termination of emergency status
3. Evacuation procedures
4. Volunteer credentialing
5. Personnel recall (chain of activation)
6. Etc.

Job action sheets (JAS)

- Standardized and easily completed forms
- A single job sheet for each position within the organizational structure (thus, anyone can quickly assume a role)
- The most important tasks are mentioned at the top
- Staff are not required to memorize the contents of JAS.

Challenges addressed by CCCC/IC:

- Coordination of stakeholders
- Application of the plan
- Activation of the Memoranda of Understanding
- Evacuation—patients transfer supplies
- Info exchange/flow
- Maintenance of surge (as long as required) and call off (at the right moment).

49.7 Conclusion

Disaster management must aim to:

- Rapid shift to disaster setting
- Rapid return to normality

The real challenge is the combination of strong leadership and strong management and the right balance between them, in executing an emergency plan trough the ICS. Sound leadership must be inspirational, visionary and persuasive.

It must be kept in mind that preparedness starts prior to the event, (during the stage of mitigation and prevention), and should include education, timely information, and emotional and psychological support of the personnel [3]. A sound communication policy will give the opportunity to better educate the personnel and to make clear the commitment of the healthcare system [4], thus making everyone a stakeholder. Only a great leadership will be able to foster a necessary "disaster culture" and to manage chaos.

References

1. McEntire, Dawson. The basics of managing emergencies. In: International humanitarian action: NOHA textbook, a cura di Hans-Joachim Heintze, Pierre Thielbörger. New York: Springer; 2007. p. 60.
2. Trainor LE, Velotti L. Leadership in crises, disasters, and catastrophes. J Leadersh Stud. 2013;7(3)., 2013 ©2013 University of Phoenix.
3. Photiou E, Delooz H. Awaiting pandemic Avian influenza: the viewpoint of Emergency Medicine Department personnel. MJEM. 2012;12:2012.

4. Photiou E. The viewpoint of ED personnel about Avian Flu: do Emergency Department Healthcare professionals feel ready to face epidemics/pandemics? Pandemics and bioterrorism. In: NATO science for peace and security series. Amsterdam: IOS Press; 2010.

Suggested Reading

5. Demiroz F, Kapucu N. The role of leadership in managing emergencies and disasters. Eur J Econ Pol Stud. 2012;5(1):91–101.
6. Russell RD, Quarantelli EL, Dennis EW. Individual and Organizational Response to the 1985 Earthquake in Mexico City, Mexico. University of Delaware DRC Book and Monograph Series 24. 1990.
7. Making Matters Worse. Naim Kapucu, Monty Van Wart. November 2008. Administration & Siciety. 40(7):711–40. https://doi.org/10.11777/0095399708323143.
8. Stern, et al. J Leadersh Stud. 7(3) https://doi.org/10.1002/jls. 39 Symposium.
9. Waugh WL, Streib G. Collaboration and leadership for effective emergency management. Public Adm Rev. 2006;66(s1):131–40.